PROGRESS IN BRAIN RESEARCH

VOLUME 53

ADAPTIVE CAPABILITIES OF THE NERVOUS SYSTEM

Recent volumes in PROGRESS IN BRAIN RESEARCH

PROGRESS IN BRAIN RESEARCH

VOLUME 53

ADAPTIVE CAPABILITIES

OF THE NERVOUS SYSTEM

Proceedings of the 11th International Summer School of Brain Research, organized by the
Netherlands Institute for Brain Research, Amsterdam, and held at the Royal Netherlands Academy
of Sciences in Amsterdam, The Netherlands on August 13–17, 1979

EDITED BY

P.S. McCONNELL

G.J. BOER

H.J. ROMIJN

N.E. van de POLL

AND

M.A. CORNER

Netherlands Institute for Brain Research,
IJdijk 28, Amsterdam, The Netherlands

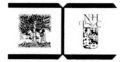

ELSEVIER/NORTH-HOLLAND BIOMEDICAL PRESS

AMSTERDAM – NEW YORK

1980

PUBLISHED BY:
ELSEVIER/NORTH-HOLLAND BIOMEDICAL PRESS
335 JAN VAN GALENSTRAAT, P.O. BOX 211
AMSTERDAM, THE NETHERLANDS

SOLE DISTRIBUTOR FOR THE U.S.A. AND CANADA:
ELSEVIER NORTH-HOLLAND INC.
52 VANDERBILT AVENUE
NEW YORK, NY 10017, U.S.A.

ISBN FOR THE SERIES 0-444-80104-9
ISBN FOR THE VOLUME 0-444-80207-X

Library of Congress Cataloging in Publication Data

International Summer School of Brain Research, 11th,
    Amsterdam, 1979.
    Adaptive capabilities of the nervous system.

    (Progress in brain research ; v. 53)
    Includes index.
    1. Brain--Congresses. 2. Neural circuitry--Adapta-
tion--Congresses. 3. Aggressive behavior in animals--
Congresses. 4. Sleep--Physiological aspects--Congres-
ses. I. McConnell, P. S. II. Nederlands Instituut
voor Hersenonderzoek. III. Title. IV. Series.
[DNLM: 1. Adaptation, Physiological--Congresses.
2. Nervous system--Physiology--Congresses. W1 PR667J
v. 53 / WL102 I658 1979a]
QP376.P7 vol. 53   612'.82s [599.01'88] 80-18276
ISBN 0-444-80207-X

WITH 197 ILLUSTRATIONS AND 38 TABLES

PRINTED IN THE NETHERLANDS

List of Contributors

K. Adam, Department of Psychiatry, University of Edinburgh, Edinburgh, Scotland, U.K.

S. Al-Maliki, Department of Zoology, University College of Swansea, Swansea, Wales, U.K.

J.L. Barker, Laboratory of Neurophysiology, National Institute of Neurological and Communicative Disorders and Stroke, National Institutes of Health, Bethesda, Md. 20205, U.S.A.

H.G. Baumgarten, Department of Anatomy, University of Berlin, Berlin, G.F.R.

J.J. Bernstein, Department of Neuroscience, University of Florida College of Medicine, Gainesville, Fla. 32610, U.S.A.

M. Berry, Department of Anatomy, University of Birmingham, Birmingham, B15 2TJ, U.K.

G.J. Boer, Netherlands Institute for Brain Research, IJdijk 28, 1095 KJ Amsterdam, The Netherlands.

K. Boer, Netherlands Institute for Brain Research, IJdijk 28, 1095 KJ, Amsterdam, The Netherlands.

B. Bohus, Rudolf Magnus Institute for Pharmacology, University of Utrecht, The Netherlands.

H.L.M.G. Bour, Netherlands Institute for Brain Research, Amsterdam, The Netherlands.

P.F. Brain, Department of Zoology, University College of Swansea, Swansea, Wales, U.K.

R.M. Buijs, Netherlands Institute for Brain Research, IJdijk 28, 1095 KJ Amsterdam, The Netherlands.

A.M.L. Coenen, Department of Comparative and Physiological Psychology, University of Nijmegen, 6525 GG Nijmegen, The Netherlands.

D.B. Cohen, University of Texas at Austin, Austin, Texas, U.S.A.

M.A. Corner, Netherlands Institute for Brain Research, Amsterdam, The Netherlands.

E. Endröczi, Central Research Division, Postgraduate Medical School, Budapest, Hungary.

W.H. Gispen, Division of Molecular Neurobiology, Rudolf Magnus Institute for Pharmacology and Laboratory of Physiological Chemistry, Medical Faculty, Institute of Molecular Biology, University of Utrecht, Padualaan 8, Utrecht, The Netherlands.

P.S. Goldman-Rakic, Yale School of Medicine, New Haven, Conn., U.S.A.

G. Hoheisel, Department of Cell Biology and Regulation, Section of Biosciences, Karl-Marx University, Leipzig, G.D.R.

O.R. Hommes, Department of Neurology, Radboud University Hospital, Nijmegen, The Netherlands.

M. Jouvet, Department of Experimental Medicine, Claude Bernard University, Lyon, France.

J.M. Koolhaas, Department of Zoology, University of Groningen, Haren, The Netherlands.

G.L. Kovács, Department of Pathophysiology, University Medical School, Szeged, Semmelweis, u.1. H-6701, Hungary.

M.R. Kruk, Leiden Medical Center, Sylvius Laboratoria, Department of Pharmacology, Leiden, The Netherlands.

A.I. Leshner, Department of Psychology, Bucknell University, Lewisburg, Pa. 17837, U.S.A.

P. McConnell, Netherlands Institute for Brain Research, IJdijk 28, 1095 KJ Amsterdam, The Netherlands.

M. Mirmiran, Netherlands Institute for Brain Research, Amsterdam, The Netherlands.

K.E. Moyer, Department of Psychology, Carnegie Mellon University, Pittsburgh, Pa. 15213, U.S.A.

W. Naumann, Department of Cell Biology and Regulation, Section of Biosciences, Karl-Marx University, Leipzig, G.D.R.

R. Olivier-Aardema, Department of Zoology, University of Groningen, Haren, The Netherlands.

T. Schuurman, Department of Zoology, State University of Groningen, The Netherlands.

J. Sievers, Department of Neuroanatomy, University of Hamburg, Hamburg, G.F.R.

T.G. Smith, Jr., Laboratory of Neurophysiology, National Institute of Neurological and Communicative Disorders and Stroke, National Institutes of Health, Bethesda, Md. 20205, U.S.A.

G. Sterba, Department of Cell Biology and Regulation, Section of Biosciences, Karl-Marx University, Leipzig, G.D.R.

D.F. Swaab, Netherlands Institute for Brain Research, IJdijk 28, 1095 KJ Amsterdam, The Netherlands.

H.B.M. Uylings, Netherlands Institute for Brain Research, IJdijk 28, 1095 KJ, Amsterdam, The Netherlands.

N.E. van de Poll, Netherlands Institute for Brain Research, Amsterdam, The Netherlands.

A.M. van der Poel, Leiden Medical Center, Sylvius Laboratoria, Department of Pharmacology, Leiden, The Netherlands.

Z.J.M. van Hulzen, Department of Comparative and Physiological Psychology, University of Nijmegen, 6525 GG Nijmegen, The Netherlands.

H.G. van Oyen, Netherlands Institute for Brain Research, Amsterdam, The Netherlands.

H.M. van Praag, Department of Psychiatry, University of Utrecht, The Netherlands.

D.N. Velis, Netherlands Institute for Brain Research, IJdijk 28, 1095 KJ, Amsterdam, The Netherlands.

W.M.A. Verhoeven, Department of Psychiatry, University of Utrecht, The Netherlands.

D.H.G. Versteeg, Rudolf Magnus Institute for Pharmacology, University of Utrecht, The Netherlands.

M.R. Wells, Veterans Administration, Medical Center, Neurochemistry Laboratories, Augusta, Ga. 30904, U.S.A.

P.R. Wiepkema, Department of Zoology, University of Groningen, Haren, The Netherlands.

M. Winick, The Institute of Human Nutrition, Columbia University College of Physicians and Surgeons, New York, N.Y., U.S.A.

Preface

"Adaptive Capabilities of the Nervous System" was the theme of the 11th in a series of International Summer Schools organized by the Netherlands Institute for Brain Research in Amsterdam. Just as the proceedings of our previous meeting (devoted to "Maturation of the Nervous System" — see Progress in Brain Research, Vol. 48, edited by M. Corner, R. Baker, N. van de Poll, D. Swaab and H. Uylings) reflected one major facet of scientific work at the "Brain Institute", so the present volume reflects its other current preoccupation. Indeed, each of the four research groups at the Institute was responsible for the organization of a session at the Summer School, relating to its own program of investigation. This explains the selection which was made from among the myriad aspects of such a wide subject as "adaptation". Corresponding to the above plan, this book is organized into four sections, each containing several invited papers which are broad in scope. In addition, a few shorter reports are included which relate specifically to problems raised in one of the invited contributions. It had been planned also to include, by way of general introduction, a paper by Hendrik van der Loos based upon his excellent public lecture during the meeting, entitled "The brain adapts . . . . to what, and how?" Serious illness, however, unfortunately prevented Professor van der Loos from preparing that talk for publication.

The first section of the book deals with the morphological responses of brain tissue to a variety of challenges, including disease, accident and malnutrition. The clinical implications of increased knowledge in these areas will be evident, but several of the papers also delve quite deeply into fundamental neurobiological questions. The second section goes in depth into a more narrowly circumscribed but currently highly active field, viz. neuropeptides and their behavioral significance. Here too, fundamental neurochemical, neurophysiological and neuroontogenetic aspects are extensively explored, nor have the considerable medical potentialities of this class of substances been ignored. The papers in the third section are exclusively concerned with sleep, a phenomenon whose biological raison d'être still has not been satisfactorily eludicated. Current serious theoretical approaches to this problem are dealt with in considerable detail, and the reader may be excused for coming away with the feeling that all of the approaches must (at least in part) be true! The concluding session emphasizes the importance of waking behaviors in the successful adaptation of higher animals to their surroundings. The choice of aggression as the focus for all of the presentations here puts the spotlight upon a highly subtle form of socio-biological fitness, one which in the human context will undoubtedly continue to be a source of intense suffering and cultural disruption for quite some time. Therefore, as a form of preventive "medicine", the importance of the topic discussed in this section can hardly be emphasized enough.

The editors hope that, at the very least, a clear picture comes across of how much remains to be learned about the phenomena dealt with in this volume.

Acknowledgements

The Summer School was generously sponsored by the International Society for Developmental Neurosciences. The editors are also pleased to acknowledge the generous financial support given to the Summer School by the C.H. van den Houten Fund, and supplementary contributions from all of the following:

K. Babajeff, Algemene Import en Export, 's-Gravenhage

L. den Boer, Foto-, Pers- en Reproductiebureau, Amsterdam

Brunschwig Chemie, Amsterdam

Mayor and Aldermen of Amsterdam

Capilux, Lelystad

Elsevier/North-Holland Biomedical Press, Amsterdam

European Training Programme in Brain and Behaviour Research, Strasbourg

Genootschap ter Bevordering van Natuur-, Genees- and Heelkunde, Amsterdam

Hoffman-La Roche, Mijdrecht

Hope Farms, Woerden

Hulskamp Metaalwarenfabriek, Alkmaar

IBM Nederland, Amsterdam

Laméris Instrumenten, Utrecht

Reisbureau Lissone Lindeman, Amsterdam

Organon-Nederland, Oss/Organon International

Peninsula Laboratories, Inc., San Carlos, Calif.

Philips-Duphar, Amsterdam

Rhodia Nederland, Amstelveen, Dutch subsidiary of the Rhône-Poulenc group

Ruco Metaalwarenindustrie Nederland, Valkenswaard

Sandoz, Uden

Shell Nederland, Rotterdam

Stag Instruments Limited, Henley-on-Thames

Substantia Nederland, Mijdrecht

P.M. Tamson, Zoetermeer

Techno Nevo, Amsterdam

Universitaire Boekhandel Nederland, Rotterdam

Zuid-Holland Instrumentenhandel, 's-Gravenhage

Dr. Saal van Zwanenbergstichting, Oss

We and the publishers would also like to acknowledge the following publishers, and all of the authors, for allowing us to use previously published figures:

Ankho Press, for one figure used in the article by Gispen (*Brain Res. Bull.*, 3, 1978); Academic Press, for four figures in the article by Bernstein (*Exp. Neurol.*, 44, 1974; ibid. 61, 1978; ibid. 64, 1979) and for one figure in the article by Berry et al. (*Exp. Neurol.*, 28, 1970); American Medical Association; for one figure in the article by Van Praag and Verhoeven (*Arch. gen. Psychiat.*, 36, 1979); American Physiological Society, for two figures in the article by Walker and Berger (*Amer. J. Physiol.*, 233, 1977); American Association for the

Advancement of Science, for two figures in the article by Walker and Berger (*Science*, 204, 1979), for two figures in the article by Barker and Smith (*Science*, 199, 1978) and for one figure in the article by Leshner (*Science*, 204, 1979); Annual Reviews Inc., for one figure in the article by Van Praag and Verhoeven (*Ann. Rev. Neurosci.*, 2, 1979); Chapman and Hall, for two figures in the article by Bernstein (*J. Neurocytol.* 6, 1977; ibid. 7, 1978); Elsevier/North-Holland Biomedical Press, for one figure in the article by Hommes (*J. Neurol. Sci.*, 33, 1977); Karger, for two figures in the article by Walker and Berger (*Brain, Behav. Evol.*, 8, 1973; ibid. 10, 1974); Little Brown, for one figure in the article by Hommes (*Ann. Neurol.*, 1, 1977); MacMillan Journals, Ltd., for two figures in the article by Barker and Smith (*Nature (Lond.)*, 253, 1975) and for one figure in the article by Hommes (*Nature (Lond.)*, 266, 1977); P. Parey, for one figure in the article by Berry et al. (*Anat. Embryol.*, 148, 1975); Pergamon Press, for one figure in the article by Coenen and Van Hulzen (*Physiol. Behav.*, 23, 1979), and for two figures in the article by Leshner (*Physiol. Behav.*, 17, 1976; ibid. 22, 1979); Plenum Press, for one figure in the article by Van Praag and Verhoeven (*Handbook of Psychopharmacology*, Iversen et al. (Eds.), 1978), for one figure in the article by Gispen (*Advanc. Exp. Med. Biol., Vol. 16*, Ehrlich et al. (Eds.), 1979), for one figure in the article by Cohen (*Consciousness and Self-regulation: Advanc. Res., Vol. 1*, Schwartz and Schapiro, (Eds.), 1976), and for one figure in the article by Hommes (*J. Neuropath. exp. Neurol.*, 24, 1965); Springer Verlag, for one figure in the article by Bernstein (from *Cerebellar Cortex, Cytology and Organization*, Palay and Chan-Palay, 1974) and for one figure in the article by Hommes (*Acta Neuropath. (Berl.)*, 43, 1978); Univ. of Chicago Press, for one figure in the article by Walker and Berger (*Physiol. Zool.*, in press); Verlag Chemie, for one figure in the article by Hommes (*Proc. Europ. Soc. Neurochem.*, V. Neuhof (Ed.), 1978); Wiley Interscience, for one figure from the article by Jouvet (*Develop. Psychobiol.*, 2, 1970), for one figure in the article by Walker and Berger (*EEG of Human Sleep: Clinical Implications*, Williams et al. (Eds.), 1974) and for one figure in the article by Berry et al. (*J. Neurobiol.*, 4, 1973); Wistar Press, for one figure in the article by McConnell (*J. comp. Neurol.*, 178, 1978) and for one figure in the article by Berry et al. (*J. comp. Neurol.*, 162, 1975).

Finally, we are once again extremely grateful to Ms. J. Sels for her meticulous attention to secretarial and organizational details during both the meeting itself and the preparation of this book. Mr. P. Wolters and Mr. R. Nooy have our thanks for their able handling of the electrotechnical side of the Summer School.

Contents

xii

SECTION I

Structural Adaptation of the Brain

(edited by P.S. McConnell)

Morphological Consequences of Prenatal Injury to the Primate Brain

PATRICIA S. GOLDMAN-RAKIC

Yale School of Medicine, New Haven, Conn., U.S.A.

INTRODUCTION

One of the most important discoveries for understanding the adaptive capabilities of the central nervous system is that under particular conditions, brain lesions can induce intact neurons and their axons to innervate structures that have lost their normal inputs. Although rearrangement of connectivity in the mammalian brain is potentially the most adaptive biological mechanism underlying recovery of function, anomalous synaptic circuitry may also be responsible for impairment of function and permanent deficits after brain injury. Consequently, detailed analysis of axonal modification and the factors that promote or prevent its expression is essential for a full understanding of the entire range of effects – the loss as well as recovery – of functional capacity following brain injury.

Until recently, most information on the nature and limits of lesion-induced neural plasticity was based largely on studies of rodents and carnivores and very little was known about the extent to which neuronal systems in a large gyrencephalic brain, like that of primates, share some or all of the neuronal resilience that has been revealed in the study of non-primate mammals. In the present report I will describe selected studies carried out in my laboratory which demonstrate that the frontal association cortex and related cortical and subcortical structures in rhesus monkeys are part of a neural system that exhibits remarkable structural and functional plasticity.

The evidence to be reviewed comes, for the most part, from studies on young monkeys that had sustained cortical ablation at some point in their embryonic development. Information on the consequences of prenatal brain injury in primates has not been available until now because of the considerable difficulties encountered in preserving pregnancy and producing viable offspring after neurosurgical manipulation of the mammalian, in particular, the primate fetus. Recent advances in the technique of prenatal surgery have enabled us to perform cortical resections in fetal monkeys at mid-gestation and obtain subsequent survival of the fetus to term (Goldman and Galkin, 1978; Goldman, 1978; Goldman-Rakic, 1980). These fetuses are temporarily exteriorized from the uterus but remain in contact with the mother via the umbilical cord. Following the neurosurgical procedure, the fetus is returned to the uterus where its intra-uterine development continues uninterrupted until delivery around the 165th day post-conception (full term in rhesus monkeys). Analysis of the long-range anatomical consequences of cortical resection performed weeks or months before birth has provided valuable and unique information on the limits of neural plasticity in primates in whom the most crucial events underlying organogenesis – neuron proliferation, cell migration and axonal and dendritic differentiation — occur to a large extent prenatally. The morphological consequences of prenatal brain injury to be discussed below include: (1) modification of the external surface of the telencephalon; and (2) alterations in afferent and efferent connections.

MODIFICATION OF THE EXTERNAL SURFACE OF THE TELENCEPHALON

In the course of our our studies on the behavioral consequences of prenatal cerebral damage, we had the opportunity to examine the brains of a number of monkeys that were given either unilateral or bilateral resections of the prospective dorsolateral prefrontal cortex at various gestational ages and to compare these with brains of animals that underwent comparable neurosurgical procedures at selected postnatal ages (Fig. 1). Structural consequences of direct or indirect injury to immature nerve cells can take a wide variety of forms ranging from gross morphological distortions of the convolutional pattern and changes in long tract

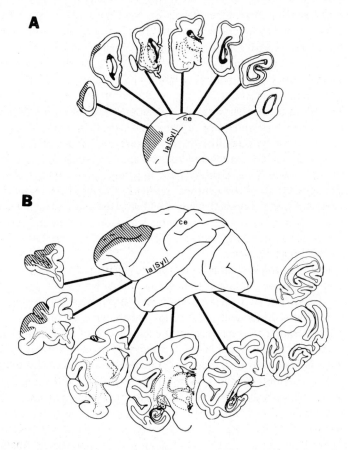

Fig. 1. A: lateral view reconstruction and selected coronal sections of a fetal brain at E106 illustrating immaturity of fissural pattern at this stage of gestation. B: lateral view and sections at comparable levels from a mature brain with fully developed sulci and gyri. Cross-hatching indicates location of dorsolateral prefrontal resections at each age. Abbreviations: ce, central sulcus; la, lateral (Sylvian) fissure.

projections to cellular and subcellular modifications of synaptic contacts and cytoplasmic organelles. The simplest and most obvious change that would attract the attention of most neuropathologists is the dramatic alteration of the cerebral surface. To our surprise, even cursory examination of the brains of prenatally operated monkeys revealed an abnormal configuration of sulci and gyri that was not a simple or direct consequence of surgery and/or removal of cortical tissue. In order to analyze the location and extent of this abnormal fissuration, full view reconstructions of the lateral and dorsal surfaces of these brains were made from drawings of serial sections. Photographs of the fixed brains viewed at different angles, obtained prior to embedding and sectioning, were used for orientation and to provide outlines for the reconstructions (for details, see Goldman and Galkin, 1978). The combination of photography, drawings and reconstructions from serial histological sections provided reliable data on the depth and regional boundaries of the ablated area in the monkeys operated before or after birth as well as on fissural patterns in intact portions of the telencephalon.

Location and bilateral symmetry of ectopic fissures

The full view reconstructions of the cerebral hemispheres revealed striking differences in sulcal pattern in the brains of monkeys operated at embryonic ages as compared with those of unoperated monkeys or monkeys operated after birth. Abnormal sulci and gyri had formed not only in areas bordering the lesion, but also in remote cortical regions. Examples of these anomalies are shown in Fig. 2, which compares lateral view reconstructions of a normal brain with a comparable reconstruction from a brain of a monkey that had both frontal lobes resected at E106 (106th embryonic day). Unusual sulci were found, for example, on the dorsolateral surface of the occipital lobe — a region which is normally smooth. Also, at the superior margin of the parietal lobe, the lunate sulcus bifurcated on the

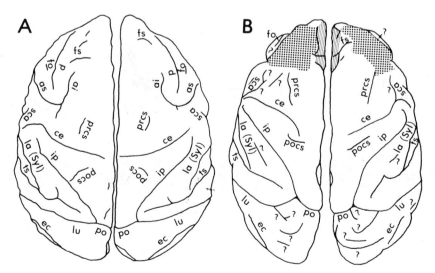

Fig. 2. A: dorsal view reconstruction of the brain of an unoperated 2.5-year-old monkey. B: dorsal view of a 2.5-year-old monkey operated at E106 illustrating size of the resection and location of the anomalous sulci punctuated by question marks. Note the preponderance of ectopic sulci in the prefrontal, temporal and occipital lobes and their relative absence in the peri-Rolandic or central portion of the cortical surface.

6

lateral surface in an unusual pattern in each hemisphere. Although in the two dimensional drawing of Fig. 2 the abnormal sulci are indicated by short lines, examination of the transverse sections on which the reconstruction is based reveals that they are often deep invaginations of cortex buried beneath the surface of the cerebrum (Fig 3).

Some of the most dramatic changes were found in regions of the frontal lobe immediately surrounding the lesion. Comparisons of coronal sections of the brain lesioned at E106 with corresponding sections from an unoperated control and from monkeys operated after birth at P50 (50th postnatal day) and P540 revealed an unusual fissural pattern on the ventral surface of the frontal lobe in the prenatal case (indicated by arrow at +27 in Fig. 3). Although the medial and lateral orbital sulci are recognizable as such, an additional unusually deep sulcus was located near the lateral border of the cortex. A sulcus of this size and configuration is never encountered in unoperated brains and also was not present in selected monkeys operated at P50 and P540. Another deep, spatially distinct, indentation of cortex was present at a more rostral level (A + 35 in Fig. 3). In contrast, it is notable that the sulcal pattern in the peri-Rolandic area on the adjacent dorsalateral convexity contained few if any aberrant sulci (Fig. 2). Thus, this portion of the frontal lobe appeared to develop normally.

The cortex lining the abnormal sulci in the frontal, temporal and occipital lobes retains the general cytoarchitectonic composition and laminar pattern characteristic of the cortical region in which it is found. For example, ectopic cortical fissures in the primary visual area had a well developed stripe of Gennari (see Fig. 13 in Goldman and Galkin, 1978). Cellular

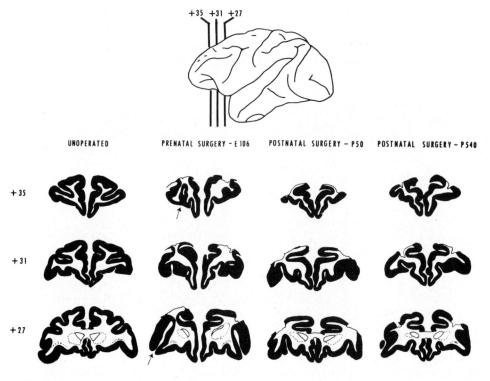

Fig. 3. Outlines of selected coronal sections cut through the frontal lobe of a control 2.5-year-old unoperated monkey and of the monkeys operated at E106, P50 and P540, respectively. Ectopic sulci are prominent in the brain of the prenatally operated monkey at the Horsley-Clarke A–P levels +35 and also at +27 (arrows).

analysis of the cortex in the anomalous sulci of the frontal lobe is more difficult because the boundaries between cytoarchitectonic subfields in the frontal granular cortex are normally less sharply delineated (Brodmann, 1925; Walker, 1940). Also, tectogenetic changes following surgery make precise cytoarchitectonic comparisons between experimental and control animals difficult. Nevertheless, the anomalous gyri in the frontal lobe appear to retain the basic characteristics of frontal granular cortex (see Fig. 15, Goldman and Galkin, 1978).

One of the striking features of the anomalous fissural pattern is its bilateral symmetry following either bilateral or unilateral lesions (Figs. 2 and 3). We found that aberrant sulci tended to develop in the same locations and had the same general orientation in all major cerebral promontories of both hemispheres. Although this bilateral symmetry might be expected in cases of bilateral brain damage, the finding that corresponding abnormalities were present in both hemispheres in monkeys with unilateral resections was surprising. As discussed in more detail below, this finding implicates a general morphogenetic mechanism of cortical dysgenesis rather than one based on the direct and local mechanical influence of surgery. If mechanical factors such as compression, distortion or cavitation were alone responsible for the ectopic gyri, they would be expected to appear in the central and opercular regions of the frontal lobe which are adjacent to the cortical lesion and would be more pronounced on the side of surgery in unilaterally operated monkeys. As mentioned, we found instead that convolutions in some adjacent areas were actually more regular in appearance than were those found in remote locations such as the occipital lobes and abnormal sulci were as prominent in the unoperated as in the operated hemisphere of monkeys with unilateral lesions. It is thus improbable that direct physical injury was the sole cause of anomalous fissuration. However, physical trauma and reduced oxygenation as a consequence of interference with cerebral blood-flow and/or alteration in cerebral spinal fluid pressure at critical stages of development, due to either unilateral or bilateral removal of tissue, cannot be ruled out as the cause of atypical fissuration throughout the brain. Indeed, disturbance of the circulatory system has been implicated in the pathogenesis of numerous cerebral cortical malformations in man (Courville, 1971).

Neogenesis of cortical neurons and the formation of abnormal fissures

One possible explanation for the sulcal and gyral abnormalities observed in prenatally operated animals is that the experimental lesions somehow induce the process of neuronal proliferation to continue beyond the normal time of termination or to resume after the relevant portion of the germinal cell matrix should normally be depleted. It is known that all prefrontal neurons in the rhesus monkey are ordinarily generated before E90 (Rakic and Wikmark, unpublished observations) but the possibility exists that neurogenesis endures beyond this time in response to injury to compensate for the loss of cells. This idea was considered tenable because prolongation of the time of Purkinje cell genesis has been reported in fetal mice treated with the protein synthesis inhibitor, 5-fluorodeoxyuridine (Andreoli et al., 1973). Also, compensatory granule cell proliferation has been observed after X-irradiation at appropriate stages of development in the rat (Altman, 1975). The hypothesis of prolonged neurogenesis was appealing because it could provide a mechanism both for the widespread changes in all lobes of the brain and for their symmetry.

To test the validity of prolonged neurogenesis, we performed unilateral prefrontal resections on two fetal monkeys at E81 and E102, respectively. Both fetuses were then subsequently exposed to pulse-label of [³H]thymidine delivered by intravenous injections of their mothers. The fetus operated at E81 was exposed to the radioactive marker more than

3 weeks later at E104; the fetus operated at E102 received the same exposure one day later at E103. In both cases, all prefrontal cortical neurons would normally be generated at the time of [³H]thymidine injection (Rakic and Wikmark, unpublished observations). The two monkey fetuses were permitted to develop in utero until close to term when, in the final step of this experiment, their brains were fixed, cut frozen and prepared for autoradiography by standard methods. Analysis of autoradiograms prepared from sections through the frontal lobes did not reveal the presence of any neurons with radioactive grains over their nuclear region. (Evidence of densely labeled neurons would indicate that these cells had undergone their last cell division at the time of [³H]thymidine injection and hence after the time when all prefrontal neurons would normally be generated.) Although analysis of the data from these experiments is not complete, the preliminary findings indicate that all labeled nuclei are those of glial cells. Thus, it seems that focal cortical resections of the size and type described above do not prolong noticeably the normal period of neuron genesis nor do they reinitiate a period of neuronal proliferation after this process normally ceases.

Given that no new neurons are generated after surgery at mid-gestation, the formation of aberrant sulci, particularly those on the lateroventral surface of the frontal lobe, may involve a redeployment of prospective dorsolateral cortical neurons that had already been generated but had not yet entered the cortical plate. There is evidence that late-generated cortical neurons in the occipital lobe of the rhesus monkey require several weeks to reach their destination in the developing cortical plate (Rakic, 1975). Our own examination of normal fetal rhesus monkeys between E100 and E119 (Goldman and Galkin, 1978) has revealed numerous immature cells in the white matter beneath the growing cortical plate similar to those described in the human fetus at comparable stages of development (Kostović and Molliver, 1974). Thus, in the monkey many neurons would not be eliminated by a resection at mid-gestation. Theoretically, the spared prospective dorsolateral neurons could change their migratory course to populate cortical regions adjacent to the ablated area. Such a redistribution would be feasible in part because resection of the developing cortex also damages the proximal segments of radial glial fibers that normally guide cortical neurons into their appropriate areal positions but also pose restraints to their lateral movement (Rakic, 1978). This and other mechanisms of cortical dysgenesis, to be discussed below, are presently under systematic examination in my laboratory. These studies should provide new insight into the origins and consequences of perinatal brain injury, particularly when such injury occurs at critical times in the morphogenesis of the external features of the brain.

Critical period of fissural development and genesis of connections

The spatial distribution of ectopic sulci can be related rather well to timetables of normal fissural development and to the outgrowth and innervation of the cortex by certain classes of its afferents. In the rhesus monkey, the general convolutional pattern of the brain begins to take shape around the end of the second-third of gestation. As in the human brain, the first primary fissures to develop are the Sylvian and Rolandic. In the monkey they appear around E100 (Goldman and Galkin, 1978). During the last-third of gestation, all other primary and most of the secondary sulci become either well delineated or at least clearly recognizable so that at the end of this period the adult cerebral fissural pattern and compartmentalization into cerebral lobes is firmly established. This period which seems to be critical for the development of the normal fissural pattern appears to coincide roughly with the time interval over which there is an influx of thalamic and corticocortical afferents into the cortex. According to the most recent studies on the development of the visual system in monkeys, the thalamocortical innervation of the occipital lobe occurs between E91 and

E124 (Rakic, 1979). Other thalamic connections in the primate brain appear to invade their cortical targets over the same period of time (Goldman and Galkin, 1978). Corticocortical and callosal fibers innervate the cortex somewhat later — roughly between E124 and E150 (Goldman-Rakic, 1980). Thus, cerebral fissuration begins about the same time that thalamo-cortical afferents invade the cortex and assumes its mature pattern during the time of major ingrowth of corticocortical connections. It is probably significant that anomalous features in the sulcal pattern can be experimentally induced only in the brains of monkeys that have been operated on before the end of this period (Goldman and Galkin, 1978; Goldman-Rakic, unpublished observations).

The correspondence in the timetable of development of fissures and the innervation of the cortical plate suggests that these two major developmental events may in some way be causally related. This hypothesis, in turn, may explain how a disruption of a rather small part of the cortex could produce widespread changes which encompass the entire cerebral surface of both hemispheres. If the prefrontal neurons are removed before their axons have reached their ipsilateral cortical targets, which are in the adjacent prefrontal cortex and in distant destinations of the temporal and parieto-occipital cortex (Goldman and Nauta, 1977b; Jacobson and Trojanowski, 1977; Künzle, 1978) these target structures will be deprived of a considerable portion of their normal input which would subject them to unusual structural forces resulting from the abnormal numbers and arrangement of ingrow-ing fibers. Furthermore, since it is known that transneuronal degeneration occurs more extensively in immature than mature brain (Cowan, 1970; Bleier, 1969), as a consequence, it may be expected that neurons in the cortical target regions that are deprived of their normal input would degenerate in greater numbers and proportions in fetal than in more mature animals. Finally, this effect would be transferred via callosal neurons to corre-sponding loci in the opposite hemisphere which would also degenerate or become rearranged — resulting in local mirror-symmetric tectogenetic changes in homotopic cortical zones.

This sequence of events is at the present time only a working hypothesis which could explain the location, the timetable of development and the symmetry of abnormal convolu-tions. Thus, the abnormal fissures tend to be located in target areas of the prefrontal cortico-cortical efferent system and are notably absent in areas such as the motor and sensorimotor cortex which are devoid of direct prefrontal projections. According to our most recent autoradiographic data on the maturation of associational and callosal connections in primate fetuses (Goldman-Rakic, 1980) the abnormal sulci develop just before these connections are fully formed. Finally, their bilateral distribution follows the circuitry that could be affected by transneuronal processes as outlined above. According to this model, protection from transneuronal degenerative processes occurs with the collateralization of afferent and efferent systems and thus would not occur to any noticeable extent after the establishment of connectivity in the brain is well advanced — presumably several weeks before birth.

This theory of fissural development suggests a number of further experiments and obser-vations, but will remain in the realm of speculation until these are carried out. It does have several implications for understanding the significance of the fissural pattern and its disturb-ance during development. Since fissures tend to separate cytoarchitectonic and functionally distinct zones of cortex (e.g. Sanides, 1969) the emergence of new fissures implies that there is also a change in the size and shape of these cytologically and functionally meaningful cortical parcels. It would be of interest to assess the new subdivisions both cytologically and behaviorally. Secondly, a more basic issue is the possibility that cortical areas may differenti-ate into different cytoarchitectonic zones on the basis of their afferent input and fissural boundaries. Thus, studies of prenatal development of a gyrencephalic brain with well-defined cytoarchitectonic fields like that of the rhesus monkey may shed light on some long-standing functional, evolutionary and ontogenetic problems.

ALTERATION IN AFFERENT AND EFFERENT CONNECTIONS

Although studies of monocular deprivation (Hubel, Wiesel and LeVay, 1977) and eye enucleation (Rakic, 1977b) indicate considerably plasticity of neural connections in the primate visual cortex, experimental data on rearrangement of connections consequent to direct brain injury have so far been obtained only in monkeys subjected to dorsolateral prefrontal resection as fetuses (Goldman and Galkin, 1978; Goldman, 1978; Goldman-Rakic, 1980). These changes have now been observed in several classes of prefrontal afferent and efferent connections (Goldman-Rakic, 1980). I will confine myself in this essay to a description of lesion-induced modifications in: (i) thalamocortical; and (ii) corticostriatal projections.

Response of the thalamocortical system to perinatal brain injury

One example of the immature primate brain's capacity to respond to injury by readjust-ment of normal neuronal relationships comes from our recent analysis of thalamocortical projections, also using monkeys whose prefrontal cortex had been resected at various pre- and postnatal ages. It should be pointed out that in the rhesus monkey, the parvocellular moiety of the mediodorsal nucleus is the principle source of thalamic afferents to the dorsolateral prefrontal association cortex, and consequently neurons in this part of the thalamus regularly degenerate following lesions in this region of the cortex in mature mon-keys (Walker, 1940a; Pribram et al., 1953; Akert, 1964).

To analyze the response of thalamoprefrontal afferents to injury at different stages of development, we performed detailed qualitative and quantitative assessment of retrograde degeneration in the mediodorsal nucleus following unilateral or bilateral dorsolateral resec-tions at fetal and neonatal ages (Goldman and Galkin, 1978). Monkeys with unilateral lesions served as their own controls. In these cases the parvocellular division of the medio-dorsal nucleus on the side of the lesion was compared with its counterpart in the unoperated hemisphere (Fig. 4). In monkeys with bilateral lesions, the relevant portion of the thalamus of monkeys operated prenatally was compared with those of unoperated animals as well as with those given similar bilateral lesions at later stages of development. Counts of neurons were made in selected loci of the magnocellular as well as the parvocellular subdivisions of the dorsomedial nucleus (Fig. 5). The latter served as a control for non-specific effects of the surgery since the cells in this part of the dorsomedial nucleus do not project to the resected area. More importantly, cell counts in an unaffected nucleus allowed us to take into account possible differences in cell density brought about by the differential shrinkage among brains that is commonly associated with processing neural tissue. Further details of the procedures and statistical analysis used to evaluate thalamic retrograde degeneration are provided in Goldman and Galkin (1978).

The results of the light microscopic analysis of sections through the thalamus in animals operated prenatally differed significantly from those of animals operated at more mature stages. The most important finding was that neurons of the parvocellular moiety of the dorsomedial nucleus in the thalamus, which degenerate following resection of the dorso-lateral cortex in adult monkeys, were nearly normal in number and remarkably well

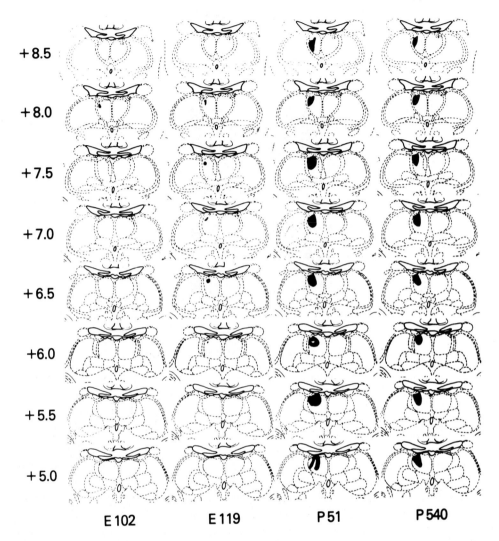

+8.5

+8.0

+7.5

+7.0

+6.5

+6.0

+5.5

+5.0

E 102   E 119   P 51   P 540

Fig. 4. Outline drawings of coronal sections cut through the mediodorsal nucleus of monkeys that sustained unilateral dorsolateral resections at E102, E119, P50 and P540. Areas of neuronal loss are marked in black.

preserved in monkeys operated before E119 (Figs. 4 and 5). Cellular degeneration was somewhat more pronounced after surgery at E119 but still considerably less than that observed following lesions in adulthood (Figs. 4 and 5). In sharp contrast, monkeys operated at the end of the second postnatal month (P50) exhibited a profile of chromatolysis and cell loss that could not easily be distinguished from that of monkeys operated as adults (Figs. 4 and 5).

The number and integrity of preserved mediodorsal neurons is somewhat surprising because both the classical (Gudden, 1870; Brodal, 1949) as well as the more contemporary (Bleier, 1969; Schneider, 1970; Leonard, 1974) literature on fiber degeneration in developing mammals indicates that thalamocortical and other projection neurons are, if anything,

12

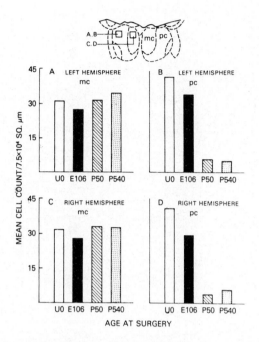

Fig. 5. Bar graph indicating mean values for cell counts through the areas denoted by squares on the diagram of the thalamus at the top of the figure. Each mean is based on counts from 7 matched sections through the relevant moiety of the mediodorsal nucleus. Abbreviations:UO, unoperated monkey (2.5 years of age); P50, representative monkey operated at P50 and sacrificed at around 2.5 years; P540, monkey operated at P540 and sacrificed as an adult: For details, see Goldman and Galkin (1978).

more susceptible to injury in the immature brain. Indeed, both primary and transneuronal degenerative processes are generally found to be more extensive after brain damage inflicted at earlier as compared with later developmental stages (for review, see Cowan, 1970). What-ever the explanation for these apparent discrepancies with data in other species and/or sys-tems, the finding in the present study that thalamic neurons survive after resection of their target cortex strongly implies that they have found some other synaptic target, since ordinarily neurons that do not establish functional synapses usually degenerate (e.g. Ham-burger, 1975; Clarke and Cowan, 1976). Such neuronal rearrangement could result from the mechanism of collateral sprouting (Raisman, 1969; Schneider, 1970; Lynch et al., 1973) in which intact axons are induced to expand their terminal distribution by injury and degenera-tion of other axon terminals in the same field. Also, it is likely that many thalamic neurons had not yet entered the developing cortical plate at E102–E106 (Rakic, 1979). Conse-quently, their growing tips would escape injury and could become rerouted into other cortical and subcortical structures in the absence of their appropriate targets. A number of alternative explanations for sparing of thalamic neurons are also possible and these are discussed fully elsewhere (Goldman and Galkin, 1978).

Response of the corticostriatal system to perinatal brain injury

A perhaps even more dramatic and certainly more direct example of the remarkable capacity of the primate brain for neuronal rearrangement comes from our recent analysis of corticostriatal connections following unilateral dorsolateral prefrontal resections on fetal and neonatal rhesus monkeys (Goldman, 1978; Goldman-Rakic, 1980). The basic design of these experiments was to remove cortical input to the neostriatum in one hemisphere by unilateral decortication and then to subsequently examine and compare the connections of the homotopic cortex in the intact hemisphere with corresponding projections in normal monkeys. The surgical procedures for prenatal cortical resection were the same as described in previous sections of this chapter. Then, the prenatally operated fetuses that survived to term and all of the animals that were first operated after birth subsequently underwent a second surgical procedure in which the homotopic cortex of the unoperated hemisphere was injected with tritiated amino acids for the purpose of tracing the corticostriatal and other prefrontal efferent projections (Fig. 6). One to 3 weeks later, the monkeys were sacrificed and their brains processed for autoradiographic tracing of neuronal connections.

The results of the autoradiographic analysis provided a particularly striking example of neuronal plasticity in response to circumscribed lesions of primate cortex, which may involve rerouting and/or expansion of intact corticostriatal projections (Fig. 7). Prefronto-caudate projections are normally directed mainly to ipsilateral caudate nucleus and putamen with only a very small number of fibers crossing the midline and innervating the contra-lateral neostriatum (Goldman and Nauta, 1977a; Künzle, 1978). In monkeys that have been deprived of prefrontal cortex from as early as 6 weeks before birth (Goldman, 1978) or as late as two months after birth (Goldman-Rakic, 1980), the projection of the prefrontal cortex to the ipsilateral caudate nucleus in the unoperated hemisphere is similar in topography and in configuration to that observed in normal monkeys. However, the projection to the contralateral caudate nucleus differs markedly from that of normal monkeys. Whereas in normal animals the contralateral caudate nucleus contains silver grains that only barely exceed background, in the previously operated monkeys, dense concentrations of label can be traced in consecutive serial sections throughout the entire extent of the contralateral nucleus, i.e. over a distance of several cm (Goldman, 1978). Significantly, the crossed projection is expanded predominantly in those areas that were deafferented by the unilateral dorsolateral lesions. Furthermore, the anomalous contralateral projections exhibit the same

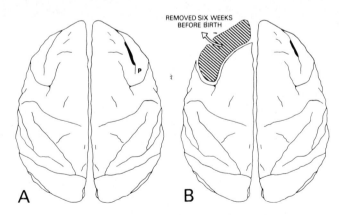

Fig. 6. Diagram illustrating experimental plan of experiment designed to reveal alterations in prefrontal efferents. In the example shown, the dorsolateral prefrontal cortex of the experimental animal was resected before birth. After birth, the right hemisphere was injected with tritiated amino acids in both (A) normal and (B) prenatally operated monkeys for the purpose of examining prefrontal cortical projections by autoradiography. Comparable injection sites in control and experimental cases are shown in black.

14

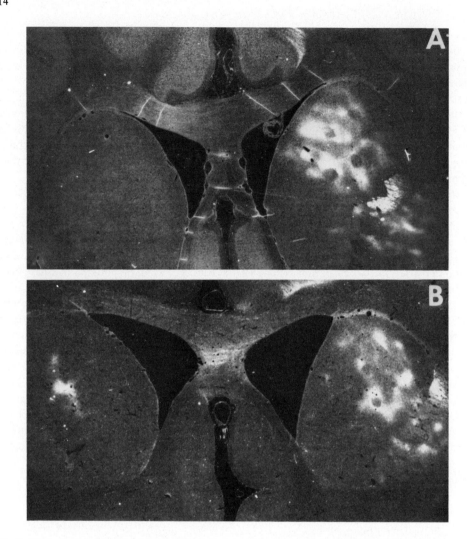

Fig. 7. Photographs of the head of the caudate nuclei in left and right hemispheres under dark-field illumination. A: a normal monkey. The autoradiogram, exposed 16 weeks, shows an intricate and dense pattern of labeling in the right (ipsilateral) caudate nucleus; the cingulum bundle, internal capsule, and putamen are also densely labeled. However, label in the contralateral nucleus is too faint to be resolved in the photograph. B: a monkey whose prospective dorsolateral prefrontal cortex in the left hemisphere was resected before birth and whose prefrontal cortex in the right hemisphere was injected with tritiated amino acids. The autoradiogram was exposed 13 weeks. Note both the intricate pattern of grains in the right (ipsilateral) caudate nucleus and also a distinct projection to the left (contralateral) caudate.

"annular" pattern of termination that characterize the normal projections described by Goldman and Nauta (1977a).

Several mechanisms may be involved in the reorganization of corticocaudate projections consequent to unilateral prefrontal resection and some of them have already been discussed (Goldman, 1978). One possibility is that the abnormally large contralateral projections result from arresting development at an embryonic stage when corticostriatal projections might normally be bilateral. It now appears that this mechanism is unlikely to be involved because of our recent autoradiographic data on prenatal development of connections (Goldman-

Rakic, 1980) which provides no evidence of strong bilateral prefrontocaudate projections at any stage of development between E60 and E155. Therefore, the phenomenon of neuronal rearrangements cannot be simply explained as a failure of selective elimination of contra-lateral projections.

A related but more likely possibility is that axons forming anomalous connections belong to the class of efferent neurons that normally issue a minor projection to the contralateral caudate nucleus. These corticostriatal neurons, which are not easy to detect by the auto-radiographic method in developing animals, may expand their terminal fields and occupy a number of synaptic spaces on caudate neurons vacated by degeneration of their ipsilateral prefrontal input. Such a mechanism has been postulated for neuronal plasticity in a variety of other systems (e.g. Hicks and D'Amato, 1970; Schneider, 1973; Lund et al., 1973; Lynch et al., 1973).

Finally we have not ruled out the possibility that the anomalous crossed corticostriatal fibers originate from callosal neurons which, in the absence of their homotopic target cells in the operated hemisphere, invade the caudate nucleus subjacent to the lesion to join with the normally meagre complement of crossed corticostriatal fibers in what is for them com-pletely foreign territory. This hypothesis is testable and, if we find that callosal fibers are rerouted to subcortical targets, it would represent a type of rewiring that is unprecedented in the mammalian nervous system. However, in order to determine the mode and mechanisms involved, further experiments are essential. The technology now available to neurobiologists allows us to examine these issues in the primate brain for the first time.

CONCLUDING REMARKS

One of the most challenging questions facing neurobiology and psychiatry is the degree of latitude that is permissible in the relationship between neural structure and functional capacity. This century has witnessed radical shifts in opinion concerning this basic question and, in particular, the matter of how experience moulds human behavior and intelligence (Sperry, 1971). Clarification of the modifiability of the mammalian nervous system, especi-ally in our own species in whom the qualities of plasticity and adaptability are paramount, will not be satisfactorily answered until we have a firm idea of the organization of the neural circuitry subserving cognitive and other higher order cerebral processes in the primate nervous system, knowledge of how and when neural connections develop, and finally, the degree of their modifiability during the course of normal and pathological development.

The studies on the consequences of prefrontal lesions in fetal rhesus monkeys described in this chapter have revealed that the primate brain is extraordinarily malleable in response to external forces and thus displays a degree of neuronal plasticity that is comparable if not greater than neuronal modifications that have been described in numerous non-primate mammals. The present findings in monkeys are particularly instructive because they reveal changes at both the gross morphological and cellular levels in a slowly developing gyren-cephalic brain which is similar to the human cerebrum. The findings therefore bear both directly and indirectly on our understanding of pediatric neuropathological disorders as well as on the normal development of the human brain.

One of the major changes described in the present report was the abnormal development of the external surface morphology of the brain after cortical lesions were induced during a "critical" period of gestation. Although interest in the subject of the convolutional pattern in primates is centuries old, very little is still known about the genetic or intra-uterine factors that govern its phylogenetic history or ontogenetic development. Experimental analyses of congenital conditions affecting brain morphology have been rare. Barron's study (Barron, 1950) on fetal sheep was the first experimental analysis of mechanical influences on the morphology of the cerebral surface. In this study extensive ablations of subcortical structures and white matter did not alter the convolutional pattern of the mature brain. Windle et al. (1967) and Myers (1969) have provided detailed descriptions of brain damage experimentally induced in monkeys by asphyxia at different stages of gestation and at parturition. Changes which include distortion of the convolutional pattern have been reported in a case of spontaneous perinatal brain damage (Myers et al., 1973). The findings described in Goldman and Galkin (1978) and additional data reviewed in the present report are the first indication of abnormal convolutions following circumscribed experimental cortical lesions in the fetal monkey.

Various patterns of abnormal fissuration have been extensively reported in the neuropathological literature (Courville, 1971; Yakovlev and Wadsworth, 1946; Larroche, 1977) including the most common disorders of brain morphology in man — porencephaly, schizencephaly, microgyria and ulegyria. Although the aberrant fissural patterns observed in these various developmental disorders do not necessarily resemble those found after focal lesions in fetal rhesus monkeys either in size, location, cellular integrity or functional consequences, an important commonality among them may be the period of gestation during which they originate. Many neuropathological conditions in man appear to arise before birth when external morphogenetic features are just begining to emerge (Courville, 1971). Although the mechanisms of formation of anomalous gyri, proposed in a previous section and by others (Yakovlev and Wadsworth, 1946; Barron, 1950; Richman et al., 1975), must at present remain in the realm of speculation, they probably involve the same interplay of genetic and extrinsic forces which guide normal development. I have tried to indicate throughout this chapter how modern neurobiological methods now available to analyze fetal brain development can be combined with prenatal surgery in infra-human primates to provide a well-controlled experimental approach to this problem.

Another example of the brain's adaptive capabilities was provided by our analysis of altered thalamo—cortical and, in particular, cortico—striatal projections. It should be emphasized that the rearrangement of central neuronal connections is not likely to be limited to just these classes of connections. Preliminary examination of other classes of prefrontal efferents already reveals equally dramatic rearrangement of connections following perinatal brain injury. For example, callosal projections can become heterotopic if the homotopic cortex has been removed at prenatal stages (Goldman-Rakic, 1980). Likewise, cortico-thalamic pathways appear to be altered by lesions performed early in gestation (Goldman-Rakic, unpublished results). The changes in these divergent classes of cortical efferents as well as those described on thalamocortical afferents in the present chapter, attest to the impressive capacity of the immature primate brain for neuronal plasticity in response to injury.

The ability of the central nervous system to reorganize its synaptic connectivity in response to deprivation or lesions is of interest not only because of its theoretical significance but also because new connections are potentially the most important biological mechanism underlying resilience of function. It is generally accepted that the severity of behavioral deficits caused by focal injury to the mammalian nervous system is strongly influenced by the age at which the lesion is sustained. Although the critical period for lesion-induced alterations in the callosal and corticostriatal connections of the primate brain is still unknown, evidence of rewiring of these cortical efferents following perinatal brain injury leads naturally to the hypothesis that anomalous connections may play an important role in restitution of function in primates. It is noteworthy that the dorsolateral prefrontal cortex, the connections of which exhibit considerable anatomical plasticity, is part of the same neural system that has been shown to exhibit modifiability in response to early experience (Goldman, 1976; Goldman and Mendelson, 1977) and hormones (Goldman and Brown, 1975), as well as a marked capacity for functional reorganization following both prenatal (Goldman and Galkin, 1978) and postnatal (Goldman, 1971) cortical injury. Although with the present state of technology, we have had to use a surgical ablation to reveal the structural plasticity of frontal-lobe connections, there is every reason to believe that these connections can also be modified in more subtle ways by relevant extrinsic stimulation and experience. Such changes in the connections of prefrontal association cortex can be expected to be of profound significance for the behavior and personality of the individual.

REFERENCES

Akert, K. (1964) Comparative anatomy of the frontal cortex and thalamocortical connections. In *The Frontal Granular Cortex and Behavior,* J.M. Warren and K. Akert (Eds.), McGraw-Hill, New York, pp. 372–396.

Altman, J. (1975) Effects of interference with cerebellar maturation on the development of locomotion. In *Brain Mechanisms in Mental Retardation,* N.A. Buchwald, and M.A. Brazier (Eds.), Academic Press, New York, pp. 41–91.

Andreoli, J., Rodier, P. and Langman, J. (1973) The influence of a prenatal trauma on formation of Purkinje cells. *Amer. J. Anat.,* 137: 87–102.

Barron, D.H. (1950) An experimental analysis of some factors involved in the development of fissure pattern of the cerebral cortex. *J. exp. Zool.,* 113: 553–573.

Bleier, R. (1969) Retrograde transsynaptic cellular degeneration in mammillary and ventral tegmental nuclei following limbic decortication in rabbits of various ages. *Brain Res.,* 15: 365–393.

Brodal, A. (1940) Modification of Gudden method for study of cerebral localization. *Arch. Neurol. Psychiat.,* 43: 46–58.

Brodmann, K. (1925) *Vergleichende Lokalisationslehre der Grosshirnrinde,* 2, Auflage, J.A. Barth, Leipzig.

Clarke, P.G.H. and Cowan, W.M. (1976) The development of the isthmo-optic tract in the chick, with special reference to the occurrence and correction of developmental errors in the location and connections of isthmo-optic neurons. *J. comp. Neurol.,* 167: 143–163.

Courville, C.B. (1971) *Birth and Brain Damage. An Investigation into the Problems of Antenatal and Paranatal Anoxia and Allied Disorders and their Relation to the Many Lesion-Complexes Residual Thereto,* N.F. Courville, Pasadena, California.

Cowan, W.M. (1970) Anterograde and retrograde transneuronal degeneration in the central and peripheral nervous system. In *Contemporary Research Methods in Neuroanatomy,* W.J.H. Nauta and S.O.E. Ebbesson (Eds.), Springer-Verlag, New York, pp. 217–251.

Goldman, P.S. (1971) Functional development of the prefrontal cortex in early life and the problem of neuronal plasticity. *Exp. Neurol.,* 32: 366–387.

Goldman, P.S. (1976) The role of experience in recovery of function following prefrontal lesions in infant monkeys. *Neuropsychologia,* 14: 401–412.

Goldman, P.S. (1978) Neuronal plasticity in primate telencephalon: anomalous crossed cortico-caudate projections induced by prenatal removal of frontal association cortex. *Science,* 202: 768–770.

Goldman, P.S. (1979) Contralateral projections to the dorsal thalamus from frontal association cortex in the rhesus monkey. *Brain Res.,* 166: 166–171.

Goldman, P.S. and Brown, R.M. (1975) The influence of neonatal androgen on the development of cortical function in the rhesus monkey. *Neurosci. Abstr.,* 1: 494.

Goldman, P.S. and Galkin, T.W. (1978) Prenatal removal of frontal association cortex in the rhesus monkey: anatomical and functional consequences in postnatal life. *Brain Res.,* 52: 451–485.

Goldman, P.S. and Mendelson, M.J. (1977) Salutary effects of early experience on deficits caused by lesions of frontal association cortex in developing rhesus monkeys. *Exp. Neurol.,* 57: 588–602.

18

Goldman, P.S. and Nauta, W.J.H. (1977a) An intricately patterned prefronto-caudate projection in the rhesus monkey. *J. comp. Neurol.,* 171: 369–386.

Goldman, P.S. and Nauta, W.J.H. (1977b) Columnar distributions of cortico-cortical fibers in the frontal association, limbic, and motor cortex of the developing rhesus monkey. *Brain Res.,* 122: 393–413.

Goldman-Rakic, P.S. (1980a) Development and plasticity of primate frontal association cortex. In *The Cerebral Cortex,* F.O. Schmitt and F.G. Worden (Eds.), MIT Press, Cambridge, in press.

Gudden, G. (1980) Experimentaluntersuchungen uber das peripherische und centrale nervensystem. *Arch. Psychiat. Nervenkr.,* 2: 693–723.

Hamburger, V. (1975) Cell death in the development of the lateral motor column of the chick embryo. *J. comp. Neurol.,* 160: 535–546.

Hicks, S.P. and D'Amato, C.J. (1970) Motor-sensory and visual behavior after hemispherectomy in newborn and mature rats. *Exp. Neurol.,* 29: 416–438.

Hubel, D.H., Wiesel, T.N. and LeVay, S. (1977) Plasticity of ocular dominance columns in monkey striate cortex. *Phil. Trans. B,* 278: 377–409.

Jacobson, S. and Trojanowski, J.Q. (1977) Prefrontal granular cortex of the rhesus monkey. I. Intrahemispheric cortical afferents. *Brain Res.,* 132: 209–233.

Kostović, I. and Molliver, M. (1974) A new interpretation of the laminar development of cerebral cortex: synaptogenesis in different layers of neopallium in the human fetus. *Anat. Rec.,* 178: 395.

Künzle, H. (1978) An autoradiographic analysis of the efferent connections from premotor and adjacent prefrontal regions (areas 6 and 9) in *Macaca fascicularis, Brain Behav. Evol.,* 15: 185–234.

Larroche, J.-C. (1977) *Developmental Pathology of the Neonate,* Elsevier, Amsterdam.

Leonard, C.M. (1974) Degeneration argyrophilia as an index of neural maturation: studies on the optic tract of the golden hamster. *J. comp. Neurol.,* 156: 435–458.

Lund, R.D., Cunningham, T.J. and Lund, J.S. (1973) Modified optic projections after unilateral eye removal in young rats. *Brain Behav. Evol.,* 8: 51–72.

Lynch, G., Stanfield, B. and Cotman, C.W. (1973) Developmental differences in post-lesion axonal growth in the hippocampus. *Brain Res.,* 59: 155–168.

Myers, R.E. (1969) Brain pathology following fetal vascular occlusion: an experimental study. *Invest. Ophthalmol.,* 8: 41–50.

Myers, R.E., Valerio, M.G., Martin, D.P. and Nelson, K.B. (1973) Perinatal brain damage: porencephaly in a cynomolgous monkey. *Biol. Neonate,* 22: 253–273.

Pribram, K.H., Chow, K.L. and Semmes, J. (1953) Limit and organization of the cortical projection from the medial thalamic nucleus in monkey. *J. comp. Neurol.,* 98: 433–448.

Rakic, P. (1975) Timing of major ontogenetic events in the visual cortex of the rhesus monkey. In *Brain Mechanisms and Mental Retardation,* N.A. Buchwald and M.A.B. Brazier (Eds.), Academic Press, New York, pp. 3–40.

Rakic, P. (1977) Effects of prenatal unilateral eye enucleation on the formation of layers and retinal connections in the dorsal lateral geniculate nucleus (LGd) of the rhesus monkey. *Neurosci. Abstr.,* 3: 573.

Rakic, P. (1978) Neuronal migration and contact guidance in the primate telencephalon. *Postgrad. Med. J.,* 54: 25–40.

Rakic, P. (1979) Genesis of visual connections in the rhesus monkey. In *Developmental Neurobiology of Vision,* R.D. Freeman (Ed.), Plenum, New York, pp. 249–260.

Richman, D.P., Steward, R.M., Hutchinson, J.W. and Caviness, V.S., Jr. (1975) Mechanical model of brain convolutional development. *Science,* 189: 18–21.

Sanides, F. (1969) Comparative architectonics of the neocortex of mammals and their evolutionary interpretation. *Ann. N.Y. Acad. Sci.,* 167: 404–423.

Schneider, G.E. (1970) Mechanisms of functional recovery following lesions of visual cortex or superior colliculus in neonate and adult hamsters. *Brain Behav. Evol.,* 3: 295–323.

Schneider, G.E. (1973) Early lesions of superior colliculus: factors affecting the formation of abnormal retinal projections, *Brain Behav. and Evol.,* 8: 73–109.

Sperry, R.W. (1971) How a developing brain gets itself properly wired for adaptive function. In *The Biopsychology of Development,* E. Tobach, L.R. Aronson and E. Shaw (Eds.), Academic Press, New York, pp. 27–44.

Walker, A.E. (1940a) The medial thalamic nucleus: a comparative anatomical physiological and clinical study of the nucleus medialis dorsalis thalami. *J. comp. Neurol.,* 73: 87–115.

Walker, A.E. (1940b) A cytoarchitectural study of the prefrontal area of the macaque monkey. *J. comp. Neurol.,* 73: 59–86.

Windle, W.F., Jacobson, H.N., deRamiriz, P., de Arellano, M.I. and Combs, C.M. (1967) Structural and functional sequelae of asphyxia neonatorum in monkeys (*Macaca mulatta*). *Res. Publ. Ass. Res. Ment. Dis.,* 39: 169–182.

Yakovlev, P.I. and Wadsworth, R.C. (1946) Schizencephalies, a study of the congenital clefts in the cerebral mantle II. Clefts with hydrocephalis and lips separated. *J. Neuropath. exp. Neurol.,* 5: 169–206.

Puromycin Induction of Transient Regeneration in Mammalian Spinal Cord

JERALD J. BERNSTEIN and MICHAEL R. WELLS

Laboratory of Nervous System Injury and Regeneration, Veterans Administration Medical Center, 50 Irving St., Washington, D.C. 20422 and Departments of Neurosurgery and Physiology, George Washington University, Washington, D.C. 20037 (U.S.A.)

INTRODUCTION

Historically, pharmacological treatments to induce regeneration of the mammalian spinal cord have met with limited or no success (Windle, 1955; Clemente, 1964; Puchala and Windle, 1977; Nesmeyanova, 1977; Bernstein et al., 1978a; 1978c). However, reports of some success (Matinian and Andreasian, 1976) and transient symptomatic improvement (Windle, 1955; Nesmeyanova, 1977; Puchala and Windle, 1977) have maintained interest in drug therapy as a viable means of inducing spinal cord regeneration.

The rationale in pharmacologic manipulation in spinal cord regeneration follows two primary directions: (1) stimulation or alteration of the neuron cell body of the intrinsic CNS neuron to enhance outgrowth; and (2) alteration of the glial and collagenous scar (cicatrix) formed at the site of a spinal lesion. In the first approach it is assumed that neurons lying entirely within the nervous system lack the ability to produce an appropriate response to axotomy and cannot regenerate their axons. Metabolic stimulation of the neuron by some means might produce a more favorable response to injury (Grafstein, 1975). The second, and by far more extensively researched approach assumes that the collagenous and glial scar forming at the site of injury is an effective barrier to the regeneration of nerve fibers (Clemente, 1955; Windle, 1955; Puchala and Windle, 1977; Matinian and Andreasian, 1976). Drugs which alter the formation of the scar to form a more suitable environment for axons appear to enhance regenerative capacity.

A major difficulty in drugs used in the above studies has been to define the manner in which the agent acts to produce even a transient enhancement of the regeneration of spinal axons. In most cases, direct action of agents applied may be obscured by their side-effects. However, such information is particularly important in the development of progressive therapy for spinal cord regeneration. The following review will outline the rationale and experimental approach in the use of the protein synthesis inhibitor, puromycin, to enhance spinal cord regeneration and discuss its effects in relation to the causes of abortive regeneration in the mammalian central nervous system.

Background and rationale

In using the adult goldfish as a model for spinal cord regeneration, (Bernstein and Bernstein, 1967; 1969) it was demonstrated that the normal regeneration of the spinal cord could be blocked mechanically with a piece of teflon inserted between the transected spinal stumps. If the teflon was implanted for 14 days and then removed, subsequent axonal

22

regeneration was severely limited. Blockage for 30 days completely halted the regenerative process. Ultrastructural analysis (Bernstein and Bernstein, 1969) of the abortive regeneration of axons rostral to the transection showed that with the teflon block, regenerating nerve fibers grew into zones next to the glial ependymal scar and formed chemical axo-axonic synapses in the region. A subsequent transection of the spinal cord, 1 to 1.5 segments rostral to the site of the teflon block and removal of the teflon resulted in the degeneration of the abnormal synapses, and nerve fibers resumed regrowth to regenerate through the scars of both transections (Bernstein and Bernstein, 1967; 1969). The lesion-induced growth of new fibers through both transection sites in the goldfish demonstrated that the glial-ependymal scar was not the factor barring axon growth. However, the regenerating nerve fibers formed axo-axonic synapses, an indication that neurons regulated their own growth by contact. The contact of the regenerating nerve fibers resulted in the concept of "contact inhibition" as a cause for the cessation of axonal growth (Bernstein and Bernstein, 1967). The possibility that a similar process might occur in mammals prompted morphological studies in the rat (J. Bernstein and Bernstein, 1973; Bernstein et al., 1978a; 1978c) and monkey (M. Bernstein and Bernstein, 1973). Contact inhibition may be active in these species as a mechanism for the control of neuron growth. When axon sprouts make synaptic contact with surrounding neurons, the growth of the sprouting neuron is inhibited (Bernstein et al., 1975; M. Bernstein and Bernstein, 1977).

Rostral to the site of spinal hemisection in the rat spinal cord, there is a cyclic reinnervation of presynaptic boutons on the soma of lamina IV and lamina IX spinal neurons (Fig. 1). This cyclic reinnervation of absolute numbers and morphology of presynaptic boutons resulted in maximal numbers of boutons at 30 days. However, the motoneuron remained chronically denervated, since the number of boutons even at 30 days was statisically less than normal. There was a spontaneous loss of boutons at 45 and 60 days, and a secondary increase in the number of boutons at 90 days (Bernstein et al., 1974; 1978a; 1978c).

In addition to bouton shifts, another property of the spinal cord after spinal hemisection in the rat and monkey was the sequential formation of varicosities along the dendritic shafts of motoneurons from the periphery of the shaft to the soma (Bernstein and Bernstein, 1971;

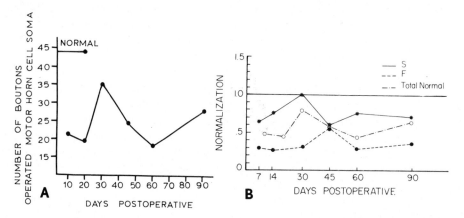

Fig. 1. A: average number of boutons on somata of motoneurons one segment rostral to a spinal hemisection over days post-operation (Bernstein et al., 1974). B: normalization of the numbers of S (spherical presynaptic vesicle) and F (flattened presynaptic vesicle) type presynaptic boutons seen ultrastructurally over days post-hemisection (M.E. Bernstein and Bernstein, 1977). Total Normal = the normalized number of boutons (seen light microscopically) from light microscopic counts (Bernstein et al., 1978a; 1978c).

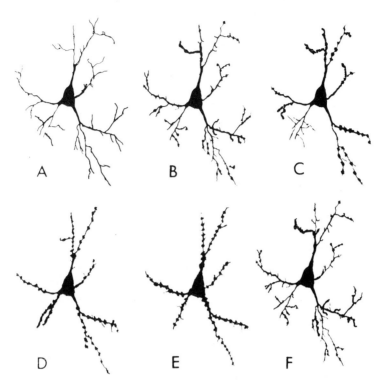

Fig. 2. Schematic diagrams of neuronal dendritic alteration 1–1.5 mm rostral to the site of hemisection in the spinal cord of rat over postoperation time (A–E) and following puromycin administration (F). In animals with spinal cord hemisection alone the number of dendritic varicosities increased over days post-operation: (A) normal, (B) 5 days, (C) 30 days, (D) 60 days and (E) 90 days. In contrast, with puromycin administration varicosities were present only on the most peripheral dendrites of motoneurons 60 days after spinal hemisection and implantation (F).

1973; Bernstein et al., 1974; 1975; 1978a; 1978c). This varicosity formation was thought to be a morphological manifestation of the partially deafferented and/or injured neuron (Fig. 2). In the rat, the formation of varicosities was progressive over time, proceeding from the peripheral to proximal dendrites (Fig. 2). In the monkey (J. Bernstein and Bernstein, 1973; M. Bernstein and Bernstein, 1973) varicosities were demonstrated on peripheral dendrites as much as 1 cm rostral to the hemisection. The formation of varicosites at such a distance, since the neurons were too far from the lesion for a direct injury model, suggests that they were, at least in part, the result of deafferentation. That varicose neurons are in fact chronically denervated was supported by the bouton counts on neurons (Fig. 1) in areas where varicose neurons are shown by the Golgi technique.

The receptivity of varicose neurons to innervation is demonstrated by the significant variation in the number of presynaptic boutons. It is possible that such neurons accept available sprouts or regrowing fibers because of their chronically denervated state. The varicose deafferented neuron might then act as a "sink" for growing or sprouting axons and halt the regenerative process, with or without interaction with the scar, in a manner perhaps not unlike the "contact inhibition" proposed for the teflon-blocked goldfish spinal cord (Bernstein and Bernstein, 1967; 1969). If varicosity formation or denervation changes could be suppressed, regeneration of axons or axon sprouts might result in the growth of axons past the denervated neurons and into the site of lesion.

Torvik and Hedding (1967; 1969) demonstrated that the morphological manifestations of the axon reaction could be suppressed by application of actinomycin D to neuron somata. It has also been shown that denervation changes in muscle may be inhibited by the application of actinomycin D or cycloheximide (Grampp et al., 1971; 1972). Since the varicosity formation on motoneurons also seems to be related to an injury-deafferentation process, protein synthesis inhibitors were chosen as candidates to prevent varicosity formation. In a series of papers on puromycin and spinal cord injury, similar results have since been found. This work will be reviewed in the following sections of this paper.

PHARMACOLOGY OF PUROMYCIN

Puromycin inhibits protein synthesis by its similarity to aminoacyl-transfer-RNA and is incorporated in a similar manner to amino acids into nascent polypeptide chains on ribosomes (Nathans, 1964). The peptidyl—puromycin chain is then released prematurely from the ribosome. Another indirect effect of puromycin on protein synthesis is alteration of ribosome metabolism to prevent completion of ribosome synthesis (Soeiro et al., 1968). This may be either a side effect of the production of peptidyl—puromycin chains (Soeiro et al., 1968) or a result of blockage of the export of ribosomal subunits from the nucleus of cells by prevention of their association with extranuclear polysomes (Lonn and Edstrom, 1977).

Side-effects of puromycin apparently not directly related to its inhibition of protein synthesis include: (1) general toxic effects of the peptidyl—puromycin chains (Gambetti et al., 1968; Barondes, 1970); (2) possible inhibition of some amino acid transport systems (Phang et al., 1975); (3) the induction of abnormal electrical activity (Barondes, 1970); and (4) inhibition of the enzymes, 3′,5′-cyclic adenosine monophosphate phosphodiesterase (Appleman and Kemp, 1966), glycogen synthetase (Sovik, 1967), and acetylcholinesterase (Zech and Domagk, 1975).

In the central nervous system of rodents, puromycin has been shown to produce a host of variable morphological alterations (mitochondrial swelling, cisternal dilation of rough endoplasmic reticulum, formation of intracisternal granules, disaggregation of polyribosomes, an increase in the number of autophagic granules and the appearance of inclusion bodies in neurons) (Gambetti et al., 1968; Kishi, 1974). Changes were not uniform across neurons even in those near the site of an intracerebral injection (Gambetti et al., 1968). Primary effects were observed over a period of 7–30 h after injection and were reversible. The mitochondrial swelling, and perhaps some of the observed alterations, were believed to be a result of the toxicity of the peptidyl—puromycin chains (Barondes, 1970). Such toxicity may persist for rather long periods of time (Flexner and Flexner, 1968).

Despite the numerous possible side-effects of puromycin at the time these experiments were initiated, the effects of its application to the nervous system had been defined to some extent morphologically, biochemically and electrophysiologically for studies of learning and memory (Barondes, 1970). In addition, puromycin can be used directly on the nervous system and its main effect is known to be protein inhibition. For this reason, despite the drawbacks, it was selected as the drug of choice for initial studies.

MORPHOLOGICAL CONSEQUENCES OF PUROMYCIN IN INJURED SPINAL CORD

Puromycin effect on dendritic varicosities

A series of rats underwent spinal cord hemisection (under the left T1-T2 vertebral segment) and a gelfoam sponge soaked in saline (vehicle control) or soaked in saline and 1 mM puromycin dihydrochloride was placed in the wound. Animals were taken at intervals up to 90 days postoperative. The spinal cord was impregnated by the tungstate modification of the Golgi–Cox technique (Ramón-Moliner, 1970). The slides were coded and the dendritic varicosities examined.

The vehicle control group (gelfoam and saline) were not different from the results expected from hemisection alone. However, there was a vast difference in varicosity formation on the dendrites of the puromycin-treated animals (Fig. 2). The pathological events that result in varicosity formation along the entire dendrite by 90 days after hemisection had been depressed. The 60-day puromycin-treated spinal cord had varicose dendrites in lamina IX that resembled neurons of 10–20-day spinal hemisected controls. A single treatment of the hemisected spinal cord with 1 mM puromycin resulted in resistance of the treated neurons to varicosity formation for approximately 60 days. The suppression of dendritic varicosities in the hemisected spinal cord suggested that the first part of a model for a spinal cord which should demonstrate enhanced regenerative capacity had been fulfilled, i.e. the morphological changes associated with denervation pathology and available innervation sites rostral to the lesion had been suppressed. However, it was necessary to demonstrate that such neurons were not still receptive to innervation. To do this, quantitative assessment of the bouton numbers on neurons rostral to a spinal hemisection and puromycin treatment were examined.

Synaptic profile of puromycin-treated neurons in hemisected spinal cord

A series of rats were spinal cord hemisected as in the former section. There were 5 animals in each of the following groups: normal; hemisection alone; hemisection with gelfoam—saline (vehicle control); and gelfoam—saline—1 mM puromycin (experimental, implantation

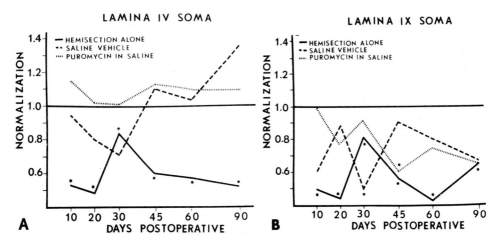

Fig. 3. Data normalized (ratio experimental : normal) from counts on lamina IV neuron soma (A) and lamina IX neuron soma (B) by days post-operation. Significant differences from normal are indicated by asterisks ($P < 0.05$). (Bernstein, 1979).

into the site of spinal cord hemisection at surgery). The tissue was impregnated for the light microscopic visualization of boutons (Bernstein et al., 1978a; 1978c). Counts were coded and subject to an analysis of variance (ANOVA) a priori and Neuman-Keuls test a posteriori.

The results are shown in the normalized data (per cent of normal) in Fig. 3. Lamina IV neurons showed an extremely interesting effect. There was a stabilization of the synaptic profile as seen by the absolute numbers of boutons. There were no statistically significant differences in the number of boutons when compared to those from normals. Lamina IX neurons showed this initial stabilization but showed a loss in absolute numbers of boutons only at 45 days postoperative.

These data show that: (1) the boutons on spinal neurons were stable for at least 45 days following puromycin treatment of spinal cord; and (2) concomitant with the suppression of varicosity formation there is an inhibition of bouton turnover, i.e. the pathology characteristically associated with denervation. If the postsynaptic sites that are available to the axonal sprouts in lamina IX are not vacated, the possibility that the axonal sprouts that would otherwise have synapsed on these cells now have few targets, and therefore grow into the lesion is an extremely tempting thought. The next series of experiments test this hypothesis.

Morphology of the spinal cord—cicatrix interface after puromcyin treatment

A series of experiments was carried out to ascertain the growth of nerve fibers into the lesion site (cicatrix) (Bernstein et al., 1978b). Groups of rats were spinal cord hemisected at the T1-T2 vertebral interface. The operated groups were: hemisection alone; hemisection with a gelfoam—saline implant; and hemisection with a gelfoam—saline—1 mM puromycin implant. The tissue was prepared for electron microscopy over a period of 90 postoperative days. The tissue examined was the spinal cord—cicatrix interface in the segment 1.0—1.5 mm rostral to the site of spinal cord hemisection and implantation (Bernstein et al., 1978a; 1978c).

Spinal cord-hemisected and saline—gelfoam-implanted animals (vehicle control) developed a dense cicatrix which interfaced with the spinal cord. The cictratix was replete with blood vessels, connective tissue and myelinated and unmyelinated nerve fibers which could only be traced to peripheral or autonomic sources.

Puromycin-treated animals showed a less dense cicatrix at 30 days than controls. However, at 60 days the cicatrix was as dense as controls with the same elements (Bernstein et al., 1978b). At 30 days the spinal cord—cicatrix interface contained interesting projections into the cicatrix (Fig. 4A). These projections were covered with basement membrane, had a cellular matrix of astrocytic projections, and contained unmyelinated nerve fibers (0.1—0.2 μm diameter) which were principally oriented in a rostrocaudal direction. Some of the nerve fibers in the projections were degenerating at 30 days and were completely absent by 60 days postoperatively. These nerve fibers also degenerated when the spinal cord was crushed (on the same side as the hemisection) 1—1.5 segments rostral to the site of spinal lesion (Bernstein et al., 1978b). These data show that the nerve fibers in the projections after a single puromycin treatment of the hemisected spinal cord result in the limited growth of centrally derived nerve fibers into the cicatrix which are derived from (or pass through) the spinal cord 1—1.5 segments rostral to the site of hemisection. In addition, at 30 days nerve fibers were also observed in the spinal cord in a zone under the basement membrane (Fig. 4B). These nerve fibers could contain growth cones and were approximately 1.0—2.0 μm in diameter. Crushing of the spinal cord resulted in degeneration of these nerve fibers (Bernstein et al., 1978b).

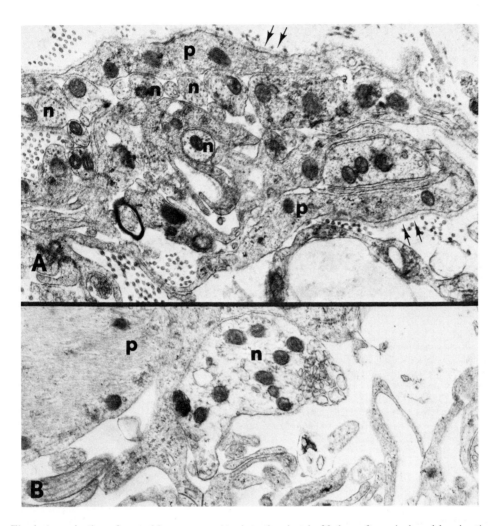

Fig. 4. A: projection of ventral horn grey matter into the cicatrix 30 days after spinal cord hemisection and puromycin administration. The projection contains unmyelinated nerve fibers (n) surrounded by astrocytic processes (p) and is central and rostral to the basal lamina (↑). Uranyl acetate and lead citrate stain; ×36,000. B: nerve fiber 0.1−0.2 μm in diameter rostral to basal lamina 30 days after hemisection and puromycin implantation. The nerve fiber (n) has increased smooth endoplasmic reticulum, increased numbers of mitochondria, and a growth cone in the form of a vacuolated tip. (p) astrocyte process. ×36,000. (Bernstein et al., 1978b).

Another interesting observation was made following puromycin treatment. It was noticed in protargol−silver stained sections that there were conglomerates of small and of large, silver-staining profiles in a zone approximately 200 μm central to where the basal lamina should occur. Electron microscopically the particles were found to be nerve terminal conglomerates of two types (Fig. 5A and B). These were conglomerates of large nerve terminals which contain mitochondria, granular and clear vesicles, and vacuoles interspersed with astrocytic processes. There were often degenerating terminals in the conglomerates (Fig. 5A). By observation these conglomerates remained about the same size from 30 days (when they were first observed) to 90 days posthemisection and puromycin treatment (the duration of the

28

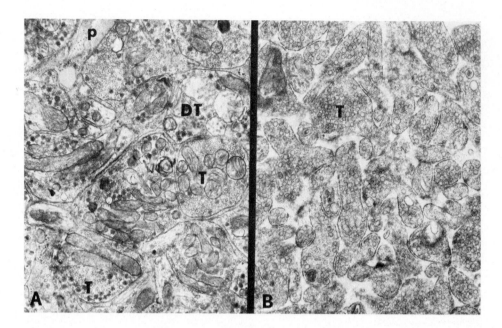

Fig. 5. A: conglomerate of bouton-like terminals (T) immediately rostral to the basal lamina 30 days after hemisection and puromycin implantation. These terminals are occasionally interspersed with astro-cytic processes (p) and contain granular and clear vesicles as well as mitochondria and vacuoles. Some of the terminals contain swollen, watery mitochondria and may be in early stages of degeneration (DT). ×27,000. B: axon terminal conglomerate immediately rostral to the basal lamina after hemisection and puromycin implantation. This conglomerate contains no astrocytic processes. The small terminals (T) contain clear and granular vesicles as well as vacuoles. ×40,000.

experiment). This is an indication that the terminals in the conglomerates were not constant in time and there could have been a process of nerve terminal renewal. The second type of conglomerate was comprised of small nerve terminals (Fig. 5B). These terminals contain clear vesicles and occasional granular vesicles. Both types of conglomerates had parent axons that passed through or were derived from a spinal cord segment 1–1.5 segments rostral to the site of hemisection since the terminals in the conglomerates degenerated when the spinal cord was crushed in that zone. There were no electrical or chemical specializations observed between the terminals in the conglomerate.

Summary of morphology

These data show that a single puromycin treatment of the spinal cord following hemisection resulted in: (a) the growth of centrally derived nerve fibers into short projections in the cicatrix for the first 30 days; (b) the growth of centrally derived axons under the basement membrane; (c) the formation of axon terminal conglomerates; (d) the stabilization of spinal neuron boutons for at least 45 days post-hemisection; and (e) the suppression of dendritic varicosity formation for approximately 60 days. One of the many possible interpretations of these data could be that the new nerve fibers in the cicatrix projection were derived from axon sprouts that grew past varicose-suppressed spinal neurons into the scar.

NEUROCHEMICAL EFFECTS OF PUROMYCIN ON INJURED RAT SPINAL CORD

Protein chemistry

With the marked morphological alterations of pathology after puromycin application, it was of great interest to study the properties of the drug, as applied, in terms of its length of action and the changes it produces in the proteins of the spinal cord.

In the first study, the depression of protein synthesis by puromycin in the treatment method described above was investigated to determine the primary time period of action (Bernstein et al., 1978d). The incorporation of [³H]lysine into the protein of rat spinal cord was measured at 3 h, 12 h, and 1, 3, 7 and 14 days after the implantation of a gelfoam sponge containing 1 mM puromycin or saline as a control into the site of a spinal cord hemisection at spinal segment T2. The procedures used were the same as for the above morphological studies. One hour prior to sacrifice animals were injected subcutaneously with 200 μCi of [³H]lysine monohydrochloride.

The time course of puromycin action on spinal cord protein compared to controls over time is shown in Figs. 6 and 7. Both groups of animals (2 per gelfoam-saline group, 5 per puromycin-treated group) show an operation-related general increase in spinal cord uptake of [³H]lysine which has been described previously (Wells and Bernstein, 1976; 1977; Bernstein et al., 1978a; 1978c) and has been attributed to the stress of anesthesia and surgery. At the site of lesion (0) with gelfoam implantation (Fig. 6), a transient depression of [³H]-lysine incorporation into protein was observed bilaterally at 3 h post-operation, presumably due to the effect of the gelfoam implant (Bernstein et al., 1978a; 1978d). By 6 h this effect had disappeared, and the reaction at the site of lesion followed essentially the same pattern of protein uptake as a similar spinal lesion without gelfoam implantation (Wells and Bernstein, 1977). There was a suggestion that the local reaction at the site of lesion at 7 days post-operation might be higher than hemisection without implantation, but this was not statistically significant. By 14 days post-operation the reaction at the site of lesion in the spinal cord was comparable to unimplanted animals (Wells and Bernstein, 1977).

In puromycin-implanted animals (Fig. 7), a depression in the uptake of [³H]lysine was noted beginning at 6 h and persisting through 12 h. Between 12 and 24 h, the incorporation at the lesion site returned to control levels. These results suggest that under the treatment methods utilized, puromycin-induced inhibition of protein synthesis is not complete, but is primarily active in the first 12–24 h post-hemisection. The increased incorporation of [³H]-lysine at 7 days in puromycin-treated animals may be due to the persistence of puromycyl peptides (Barondes, 1970) or the reaction of the tissue to other toxic effects of puromycin.

SDS polyacrylamide gel electrophoresis

The protein composition of the spinal cord of puromycin-treated animals was also studied on SDS polyacrylamide slab gels (Figs. 8 and 9) on an 8%–20% acrylamide linear gradient. Samples were taken which included the lesion site and 2 mm rostral and caudal on the left side of the spinal cord and processed according to published procedures (Wells, 1978) for analysis on polyacrylamide slab gels. Two animals were perfused with saline at time periods of 6, 12 and 24 h, and 3, 7, 14, 30, 45 and 60 days after a spinal cord hemisection at T2 and implantation of a gelfoam sponge soaked in saline or 1 mM puromycin as in the studies mentioned above. The approximate molecular weights of proteins were determined by comparisons to known molecular weight standards run on the same gel.

The protein patterns of the gelfoam–saline- (Figs. 8 and 9) implanted animals over the time periods studied exhibited patterns essentially the same as those of animals with spinal

30

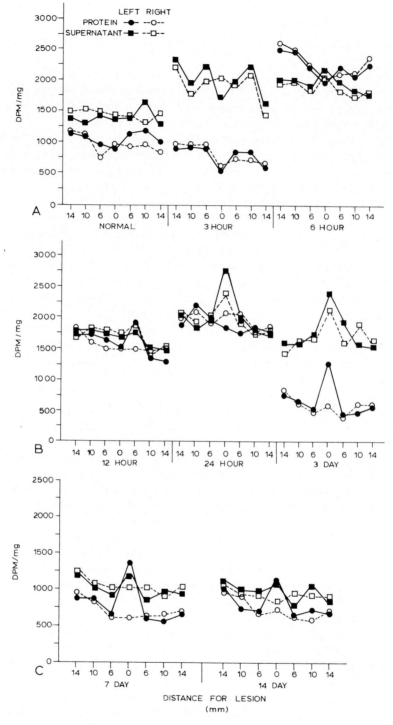

Fig. 6. Incorporation of [^{3}H]lysine into the trichloroacetic acid (TCA)-precipitable protein and soluble fractions of spinal cord from normal and from gelfoam—saline-implanted, left spinal hemisected rats over time post-operation. A: normal animals (n = 5) and gelfoam-implanted, spinal hemisected animals (n = 5 per group) at 3 and 6 h post-operation. B: at 12 h, 1 and 3 days post-operation. C: at 7 and 14 days post-operation. Rostral (left) and caudal (right) distances from the site of spinal hemisection (0) are expressed in mm. Solid symbols represent the left half of the spinal cord. Open symbols represent right half. Protein radioactivity is expressed as dpm/mg protein; soluble fraction radioactivity is expressed as dpm/mg dry weight of tissue. (Bernstein et al., 1978d).

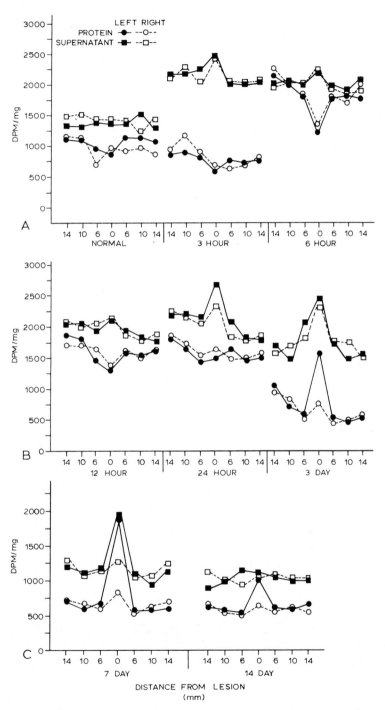

Fig. 7. Incorporation of [³H]lysine into TCA-precipitable protein and soluble fractions of spinal cord of normal animals (n = 5) and puromycin-implanted animals with a left spinal hemisection (n = 5 per group). A: normal animals and puromycin-implanted animals 3 and 6 h post-implantation. B: at 12 h, 1 and 3 days after spinal hemisection and implantation. C: at 7 and 14 days. Rostral (left) and caudal (right) distances from the site of spinal hemisection (0) are expressed in mm. Protein and soluble fraction radioactivities are expressed as in Fig. 6 (Bernstein et al., 1978d).

hemisections alone (Wells, 1978). This consisted of increases in the intensities of protein bands in the regions of 70,000 mol. wt., 30,000 mol. wt., and 15,000 mol. wt., representing serum albumin and components of blood cells respectively. The amount of these proteins present, as well as the rostrocaudal extent of the serum albumin varied between animals. The bands decreased in intensity 3–7 days after a spinal hemisection. The presence of these proteins at the lesion site and in adjacent areas to the spinal lesion has been attributed to hemorrhage and vasogenic edema (Wells, 1978). Another aspect of the spinal cord protein composition in spinal hemisected gelfoam-implanted animals (Figs. 8 and 9) and in spinal hemisection-alone animals, was a reduction in the comparative intensity of proteins in regions of 150,000 mol. wt., 45,000–60,000 mol. wt. and 18,000–25,000 mol. wt. These losses in intensity have been attributed to degenerative processes (Wells, 1978).

In puromycin-treated animals (Figs. 8 and 9) the same general changes which occurred in hemisected and gelfoam-implanted animals were present with some interesting modifications. The reduction in proteins in the region of 45,000–60,000 mol. wt. was much greater in puromycin-treated animals than in gelfoam-implanted controls in time intervals of 14–60 DPO (Figs. 8 and 9). Proteins which increased in relative intensity in puromycin-treated ani-

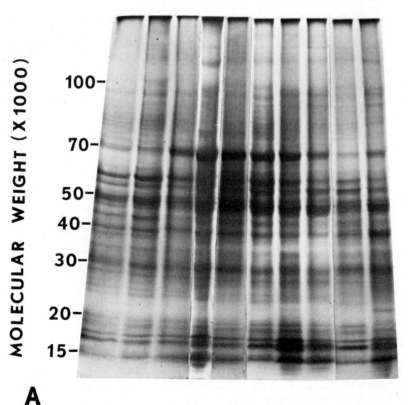

TIME POSTHEMISECTION

N 6 12 1 3 7 14 30 45 60

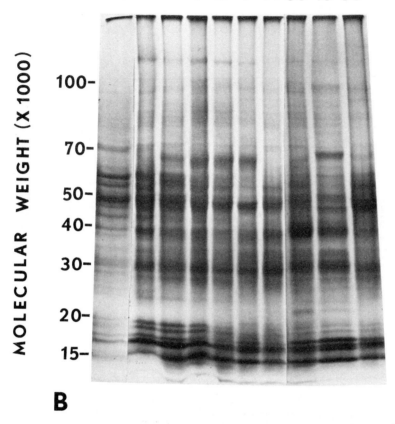

MOLECULAR WEIGHT (X 1000)

100-
70-
50-
40-
30-
20-
15-

B

Fig. 8. A: SDS polyacrylamide slab-gel (8–20% acrylamide linear gradient) electrophoresis of spinal cord from the lesion site (2 mm rostral and caudal to the center of the lesion) of gelfoam–saline implanted spinal hemisected animals. From left to right time periods are 6 and 12 h, 1, 3, 7, 14, 30, 45 and 60 days post-operation. The approximate molecular weight (determined from known standards) is given on the vertical axis. B: SDS polyacrylamide slab-gel (8–20% linear gradient) of spinal cord from the lesion site of gelfoam–puromycin implanted animals. Time periods and molecular weight markings are the same as in A.

mals occurred at 40,000 mol. wt. (45, 60 DPO) and 27,000 mol. wt. Other differences were present in some animals, but were not consistent. The 27,000 mol. wt. protein also increased in intensity in a gelfoam-implanted control at 60 DPO.

Despite a considerable variability in the protein composition of the scar region of the spinal cord, particularly in puromycin-treated animals, the consistent changes which did occur suggest that relative concentration of proteins in puromycin-treated animals differed from controls. The reduction of proteins in the region of 45,000–60,000 mol. wt. indicates that degenerative processes in puromycin-treated animals vs controls may proceed more rapidly. The increases in specific proteins in the face of the loss of others is difficult to interpret. However, these data suggest that, as early as 14 DPO, the protein composition of the

34

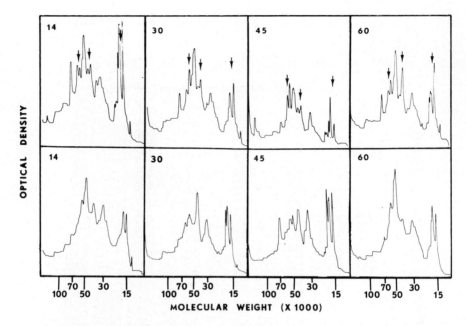

Fig. 9. Optical density reading from SDS polyacrylamide gels shown in Fig. 8. Samples shown are from the site of spinal hemisection from gelfoam–saline-treated animals (top) and puromycin-treated animals (bottom) at 14, 30, 45 and 60 days post-hemisection. Arrows indicate regions of consistent change between treatments mentioned in the text. Large variation in the region of 15,000 mol. wt. (also indicated by an arrow) are due to varying amounts of non-perfusable blood in the lesion.

region surrounding the lesion in puromycin-treated animals differs significantly from control values.

Summary of protein chemistry

The above data indicate that the puromycin implant in the dosage and method given partially inhibits protein metabolism over a period of 6–24 h after implantation. There is some evidence to indicate that the local increase in amino acid incorporation at the lesion site in spinal hemisected animals is increased by puromycin treatment at 7 days post-operation. The analysis of the protein composition of gelfoam-implanted and puromycin-treated animals indicated differences in the area of the lesion detectable beginning 14 days post-hemisection. This consists of a greater loss of 45,000–60,000 mol. wt. proteins and a relative increase in proteins at 40,000 and 27,000 mol. wt. These data are consistent with the morphological data demonstrating long-term effects of puromycin in spite of evidence of its short-term of action.

DISCUSSION

These data indicate that 6–24 h of inhibition of cellular function after spinal cord hemisection, the major portion of which is protein synthesis, results in transient regrowth of nerve fibers into the cicatrix, dendritic varicosity suppression, inhibition of synaptic renewal, stabilization of synaptic profile and alteration in the protein content in the region of the scar. The proportion of these phenomena not directly related to the inhibition of protein synthesis by puromycin, or due to its side-effects, is difficult to ascertain on the basis of these data alone. However, preliminary results of experiments using cycloheximide (100 μg/ml) in the same experimental design (Bernstein, in preparation) indicate that a similar time period of protein synthesis inhibition using this drug (6—24 h) produces similar morphological sequelae.

If the assumption is made that protein synthesis inhibition is the key to the observed suppression of pathological changes in the CNS, how can 6—24 h of protein synthesis inhibition from a single dose of inhibitor have such long-lasting effects? One must assume that critical pathological and regenerative events in the central nervous system, which are protein synthesis linked, occur during this time period and are linked to the subsequent regenerative capacity. These data indicate that the events in the spinal cord that occur after spinal cord injury are linked to growth. There are mechanisms that cause dedifferentiation of the neuron to the degree that it can accept and form new multiple synaptic connections (Bernstein and Bernstein, 1973; Bernstein et al., 1978a; 1978c), form varicosities, which are characteristic of early stages in neuronal development (Purpura et al., 1964), and can increase its metabolism from this growth process. The concept that the neuron is in a state of continual growth was supported recently by the work of Lasek and Hoffman (1976; 1979), showing that there are at least two components in the slow fraction of axoplasmic transport. These components are parts of the axonal cytoskeleton and are continuously produced at a constant rate. The rate of transport of these slow component substances is the same as the rate of peripheral nerve regeneration (1—4 mm per day). From these observations it appears that peripheral nerves are in a continual state of growth, and that therefore, the neuron as a whole must be in a similar state. It appears from this line of reasoning that the entire neuronal population of the nervous system is in a state of growth since all neurons must have active axoplasmic and dendroplasmic transport processes. When the nervous system is injured, metabolic processes are brought into effect both at 3 h whereby the soluble pools of radiolabeled amino acids increase, and at 6 h, when the protein metabolism of the entire nervous system increases. This general effect peaks at 24 h and is gone by 3 days postoperation (Wells and Bernstein, 1977). The effect has been considered to be a stress effect, but the present puromycin data could be interpreted as a cellular growth mobilization effect which prepares the entire nervous system for the pathological events that will occur up to 90 days postoperative. If the metabolic mobilization is not triggered by the injury (due to suppression of protein synthesis) then the specific pathological responses (dendritic varicosity formation, etc.) do not occur and spinal neurons can continue in their normal state, which is a growth pattern.

The concept of "contact inhibition" as a mechanism for the cessation of neuronal growth has been postulated (Bernstein and Bernstein, 1967; 1969). This concept requires that neurons carry a finite number of terminals. When the number of terminals of a neuron is decreased by injury to the axon or when new local sites become available, the neuron will then expand its synaptic field. In addition, inhibition of protein synthesis by puromycin in some manner decreases "cellular recognition" of injury (Lieberman et al., 1970; Farber et al., 1971). Then the neuron does not make a pathological response, but there are still markers "telling" that connectivity is lost or that new synaptic sites have become available following injury. Since the neuron is in a state of continual growth, axon sprouts could be produced. Some usual sites of termination of these axons are the denervated lamina IX and lamina IV neurons following injury. However, these cells are not available for renervation after puromycin administration (puromycin prevents or suppresses bouton turnover for at least 45 days) since the spinal neurons have retained their numbers of dendritic terminals.

The axon sprouts could then grow towards and into the cicatrix. In fact, centrally derived nerve fibers are found growing for short distances (~5 μm) in the cicatrix at 30 days after spinal cord injury and puromycin treatment (Bernstein et al., 1978b). However, this growth is not sustained. Perhaps nerve fibers require secondary growth processes that are not maintained by the neuron if a target is not encountered and no intercellular communication exists. This assumption predicts that the axons would be retracted and, by some method, communicate with other growing or developing processes. This may be the basis for bouton neuroma formation which is seen between 30 and 90 days after spinal cord hemisection and puromycin administration (Bernstein et al., 1978b).

This model of the nervous system postulates the system as a continuously growing entity. Suppression of processes which allow for pathological responses results in the continuation of normal growth and regenerative processes which may or may not be maintained, since such growth requires feedback from other cells within the nervous system. Therefore, the method of studying the regenerative capacity of this system should be the study of the normal growth characteristics of the system and not the study of artifact or pathology in the system after injury.

SUMMARY

The action of puromycin in the injured spinal cord has been reviewed. Inhibition of protein synthesis for a period of 6–24 h after spinal cord injury has long-lasting consequences. These data indicate that the central nervous system is in a continual state of growth. Inhibition of protein synthesis results in suppression of pathological responses but allows for the continuation of the normal growth processes in the injured spinal cord resulting in transient growth of nerve fibers into the site of spinal cord injury.

ACKNOWLEDGEMENTS

This work was supported by a grant from the National Institutes of Health (NS-06164) and a grant from the Paralyzed Veterans of America (P-45).

The authors wish to thank N. Standler, M. Davis and Dr. S. Matthews for their aid.

REFERENCES

Appleman, M.M. and Kemp, R.G. (1966) Puromycin: a potent metabolic effect independent of protein synthesis. *Biochem. biophys. Res. Commun.*, 24: 564–568.

Barondes, S.H. (1970) Cerebral protein synthesis inhibitors block long term memory. *Int. Rev. Neurobiol.*, 12: 177–205.

Bernstein, J.J. (1979) Effect of puromycin administration on presynaptic bouton regeneration after hemisection of rat spinal cord. *Exp. Neurol.*, 64: 76–82.

Bernstein, J.J. and Bernstein, M.E. (1967) Effect of glial-ependymal scar and teflon arrest on the regenerative capacity of goldfish spinal cord. *Exp. Neurol.*, 19: 25–32.

Bernstein, J.J. and Bernstein, M.E. (1967) Ultrastructure of normal regeneration and loss of regenerative capacity following teflon block of the goldfish spinal cord. *Exp. Neurol.*, 24: 538–557.

Bernstein, J.J. and Bernstein, M.E. (1971) Axonal regeneration and formation of synapses proximal to the site of lesion following hemisection of the rat spinal cord. *Exp. Neurol.*, 30: 336–351.

Bernstein, J.J. and Bernstein, M.E. (1973) Neuronal alteration and reinnervation following axonal regeneration and sprouting in the mammalian spinal cord. *Brain Behav. Evol.*, 8: 135–161.

Bernstein, M.E. and Bernstein, J.J. (1973) Regeneration of axons and synaptic complex formation rostral to the site of hemisection in the spinal cord of the monkey. *Int. J. Neurosci.*, 5: 15–26.

Bernstein, J.J., Gelderd, J. and Bernstein, M.E. (1975) Alteration of neuronal synaptic complement during axonal sprouting and regeneration of rat spinal cord. *Exp. Neurol.*, 45: 634–637.

Bernstein, M.E. and Bernstein, J.J. (1977) Synaptic frequency alteration on rat ventral horn neurons in the first segment proximal to spinal cord hemisection: an ultrastructural statistical study of regenerative capacity. *J. Neurocytol.*, 6: 85–102.

Bernstein, J.J., Bernstein, M.E. and Wells, M.R. (1978a) Spinal cord regeneration in mammals: neuroanatomical and neurochemical correlates of axonal sprouting. In *Physiology and Pathobiology of Axons*, S.G. Waxman (Ed.), Raven Press, New York, pp. 407–420.

Bernstein, J.J., Gelderd, J. and Bernstein, M.E. (1974) Alteration of neuronal synaptic complement during regeneration and axonal sprouting of rat spinal cord. *Exp. Neurol.*, 44: 470–483.

Bernstein, J.J., Wells, M.R. and Bernstein, M.E. (1975) Dendrites and neuroglia following hemisection of rat spinal cord: effects of puromycin. *Adv. Neurol.*, 12: 439–451.

Bernstein, J.J., Wells, M.R. and Bernstein, M.E. (1978b) Effect of puromycin treatment on the regeneration of hemisected and transected rat spinal cord. *J. Neurocytol.*, 7: 215–228.

Bernstein, J.J., Wells, M.R. and Bernstein, M.E. (1978c) Mammalian spinal cord regeneration: synaptic renewal and neurochemistry. In *Neuronal Plasticity*, C. Cotman (Ed.), Raven Press, New York, pp. 49–71.

Bernstein, J.J., Wells, M.R. and Zanakis, M.F. (1978d) Effects of puromycin on incorporation of [^{3}H]-lysine into protein following hemisection of rat spinal cord. *Exp. Neurol.*, 61: 537–548.

Clemente, C.D. (1955) Structural regeneration in the mammalian central nervous system and the role of neuroglia and connective tissue. In *Regeneration in the Central Nervous System*, W.R. Windle (Ed.), C.C. Thomas, Springfield, Ill., pp. 147–161.

Clemente, C.D. (1964) Regeneration in the vertebrate central nervous system. *Rev. Neurobiol.*, 6: 257–301.

Farber, E., Verbin, R.S. and Lieberman, M. (1971) Cell suicide and cell death. In *Mechanisms of Toxicity*, W.N. Alarige (Ed.), MacMillan, London, pp. 163–173.

Flexner, L.B. and Flexner, J.B. (1968) Studies on memory: the long survival of peptidyl-puromycin in mouse brain. *Proc. nat. Acad. Sci. (Wash.)*, 60: 923–927.

Gambetti, P., Gonatas, N.K. and Flexner, L.B. (1968) The fine structure of puromycin-induced changes in mouse entorhinal cortex. *J. Cell Biol.*, 36: 379–390.

Grafstein, B. (1975) The nerve cell body response to axotomy. *Exp. Neurol.*, 48: 32–51.

Grampp, W., Harris, J.B. and Thesleff, S. (1971) Inhibition of denervation changes in mammalian skeletal muscle by actinomycin D. *J. Physiol. (Lond.)*, 217: 47–48.

Grampp, W., Harris, J.B. and Thesleff, S. (1972) Inhibition of denervation changes in skeletal muscle by blockers of protein synthesis. *J. Physiol. (Lond.)*, 221: 743–754.

Kishi, K. (1974) Electron microscope studies on puromycin-induced changes in nerve cells of the medulla oblongata. *J. Cell Biol.*, 63: 1091–1097.

Lasek, R.J. and Hoffman, P.N. (1976) The neuronal cytoskeleton, axonal transport and axonal growth, *Cold Spr. Harb. Conf. on Cell Proliferation, Cell Motility*, 3: 1021–1049.

Lieberman, M.W., Verbin, R.S., Landay, M., Liang, H., Farber, E., Lee, T. and Starr, R. (1970) A probable role for protein synthesis in intestinal epithelial cell damage induced in vivo by cytosine arabinoside, nitrogen mustard, or X-irradiation, *Cancer Res.*, 30: 942–951.

Lonn, U. and Edstrom, J.E. (1977) Protein synthesis inhibitors and export of ribosomal subunits, *Biochim. biophys. Acta (Amst.)*, 475: 677–679.

Matinian, L.A. and Andreasion, A.S. (1976) *Enzyme Therapy in Organic Lesions of the Spinal Cord.* E. Tanasecu (trans.), Brain Information Service, University of California, Los Angeles, Calif., 156 pp.

Nathans, D. (1964) Puromycin inhibition of protein synthesis: Incorporation of puromycin into peptide chains. *Proc. nat. Acad. Sci. (Wash.)*, 51: 585–592.

Nesmeyanova, T.N. (1977) *Experimental Studies in Regeneration of Spinal Neurons,* V.H. Winston, Washington, D.C., 267 pp.

Phang, J.M., Valle, D.L., Fisher, L. and Granger, A. (1975) Puromycin effect on amino acid transport: differential rates of carrier protein turnover. *Amer. J. Physiol.*, 228: 23–26.

38

Puchala, E. and Windle, W.F. (1977) The possibility of structural and functional restitution after spinal cord injury. A review. *Exp. Neurol.*, 55: 1–42.

Purpura, D., Shofer, R., Housepain, E. and Noback, C. (1964) Comparative ontogenesis of structure-function relations in cerebral and cerebellar cortex. In *Growth and Maturation of the Brain, Progress in Brain Research, Vol. 4,* D.P. Purpura and J.P. Schadé (Eds.), Elsevier, Amsterdam, pp. 187–221.

Ramón-Moliner, E. (1970) The Golgi-Cox technique. In *Contemporary Research Methods in Neuroanatomy,* W.J.H. Nauta and S.O.E. Ebbesson (Eds.), Springer, New York, pp. 32–55.

Soeiro, R., Vaughan, M.H. and Darnell, J.E. (1968) The effect of puromycin on intracellular steps in ribosome biosynthesis. *J. Cell Biol.*, 36: 91–101.

Sovik, O. (1967) The effect of puromycin on glycogen synthetase, *Biochim. biophys. Acta (Amst.)*, 141: 190–193.

Torvik, A. and Hedding, A. (1976) Histological studies on the effect of actinomycin D on retrograde nerve cell reaction in the facial nucleus of mice. *Acta neuropath.*, 9: 146–157.

Torvik, A. and Hedding, A. (1969) Effect of actinomycin D on retrograde nerve cell reaction. Further observations. *Acta neuropath.*, 14: 62–71.

Wells, M.R. and Bernstein, J.J. (1976) Early changes in protein synthesis following spinal cord hemisection in the cebus monkey *(Cebus apella). Brain Res.*, 111: 31–40.

Wells, M.R. and Bernstein, J.J. (1977) Amino acid uptake in the spinal cord and brain of the short term spinal hemisected rat. *Exp. Neurol.*, 57: 900–912.

Wells, M.R. (1978) Protein composition of spinal cord and cortex from short-term spinal hemisected rats. *Exp. Neurol.*, 62: 708–719.

Windle, W.F. (1955) Comments on regeneration in the human central nervous system. In *Regeneration in the Central Nervous System,* W.F. Windle (Ed.), C.C. Thomas, Springfield, Ill., pp. 265–272.

Zech, R. and Domagk, G.F. (1975) Puromycin and cycloheximide as inhibitors of human brain acetylcholinesterase. *Brain Res.*, 86: 339–342.

Remyelination in Human CNS Lesions

O.R. HOMMES

Department of Neurology, Radboud University Hospital, Nijmegen, The Netherlands

INTRODUCTION

Medical prognosis with regard to human CNS lesions has been poor, the general view being that most of these lesions show no tendency to functional recovery. Studies on Wallerian and retrograde degeneration, in particular, gave the impression that repair in the CNS is a rare phenomenon, since the axon as well as the myelin sheath disintegrates.

One specific class of pathological processes in the CNS is demyelination: the myelin sheath is destroyed while the nerve fibre usually remains intact. Several demyelinating diseases of the human CNS are now known, the most frequent of which is multiple sclerosis. In some European countries, one out of every 10,000 people is affected by the disease. Usually these patients acquire it in their twenties. This disease runs a progressive course, so that a great number of the patients show more or less disability within 10 years after the first symptoms and signs (Poser, 1978).

In the peripheral nervous system (PNS), remyelination is well known. Here the Schwann cell produces myelin by wrapping its cell membrane around the nerve fibre, and it is able to remyelinate even after complete or extensive destruction of the myelin sheath. In the central nervous system (CNS) the myelin-forming cell is the oligodendrocyte and its relation to the nerve fibre differs from that of the Schwann cell. The oligodendrocyte ensheaths regions (internodes) of several nerve fibres, whereas one Schwann cell is related to one internode of a single nerve fibre (Bunge, 1964). Until recently, phenomena of remyelination in the CNS were unknown. However, in the last two decades an increasing number of reports have been published describing remyelination in the CNS not only in experimental animals, but also human demyelinating diseases. The present paper is a review of the results of published investigations, with a discussion of their implications.

STRUCTURE OF MYELIN IN THE CNS AND PNS

In the PNS the nerve fibre is invaginated in the Schwann cell body, trailing a bi-layer of the Schwann cell membrane and the mesaxon, behind it. This, in principle, is the position of every nerve fibre, including those which we call unmyelinated (Fig. 1).

The mesaxon in most instances is wrapped around the nerve fibre in more or less frequent turns. Hardly any cytoplasm remains between the several layers of Schwann cell membrane, thus producing a compact structure of bilayers called myelin (Sjöstrand, 1963). The ultra-

40

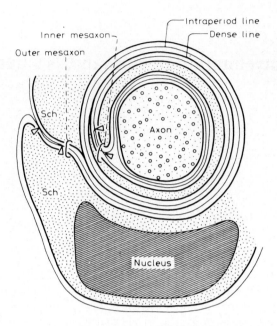

Fig. 1. Relationship between Schwann cell and peripheral nerve fibre. The proportionate thickness of the myelin layers is enlarged for clarity of the diagram. The intraperiod line is derived from two outer layers of the cell membrane, the dense line from two inner layers of the membrane. Sch, Schwann cell cytoplasm. (From Sandri, van Buren and Akert, 1977)

structure of this type of myelin in osmium-stained material shows "major dense lines" of about 2–3 nm thick regularly spaced by a distance of 17 nm. The major dense lines are the composite structure of the inner, protein part of two cell membranes, and the unstained space in-between contains a bi-layer of the outer, lipid parts of two Schwann cell membranes (Fig. 2), called the intraperiod lines. The major dense lines contain around 30% basic protein, a protein with antigenic properties important in the induction of experimental allergic encephalomyelitis (see later).

The Schwann cell is covered externally by a basement membrane. The cell's cytoplasm provides both an inner and an outer collar of cytoplasm in relation to compact myelin. The segment of the nerve fibre covered by one Schwann cell is separated from the adjacent seg-

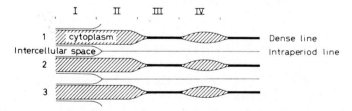

Fig. 2. Stages in formation of periodic lines in myelin. I: three cytoplasmic loops of a Schwann cell. II: fusion of the outer layers of cell membrane to form the intraperiod line. III. fusion of the inner layers of the cell membrane to form the dense line. IV: residual cytoplasma between compacted cell membranes form the Schmidt-Lantermann incisures. (From Sandri, van Buren and Akert, 1977)

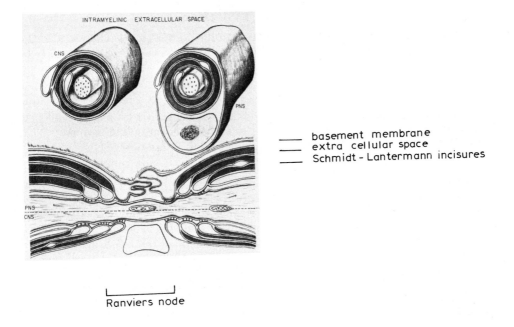

INTRAMYELINIC EXTRACELLULAR SPACE

CNS

PNS

_____ basement membrane
_____ extra cellular space
_____ Schmidt-Lantermann incisures

PNS
CNS

Ranviers node

Fig. 3. Diagrammatic representation of PNS and CNS nodal regions of myelin. The drawing has left open the extracellular space (dark) that is normally obliterated to form the intraperiod line. Interdigitation of outer cytoplasmic rims at Ranvier's node is shown in the upper Schwann cell diagram. In the lower oligodendrocyte diagram, the unmyelinated part of the nerve fibre at Ranvier's node is covered by astrocytic feet. The spiraling cytoplasmic loops of Schwann cells and of oligodendrocytes contact the nerve fibre with "tight junctions" that are more numerous in the PNS than in the CNS myelin. (From Mugnaini, 1978)

ments by strictures called Ranvier's nodes, composed of interdigitating and spiraling collars of protoplasm, left between the ends of compacting cell membrane layers (Fig. 3). The Schmidt-Lantermann incisures are spiraling rims of cytoplasm at places where cell membrane layers did not compact. The cytoplasm of Schmidt-Lantermann incisures is in contact with that of Ranvier's nodes and thus could have comparable functional activities. The length of the internodes is directly proportional to fibre diameter. In adult animals, the same is also true of myelin thickness.

Central myelin is formed by the oligodendrocytes, several nerve fibres usually deriving their myelin sheath from a single oligodendrocyte (Bunge, 1964: Hirano and Dembitzer, 1967). The number of fibres served by one oligodendrocyte is estimated in vertebrates to be, at maximum, 3 to 4 (Prineas, Raine and Wisniewski, 1969). The compactness of central myelin differs from that of myelin in the PNS. The distance between the major dense lines is 15 nm, that is around 10% less than in the PNS (Sandri, van Buren and Akert, 1977). In addition, central myelin has only a thin, inner cytoplasmic collar and no outer one. It has no basement membrane, hardly any Schmidt-Lantermann incisures and fewer tight junctions than PNS myelin (Fig. 3). The node of Ranvier in the CNS leaves part of the nerve fibre unmyelinated. The considerable extracellular space at this site is usually partly filled by astrocytic feet.

From this description, it is clear that there are considerable differences in CNS and PNS myelin. These are not only structural but also biochemical differences that have con-

TABLE I

BIOCHEMICAL, ULTRASTRUCTURAL AND STAINING DIFFERENCES BETWEEN CENTRAL AND PERIPHERAL TYPE OF MYELIN

	Peripheral type	Central type
Biochemical:		
diphosphoinositide ratio	1,5	1
proteolipids	absent	present in small quantities
glycolipids	resist extraction	easily extractable
glycoproteins	present in higher quantities than in central type	
lipid composition *:		
cholesterol	+	−
glycerides	+	−
sphyngomyelin	−	+
Staining properties:		
Luxol fast blue−PAS **	deep blue	blue-green
*Ultrastructure ***:*		
	−one Schwann cell for one internode on one nerve fibre	one oligodendrocyte for up to 4 nerve fibres and 40 internodes
	−many Schmidt-Lantermann incisures	fewer S.-L. incisures
	−broad cytoplasmic outer and inner rim	compacted inner and outer mesaxon
	−period 17 nm	period 11 nm
	−basement membrane present	basement membrane absent
microvilli at node of Ranvier	present	absent
axolemma at node of Ranvier	covered by Schwann cell	not covered by oligodendrocyte
tight junctions	less numerous	numerous

* Horrocks, 1967.
** Feigin and Popoff, 1966.
*** Mugnaini, 1978.

sequences for the staining properties of peripheral and central myelin. The differences, summarized in Table I, make it possible to distinguish between the two types of myelin by both light and electron microscopy. In remyelination, the thickness of the myelin sheath is also important in making this distinction. It is therefore appropriate to discuss first the normal growth of the myelin sheath during development and to compare this with phenomena of demyelination and remyelination.

NORMAL MYELOGENESIS COMPARED WITH DEMYELINATION AND REMYELINATION

During development, nerve fibres are covered by a myelin sheath which increases in thickness by increasing the number of mesaxon turns. Electron microscopy and [^{3}H]-thymidine labelling have left no doubt that, in the rat optic nerve, all oligodendrocytes undergo their final cell division during postnatal development, and that these oligodendrocytes are responsible for subsequent myelination (Skoff, Price and Stocks, 1976). In the following period the thickness of the myelin sheath increases, the increase being greatest

TABLE II

ARGUMENTS FOR REMYELINATION CNS LESIONS

–configuration of membranes in adult CNS resembling early stages in the development of myelin
–appearance of compacting of membranes resembling myelin structure
–appearance of myelin on demyelinated fibres
–abnormally short and thin internodes in a lesioned CNS region
–presence of Schwann cell myelin in CNS

around thicker fibres. This results, in the adult CNS, in a close correlation between fibre-diameter and myelin sheath thickness. A thick fibre with a thin myelin sheath in an adult CNS may thus be strongly suspected of indicating remyelination. The same holds if an axon–glial relation is found in adult CNS that closely resembles developmental stages of myelination. A continuous membrane, traceable from the surface of an oligodendrocyte, through a spiral around the nerve fibre and back to the surface again, demonstrates remyelination in adult CNS. These characteristics are not found in early demyelination. In this latter situation, the myelin appears fractured and discontinuous and its compactness is severely disturbed (Harrison, McDonald and Ochoa, 1972; Harrison and McDonald, 1977). The presence of such alterations very shortly after the occurrence of a lesion is most strongly indicative of demyelination.

If serial studies establish that thinly myelinated fibres appear after a period of complete demyelination, then remyelination is certain. The occurrence of internodes which are inappropriately short for the diameter of the nerve fibres in a certain region of the CNS is another argument for remyelination. There is a positive correlation between length of internode and fibre diameter in definite regions of the CNS, thus thinly myelinated and short internodes are probably remyelinated internodes (Gledhill, Harrison and McDonald, 1973).

Thick layers of cytoplasm in the paranodal region, the presence of a basement membrane enclosing the whole internode, and an abnormally large distance between major dense lines suggest the presence of a Schwann cell-myelinated internode in the CNS. As myelination by Schwann cells never occurs in normal CNS but is frequently found after lesions of the CNS (see later), this can also be taken as a sign of remyelination (Gledhill, Harrison and McDonald, 1973). Usually the combination of the above mentioned arguments is needed for the acceptance of remyelination in CNS lesion (Table II). Negative arguments can usually be added to this, so that, finally, nearly absolute certainty of remyelination can be reached (Harrison, McDonald and Ochoa, 1972; McDonald, 1974).

DEMYELINATION IN ANIMAL EXPERIMENTS

The first report of remyelination in the CNS is that of Duncan (1950, 1954). Compression of the rat spinal cord resulted, in the lesioned part of the cord, in the frequent occurrence of patches of fibres that stained excessively by the Weigert method. This phenomenon was invariably accompanied by an equally distinct alteration and increase in the number and nature of supporting cells (Duncan, 1955). The excessive staining with Weigert's method indicated heavy myelination. The hypermyelinated fibres were found close to the root areas but also in the ventral and lateral white columns. "Characteristically and without a single discovered exception the hypermyelinated areas were separated from the normal by a narrow zone in which stainable myelin was absent or very nearly so. This fact suggests that

TABLE III

TYPES OF LESIONS AND THEIR SITES IN THE CNS OF EXPERIMENTAL ANIMALS PRODUCING
DEMYELINATION FOLLOWED BY REMYELINATION

Type of lesion	Site of lesion	Animal	Remyelinating cell	Authors
Mechanical				
compression by sarcoma	spinal cord	rat	Schwann cell	Duncan, 1950, 1954
spinal fluid barbotage	spinal cord	cat	oligodendrocyte	Bunge, Bunge and Ris, 1961
	spinal cord	cat	oligodendrocyte	Gledhill, Harrison and McDonald, 1973
pressure	spinal cord	cat	oligodendrocyte	Gledhill, Harrison and McDonald, 1973
			Schwann cell	Harrison, Gledhill and McDonald, 1975 McDonald, 1975 Harrison and McDonald, 1977 Gledhill and MacDonald, 1977
transection followed by autogenous grafts	spinal cord	dog	not mentioned but probably Schwann cell	Kao, 1974
transection	spinal cord	rat	Schwann cell oligodendrocyte	Lampert and Cressman, 1964
transection and crush	optic nerve	tadpole	oligodendrocyte	Reier and Webster, 1974
Experimental allergic ence-phalomyelitis	spinal cord, medulla, cerebellum	rat	oligodendrocyte	Lampert, 1965
	spinal cord lumbar region	rabbit	oligodendrocyte	Prineas, Raine and Wisniewski, 1969
	spinal cord *tissue culture*	mouse	oligodendrocyte	Raine and Bornstein, 1970
	spinal cord lumber, sacral region	guinea pig	not mentioned probably oligodendrocytes	Raine, Snyder, Stone and Bornstein, 1972
	spinal cord	guinea pig	oligodendrocytes	Raine, Traugott and Stone, 1978
Thiamine deficiency	brain stem	rat	very probably Schwann cell	Collins, 1966
Viral infection	spinal cord	mouse	oligodendrocyte	Herndon, Price and Weiner, 1977
JHM strain of mouse hepatitis				Herndon, Griffin, McCormick and Weiner, 1975 Lampert, Sims and Kniazeff, 1973
Theiler's murine encephalo-myelitis	spinal cord	mouse	Schwann cell, oligodendrocyte	Dal Canto and Lipton, 1979

TABLE III (continued)

Type of lesion	Site of lesion	Animal	Remyelinating cell	Authors
Cold injury	parietal cortex	rat	oligodendrocyte	Estable-Puig and Estable-Puig, 1972
	cerbral white matter	rat	not mentioned, probably oligodendrocyte and Schwann cell	Hirano and Dembitzer, 1967
Chemical				
6-aminonicotin-amide	dorsal column of spinal cord	rat	oligodendrocyte Schwann cell	Blakemore, 1975
cyanide	systemic	rat	not mentioned	Hirano and Dembitzer, 1967
	systemic, forebrain	rat	Schwann cell oligodendrocyte	Hirano, Zimmerman and Levine, 1969
	corpus callosum	rat	oligodendrocyte, probably Schwann cell	Hirano, Levine and Zimmerman, 1968
lysolecithin	spinal cord	rat	oligodendrocyte Schwann cell	Blakemore, 1976
	dorsal column	cat	oligodendrocyte Schwann cell	Blakemore, Eames, Smith and McDonald, 1977
	dorsal column lateral column	rabbit	oligodendrocyte Schwann cell	Blakemore, 1978
diphtheria toxin	subcortical frontal, parietal, occipital, spinal cord	rabbit	oligodendrocyte	Wisniewski and Raine, 1974
	dorsal column	cat	occasional Schwann cell oligodendrocyte?	Harrison, MacDonald and Ochoa, 1972
	optic chiasm	cat	oligodendrocyte? almost absent	Eames, Jacobson and McDonald, 1977
Transplantation optic nerve	sciatic nerve	?	oligodendrocyte	Weinberg and Spencer, 1978

local demyelination preceded the appearance of the altered and peripheral type of myelin" (Duncan, 1955, page 257).

In this way, not only remyelination but also the appearance of a peripheral type of myelin in a lesion of the CNS was clearly described. The significance of these findings at the light microscopic level was only understood following a systematic EM study of remyelination in spinal fluid exchange (barbotage) lesions of the cat spinal cord by Bunge et al. (1961). In these experiments, no stainable myelin was present 14 days after production of the lesion. The nerve fibres showed a normal pattern, indicating that this was a purely demyelinating lesion. Around 19 days after production of the lesion the deposition of new myelin began, probably produced by oligodendrocytes derived from the adjacent normal white matter (Koenig et al., 1962; Bunge and Glass, 1965). Since that time, a number of experimental reports have appeared which clearly describe remyelination after various types of central lesions in different animal species. The relevant data are set out in Table III.

It can be seen that remyelination in central nervous system has been demonstrated after

46

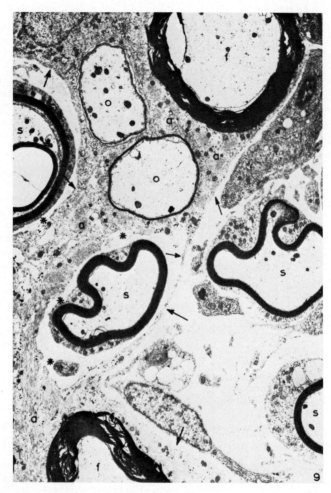

Fig. 4. Remyelination in the spinal cord of the cat one month after a lysolecithin injection. Two oligo-dendrocyte-remyelinated axons (o) lie within an area containing astrocyte cytoplasm (a), as do two fibres (f) that were not demyelinated. Schwann cells (s) have remyelinated 4 other axons and the astrocyte surface apposed to these cells is covered with basement membrane in the areas indicated by arrows, but not where indicated by asterisks. ×7000. (From Blakemore, Eames, Smith and McDonald, 1977)

mechanical, freezing, chemical, immunological, deficiency, viral and transplantation lesions. It has been demonstrated in the spinal cord, in the parietal, frontal and occipital cortex, in the optic nerve and chiasm, in the cerebral white matter and in the brain stem. Remyelina-tion occurred in rat, cat, dog, rabbit, mouse, guinea pig and also in the tadpole. Very impor-tant, and highly remarkable, is the confirmation of Duncan's first observation that remyeli-nation in various parts of the CNS takes place by Schwann cells (Fig. 4). As we have seen, light and electron microscopic features of the peripheral and central type of myelin can readily be distinguished. The type of remyelination may be related to the type of lesion. Schwann cell remyelination is clearly present in mechanical and in some chemical lesions, but in lesions by diphtheria toxin, experimental allergic encephalomyelitis and viral infec-tions, the preference is for remyelination with oligodendrocytes. Other factors may also influence the remyelinating cell type, however. Several experimental studies have attempted to elucidate the nature of such factors and these will be discussed in the following sections.

ORIGIN OF REMYELINATING OLIGODENDROCYTES

Most of the authors studying remyelination have accepted the EM evidence that remyelinating cells in the CNS are usually oligodendroglia (Table III). It was not known whether the remyelination resulted from the surviving oligodendrocytes extending their territory, or from the generation of new oligodendroglia from glial stem cells. Recently, it was established that fully differentiated glial cells can still divide and that during neonatal glial development, oligodendroblasts either divide to form daughter oligodendroblasts or continue their differentiation into oligodendroglia. Proliferating oligodendroblasts may have already started the process of myelination during the neonatal period, and conversely, myelinating cells may conceivably regress to the stage of proliferation (Skoff, Price and Stocks, 1976).

Following infection of mice with the JHM strain of mouse hepatitis virus, demyelinating lesions occur in the CNS as a result of a cytolytic infection of oligodendroglia by the virus (Weiner, 1973; Lampert et al., 1973; Herndon et al., 1975). In autoradiographic EM studies of remyelination in encephalitis (Herndon et al., 1977), it was demonstrated that, in the areas of remyelination, silver grains were present over the nuclei of oligodendroglia, astroglia, inflammatory cells and endothelial cells. Oligodendroglia were identified by their round nuclei containing clumps of heterochromatin, and by their dense cytoplasm containing many free polyribosomes and microtubules (Skoff et al., 1976). Labelled oligodendrocytes were conspicuous in, and adjacent to, areas of active remyelination, but were rarely seen in areas remote from demyelinated foci. In some of the more actively remyelinating areas, more than 50% of the oligodendroglia were labelled. In control animals, no such labelled oligodendrocytes could be identified. This study, therefore, demonstrated the regeneration of oligodendrocytes by cell division, although the stem cell could not be identified. However it is probable that these stem cells are either oligodendrocytes or partially differentiated oligodendroblasts. By sulfate labelling the same authors (Herndon et al., 1976) demonstrated that only the newly formed myelin sheath contained sulfate, with no labelling of older myelin. This indicates that newly formed oligodendrocytes were the actively remyelinating cells. As remyelination is found not only in infectious lesions of the CNS, but also in all other types of lesions (Table III), we may conclude that in and around lesions, division of oligodendrocytes gives rise to new generations of actively myelinating cells. Local irradiation of rat and cat spinal cords, prior to the production of an area of demyelination by injection of lysolecithin, inhibits this process of remyelination. The type of remyelination taking place depended on the dose of irradiation – with lower doses oligodendrocyte remyelination occurred, with higher doses remyelination was mainly produced by Schwann cells. The results also show that not only the remyelinating oligodendrocytes, but also the remyelinating Schwann cells are derived from a local source, in or around the spinal cord (Blakemore and Patterson, 1978).

ORIGIN OF REMYELINATING SCHWANN CELLS

Schwann cell myelin is not normally found in the CNS. In remyelinating lesions, however, the presence of Schwann cell myelin is frequently observed. The occurrence of this type of myelin was mentioned in the first description of remyelination and its origin was discussed (Duncan, 1950). A relationship to the dorsal roots was suggested. More recently, in a central diphtheria toxin lesion in the spinal cord of the cat, groups of fibres with peripheral-type myelin were seen in the posterior column, close to the dorsal root entry zone, and at the

48

periphery of the spinal cord (Harrison et al., 1972; Harrison et al., 1975). It therefore seemed most likely that the myelin-forming cells were invading the cord from the dorsal roots and the pial surface. This was confirmed by local irradiation of the central lesion, which inhibited the Schwann cell remyelination (Blakemore and Patterson, 1978) and was supported by studies of irradiated, neonatal rat spinal cord (Gilmore and Duncan, 1968).

It was further suggested that in the cat, Schwann cells can only invade the CNS if the astrocytes covering the spinal cord, the so-called glial-limiting membrane, is destroyed. Their invasion ceases once this structure is reconstituted (Blakemore, 1975; Blakemore et al., 1977). In the rat, however, the same authors found that Schwann cell remyelination was limited to the *centre* of the lesion and to the pial surface, with oligodendrocytes remyelinating the remaining axons (Blakemore, 1976). In the early stages of remyelination, Schwann cells and oligodendrocytes were intermingled, as in the cat, but later the two cell types segregated. The different types of cell were then separated by astrocyte processes, covered on the side nearer the Schwann cell by astrocyte-derived basement membrane, as is found in the root entry zone (Blakemore, 1976). Such basement membranes are only found when astrocyte feet touch on non-neural tissue, like pia and blood vessels, and they are thus called "glial-limiting membranes". It was therefore suggested that the amount and spatial organiza-

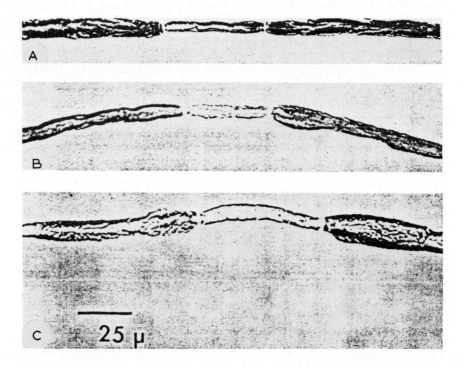

Fig. 5. Demyelination, produced by transient spinal cord compression in the cat, is followed by remyelination. A single fibre study of central fibres shows remyelinated internodes at 5 weeks (A), 3 months (B) and 6 months (C). The remyelinated internodes are shorter and thinner than normal. The thickness of the remyelinated internode increases with remyelination-time. (From Gledhill and McDonald, 1977)

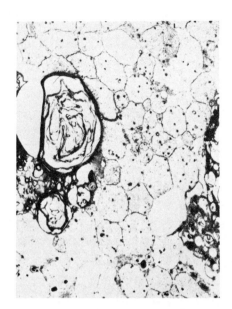
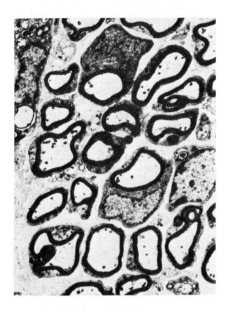

Fig. 6. Persistently demyelinated axons in the dorsal column following lysolecithin injection into the X-irradiated spinal cord of the rat. ×4400.

Fig. 7. Schwann cell remyelination of axons of X-irradiated, lysolecithin-demyelinated rat spinal cord. ×4400. (From Blakemore, 1977)

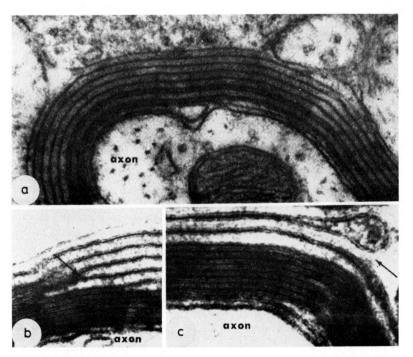

Fig. 8. Splitting of myelin lamellae as initial phase of experimental allergic encephalomyelitis in the presence of mononuclear cells (a, ×8500). The splitting occurs at the intraperiod lines (b, ×120,000) and is continuous with the extracellular space through the outer mesaxon (c, ×150,000) (arrow). (From Lampert, 1965)

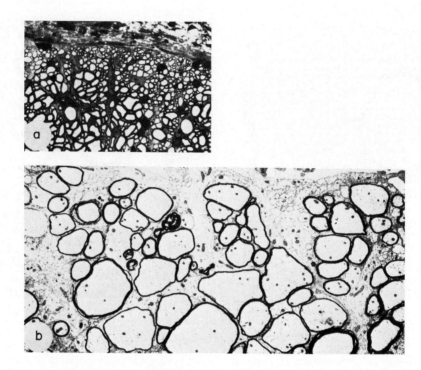

Fig. 9. Suppressed chronic EAE 8 weeks after inoculation. a: a subpial lesion shows remyelination of all fibres and fibrotic changes in the leptomeninges. ×480. b: EM appearance of (a). Leptomeninges are not shown at the top of the figure. Sub-pial fibres show early remyelination. ×4300. (From Raine, Traugott, and Stone, 1978)

tion of Schwann cell remyelination in the CNS depends on the presence and activity of astrocytes (Blakemore, 1975). If astrocytes are inhibited by irradiation or by chemical destruction, Schwann cells can invade the white and grey matter freely and in large numbers (Gilmore and Duncan, 1968; Blakemore, 1975; Blakemore and Patterson, 1975). The proliferative activity of Schwann cells seems to be much greater than of oligodendrocytes (Raine et al., 1969), which may partly explain the strong tendency of Schwann cells to remyelinate the CNS under certain conditions.

Another factor governing the entry of Schwann cells into the CNS is probably the severity of the lesion. Schwann cells were obviously absent in compression lesions that left axons intact, but they were present predominantly in lesions with complete degeneration of nerve fibres (Harrison et al., 1975). As already discussed, the proximity of the lesion to the root entry zone might also influence the degree of Schwann cell remyelination, although the presence of remyelinating Schwann cells has been reported in areas of the CNS, such as the cerebral hemispheres, with no roots entering (Table III; Hirano et al., 1969; Hirano and Dembitzer, 1967).

The remyelinated internodes of Schwann cells and oligodendrocytes are definitely shorter and thinner than normal, as shown in a teased fibre study (Fig. 5) (Gledhill and McDonald, 1977). If the source of Schwann cells for remyelination is destroyed by X-irradiation of 4000 rads in rats and cats, remyelination does not occur, leaving large numbers of persistently demyelinated axons in the spinal cord lesions. If a teased mass of autologous sciatic nerve is then placed over the surface of the lysolecithin-lesioned spinal cord, this demyelination is no longer seen, Schwann cell remyelination of the central fibres having again occurred (Figs. 6 and 7). The extent of remyelination is greater in rats than in cats, and occurs principally on the surface rather than deeper in the spinal cord (Blakemore, 1977). This seems to prove decisively that even with lesions where there is no tendency to remyelinate, this can occur under the influence of an external source of Schwann cells. Thus, the question arises: why does remyelination fail to occur in certain lesions of the CNS, despite the general tendency of all types of animal and most types of lesion to display remyelination.

DEMYELINATION AND REMYELINATION IN EXPERIMENTAL ALLERGIC ENCEPHALOMYELITIS (EAE)

In some aspects, EAE resembles multiple sclerosis and other demyelinating diseases of the human CNS. It is a demyelinating disease of laboratory animals that has been intensively studied with respect to demyelination and remyelination. It is discussed here separately because the immunological aspects of de- and remyelination are of the utmost importance for the understanding of human desease.

Electron and light microscopic studies on the pathogenesis of EAE have shown that the initial lesion is a perivenous infiltration of mononuclear cells. These cells penetrate the myelin sheaths at the node of Ranvier or at the outer mesaxon, i.e. the extracellular part of myelin, and thence destroy the myelin lamellae. In the presence of mononuclear cells, a cluster of myelinated nerve fibres shows widened spaces between major dense lines (extracellular space), caused by a split of the intraperiod or intralamellar lines. In fact, this results from the widening of the extracellular space continuous with the outer mesaxon and the terminal loops at the node of Ranvier (Fig. 8; Lampert, 1965). The widening continues so that the myelin becomes vesicular in appearance. The mononuclear cells then either displace the myelin from the axon or else the dissolution of this vesicular material occurs in the presence of mononuclear cells. Evidence from serial sections has indicated that the oligodendrocytes are phagocytosed by cytoplasmic processes of mononuclear cells before showing any visible alteration. This probably signifies the first phase of the demyelinating lesion. The phagocytosing mononuclear cell showed a clear rim of cytoplasm around the cell to be phagocytosed (Lampert, 1965). In later phases of the disease, numerous oligodendrocytes start to wrap demyelinated axons in a thin myelin sheath, indicating the beginning of remyelination. It was clear that, at this stage, oligodendrocytes are no longer phagocytosed by mononuclear cells. It was therefore concluded that the mononuclear cell plays an important role in the early phases of the pathogenesis of EAE. The splitting of the myelin membranes is probably secondary to a disturbance of oligodendrocyte function by the mononuclear cell, as this phenomenon is also found in edema and in intoxication with silver nitrate and triethyl tin (Lampert, 1965), as well as in viral encephalomyelitis (Lampert et al., 1973).

In recent years, the experimental model provided by EAE has been refined. Not only acute, but also chronic relapsing types of EAE have been described, showing close similarity with even the minor clinical and morphological details of human demyelinating disease (Raine et al., 1977; Raine et al., 1978; Weiner, 1973; Lampert et al., 1973; Herndon et al., 1975). In the chronic, subacute and recurring types of encephalomyelitis, in particular, extensive remyelination was found. Remyelination in general was a phenomenon occurring from one to two months after initial demyelination. It occurred rapidly in lesions which underwent only one demyelinating assault, and was characterized by an abundance of oligodendrocytes (Raine, Traugott and Stone, 1978). These oligodendrocytes are probably derived from mitotic activity around the lesion (Herndon, Price and Weiner, 1977). In old lesions remyelination was found not only in the periphery but also deep inside the lesion. If the encephalomyelitis was suppressed by injections with myelin basic protein (MBP), the remyelination was more pronounced (Fig. 9).

During the latent periods of acute and chronic EAE in strain 13 guinea pigs, the percentage of circulating early T-cells was found to increase. It decreased immediately before the onset of clinical signs (Traugott and Raine, 1977). The T-cells are responsible for the cell-mediated immune reactions and, prior to the onset of clinical signs, they migrate from the blood into the CNS (Traugott, Stone and Raine 1978; Traugott and Raine, 1979). It is not completely clear that these cells form the perivenous mononuclear infiltrates nor that they produce the mononuclear phagocytosing cells, but it seems very likely that this is the case (Prineas, Raine and Wisniewski, 1969). If this could be proven, the morphological circle of events in EAE leading to demyelination would be closed. It suggests that extensive remyelination is only possible if the migration of these cells into the CNS can be inhibited, and that the extent of remyelination increases, as the number of migrating cells and the frequency of the clinical exacerbations are reduced (Raine, Traugott and Stone, 1978).

FACTORS INFLUENCING REMYELINATION IN THE CNS

The remyelinating activity of the oligodendrocyte seems to be slower than that of the Schwann cell. This probably depends on the difference in the mobility of the two types of cells. Another factor may be the difference in the ratio of oligodendrocytes to CNS internodes (1 to 3 or 4), compared with the one-to-one ratio of Schwann cells to internodes in the PNS (Bunge, 1964). The demand made on the growth and remyelination capacity of each cell is presumably much greater in the case of the oligodendrocytes than in the Schwann cells (Pineas, Raine and Wisniewski, 1969). A further inhibiting factor may be the number of astrocytic processes covering the demyelinated axons, and the presence of myelin debris around these axons (Blakemore, 1978).

Still another factor which affects the remyelination is the type of lesion. Spinal fluid exchange lesions remyelinate faster than do EAE lesions (Prineas, Raine and Wisniewski, 1969), while diphtheria toxin lesions show even slower, or hardly any, remyelinating activity (Wisniewski and Raine, 1971; Harrison et al., 1972; Eames et al., 1977). It was suggested that viral infections may specifically inhibit or arrest myelination by infesting the oligodendrocytes, and the same may hold for remyelination (Kristensen and Wisniewski, 1978). The site of the demyelinating lesion may also be of importance in remyelination. Although in cortical lesions remyelination was observed (Estable-Puig and Estable-Puig, 1972), it seems to be less extensive than in the subcortical white matter of the cerebral hemispheres (Hirano and Dembitzer, 1967; Hirano, Levine and Zimmerman, 1968; Hirano, Zimmerman and Levine, 1969). The remyelinating activity of both sites is, however, inferior to that of the spinal cord (see Table III).

Species differences may also have a decisive influence on the amount of remyelination observed. Clear differences were found between rat and cat (Blakemore, Eames, Smith and McDonald, 1977), and these were related to differences in the astrocytic response to the lesion and in the amount of fibrosis which occurred. Species differences also seem to play a role in the amount of central remyelination by Schwann cells as compared to oligodendrocytes (Blakemore, 1978).

The fact that oligodendrocytes at the site of the lesion are replaced by new ones, does not necessarily indicate that remyelination will occur (Blakemore, 1975; Blakemore, 1978). Some authors consider inhibition of remyelinating activity to be an effect of the absence or paucity of astrocytes suggesting that for myelination and remyelination to take place an "active astrocyte–oligodendrocyte relation" with the nerve fibre is necessary (Bunge, Bunge and Ris, 1961; Reier and Webster, 1974).

All these factors, together with those discussed earlier in this review are listed in Table IV. The resulting picture is a complicated one, that in this review will be brought together with what is known about the pathology of human demyelinating disease, especially multiple sclerosis.

FUNCTIONAL SIGNIFICANCE OF REMYELINATED AXONS

Remyelinated internodes are usually short and have a thin myelin sheath in relation to the nerve fibre diameter (Blakemore, 1978; Gledhill and McDonald, 1977; Gledhill, Harrison and McDonald, 1973). Both factors are thought to decrease conduction velocity, thus raising the question of whether the newly-formed myelin is functionally active. As discussed earlier, many of the known ultrastructural specializations which appear to be necessary for conduction are present in the newly-formed internodes. From computer simulation of demyelinated fibres, it was calculated that newly-formed myelin sheaths are thick enough to support conduction after 2 or 3 months (Koles and Rasminsky, 1972; McDonald, 1974; McDonald, 1975) and that 3% of normal myelin thickness may ensure saltatory conduction. In a recent study full restoration of conduction through a remyelinated area of the cat dorsal column was convincingly demonstrated (Smith, Blakemore and McDonald, 1979).

It therefore seems possible that remyelination is accompanied by incomplete or complete functional restitution. All of these findings bring to the fore an extremely important question: does remyelination occur in human disease? In the next section the evidence for this will be discussed, with emphasis on demyelinating diseases, especially multiple sclerosis. At least from the review of experimental data, remyelination of central nervous system lesions is a normal occurrence. Of particular note is the observation that remyelination is definitely present in EAE, the experimental counterpart of MS. From these data a positive response to the above question may be expected.

TABLE IV

FACTORS INFLUENCING REMYELINATION IN THE CNS

—oligodendrocyte to internode ratio
—mobility of oligodendrocyte
—mitotic activity of oligodendrocyte and Schwann cell population
—astrocyte–oligodendrocyte relation to nerve fibre
—myelin debris around demyelinated fibres
—type of lesion
—size of lesion
—place of lesion in the CNS
—animal species
—availability of Schwann cells
—presence of glial limiting membrane
—viral infection

REMYELINATION IN HUMAN CNS LESIONS, ESPECIALLY MULTIPLE SCLEROSIS

Evidence of structural and functional regeneration of the central nervous system in man has been reviewed by Lockhart (1955) and by Windle (1955). In both of these reviews, the question of regeneration of nerve fibres was under discussion, but the aspect of remyelination did not even reach the level of speculation.

However, in one case of syringomyelia and two cases of spinal cord compression, aberrant regenerating nerve fibres, covered with Schwann cell myelin, were found close to blood vessels. This phenomenon had already been described in normal human spinal cords (Staemmler, (1939), cited by Druckman and Mair, 1953). The subject was revived in the study by Hughes and Brownell (1963) of 9 cases of long-standing lesions of the human spinal cord, two of which certainly showed evidence of a demyelinating disease. In these, the spinal cord was invaded by abnormal myelinated fibres of peripheral type, arising from the posterior nerve roots or from the anterior horn neurons.

Prior to 1965, abnormal nerve fibres and myelination were described in syringomyelia, various types of compression of the spinal cord, demyelinating disease, various types of viral and bacterial infections of the CNS and diabetes mellitus (Hughes and Brownell, 1963; Klintworth, 1964). These abnormal nerve fibres were frequently arranged in whorls, called intraspinal neuromata. Their possible origin from perivascular nerves was discussed. As much of the bulk of the "neuroma" was thought to result from hyperplasia of sheath elements, and of neurolemmal elements, in particular, regeneration of long tract nerve fibres with Schwann cell remyelination was suggested (Druckman and Mair, 1953; Hughes and Brownell, 1963).

In 1965, Périer and Grégoire published an EM study of 3 cases of multiple sclerosis. They found that internodes as a whole were demyelinated, that myelin lamellae underwent cleavage during the first stages of demyelination, and that nerve fibre regions with a normal myelin sheath became naked at Ranvier's node, without ultrastructural alteration. They also gave what seems to be the first EM description of remyelination of axons by oligodendrocytes, occurring at the edge of the lesion but not at the center. The center of the lesion seemed to be filled with astrocytic elements. In regions of apparently "normal" white matter, also, internodes showed cleavage of myelin lamellae, suggesting that this white matter was probably in the first phase of demyelination.

Since then there have been several reports of remyelination in human CNS lesions, especially in MS. Together with the experimental data that were forthcoming at the same time (see above), they form a strong body of evidence for remyelination, and they have directed attention to unexpected fields.

The literature concerning diseases *other than MS* was reviewed by Koeppen, Ordinario and Barron (1968) and they added two cases themselves, one of a meningeoma and one of coal gas intoxication. They concluded that aberrant nerve fibres, with peripheral type myelin, were frequently associated with various diseases of the spinal cord or other parts of the CNS. Abnormally myelinated fibres were usually found in close association with blood vessels. The myelinating cells were usually thought to be Schwann cells. Feigin and Ogata (1971) demonstrated with the Luxol blue—Periodic Acid Schiff (LBPAS) technique, peripheral type myelin under the following conditions: traumata, infarcts, myelopathy, hemorrhage, post-operative state, diabetes mellitus, lipoma and hamartoma.

In 25% of autopsies carried out on 684 patients of 16 years and older, Adelman and Aronson (1972) found focal "Schwannosis" of the spinal cord using light microscopic staining techniques. Two hundred and seventy-nine such areas were present in 174 patients,

TABLE V

REMYELINATION IN HUMAN DEMYELINATING DISEASES

Author	Year	Disease	Remyelination type	Part of CNS	Suggested origin of remyelinating cell	Type invest
Hughes and Brownell	1963	necrotizing myelitis necrotizing myelitis and MS neuromyelitis optica	probably Schwann cells	spinal cord	nerve roots	LM
Périer and Grégoire	1965	3 cases of MS	oligodendrocyte	occipital and frontal lobe of one patient	not indicated	EM
Feigin and Popoff	1966	5 cases of MS	Schwann cells	spinal cord, medulla, pons, mesencephalon, occipital lobe	heterotopic peripheral tissue in CNS, mesenchymal cells	LM
Howell, Jellinek and Gravilescu	1968	1 case of "demyelinating" disease resembling MS	Schwann cells	spinal cord	not indicated	LM
Suzuki, Andrews, Waltz and Terry	1969	6 cases of MS biopsies	oligodendrocytes	frontal lobe in all cases	not indicated	EM
Feigin and Ogata	1971	15 cases of MS	Schwann cell	pyramidal tract, corpus callosum	mesenchymal cell	LM
Ghatak, Hirano, Doron and Zimmerman	1973	1 case of MS	Schwann cell	spinal cord		LM EM
Prineas and Connell	1979	2 cases of MS	Schwann cell oligodendrocytes	spinal cord, hemispheres	not indicated	EM

17 in the cervical, 194 in the thoracic, 53 in the lumbar and 15 in the sacral regions. The areas were more frequently present in men than in women, increasing in frequency with age up to 34% in men and 26% in women over 76 years of age. The "Schwannosis" was about twice as frequent in patients with diabetes mellitus, regardless of age and sex compared to non-diabetics, thus confirming the finding of Budzilovich (1970). The levels reached 48% in male and 34% in female diabetic patients.

The reports on remyelination in MS and other demyelinating diseases are set out in Table V and will be discussed in more detail below.

Feigin and Popoff (1966) demonstrated, in demyelinated MS plaques, a type of fibre that stained like peripheral myelin with LBPAS. It was found in 5 out of 18 MS patients, all of whom were younger than the other 13 patients and 4 of whom were women. Positive staining was demonstrated only in quiescent plaques. No EM study of the material was presented, nor were any other details given.

The case reported by Howell, Jellinek and Gravilescu (1968) showed darkly staining myelin sheaths, identified with light microscopic staining techniques as being of the peripheral type. An electron microscopic study was published by Suzuki, Andrews, Waltz and Terry in 1969. They investigated frontal lobe biopsies obtained during cryosurgical, stereotaxic procedures in 6 patients with MS. Their findings are given in TableVI. The study was limited by the amount of tissue available and by the type of tissue studied, since the frontal, subcortical areas may not be the sites at which the large plaques, active as well as

TABLE VI

SUMMARY OF EM FINDINGS IN MS ACCORDING TO SUZUKI et al., 1969

Myelin sheath
    Primary demyelination, but no cells peeling away myelin lamellae
    Segmental demyelination
    Short internodes
    Wide nodes of Ranvier
    Thin sheaths in relation to axon diameter
    Remyelination, including unusual node of Ranvier structures
    No definite Schwann cell remyelination

Oligodendroglia
    Accumulation of dense bodies and myelin figures
    Vacuolization of cytomembrane systems

Astrocytes
    Accumulation of dense bodies and myelin figures
    Increased glial filaments
    Scattered cytoplasmic vacuoles

Phagocytes

Blood vessels
    Dense bodies and "lipid" droplets in endothelium
    Dense bodies in perivascular cells
    No structural abnormalities of capillary or basement membrane
    No platelet or other thrombi

Miscellaneous
    Axonal dense bodies (axonal degeneration) rare
    Increased extracellular space
    Intranuclear inclusions (rare) no unequivocal virus particles

inactive, are commonly found. However, combining their observations with the more extensive knowledge of remyelination available from experimental lesions, the authors suggested that short internodes, wide nodes of Ranvier, tortuous outermost lamellae at nodes of Ranvier, and thinly myelinated axons could all be interpreted as signs of remyelination (Andrews, 1972). In spite of an extensive search, the authors did not see profiles with the characteristics of peripheral type myelin, i.e. the presence of large, outer tongues of cytoplasm and several Schmidt-Lantermann incisures (see Table I).

Feigin and Ogata (1971) were able to demonstrate, with the light microscope and the LBPAS stain, only peripheral type of myelin within the plaques of 15 MS patients. This involved lesions in the spinal cord in 8 of the cases, in the brain stem in 6, and in the cerebral white matter in 7 cases. "The peripheral myelin was formed about segments of axons which had lost their original central myelin within the plaque, but which were still covered by central myelin beyond the plaque; this was most readily recognized in longitudinally-oriented sections of the pyramidal tracts, the corpus callosum, or similar areas. Occasionally, an abrupt junction between central and peripheral myelin segments was seen about an axon at the margin of the plaque. The segments of peripheral myelin were often isolated or scattered in small clusters and were present only rarely in large numbers in a given area."

The next study on remyelination, in a 43-year-old patient with MS of 11 years duration, appeared in 1973 (Ghatak, Hirano, Doron and Zimmerman, 1973). In light microscopy of the spinal cord, a major portion of the myelinated areas stained purplish blue with the LBPAS stain, indicating a peripheral type of myelin. The zones of peripheral type myelin were usually connected with the zone of entrance of a spinal nerve root. All the EM characteristics of peripheral type myelin were present (see Table I). Desmosome-like structures and frequent Schmidt-Lantermann incisures were also seen. Two myelinated axons were occasionally found in the cytoplasm of one Schwann cell. In this case report, the distribution of the remyelinated areas closely resembled the distribution of plaques, indicating that remyelination was nearly complete, although some of the nerve fibres in the plaques were probably damaged since areas of Wallerian degeneration were observed above and below the remyelinated areas. The latest report on remyelination was an EM study by Prineas and Connell (1979) of two patients with long-standing MS. Oligodendrocyte remyelination was found in most cerebral and spinal plaques studied. In sub-pial, spinal cord plaques of both patients, occasional axons were myelinated by Schwann cells.

In summary, there can be no reasonable doubt that remyelination occurs in the demyelinating disease, MS. It can be of an oligodendrocytic or a Schwann-cell type. In other diseases of the CNS and even in apparently normal CNS, the presence of peripheral Schwann cell-type myelin has been reported so frequently that it almost seems to be a regular phenomenon rather than a peculiar finding. In view of the relatively few LM and EM investigations of MS which have so far been carried out, it is difficult to determine the frequency with which remyelination occurs; it may be much more common than is presently thought. Investigations of this type should have priority, in order to demonstrate the real frequency of the phenomenon in relationship to age, sex, type of lesion and type of myelin. An attempt should also be made to correlate the extent of remyelination with the course of the disease. Furthermore, since improvement of MS is produced by immuno-suppressive therapy (Frick, Angstwurm and Strauss, 1974; Hommes, Prick and Lamers, 1975; Gonsette, Demonty and Delmotte, 1977; Delmotte, Hommes and Gonsette, 1977; Hommes, Lamers and Reekers, 1978 a and b) it is of great importance to know if the finding in EAE, viz. that remyelination is more complete in animals given myelin basic protein, is also true of MS (Raine, Snyder, Stone and Bornstein, 1977; Raine, Traugott and Stone, 1978). Since post-mortem or biopsy studies are not usually possible in MS, neurophysiological approaches via the visual-evoked response (VER), the auditory-evoked response (AER) and the somatosensory-evoked response (SER) are of prime importance, in order to be able to demonstrate any improvements in conduction time after various treatments. That such an approach is possible was demonstrated by Namerow (1972), who reported evidence for remyelination in MS from neurophysiological studies. In these studies latencies of the SER were measured, during and following an exacerbation. At a time when the patients had returned to normal clinical functioning, latencies were still abnormal in 7 out of 8 patients. The sensory deficits disappeared over the course of several weeks in each individual case. However, latency values continued to shorten for several months following the disappearance of symptoms. It was concluded that long-term "repair" or remyelination probably occurs in MS, and that it can be demonstrated by neurophysiological methods.

CONCLUSIONS

From the data reviewed in this chapter, it can be concluded that, in a demyelinating disease like multiple sclerosis, remyelination is possible. This remyelination may be brought about by both oligodendrocytes and by Schwann cells. All other information concerning remyelination in the human CNS is absent, although it is clinically relevant. All speculation concerning remyelination in the human CNS must be directed by the information derived from experimental studies.

One of the first questions in this respect is why the demyelinated lesion in MS does not more commonly remyelinate. The factors influencing remyelination of CNS in experimental studies (Table IV) are many and varied. Certainly the type of lesion plays an important role. In MS, the presence of a serum factor and a spinal fluid factor causing demyelination have been demonstrated (Tabira, Webster and Wray, 1976; Ulrich and Lardi, 1978). The same serum factor might also inhibit remyelination in MS, and such a sequence has, in fact, been demonstrated in EAE (Raine and Bornstein, 1970). In EAE, the presence of mononuclear cells close to the oligodendrocyte must be considered as one of the initiating phenomena of demyelination. Possibly these immunologically competent, mononuclear cells, which are thought to be derived from the blood, might produce the above-mentioned substance which attacks the oligodendrocytes, thus initiating the demyelination of the internodes served by the oligodendrocytes. In EAE, the "bouts" of demyelination and the limits to remyelination are both correlated with the presence of these mononuclear cells.

The absence of oligodendrocytes from the demyelinated lesion of MS (Andrews, 1972; Ghatak, Hirano, Doron and Zimmerman, 1973) may be the factor which limits remyelination by oligodendrocytes. The proliferation of oligodendrocytes and Schwann cells is a normal phenomenon in lesions of the animal CNS. The absence of oligodendrocytes from the MS lesion, and the absence of an increased number of oligodendrocytes around the MS lesion (Andrews, 1972), may therefore be a phenomenon specific to this disease. In MS an oligodendrocyte destroying or inhibiting substance or cell seems very probable.

In experimental studies remyelination by Schwann cells occurs preferentially if the proliferation of oligodendrocytes is inhibited. Such a situation may occur naturally in MS, which could explain those instances in which remyelination was predominantly of the Schwann cell type. Such Schwann cell remyelination in experimental lesions is, in turn, inhibited by the formation of an external glial-limiting membrane and by the presence of astrocytes. The predominance of astrocytes in the MS lesion might, therefore, be an important factor in the prevention of remyelination by peripheral type myelin, possibly blocking the infiltration of the CNS lesion by Schwann cells.

In this context, it is important to determine the origin of the remyelinating Schwann cell. Experimental studies indicate that the peripheral nerve roots play a role as a source of Schwann cells. On the other hand, implantation of Schwann cells from a peripheral source leads to extensive remyelination. Furthermore, Schwann cell remyelination is also found deep inside the CNS. The origin of remyelinating Schwann cells from blood-vessel walls or other parts of the CNS remains an important possibility (Feigin and Ogata, 1971). That this may indeed play an important role in regeneration of the human CNS, is indicated by studies on the occurrence of "neuromata" or "Schwannosis" in various types of diseases of the human CNS. The evidence for these phenomena is so overwhelming that they are probably regular features in all long-standing lesions of the human CNS (Adelman and Aronson, 1972). It is intriguing that diabetes mellitus seems to strongly enhance this regenerative activity. The well-known presence of hypertrophic neuropathy in diabetes seems to point to a specific effect on Schwann cell myelinating activity. Experimental studies are, therefore, needed to provide more insight into the factors which cause this "hyperactivity" of Schwann cells in diabetes mellitus. Speculations with regard to the role of growth hormone are appropriate, since this hormone plays a key role in diabetes mellitus.

There remains another very important question about which experimental information is extremely scarce: what determines the amount of myelin around an axon? The thickness of the myelin sheath is positively correlated with the size of the nerve fibre. Nerve fibres which are too thinly myelinated for their size are a hall-mark of remyelination. In EAE, it takes several months for a demyelinated nerve fibre to remyelinate to its normal extent. It is not known whether it is the nature of the fibre or the nature of the myelinating cell which determines the amount of myelination. Therefore, investigations are needed to clarify the nature of the stimuli for myelination and remyelination in the PNS and the CNS.

From this review, it can be concluded that in MS the possibility of remyelination exists. In experimental demyelination, remyelination is so common and so complete that investigations in MS should be directed to the question of why remyelination does not occur regularly and completely.

However, the spontaneous dramatic improvement of symptoms in MS within several hours or days, cannot be explained by remyelination. From all experimental evidence, it is clear that remyelination is a phenomenon that starts around 6 days after the demyelinating lesion, and is completed only after several months. This indicates that there are other factors responsible for the very quick improvement often observed in MS. One of these factors may be a decrease of the edema of the demyelinating lesion. The removal of serum blocking factors, said to be present in MS, might also play a role.

With respect to this last factor, a very important question is, whether or not the remyelinated nerve fibres in MS are functionally active. We have reviewed data suggesting that this may be the case, but definite experimental proof is lacking. In the meantime, however, we should certainly direct our attention to longitudinal studies of MS patients using neurophysiological methods, to determine whether conduction velocities improve over periods of months. Such findings would strongly suggest extensive remyelination. Therapeutic schemes in MS could then be studied by neurophysiological methods. Recently the restoration of conduction by remyelination has been demonstrated very convincingly after lysophosphatidylcholine injection in the dorsal columns of the cat spinal cord (Smith, Blakemore and McDonald, 1979).

REFERENCES

Adelman, L.S. and Aronson, S.M. (1972) Intramedullary nerve fibre and Schwann cell proliferation within the spinal cord (Schwannosis). *Neurology*, 22: 726–731.

Andrews, J.M. (1972) The ultrastructural neuropathology of multiple sclerosis. In *Multiple Sclerosis, Immunology, Virology and Ultrastructure*, F. Wolfgram, G. Ellison, J. Stevens and J. Andrews (Eds.), Academic Press, N.Y., pp. 23–49.

Blakemore, W.F. (1975) Remyelination by Schwann cells of axons demyelinated by intraspinal injection of 6 aminonicotinamide in the rat. *J. Neurocytol.*, 4: 745–757.

Blakemore, W.F. (1976) Invasion of Schwann cells into the spinal cord of the rat following local injections of lysolecithin. *Neuropath. appl. Neurobiol.*, 2: 21–39.

Blakemore, W.F. (1977) Remyelination of CNS axons by Schwann cells transplanted from the sciatic nerve, *Nature (Lond.)*, 266: 68–69.

Blakemore, W.F. (1978) Observations on remyelination in the rabbit spinal cord following demyelination induced by lysolecithin. *Neuropath. appl. Neurobiol.*, 4: 47–59.

Blakemore, W.F. Eames, R.A., Smith, K.J. and McDonald, M.I. (1977) Remyelination in the spinal cord of the cat following intraspinal injection of lysolecithin. *J. neurol. Sci.*, 33: 31–43.

Blakemore, W.F. and Patterson, R.C. (1975) Observations on the interactions of Schwann cells and astrocytes following X-irradiation of neonatal rat spinal cord. *J. Neurocytol.*, 4: 573–585.

Blakemore, W.F. and Patterson, R.C. (1978) Suppression of remyelination in CNS by X-irradiation. *Acta neuropath. (Berl.)*, 42: 105–113.

Budzilovich, G.N. (1970) Diabetic neuropathy complex. *Virchows Arch. path. Anat.*, 350: 105–122.

Bunge, M.B., Bunge, R.P. and Ris, H. (1961) Ultrastructural study of remyelination in an experimental lesion in adult cat spinal cord. *J. Biophys. Biochem. Cytol.*, 10: 67–94.

Bunge, R.P. (1964) Glial cells and central myelin sheath. *Physiol. Rev.*, 48: 197–251.

Bunge, R.P. and Glass, P.M. (1965) Some observations on myelin glial relationships and on the etiology of the cerebrospinal fluid exchange lesion. *Ann. N.Y. Acad. Sci.*, 122: 15–28.

Collins, G.H. (1966) An electron microscopic study of remyelination in the brainstem of thiamin deficient rats. *Amer. J. Path.*, 48: 259–276.

Dal Canto, M.C. and Lipton, H.L. (1979) Recurrent demyelination in chronic central nervous system infection produced by Theiler's murine encephalomyelitis virus. *J. neurol. Sci.*, 42: 391–405.

Delmotte, P., Hommes, O.R. and Gonsette, R. (1977) *Immunosuppressive Treatment in Multiple Sclerosis*, European Press, Gent, Belgium, 224 pp.

Druckman, R. and Mair, W.G.P. (1953) Aberrant regenerating nerve fibres in injury to the spinal cord. *Brain*, 76: 448–454.

Duncan, D. (1950) Alteration of nerve fibres and supporting cells of the spinal white matter to peripheral types. *Anat. Rec.*, 106: 102–103.

Duncan, D. (1954) Additional observations on hyperstaining myelin and alterations of neurologia induced by restricting the growth of the spinal cord. *Anat. Rec.*, 118: 296.

Duncan, D. (1955) Experimental compression of the spinal cord. In *Regeneration in the Central Nervous System*, W.F. Windle (Ed.), Thomas, Springfield, pp. 247–258.

Eames, R.A., Jacobson, S.G. and McDonald, W.I. (1977) Pathological changes in the optic chiasm of the cat following local injection of diphtheria toxin, *J. neurol. Sci.*, 32: 381–393.

Estable-Puig, J.F. and de Estable-Puig, R.F. (1972) Paralesional reparative remyelination after chronic local cold injury of the cerebral cortex. *Exp. Neurol.*, 3: 239–253.

Feigin, I. and Popoff, N. (1966) Regeneration of myelin in multiple sclerosis. The role of mesenchymal cells in such regeneration and in myelin formation in the peripheral nervous system. *Neurology*, 16: 364–372.

Feigin, I. and Ogata, J. (1971) Schwann cells and peripheral myelin within human central nervous tissues: the mesenchymal character of Schwann cells. *J. Neuropath. exp. Neurol.*, 30: 603–612.

Frick, E., Angstwurm, H. and Strauss, G. (1974) Immunosuppressive Therapie der Multiple sklerose. 3 Mitteilungen: Eigene Behandlungsergebnisse mit Azathioprin und Antilymphozytenglobulin. *Münch. Med. Wschr.*, 116: 2105.

Gilmore, S.A. and Duncan, D. (1968) On the presence of peripheral like nervous and connective tissue within irradiated spinal cord. *Anat. Rec.*, 160: 675–690.

Gledhill, R.F., Harrison, B.M. and McDonald, W.I. (1973) Pattern of remyelination in the CNS. *Nature (Lond.)*, 244: 443–444.

Gledhill, R.F. and McDonald, W.I. (1977) Morphological characteristics of central demyelination and remyelination: a single-fibre study. *Ann. Neurol.,* 1: 552–560.

Ghatak, M.R., Hirano, A., Doron, Y. and Zimmerman, H.M. (1973) Remyelination in multiple sclerosis with peripheral type myelin. *Arch. Neurol.,* 29: 262–267.

Gonsette, R.E., Demonty, L. and Delmotte, P. (1977) Intensive immunosuppression with cyclophosphamide in multiple sclerosis. *J. Neurol.,* 214: 173–181.

Harrison, B.M., Gledhill, R.F. and McDonald, W.I. (1975) Remyelination after transient compression of the spinal cord. *Proc. Austr. Ass. Neurol.,* 12: 117–122.

Harrison, B.M. and McDonald, W.I. (1977) Remyelination after transient experimental compression of the spinal cord. *Ann. Neurol.,* 1: 542–551.

Harrison, B.M., McDonald, W.I. and Ochoa, J. (1972) Remyelination in central diphtheria toxin lesion. *J. Neurol. Sci.,* 17: 293–302.

Herndon, R.M., Griffin, D.E., McCormick, U. and Weiner, L.P. (1975) Mouse hepatitis virus-induced recurrent demyelination. A preliminary report. *Arch. Neurol.,* 32: 32–35.

Herndon, R.M., Price, D.L. and Weiner, L.P. (1977) Regeneration of oligodendroglia during recovery from demyelinating disease. *Science,* 195: 693–694.

Herndon, R.M., Weiner, L.P. and Price, D.L. (1976) Oligodendrocyte proliferation following THM virus infection. *J. Neuropath. exp. Neurol.,* 35: 330.

Hirano, A. and Dembitzer, H.M. (1967) A structural analysis of the myelin sheath in the central nervous system. *J. Cell Biol.,* 34: 555–567.

Hirano, A., Levine, S. and Zimmerman, H.M. (1968) Remyelination in the central nervous system after cyanide intoxication. *J. Neuropath. exp. Neurol.,* 27: 234–245.

Hirano, A., Zimmerman, H.M. and Levine, S. (1969) Electronmicroscopic observations of peripheral myelin in a central nervous system lesion. *Acta neuropath. (Berl.),* 12: 348–365.

Hommes, O.R., Lamers, K.J.B. and Reekers, P. Assessment of process activity in multiple sclerosis and changes in spinal fluid. *Proceedings of the MS Symposium, Göttingen 1978,* Springer, Berlin, in press.

Hommes, O.R., Lamers, K.J.B. and Reekers, P. Prognostic factors in intensive immunosuppressive treatment of chronic progressive MS, *Proceedings of the MS Symposium, Göttingen 1978,* Springer, Berlin, in press.

Hommes, O.R., Prick, J.J.G. and Lamers, K.J.B. (1975) Treatment of the chronic progressive form of multiple sclerosis with a combination of cyclophosphamide and prednisone. *Clin. Neurol. Neurosurg.,* 78: 59–72.

Horrocks, L.A. (1967) Composition of myelin from peripheral and central nervous system of squirrel monkey. *J. Lipid Res.,* 8: 569–576.

Howell, D.A., Jellinek, E.H. and Gravilescu, K. (1968) Demyelinating disease in a woman from tropical South America with features of multiple sclerosis and neuromyelitis optica. Clinical protein chemistry and pathological findings. *J. neurol. Sci.,* 7: 115–135.

Hughes, J.T. and Brownell, B. (1963) Aberrant nerve fibres within the spinal cord. *J. Neurol. Neurosurg. Psychiat.,* 26: 528–534.

Kao, C.C. (1974) Comparison of healing process in transected spinal cords grafted with autogenous brain tissue, sciatic nerve and nodose ganglion. *Exp. Neurol.,* 44: 424–441.

Klintworth, G.K. (1964) Axon regeneration in the human spinal cord with formation of neuromata. *J. Neuropath. Exp. Neurol.,* 23: 127–134.

Koenig, H., Bunge, M.B. and Bunge, R.P. (1962) Nucleic acid and protein metabolism in white matter. *Arch. Neurol.,* 6: 177–193.

Koeppen, A.H., Ordinario, A.T. and Barron, K.D. (1968) Aberrant intramedullary peripheral nerve fibres. *Arch. Neurol.,* 18: 567–573.

Koles, Z.J. and Rasminsky, M. (1972) A computer simulation of conduction in demyelinated nerve fibres. *J. Physiol. (Lond.),* 227: 351–364.

Kristenson, K. and Wisniewski, H.M. (1978) Arrest of myelination and demyelination in rabbit retina induced by herpes simplex virus infection. *Neuropath. appl. Neurobiol.,* 4: 71–82.

Lampert, P.W. (1965) Demyelination and remyelination in experimental allergic encephalitis. Further electron microscopic observations. *J. Neuropath. exp. Neurol.,* 24: 371–385.

Lampert, P. and Cressman, M. (1964) Axonal regeneration in the dorsal columns of the spinal cord of adult rats. An electron microscopic study. *Lab. Invest.,* 13: 825–839.

Lampert, P.W., Sims, J.K. and Kniazeff, A.J. (1973) Mechanism of demyelination in JHM virus encephalomyelitis. Electron microscopic studies. *Acta neuropath. (Berl.),* 24: 76–85.

Lockhart, W.S. (1955) Evidence of structural and functional regeneration of the central nervous system in man. In *Regeneration in the Central Nervous System,* W.F. Windle (Ed.), Charles Thomas, Springfield, pp. 259–264.

McDonald, W.I. (1974) Remyelination in relation to clinical lesions in the central nervous system. *Brit. Med. Bull.,* 30: 186–189.

McDonald, W.I. (1975) Mechanisms of functional loss and recovery in spinal cord damage. *Ciba Found. Symp.,* 34: 23–33.

Mugnaini, E. (1978) Fine strucutre of myelin sheaths. In *Proceedings of the European Society for Neurochemistry, Vol. 1,* V. Neuhoff (Ed.), Verlag Chemie Weinheim, N.Y., pp. 3–31.

Namerow, N.S. (1972) The pathophysiology of multiple sclerosis, In *Multiple Sclerosis. Immunology, Virology and Ultrastructure,* F. Wolfgram, G.W. Ellison, J.G. Stevens and J.M. Andrews (Eds.), Academic Press, N.Y., London, pp. 143–172.

Périer, O. and Grégoire, A. (1965) Electron microscopic features of multiple sclerosis lesions, *Brain,* 88: 937–952.

Poser, S. (1978) *Multiple Sclerosis. An Analysis of 812 Cases by Means of Electronic Data Processing,* Springer Verlag, Berlin, 93 pp.

Prineas, J.W. and Connell, F. (1979) Remyelination in multiple sclerosis. *Ann. Neurol.,* 5: 22–31.

Prineas, J., Raine, C.S. and Wisniewski, H. (1969) An ultrastructural study of experimental demyelination and remyelination. III Chronic experimental allergic encephalomyelitis in the central nervous system. *Lab. Invest.,* 21: 472–483.

Raine, C.S. and Bornstein, M.B. (1970) Experimental allergic encephalomyelitis: a light and electron microscope study of remyelination and "sclerosis" in vitro. *J. Neuropath. exp. Neurol.,* 29: 552–574.

Raine, C.S., Snyder, D.H., Stone, S.H. and Bornstein, M.B. (1977) Suppression of acute and chronic experimental allergic encephalomyelitis in strain 13 guinea pigs. A clinical and pathological study. *J. neurol. Sci.,* 31: 355–367.

Raine, C.S., Traugott, U. and Stone, S.H. (1978) Chronic relapsing experimental allergic encephalomyelitis: CNS plaque development in unsuppressed and suppressed animals. *Acta neuropath. (Berl.),* 43: 43–53.

Raine, C.S., Wisniewski, H. and Prineas, J. (1969) An ultrastructural study of experimental demyelination and remyelination. II Chronic experimental allergic encephalomyelitis in the peripheral nervous system. *Lab. Invest.,* 21: 316–321.

Reier, P.J. and Webster, H. de F., (1974) Regeneration and remyelination of Xenopus tadpole optic nerve fibres following transection or crush. *J. Neurocytol.,* 3: 591–618.

Sandri, C., Buren van, J.M. and Akert, K. (1977) Membrane morphology of the vertebrate nervous system. A study with freeze-etch technique. In *Membrane Morphology of the Vertebrate Nervous System, Progr. Brain Res., Vol. 46,* C. Sandri, I.M. van Buren and K. Akert (Eds.), Elsevier, Amsterdam, 384 pp.

Sjöstrand, F.S. (1963) The structure and formation of the myelin sheath. In *Mechanisms of Demyelination.* A.S. Rose and C.M. Pearson (Eds.), McGraw-Hill, N.Y., pp. 1–43.

Skoff, R.P., Price, D.L. and Stocks, A. (1976) Electron microscopic autoradiographic studies of gliogenesis in rat optic nerve. I Cell proliferation. *J. comp. Neurol.,* 169: 291–312.

Smith, K.J., Blakemore, W.F. and McDonald, W.I. (1979) Central remyelination restores secure conduction. *Nature (Lond.),* 280: 395–396.

Suzuki, K., Andrews, J.M., Waltz, J.M. and Terry, R.D. (1969) Ultrastructural studies of multiple sclerosis, *Lab. Invest.,* 20, 444–454.

Tabira, T., Webster, H. de F., and Wray, S.H. (1976) Multiple sclerosis cerebrospinal fluid produces myelin lesions in tadpole optic nerve, *N. Engl. J. Med.,* 295, 644–649.

Traugott, U. and Raine, C.S. (1977) Experimental allergic encephalomyelitis in inbred guinea pigs. Correlation of decrease in early T cells with clinical signs in suppressed and unsuppressed animals, *Cell Immunol.,* 34: 146–155.

Traugott, U. and Raine, C.S. (1979) Acute experimental allergic encephalomyelitis – myelin basic protein – reactive T cells in the circulation and in meningeal infiltrates, *J. Neurol. Sci.,* 42: 331–336.

Traugott, U., Stone, S.H. and Raine, C.S. (1978) Experimental allergic encephalomyelitis: T cell migration to the central nervous system, *J. Neurol. Sci.,* 36: 55–61.

Ulrich, J. and Lardi, H. (1978) Multiple sclerosis: demyelination and myelination inhibition of organotypic tissue cultures of the spinal cord by sera of patients with multiple sclerosis and other neurological disease, *J. Neurol.,* 218: 7–16.

Weiner, L.P. (1973) Pathogenesis of demyelination induced by mouse hepatitis. *Arch. Neurol.*, 28: 298–303.

Weinberg, E. and Spencer, P.C. (1978) Experimental induction of CNS myelination by regenerating PNS axons, *Neurology,* 28: 356.

Windle, W.F. (1955) Comments on regeneration in the human central nervous system. In *Regeneration in the Central Nervous System,* W.F. Windle (Ed.), Charles Thomas, Springfield, pp. 264–271.

Wisniewski, H. and Raine, C.S. (1974) An ultrastructural study of experimental demyelination and remyelination. V Central and peripheral nervous system lesions caused by diphtheria toxin, *Lab. Invest.,* 25: 73–80.

Adaption of the Cerebellum to Deafferentation

M. BERRY, J. SIEVERS and H.G. BAUMGARTEN

Department of Anatomy, University of Birmingham, Birminghem, B15 2TJ, U.K., (J.S.) Department of Neuroanatomy, University of Hamburg, Hamburg and (H.G.B.) Department of Anatomy, University of Berlin, Berlin, G.F.R.

INTRODUCTION

Until recently it was thought that the post-injury response of the central nervous system (CNS) was very limited indeed, and this view was perpetuated by the observation that recovery of function is consistently poor. But, more recently, as research has intensified, it has become clear that the reactions of the CNS to injury are, in fact, legion and that many of the changes could be interpreted as attempts by the system to adapt to circuit failure, albeit abortively. Such plastic responses to injury by the CNS occur more readily during development than in adulthood and this may account for the enhanced functional recovery of young compared with mature animals.

The sequelae of injury to the CNS include true axonal and dendritic regeneration, collateral sprouting, heterologous synaptogenesis, dendritic proliferation, changes in glia and alterations in synaptic function (for reviews see Berry, 1979; Björklund and Steveni, 1979; Kiernan, 1979). These discoveries have generated an immense surge of research activity in two separate but overlapping fields. In developmental neurobiology, concepts relating to the mechanisms of axon growth and guidance and the specificity of formation of connections have been challenged, whilst in neuropathology the findings have engendered a more optimistic outlook on recovery of function than has prevailed hitherto, because it now seems conceivable that such plasticity could be harnessed to greatly improve prognosis after CNS damage in man.

Of course, the CNS is capable of responding adaptively in circumstances other than those of organic disease and trauma. The most dramatic examples are seen following sensory deprivation or enhancement in young animals, (Rosenzweig et al., 1962; Blakemore and Cooper, 1970) before or during the sensory period when neural circuits demonstrate their greatest powers of reorganization (Hubel, Wiesel and Le Vay, 1977). This manipulation of the CNS by environmental influences could be used clinically to increase the connectivity potential of damaged brains, particularly those of very young patients.

When studying the adaptive capabilities of the nervous system it is important to use a model in which intrinsic structure is well understood, so that reorganization can be easily detected, and in which afferent connections are thoroughly documented, so that the postsynaptic sites affected by manipulation are readily identifiable. It was attention to such details, in Raisman and Field's (1973) work on the mammalian septal region, which first detected, in a partially denervated target area, a degree of plasticity which had not previously been envisaged in the adult CNS. Like the septal region, the organization of the

66

cerebellum is extremely well documented (Eccles et al., 1967; Palay and Chan-Palay, 1974) as is the origin and course of individual afferent fibre tracts. Accordingly, specific cerebellar afferent systems can be separately ablated and repercussions in intrinsic organization followed precisely both in the developing and mature animal.

STRUCTURE AND DEVELOPMENT OF THE CEREBELLUM

The mature cerebellum is a beautifully uniformly organized structure made up of 4 layers: the molecular layer (ML), Purkinje cell layer (PCL), granular layer (GL) and a medullary layer (Fig. 1). The latter contains all of the afferent fibres projecting into the cortex, and the axons of Purkinje cells (PCs), the only efferent system projecting to the deep cerebellar nuclei (DCN). The GL contains granule cells (GCs) and Golgi cells (GoCs). The former have a few short dendrites and long axons which ascend through the GL and PCL to bifurcate within the ML where they run along the long axes of folia forming axodendritic contacts with the spines of PCs. GoCs are large neurons, with massive dendritic trees mainly extending into the ML, which receive contacts from parallel fibres (PFs) and climbing fibres (CFs). A few dendrites ramify within the GL and are contacted by mossy

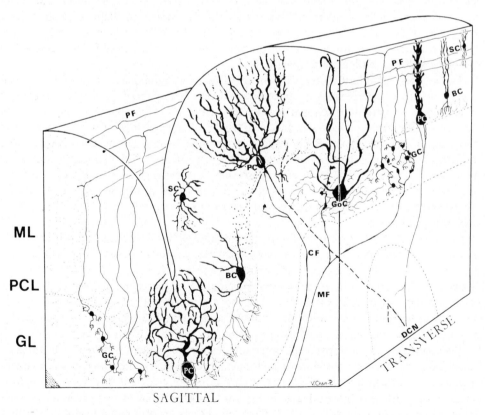

Fig. 1. Diagrammatic representation of the disposition of elements within a folium of the cerebellum. ML, molecular layer; PCL, Purkinje cell layer; GL, granular layer; PC, Purkinje cell; GC, granule cell; PF, parallel fibre; CF, climbing fibre; MF, mossy fibre – see text. (From Palay and Chan-Palay, 1974).

fibres (MFs), CFs and PC recurrent collaterals. MFs and CFs also make contact with the somata of GoCs at specialized "en marron" synapses (Chan-Palay and Palay, 1971a and b). PCs have enormous dendritic expansions extending through the entire depth of the ML. They are fan-shaped, orientated at right angles to the long axes of folia, and receive axo-dendritic contacts from PFs and stellate cell (SC) axons. Thus, the ML contains PFs and the axons of SCs, the dendrites of PCs, SCs and GoCs and the somata of SCs. SCs can be divided into SCs proper and basket cells (BCs). The former are generally smaller than the latter, which have a specialized axonal network engaging the initial segment and soma of the PC.

The macroneurons of the DCN, PCs and GoCs are formed prenatally and migrate into the deep part of the primitive cerebellum. SCs and GCs are formed from a layer of germinal cells called the external granular layer (EGL), which lies under the pial surface. All these micro-neurons attain their definitive position postnatally. In the rat, BCs are the first cells to be formed by the EGL over the first week (Altman, 1969). Thereafter, GCs and SCs are formed contemporaneously over the 2nd and 3rd week. GCs migrate through the ML to establish the GL, depositing their axons before moving. Thus, PFs are stacked in the ML in a chronological sequence from below outwards. SCs fail to migrate and elaborate their axons and dendrites in situ (Altman, 1972a and b).

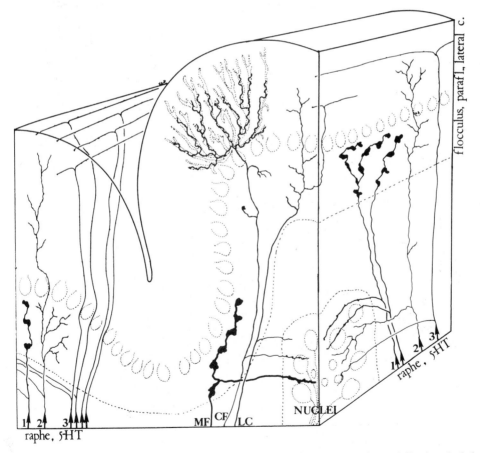

Fig. 2. Distribution and character of 5-HT fibres in the cerebellum. Presynaptic specializations include typical MF(1) and PF(3) terminals, in addition a diffuse system exists which has a similar distribution to NA fibres from the LC (Fig. 3). (From Chan-Palay, 1975).

AFFERENT FIBRES TO THE CEREBELLUM

Three groups of afferent fibres converge on the cerebellum (Fig. 1). MFs originate from multiple sources in the CNS and innervate GC dendrites in the GL. A single MF contacts several groups of GC dendrites within a synaptic complex called a glomerulus. CFs originate in the inferior olive and innervate GCs and PCs. In the adult mammal, one CF contacts one PC (Eccles et al., 1967; Palay and Chan Palay, 1974; Crépel et al., 1976) by ascending over the proximal thick branches of the dendritic tree and forming multiple contacts with low spines or thorns. They also innervate GCs in glomeruli similar to those of MFs. Mono-aminergic (MA) fibres constitute noradrenergic (NA), serotoninergic (5-HT) and dop-aminergic (DA) systems. The DA system within the cerebellum is not extensive, indeed, some authors believe it to be non-existent in the cerebellum of the rat. 5-HT fibres take origin from the raphe nuclei and ramify within the cerebellar cortex as is typical of MFs and PFs (Chan-Palay, 1975; 1977) (Fig. 2). NA axons originate in the nucleus of the locus coeruleus (LC), pass through the superior cerebellar peduncle and ramify within the GL and ML, with a high density of fibres about PC somata and their proximal dendrites (Lindvall and Björklund, 1978) (Fig. 3). The only established synaptic connections of NA fibres in the cerebellum are with PC somata and dendrites (Bloom et al., 1971), which seem to modify

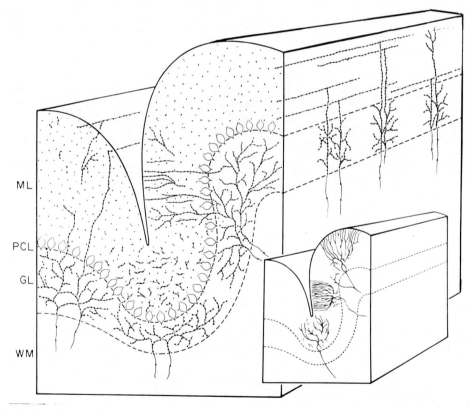

Fig. 3. Distribution of NA fibres form the LC to the cerebellum of the chick (from Mugnaini and Dahl, 1975). Varicose NA fibres form a highly branched network in the GL and a perpendicularly and horizontally running system in the ML. The course of fibres is similar in mammals (Chan-Palay, 1977). The inset shows the normal disposition of PCs in the cerebellar cortex.

the rate of spontaneous discharge of PCs (Hoffer et al., 1971; Siggins et al., 1971). Although all MA axons possess vesicle-filled expansions at regular intervals along their length, only a few of these appear to contact other elements synaptically. This has led to the concept that MA varicosities may secrete transmitters into the extracellular space where they act as neuro-humors.

EFFECTS OF ABLATION OF EXTRINSIC FIBRE SYSTEMS

Mossy fibres

MFs probably begin to form connections with GC dendrites in typical glomeruli in the 2nd and 3rd week in the rat (Altman, 1972a and b). It has been suggested that the growth of MF rosettes into the presumptive GL at this time arrests GC migration (Ebels, 1972). According to this hypothesis, cases of GC ectopia in the ML are attributable to MFs over-shooting the GL and meeting migrating GCs in the ML where they become arrested. How-ever, GC ectopia is, in most cases, associated with a failure of migratory mechanisms, and MF invasion of ectopic GC nests is a secondary event, except in rabbits where ectopic ML GoCs are contacted by MFs and GCs may be arrested about them during their migration (Špaček et al., 1973). Normally, MFs preferentially contact GC dendrites in typical glomer-uli wherever the GCs may be located, i.e. in the GL, ectopically placed in the ML (Špaček et al., 1973; Chan-Palay, 1972), subarachnoid space (Stroughton et al., 1978) or disorganized in organ culture (Privat and Drian, 1975). However, when these postsynaptic targets are absent, MFs can form contacts with almost any other element. Thus, in the murine mutant Weaver (Sotelo, 1975), in the deep cerebellar cortex of the mutant Reeler (Mariani et al., 1977) and in rats after irradiation (Hámori, 1969; Altman and Anderson, 1972) or infection with panleucopenic virus (Llinás et al., 1973), almost all GCs are absent and MF rosettes are found throughout the depths of the entire cortex, where they make synaptic contact with GoC dendrites, PC somata and dendritic spines and with BCs (Fig. 4). In all cases, the postsynaptic membrane is not affected by the presence of the presynaptic MF terminal (Altman and Anderson, 1972). For example, MF contacts on PC spines are asymmetrical, but on PC somata they are symmetrical. Assuming that the different postsynaptic specializa-tions possess the receptors for the excitatory transmitter in MF terminals (probably acetyl-choline – Altman and Das, 1970), MF contacts will generate EPSPs universally. This has been confirmed by the neurophysiological work of Llinás et al. (1973), Woodward et al. (1974), Crépel et al. (1976) and Mariani et al. (1977), since MF stimulation induces PC firing and inhibition in the DCN. Thus, MF synaptic reorganization within the degranulated cerebellar cortex maintains an excitable drive on PCs, but dispersion of MF activity through GCs and SCs is lost together with the inhibitory effects of the latter two interneuron if these are also absent (Fig. 4).

In the homozygous Weaver murine mutant, MFs develop typical rosettes, in areas where GCs are completely absent (Rakic and Sidman, 1973b), which make abnormally large synaptic contacts with GoC dendrites. Early MF contacts with PC dendrites are temporary, disappearing as astrocyte cytoplasm inserts between appositions (Rakic, 1976). MFs also invade the ML and synapse with GoC dendrites and occasional ectopic GCs, but not with the PC dendritic membrane (Rakic and Sidman, 1973b). Differences between synaptogenesis in experimentally-induced granuloprival animals and the Weaver mutant could be explained if the experimental procedure in the former altered membrane specificity and thus the cell recognition process. On the other hand, the reaction of MFs to loss of their specific target

70

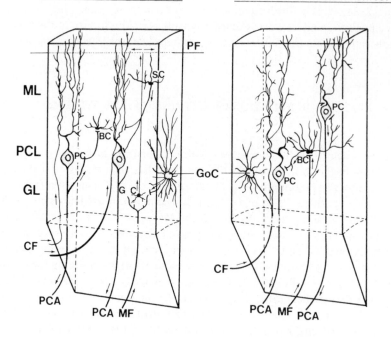

NORMAL CEREBELLAR CIRCUIT   AGRANULAR CEREBELLAR CIRCUIT

Fig. 4. Typical reorganization of cerebellar circuitry after destruction of GCs. Note the relationship of MFs with BCs and PCs. PCA, Purkinje cell axon. (From Llinás et al., 1973)

cells may not represent a reorganization per se, but the persistence of a primitive synaptology which existed in ontogeny before GCs appeared. Thus, Altman and Das (1970), using the acetylcholinesterase (AChE) technique, suggested that MFs first contact the perisomatic processes of PCs in the second half of the first week. But, in the first half of the second week, as GCs are established and perisomatic PC processes resorbed, MFs are rerouted to GL glomeruli (Fig. 5). In the absence of GCs, MFs may maintain their somatic contact with PCs. In the first week of life PCs are temporarily AChE-positive and Altman and Das (1970) argued that this is due to the presence of enzymes supporting a cholinoceptive function. The persistence of cholinoceptive mechanisms within the PCs of agranular animals could account for the invasion of cholinergic MFs onto denuded spines. The fragility of the MF/PC connection recorded by some workers (Rakic, 1976) might be related to a variable deterioration of enzyme levels in different species. Unfortunately, there is no information on the effects of degranulation in the mature animal to know if MF plasticity is as extensive in the adult as it is during development.

A reduction of MF input to the cerebellar cortex can be achieved by ablating a major MF source through the corticopontine system (Snider, 1936; Mettler and Lubin, 1942). Anwar and Berry (1980) destroyed both cerebral hemispheres on the day of birth in the rat, and studied the development of GC acquisition and PC dendritic growth in an attempt to detect reorganization. GC numbers are normal in neonatally hemispherectomized rats at 30 days post partum (dpp), but PC dendrites have abnormal branching patterns although the size of their trees is normal. The abnormal PC branching pattern was attributed to remodelling as a consequence of changed MF-PF input (see later). Hámori (1969) observed

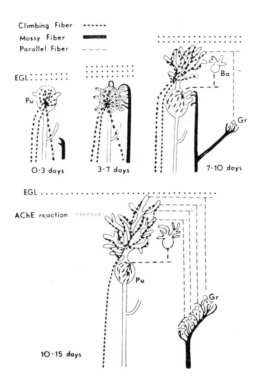

Fig. 5. Schematic diagram of the development of CFs, MFs, PFs and BC axons. Note the multiple inner-vation of PCs and a MF input to PCs during early development. (From Altman and Das, 1970).

atrophy of the cerebellar hemispheres in kittens 6 weeks after extensive ablation of the contralateral convex surface of the cerebral hemisphere as well as the frontal and occipital poles. The size of glomeruli in the GL was reduced as was the number of GC dendrites engaging them. Interpretation of these experiments is complicated by the fact that pontine nuclei do not degenerate after hemispherectomy (Hicks and D'Amato, 1970) and although the pontocerebellar projection may be non-functional in such animals, the possibility that 5-HT MFs (Chan-Palay, 1977) could hypertrophy and take over non-functional or vacated MF postsynaptic sites in hemispherectomized animals has never been investigated.

Climbing fibres

As observed by Cajal (1960), CFs grow into the cerebellum in the immediate neonatal period. In the rat, CF responses can be elicited from PCs by 3 dpp (Crépel, 1971). Early innervation is from multiple CFs (Crépel et al., 1976) but by 15 dpp the adult one-to-one relationship is obtained (Eccles et al., 1967; Palay and Chan-Palay, 1974). It is interesting that in the agranular animal CF varicosities have a higher density than normal in the ML (Sotelo, 1975) and CF multiple innervation of PCs persists (Crépel et al., 1976; Hámori, 1969; Puro and Woodward, 1977; Crépel and Mariani, 1976; Woodward et al., 1974; Crépel and Delhaye-Bouchaud, 1979). This situation appears analogous to MF innervation of PCs in the agranular cerebellum. CFs also innervate PC spines and GoCs in agranular cortex (Hámori, 1969; Altman and Anderson, 1972; Sotelo, 1975) and these constitute true heter-ologous synapses. If the cerebellum is degranulated later in development during the second post-natal week some GCs attain the GL and multiple innervation of PCs by CFs does not persist. Thus, synaptic contacts established between early PFs and PC dendrites could be important in specifying olivocerebellar connections (Delhaye-Bouchaud et al., 1978).

Specification of connectivity was also suggested as a role of CFs by Hámori (1973). He proposed that CFs induce the formation of spines on the distal branches of PC dendrites. However, experimental testing of this hypothesis has shown that PC spine production proceeds independently of CF innervation. Thus, when CFs are absent, spines still develop on PC dendrites (Calvet et al., 1976; Privat et al., 1973, 1974; Privat, 1975; Kawaguchi et al., 1975; Bradley and Berry, 1976a and b; Sotelo and Arsenio-Nunes, 1976; Sotelo et al., 1975). Indeed, when CFs are destroyed in adult animals spine degeneration does not ensue but, on the contrary, new spines appear over the proximal PC dendritic membrane previously engaged by CFs. These latter results suggest that CFs compete for PC dendritic membranes with PFs and that CFs suppress the formation of spines. CFs may also have a trophic influence on PC growth since in their absence PC dendritic fields are smaller than normal (Bradley and Berry, 1976a). The specific postsynaptic targets of CFs and PC dendritic thorns and GC dendrites. As yet, there is no information about the fate of CFs in animals which have no PCs, like for example, the murine mutants "Purkinje-cell-degeneration" (PCD), Nervous and Lurcher or, indeed, of the fate of CF glomeruli in agranular animals.

Noradrenergic fibres

The NA fibre system is the first extrinsic group of axons to invade the developing cerebellum between embryonal days 16 and 17 (Seiger and Olson, 1973; Sievers et al., 1980). By birth they ramify mainly within the primordial GL and the PCL. The EGL receives only a few NA axons.

The function of NA fibres in the immature cerebellum is largely unknown, but, as in other brain regions which receive NA input at comparably early stages of ontogeny, NA axons may regulate within their target areas developmental processes such as proliferation, migration or differentiation of neurons (Seiger and Olson, 1973; Maeda et al., 1974; Schlumpf et al., 1977; Lauder and Krebs, 1976; Kasamatsu and Pettigrew, 1976; 1979; Kasamatsu et al., 1979; Pettigrew and Kasamatsu, 1978). Such effects could be initiated and maintained by NA activation of intracellular cyclic adenylase, which in turn could lead to increased levels of c-AMP and ultimately to the expression of genetic information controlling neuronal differentiation (McMahon, 1974; Bloom, 1974). In this model, NA could act on target cells either through synaptic contacts, as a conventional neurotransmitter, or through specific surface NA receptors as a neurohumor, after release from axonal varicosities (Bloom, 1974; Chan-Palay, 1977).

We have performed a number of experiments to test the hypothesis that the NA system controls neural development, and to study the adaptive responses of the developing cerebellum to the loss of NA fibres. The achievement of a selective ablation of NA innervation is complicated by numerous methodological limitations. Electrolytic destruction of the LC, on both sides of the brain stem, is impracticable in newborn rats because stereotactic maps are incompletely developed (Maeda et al., 1974; Wendlandt et al., 1977) and also because the electrode tracts pass through the developing cerebellum. We have therefore resorted to the use of the neurotoxin, 6-hydroxydopamine (6-OHDA). This substance acts selectively on CA axon terminals and cell bodies, but its use in the newborn has considerable limitations.

Subcutaneous (s.c.) administration of 6-OHDA to neonates, in doses that are sufficient to permanently destroy the NA axons of the cerebral neocortex, leads to paradoxical effects in the cerebellum. After an initial decrease in NA content and uptake capacity, NA fibres display a fulminant regrowth, and ultimately an overgrowth, resulting in an uptake capacity which is more than twice as high as in control animals of the same age (see below). This reaction is, in fact, a demonstration of the great regenerative properties of LC neurons in the early postnatal period. Thus, the most effective way of ablating the NA innervation of the neonatal rat cerebellum is to destroy the entire LC by neurotoxicological means. In adult rats, the successful neurotoxic destruction of the LC by i.c. injection of 6-OHDA has been reported by Descarries and Saucier (1972), but in neonates higher doses of 6-OHDA are needed to produce the same effect.

In our first experiment, newborn rats received one intracisternal (i.c.) injection of 100 µg (free base) of 6-OHDA. The effects of this treatment on cerebellar NA innervation were monitored by biochemical measurements of the uptake capacity for NA and tissue NA levels, as well as the histochemical demonstration of NA fibres. All of these parameters showed that the number of NA fibres in the cerebellum was reduced by more than 90% between 1 and at least 15 days post-injection (dpi), which is the duration of the most active period for cerebellar development. After that period, the NA innervation slowly recovered to about 50% of control values by 60 dpi (Fig. 6).

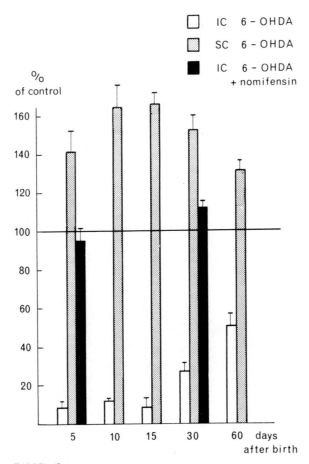

Fig. 6. Time course of dimethyl imipramine-sensitive [³H]NA uptake after different modes of injection of 6-OHDA on the day of birth expressed as per cent of age-matched, control-injected animals.

74

Morphological analysis revealed that most of the neurons in the caudal and middle parts of the LC were severely damaged and degenerated. By 5 dpi many of these cells had completely disintegrated and were surrounded by numerous macrophages, containing large vacuoles filled with masses of fragmented membranes and pyknotic nuclei. A second type of degeneration was characterized by the accumulation of large osmiophilic precipitates, myelinoid inclusions and numerous vacuoles with an electron-dense content. In the rostral part of the LC, especially its dorsal portion, most of the neurons exhibited a retrograde axon reaction: their nuclei were displaced to the periphery of the perikarya, many of the normally large Nissl bodies were decomposed, and lipoid inclusions of various sizes were seen in different parts of the cytoplasm. Electron microscopic examination of the effects of 6-OHDA on the different cerebellar elements showed that, in addition to the destruction of the NA fibres, neurons in the GL and neuroblasts in the EGL, as well as glial cells and the fibroblasts of the pial coverings were damaged (Fig. 7). This, in turn, resulted in a complex pattern of permanent changes in the architecture of the cerebellum 30 dpi. The fissures between individual vermal folia, with the exception of those between nodulus and uvula, either became obliterated some distance from their bases or disappeared altogether, leading to a primitive form of foliation (Fig. 8). The posterior sulci were less affected than the anterior, although the latter were closer to the site of injection. A severe alteration was seen in the GC population (Fig. 9). The most striking finding was a massive ectopia of GCs along the line of fusion of folia, (Fig. 8) and also in the subarachnoid space of the surface of the cerebellum (Fig. 10).

Dendritic field analysis of PCs, which are the only cerebellar cells with an established NA

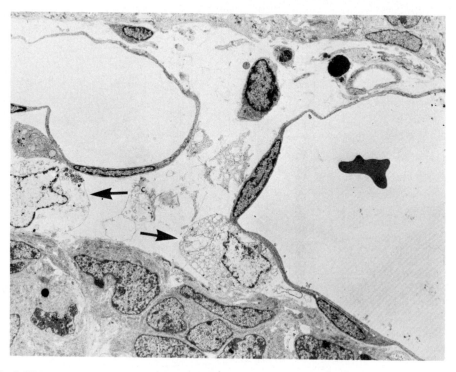

Fig. 7. Electron micrograph of a cerebellar sulcus of a neonatal rat 24 h after i.c. 6-OHDA on the day of birth. Note the degenerating pial fibroblasts (↑). ×2275.

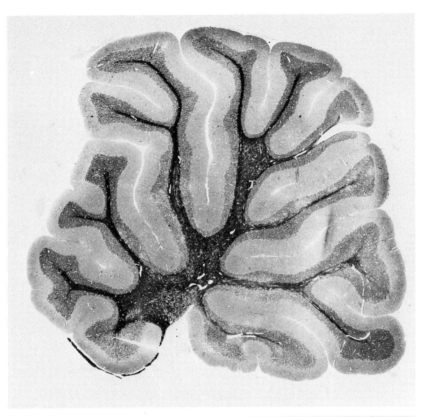

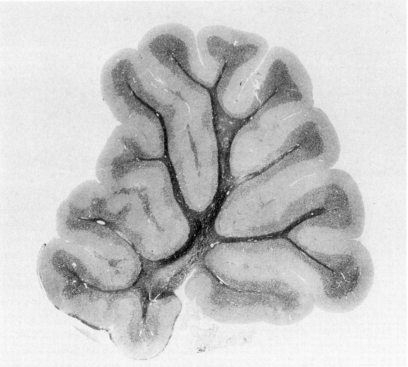

Fig. 8. Mediosagittal sections of the cerebella of control (upper) and i.c. 6-OHDA-treated (lower) rats 30 dpi. Note the defects in foliation and fissuration as well as the large ectopic GC groups in the treated cerebellum.

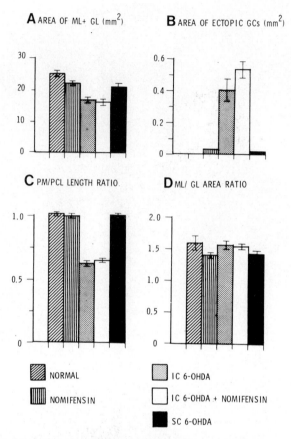

A AREA OF ML+ GL (mm^2) **B** AREA OF ECTOPIC GCs (mm^2)

C PM/PCL LENGTH RATIO **D** ML/ GL AREA RATIO

NORMAL   IC 6-OHDA

NOMIFENSIN   IC 6-OHDA + NOMIFENSIN

SC 6-OHDA

Fig. 9. Values for the areas of parasagittal vermal sections from normal rats and those treated with nomifensin; i.c. 6-OHDA; i.c. 6-OHDA and nomifensin; and s.c. 6-OHDA. The ratio of the length of the pia mater (PM) and length of the PCL (C) is a measure of fissuration. The ratio ML/GL (D) shows that the relationship of these two layers remains the same despite reductions in area seen in A. GC ectopia (B) is only a feature in animals receiving heavy i.c. doses of 6-OHDA.

synaptic connection (Bloom et al., 1971), showed that the size of the dendritic trees, as well as the total number of segments, was reduced while internodal segment lengths were elongated. These changes are thought to be consistent with the decreased number of PFs subsequent to GC loss (Berry et al., 1978). The number of PCs in treated animals did not differ from that of controls.

In the course of the evaluation of our first experiment it had become apparent that the high doses of 6-OHDA used had damaged non-NA elements of the cerebellum so that a conclusive result of the effects of NA-deprivation on the differentiation of the cerebellum could not be obtained. In order to separate NA-mediated from non-specific side-effects of 6-OHDA on other cerebellar elements, a control experiment was designed, in which the same dose of neurotoxin was given as before, but its uptake into NA axons was prevented by the concomitant administration of the highly selective NA and DA uptake-blocker, nomifensin (Sievers et al., 1980). The NA fibre protection by nomifensin was confirmed by measurements of [^{3}H]NA uptake, which showed that both in the acute and long-term period after

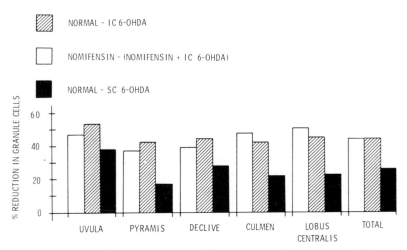

Fig. 10. Per cent reduction in GCs in representative folia of the cerebellum after i.c. 6-OHDA; i.c. 6-OHDA and nomifensin and after s.c. 6-OHDA. There is statistically no significant difference between the i.c. 6-OHDA and i.c. 6-OHDA and nomifensin reductions, indicating that destruction of GCs is not related to the ablation of NA terminals but to direct effects of 6-OHDA on GCs. The small reduction of GCs in the hyperinnervated NA cerebellum is probably related to the toxicity of the small dose of 6-OHDA given s.c.

injection, NA uptake sites in the brain stem and cerebellum were unaffected by 6-OHDA (Fig. 6).

The cerebellar defects seen at 30 dpi were qualitatively identical to those seen in the previous experiment using 6-OHDA alone (Fig. 8). A detailed morphometric analysis of the results showed that, in addition to such gross defects as decreases in cerebellar weight, vermal area and total ML area (Fig. 9), the number of GCs was also reduced in relation to control values, showing an average decrease of about 50% in the individual folia (Fig. 10). It was therefore concluded that, in our first two experiments, the effects of 6-OHDA on the development of the cerebellum are largely, if not entirely, attributable to toxic effects on non-NA elements which include pial fibroblasts, glial cells and GCs.

Taking into account that the gross toxicity of 6-OHDA could have masked subtle trophic and/or inductive effects mediated by NA fibres, a third experiment was conducted to test the hypothesis of NA regulation of cerebellar development. It was argued that, if the normal sequence of developmental events such as cell proliferation, migration and outgrowth of processes, is controlled by NA innervation, alterations in any of these events should result from either a reduction or an increase of the cerebellar NA fibre supply. As our experiments on NA ablation had produced little evidence in favour of this hypothesis (possibly because of the difficulties connected with using high doses of 6-OHDA) we proceeded to markedly increase the cerebellar NA innervation over the period of morphogenesis in the postnatal period.

An established experimental procedure for achieving NA hyperinnervation is the administration of a low s.c. dose of 6-OHDA to neonatal rats (Sachs and Jonsson, 1975; Schmidt and Bhatnagar, 1979a and b). In agreement with previous reports, we found that the uptake capacity for [3H]NA in the cerebellum started to rise considerably in the first 5 dpi, increased to 160% of control by 10 dpi, and was maintained at this level thereafter (Fig. 6). NA content had reached 220% of control values by 15 dpi and this high level remained at least until 60 dpi.

Qualitative morphological and quantitative morphometric examination of the cerebellum of treated animals 30 dpi showed that vermal area was reduced by 25% (Fig. 9), and this was reflected by a reduction of 25% in GC numbers (Fig. 10), whereas all other parameters were normal. It was concluded that the small dose of 6-OHDA, given s.c., was causing some toxicity to GCs but that there was no demonstrable effect of NA hyperinnervation on cerebellar development.

Taken together, the results of our 3 experiments testing the hypothesis that NA fibres control cerebellar development, exclude a decisive influence of this axonal projection on major postnatal events in cerebellar morphogenesis, such as the differentiation of individual cerebellar elements, the development of intrinsic and extrinsic fibre systems, foliation and fissuration. They do not, of course, exclude a role in prenatal cerebellar development. These results complement those of Wendlandt et al. (1977) in which a 70% reduction in NA content, after neonatal LC ablation, was associated neither with any change in the anatomy of neocortical and hippocampal neurons nor with any effect on GC replication and acquisition in the dentate gyrus. These latter findings were not, however, substantiated by Lewis et al. (1977) and Patel et al. (1977) using reserpinized animals. In these studies the cell kinetics of the EGL were found to be markedly abnormal. Maeda et al. (1974) reported that the development of neocortical apical dendrites was retarded after neonatal LC ablation, although this was a qualitative judgement on Golgi–Cox preparations from only 2 animals.

The adaption of the cerebellum to NA denervation or hyperinnervation by the redistribution of NA axons into different layers of the cerebellar cortex is of special interest in the light of a recent hypothesis (Schmidt et al., 1979) which suggests that the potential for growth and regeneration of NA axons, lesioned at different times after birth, is not inherent in the parent LC neurons but depends on as yet unidentified extrinsic factors released from individual target tissues differentially according to age. These factors act on the LC to stimulate or to stop axonal growth. This hypothesis, which is analogous to the induction of growth of sensory neurons and sympathetic postganglionic fibres by nerve growth factor (NGF), is supported by findings which show that displaced neurons in both the immature and the adult LC are capable of regenerating axons into peripheral or central target areas and replicating the normal pattern of innervation and normal function (Björklund and Stenevi, 1979; Olson and Seiger, 1976). Schmidt et al. (1979) formulated their hypothesis to explain the results of experiments in which NA regeneration was studied in the cerebella of rats treated with 6-OHDA at different times after birth. It was shown that NA regrowth declined progressively with increasing age and was absent when the animals were treated from 12 dpp (Schmidt et al., 1979). Their interpretation of these findings took into account the propensity of the adult LC to form new axons after transplantation to ectopic sites (Björklund and Stenevi, 1979; Seiger and Olson, 1977) and focussed on the possible regulation of regeneration by the innervated target area, in this case the cerebellum, in addition to an intrinsic growth potential of NA neurons.

In our experiments, after 6-OHDA injection at birth, biochemical and fluorescence histochemical findings showed that NA fibres were practically absent from the cerebellum at least up to 15 dpp. NA fibre density recovered to 50% of control values by 30 and 60 dpp in all parts of the cerebellar vermis, especially in the anterior folia, forming a loose plexus in all 3 cortical layers accentuated in the PCL and the lower ML as normally. However, irregularly oriented fibres were seen in the ML, especially at the pial surface and at the bases of sulci. All the fibres displayed larger varicosities than normal and a higher intensity of fluorescence suggesting the occurrence of collateral accumulation (Sachs and Jonsson, 1975; Schmidt and Bhatnager, 1979b). Interestingly, fluorescent fibres were also found in groups of ectopic

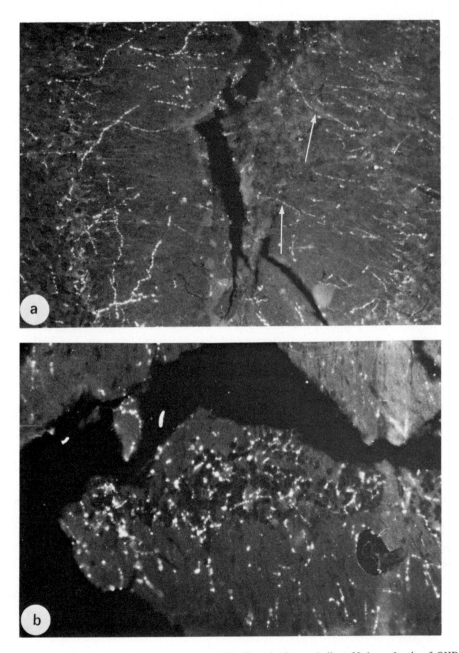

Fig. 11. a: fluorescence micrograph of regenerated NA fibres in the cerebellum 60 days after i.c. 6-OHDA. Strongly fluorescent axons are seen in an organotypic distribution in the GL, PCL and ML. Some of them are invading ectopic GC nests (↑). ×350. b: higher magnification of NA innervation of ectopic GCs in the same animal as in Fig. 11a. ×560.

GCs where they formed dense plexuses around invidual cells (Fig. 11).

The source of these regrown NA axons were the neurons of the dorsorostral part of the LC that had survived the treatment, while the caudal LC had completely degenerated. Thus, LC neurons damaged by 6-OHDA shortly after birth either degenerate or recover slowly over the first two weeks post-injection and then, after this latent period, form new axons which innervate the cerebellum. In this light, the regeneration of NA fibres into different parts of the brain after neonatal 6-OHDA treatment might be related primarily to the differential survival of LC neurons and their inherent capacity of projecting axons to these regions, rather than to the presence of target-elicited factors which, according to Schmidt and Bhatnagar (1979) are not found in the cerebellum beyond 12 dpp.

In summary, our results suggest that the cerebellum adapts to NA fibre deafferentation by providing postsynaptic sites for regenerating NA axons, which can innervate both normally located and ectopic cerebellar elements. At present it cannot be decided whether regeneration is achieved by the release from target areas of specific factors that stimulate a regenerative response in NA axons after a prolonged latency period, or whether regrowth is solely dependent on factors inherent in LC neurons. Reinnervation of the cerebellum is reduced by 50% and this is correlated with massive destruction of caudal LC neurons, although the density of innervation to all folia is uniform.

5-HT system

An extensive 5-HT system has recently been discovered in the cerebellum (Bloom et al., 1972; Chan-Palay, 1975; Chan-Palay, 1977). Like the NA system, many 5-HT vesicle-filled varicosities are synaptic in the classical sense of engaging a postsynaptic specialization, but many do not form synaptic junctions and are thought to release transmitter into the parenchyma where it could act as a neurohumor engaging indolamine receptors. The 5-HT system is of special interest because it appears to be selectively involved in the pathogenesis of some of the neurological manifestations of thiamine deficiency. Thiamine deficiency in animals simulates Wernicke's encephalopathy in man (Dreyfus and Victor, 1961). Thiamine deficient rats exhibit a greatly reduced 5-HT axon system which can be demonstrated within the cerebellum using radioactive exogenous 5-HT labelling and neurochemical techniques (Chan-Palay et al., 1977; Plaitakis et al., 1977). MF and PF 5-HT fibres are the most severely affected with some sparing of the diffuse branching system suggesting that synaptic indolamine axons are more susceptible to thiamine deficiency than the non-synaptic system (Chan-Palay et al., 1977; Chan-Palay, 1977).

Like NA axons, 5-HT fibres possess remarkable powers of regeneration and thus many of the effects of thiamine deficiency might be reversed by early dietary correction. However, it is still uncertain whether the thiamine-associated changes in uptake of [^{3}H]serotonin represent functional membrane changes or true neural destruction (Chan-Palay et al., 1977). Moreover, like NA fibres, 5-HT axons have also been implicated in the control of CNS development by mobilizing intracellular c-AMP. Lauder and Krebs (1976) have found that after p-chlorophenylalanine administration to pregnant rats, their offspring show delayed differentiation in 5-HT target areas. However, in this investigation the cerebellum was not included for study and 5-HT levels were not monitored.

ABLATION OF INTRINSIC SYSTEMS

Effects on microneurons: basket and stellate cells (BCs and SCs)

The microneurons of the cerebellar cortex are all formed from the EGL and include BCs, SCs and GCs. They form a link in the circuit between MFs and PCs and GoCs. BCs are formed in the first week pp, SCs and GCs over the following 2 weeks (Altman, 1969). It is possible that BCs may by responsible for the resorption of PC perisomatic spines in the latter part of the first week pp (Altman, 1976) and they could thus displace MFs from PC somata at this time (Altman and Anderson, 1972).

As mentioned above, in partially agranular cortex MFs invade the ML and make heterologous synaptic connections with BCs and SCs (Altman and Anderson, 1972; Llinás et al., 1973). This implies that true circuit reorganization does develop in agranular cortex since primary afferents engage inhibitory interneurons in the absence of the intermediary GC link. On the other hand, this degree of reorganization after neonatal injury may only be found in the developing CNS and could be effected through a process of functional stabilization of synapses as the animal matures (Changeux and Danchin, 1976). At present, we know too little of the effects of degranulation in the adult cerebellum (Herndon, 1968; Bradley and Berry, 1979) to decide if the neonatal response is true reorganization or achieved through functional stabilization. A prerequisite for the latter hypothesis is that all afferents initially contact a more dispersed target quantitatively and, possibly, qualitatively (Changeux and Danchin, 1976) but that this becomes contracted by function. Unlike the MF—PC connection, we have no evidence that MFs normally contact BCs and SCs during development.

In the Weaver mouse, SCs and BCs do not expand their axonal arbors to synaptically engage bare PC dendritic spines. They maintain their specificity, making only homologous synaptic relationships with smooth PC dendritic membranes (Rakic, 1976). Large postsynaptic areas are elaborated on interneuronal dendritic membranes which are not engaged by presynaptic elements, and BCs do not form typical perisomatic baskets or the pinceau formation about the initial axonal segment (Sotelo, 1975). In the PCD mutant the targets of SCs and BCs — the PCs — are absent. Our own observations on PCD show BC axons persisting and forming a diffuse axon network in the superficial GL but no electron microscope study has been done so far.

GCs. GCs normally migrate from the EGL, through the ML to establish the GL where their dendrites synapse with MFs. If migration fails, ectopic groups of GCs are found within the ML. In normal animals, small nests of GCs are seen below the pia within the ML and sometimes outside the CNS resting on the pial surface in the subarachnoid space (Pfaffenroth and Das, 1974; Chan-Palay, 1972; Stoughton et al., 1978). The synaptology of ectopically placed cells is intriguing because it offers a means of investigating the specificity of contacts and the mechanism by which afferent axons find their targets. A universal finding is that GCs differentiate normally (e.g. Sosa et al., 1971) and their synaptology is normal. Thus, MFs course through the ML and innervate GC dendrites in typical glomeruli (Landis, 1973; Ebels, 1972; Altman and Anderson, 1972; Chan-Palay, 1972; Špaček et al., 1973) as do CFs (Landis, 1973). Occasional SCs are seen within the ectopic nests and these also have normal synaptology. Sometimes GCs form somadendritic and dendrodendritic contacts with PCs (Špaček et al., 1973) but this is unusual.

Perhaps the most remarkable site of GC ectopia is the subarachnoid space over the surface of the cerebellum. A few cells are seen here in normal animals probably resulting from escape through the basement membrane during development (Stoughton et al., 1978). The numbers of subarachnoid GCs can be greatly increased by i.c. administration of 6-OHDA on day 1 pp. As mentioned above, 6-OHDA destroys glial and pial elements, with the result that the basement membrane over the pial surface fractures because the cerebellum continues to expand without producing sufficient basement membrane to accommodate the increase in surface area (Fig. 7). Under such circumstances germinal microneurons escape from the EGL and spill into the subarachnoid space through breaches in the basement membrane both within the fissures and over the surfaces of folia. Ectopic EGL cells proliferate and those in the sulci migrate into the subarachnoid space on the crest of the folia or into the cisternae

82

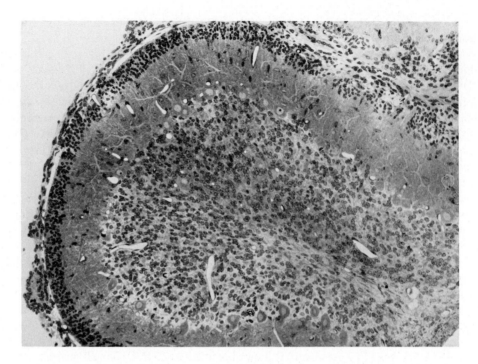

Fig. 12. Sagittal section of the cerebellum of a young rat 15 days after i.c. 6-OHDA. Neuroblasts are seen migrating out of the depth of a sulcus onto the crest of the folium (left part of the photograph) where they are separated from the cerebellar cortex by intervening blood vessels and pial cells. ×140.

between folial apices (Fig. 12). These show many of the typical morphological features of migrating neuroblasts, such as bipolarity of the cell body, elongated dendritic and axonal processes with growth cones at their tips, lamellipodia and filopodia.

In contrast to these migratory stages in the first two weeks pi, when the ectopic cells were scattered singly or in small groups over the surface of the cerebellar folia, at 30 dpi we found numerous large cell colonies of ectopic cells and at 90 dpi the number of colonies and their size had increased even further. Colonies consisted chiefly of GCs but SCs, BCs and glial cells were also present (Fig. 13). SCs and BCs were also seen lying singly in the sub-arachnoid space. The histotypic organization of colonies suggests that the aggregation mechanisms operating in the establishment of specific cell associations in certain stages of neural differentiation (Garber and Moscona, 1972) are maintained by these ectopic cell groups located outside the CNS. The possibility that each colony represents a clone of cells derived from a single EGL stem cell demonstrates the potential of this ectopic cell model for studies of neuronal cell lineage.

Using the SEM, numerous nerve fibres of various diameters were seen interconnected with cell colonies or disappearing into the underlying cerebellar cortex. These could be separated into two distinct groups, which differed not only in their diameter but also in their type of termination and connection. Easily identifiable were PFs because they originated from GCs and could often be traced to T-junctions, the arms of which had a diameter of 1 μm or less. PFs displayed varicosities of various diameters and often tended to run in fibre bundles which traversed the subarachnoid space in parallel formations. PFs were often seen to converge and terminate in clusters of bulbous, club-shaped endings on either the dendrites or

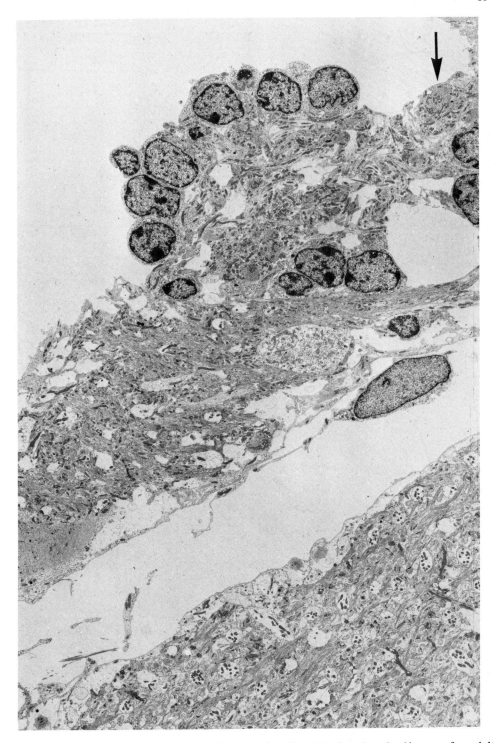

Fig. 13. Low power electron micrograph of an ectopic cell nest in the subarachnoid space of an adult rat 90 days after i.c. 6-OHDA. This cell-and-neuropil aggregation is separated from the underlying cerebellar cortex by two basement membranes, a pial fibroblast and a solid sheath of glia. Besides the typical mature GCs, a peripheral part of BC cytoplasm is visible in the lower part of this ectopic cell group. A typical MF glomerulus is situated on top of the neuropil (↑). A higher magnification of this structure is shown in Fig. 14b. ×2400.

84

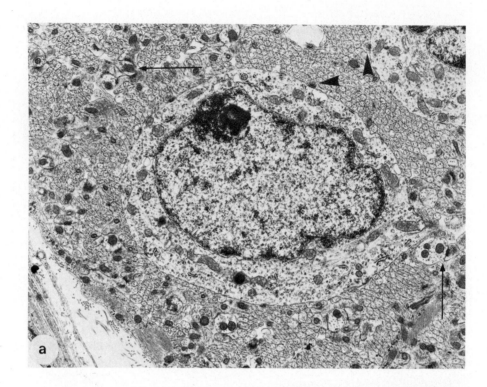

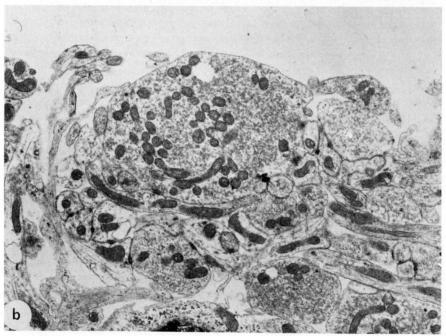

Fig. 14. a: ectopic SCs surrounding by large bundles of PFs (same animal as in Fig. 13), lying on top of a pial blood vessel (left part of the photograph). Specific cerebellar synapses between PF varicosities and SC dendrites (↑) and PFs and SC somata (▲) are pointed out. ×8970. b: higher magnification of a part of Fig. 13. Typical MF glomerulus making synaptic contacts with several GC dendrites. ×11,000.

somata of GCs or on larger, isolated round-to-oval cells which were tentatively identified as SCs or BCs. These latter cells and their synaptic complexes were often covered with glial laminae. In addition to these terminal synaptic complexes, synapses en passant between PF varicosities and SC dendrites were regularly seen. The high frequency of synapses between SCs or BCs and PFs may indicate a greater than normal innervation of these cells by ectopic GC PFs. The SEM identification of PFs and the nature and specificity of their synaptic connections were verified with the TEM. Thus, axodendritic synapses between PFs and SCs and BCs, as well as axosomatic contacts between the same elements, were observed (Fig. 14A). Thus, the same intrinsic fibre connections existed in ectopic colonies as are found within the cerebellar cortex, suggesting that a stable mechanism is operating in the establishment of synaptic connections between cerebellar cells.

The second group of fibres was more heterogeneous, varying considerably in diameter with a range of 0.5–1.5 μm. A common feature was their termination at the dendrites of GCs where they often formed large synaptic conglomerates, apparently equivalent to cerebellar glomeruli. Usually, these were characterized by the presence of large bulbous structures lying in the peripheral regions of the glomerulus on top of the GC dendrites. In the TEM, the bulbous enlargements of the afferent fibres were readily identified as typical MF terminals, which were engaged in characteristic MF glomeruli with GC dendrites (Fig. 14B). CF terminals were also seen in the ectopic GC groups, although glomerular connections with GC dendrites have not yet been observed.

We conclude the following: (1) EGL cells move out of their normal position into the subarachnoid space when the glial/pial barrier is damaged; (2) EGL cells can migrate within the subarachnoid space and proliferate to form colonies of cells, which in some cases may represent true clones derived from a single stem cell. During normal development, stem cell proliferation in the EGL of the rat is complete by about 21 dpp (Addison, 1911; Altman, 1969). In the subarachnoid space, however, proliferation appears to continue at least up to 90 dpp (as judged by the increase in size of ectopic nests seen in the SEM), suggesting that EGL stem cells have escaped from the proliferative controls exerted by structures in the cerebellum, and exhibit free-running mitotic acitivity; (3) most ectopic cells are able to differentiate and survive in their abnormal environment, in spite of a defective migratory stage. This observation challenges concepts in cerebellar developmental neurobiology which suggest that: (i) GC migration is a prerequisite for GC survival, an explanation often proffered to account for the Weaver defect (Rezai and Yoon, 1972; Rakic and Sidman, 1973a), and (ii) GC survival is trophically dependent on PF/PC dendritic contact (probably not present in most subarachnoid ectopic GCs), an explanation put forward to account for GC death in the Staggerer mutant (Sotelo and Changeux, 1974) and in starved animals (McConnell and Berry, 1980); and (4) the specificity of connections in ectopic GC colonies in the subarachnoid space appears to argue strongly in support of a "preformist" point of view (Cajal, 1911) since it seems inconceivable that MFs can seek out GC dendrites in the subarachnoid space except by some specific trophic cue which is effective over considerable distances of neuropil. Similarly, since most of the ectopic PFs probably do not make contact with PC dendrites there is not likely to be any output for GC activity. Thus, there is no possible means by which the system can stabilize meaningful synapses according to functional activity (Changeux and Danchin, 1976). But, in the absence of function, synaptic connections are completely homologous and there are few, if any, abnormal connections.

A similar condition is seen in PCD and Nervous mutant mice in which PCs completely degenerate. Under these circumstances GCs do not degenerate but, in the PCD mutant at least, survive normally into old age. The synaptology of the PCD and Nervous cerebellum has not been reported in any detail so there is no information on circuit alterations, but GC longevity in these mutants clearly demonstrates that maintained GC contact with PCs is not essential to the survival of GCs.

Effects on macroneurons: Purkinje cells (PCs)

These massive neurons represent the "final common path" of cerebellar activity, since their axons are the only ones that leave the cortex. PCs receive a large excitatory input from PFs over their spiny distal branches and from CFs over thorns on proximal thick dendrites. Inhibitory SC and BC axons converge on PC smooth dendritic membrane, soma and initial axonal segment respectively (Eccles et al., 1967). MFs normally make no direct contact with PCs except a possible transitory connection during early development (Altman and Das, 1970).

It has been suggested that during normal development PFs have a major influence on PC dendritic growth (Berry et al., 1978; 1980a and b) PFs could maintain PC dendritic growth by mediating an inductive stimulus, via axon—spinous synapses which activates metabolism to support growth. After PF induction the tips of PC dendrites advance through the neuropil of the ML at a constant speed and dendritic branching is controlled by interaction between PFs and dendritic growth cone filopodia (Berry et al., 1978; 1980a and b).

The mutant mice, Staggerer and Weaver, do not develop PF spinous contacts with PCs. In the former case, this is because spines fail to develop (Sidman, 1968; 1972; 1974; Sotelo, 1973; 1975; Landis, 1971; Yoon, 1976; Mallet et al., 1976; Sotelo and Changeux, 1974) and, in the latter, bacause GCs die in the EGL before migration occurs, so that no PFs are deposited (Sidman, 1968; Rakic and Sidman, 1973a and b; Sidman et al., 1965; Rezai and Yoon, 1972). In these mutants the PC dendritic free attains only some 12% of its normal size (Bradley and Berry, 1978a). Growth is arrested on about the 7th dpp possibly because PFs fail to make the required number of contacts on PC dendritic spines mandatory for the continuation of dendritic growth (Berry et al., 1980a and b). Berry et al. (1980a and b) were able to calculate that PC/GC ratio must attain a value of at least 1 : 80 in order for PF induction to occur. Thereafter, dendritic growth cones advance through the neuropil of the ML at a constant speed, the rate of advance being measured from the increments in the mean dendritic path length with age. We have found that, over the period of PF deposition, path lengths increase linearly. The growth of dendrites stops when PF formation ceases, but the mechanism of this arrest is as yet unknown. One factor might be that growth cones interact over finite distances to mutually inhibit their further outgrowth.

The mechanisms by which PFs could influence dendritic growth are not understood, but it has been suggested that there exists in the cerebellum a specific adhesive affinity between SC and PC dendritic growth cone filopodia and PFs (Berry et al., 1978, 1980a and b). According to this hypothesis, the number of segments generated and the frequency of different orders of branching (dichotomy, trichotomy, etc.) are directly proportional, while segment lengths are inversely proportional, to the frequency of adhesive sites about the growing tree. Since growth cones are mainly located at the tips of growing dendrites, arborization patterns will be elaborated by terminal rather than by segmental branching. Dendritic trees will grow into areas of neuropil where the density of adhesive sites is greatest.

Several observations support this hypothesis. Rakic (1972) has shown that the dendritic trees of SCs in the ML of the rat grow preferentially towards PFs. In partially agranular cerebellar cortex the number of PFs is reduced. Predictably, PC dendritic trees have fewer branches than normal and the frequency of trichotomy is reduced, but segment lengths are increased although overall path lengths are normal (Hámori, 1969; Bradley and Berry,

1976a, 1978b; Berry and Bradley, 1976c; Crépel and Mariani, 1976). The normal PC dendritic path length in partially agranular cerebellar cortex supports the contention that a sufficient number of parallel fibres is deposited to induce dendrites to grow at a constant rate. Mean path lengths will be normal if growth stops at the same time as normally, but fewer branches will be formed.

If dendritic branching is causally related to the density of deposition of PFs, a positive correlation should exist between the number of dendritic segments formed and the number of PFs deposited in the ML throughout development. In fact, this correlation is tightly maintained (Hollingworth and Berry, 1975; Berry et al., 1980a and b) even if the number of GCs is reduced (McConnell and Berry, 1980). The prediction that dendritic networks grow by terminal branching has the corollary that PC trees will exhibit random terminal branching because the ML density of PFs is uniform. The frequencies of distinct PC branching topologies at 30 dpp are distributed in a pattern indistinguishable from that established by random terminal branching (Hollingworth and Berry, 1975; Berry and Bradley, 1976a and b). During development, however, some non-random branching does occur as denditic trees become oriented towards the pial surface (Berry and Bradley, 1976b).

There is now some evidence that remodelling of circuits occurs in later stages of cerebellar development as the animal grows and acquires a full repertoire of motor skills. Thus, Weiss and Pysh (1978) have observed an increase in PC dendritic segment lengths accompanied by a reduction in segment number after 20 dpp in mice. McConnell and Berry (1978) observed an increase in PC segment lengths in rats at the end of some 50 days of rehabilitation, after starving the animals for the first 30 days of life. They also detected marked changes in PC dendritic branching patterns, not only in starved animals which were subsequently rehabilitated, but also in normal rats, over the period from 30 to 80 dpp. These findings suggest that PC dendritic trees are responding both to changes in MF input and to PF readjustments as GCs die after the migratory period (McConnell and Berry, 1980), a phenomenon which could be a manifestation of weeding out redundant or inappropriate PF connections. Destruction of PFs in adults, either by degranulation (Bradley and Berry, 1979) or by surgical transectioning (Mouren-Mathieu and Colonnier, 1969), also causes a reduction in the size of PC trees by a pruning of distal branches.

CONCLUSIONS

The reaction of the cerebellum to deafferentation differs with age and according to the type of fibre system interrupted. In general, the response of the young CNS is more plastic than that of the ageing brain although there is insufficient experimental evidence substantiating this proposition. The development of the cerebellum in the absence of major afferent input, like MFs, CFs or MA fibres, does not appear to produce repercussions in target cells, as might be expected if these systems are mediating trophic or inductive cues. Experimental reduction of MA axons and MF input into the neonatal cerebellum, for example, has produced little detectable alteration in gross organization, whereas without CFs, PCs are smaller and spine distribution is abnormal. If, however, the target cells of afferent fibres are absent, major connectivity disturbances ensue as incoming axons "seek out" alternative postsynaptic sites. Thus, when GCs are absent, MFs make contact with other elements throughout the depth of the cortex — but, there is some doubt about the permanence of these connections, their functional integrity and the possibility of damage to membranes by experimental manipulation which could interfere with membrane recognition, presumed to be the basis of synaptic specificity. Such reorganization might also be explained by invoking the hypothesis of functional stabilization of synapses. Indeed, there is some evidence that the synaptology of MFs in agranular animals could reflect a primitive pattern existing before the GCs were formed. However, changes in the positions of target cells in the cerebellar cortex do not interfere with synaptology even if cells occupy the subarachnoid space, an observation which supports the contention that throughout ontogeny, synaptogenesis is very specific.

If GCs do not make contact with PCs, the dendritic field of the latter fails to develop normally. There is a direct correlation between the number of PFs and the number of PC dendritic segments elaborated. The relationship is not dependent on function since when MF input is reduced the frequency of dendritic segments remains normal, as does the number of GCs formed. The correlation appears to be established by adhesive interaction of PFs with PC dendritic growth cone filopodia. In the adult, GC reduction appears to be associated with a decrement in the size of the PC tree indicating that dendritic fields might be maintained by the presence of afferent fibres and/or the firing level (or pattern) of their input.

MA fibres are the only system of axons to regenerate into the cerebellum after damage, but their ability to do so may be related to: (1) age; (2) differential survival of LC neurons; (3) intrinsic potential to regenerate; and (4) trophic cues passing to the LC from target areas. There are no structural alterations in the cerebellum after postnatal NA deafferentation.

REFERENCES

Addison, W.H.F. (1911) The development of the Purkinje cells and of the cortical layers in the cerebellum of the albino rat. *J. comp. Neurol.*, 21: 459–488.

Altman, J. (1969) Autoradiographic and histological studies of postnatal neurogenesis III. Dating the time of production and onset of differentiation of cerebellar microneurones in rats. *J. comp. Neurol.*, 136: 269–294.

Altman, J. (1972a) Postnatal development of the cerebellar cortex of the rat. I. The external granular layer and the transitional molecular layer. *J. comp. Neurol.*, 145: 353–398.

Altman, J. (1972b) Postnatal development of the cerebellar cortex in the rat. II. Phases in the maturation of Purkinje cells and of the molecular layer. *J. comp. Neurol.*, 145: 399–464.

Altman, J. (1976) Experimental reorganisation of the cerebellar cortex. V. Effects of early X-irradiation schedules that allow or prevent the acquisition of basket cells. *J. comp. Neurol.*, 165: 31–48.

Altman, J. and Anderson, W.J. (1972) Experimental reorganisation of the cerebellar cortex. I. Morphological effects of elimination of all microneurons with prolonged X-irradiation started at birth. *J. comp. Neurol.*, 146: 355–406.

Altman, J. and Das, G.D. (1970) Postnatal changes in the concentration and distribution of cholinesterase in the cerebellar cortex of rats. *Exp. Neurol.*, 28: 11–34.

Anwar, A. and Berry, M. (1980) Effects of hemispherectomy on Purkinje cell dendritic growth in the rat. *Neurosci. Lett.*, in press.

Berry, M. (1979) Regeneration in the central nervous system. In *Recent Advances in Neuropathology*, W. Thomas Smith and J.B. Cavanagh (Eds.), Churchill Livingstone, Edinburgh, London and New York, pp. 67–111.

Berry, M. and Bradley, P. (1976a) The application of network analysis to the study of branching patterns of large dendritic fields. *Brain Res.*, 109: 111–132.

Berry, M. and Bradley, P. (1976b) The growth of the dendritic trees of Purkinje cells in the cerebellum of the rat. *Brain Res.*, 112: 1–35.

Berry, M. and Bradley, P. (1976c) The growth of Purkinje cells in irradiated agranular cerebellar cortex. *Brain Res.*, 116: 361–387.

Berry, M., Bradley, P. and Borges, S. (1978) Environmental and genetic determinants of connectivity in the central nervous system. An approach through dendritic field analysis. In *Maturation of the Nervous System, Progr. Brain Res. Vol. 48*, M.A. Corner, R.E. Baker, N.E. van de Pol, D.F.

Swaab and H.B.M. Uylings (Eds.), Elsevier/North-Holland Biomedical Press, The Netherlands, pp. 133–148.

Berry, M., McConnell, P. and Sievers, J. (1980a) Dendritic growth and the control of neuronal form. In *Current Topics in Developmental Biology,* R.K. Hunt, A. Monroy and A.A. Moscona (Eds.), Academic Press, New York.

Berry, M., Sievers, J. and Baumgarten, H.G. (1980b) The influence of afferent fibres on the development of the cerebellum. In *A multidisciplinary Approach to Brain Development,* C. Di Benedetta (Ed.) Elsevier/North-Holland Biomedical Press, The Netherlands.

Björklund, A. and Stenevi, V. (1979) Regeneration of monoaminergic and cholinergic neurons in the mammalian central nervous system. *Physiol. Rev.,* 59: 62–100.

Blakemore, C. and Cooper, G.F. (1970) Development of the brain depends on the visual environment. *Nature (Lond),* 228: 477–478.

Bloom, F.E. (1974) The role of cyclic nucleotides in central synaptic function. *Rev. Physiol. Biochem. Pharmacol.,* 74: 1–103.

Bloom, F.E., Hoffer, B.J. and Siggins, G.R. (1971) Studies on norepinephrine-containing afferents to Purkinje cells of rat cerebellum. I. Localization of the fibers and their synapses. *Brain Res.,* 25: 501–521.

Bloom, F.E., Hoffer, B.J., Siggins, G.R., Barker, J.L. and Nicoll, R.A. (1972) Effects of serotonin on central neurons, microiontophoretic administration. *Fed. Proc.,* 31: 97–106.

Bradley, P. and Berry, M. (1976a) The effects of reduced climbing and parallel fibre input on Purkinje cell dendritic growth. *Brain Res.,* 109: 133–151.

Bradley, P. and Berry, M. (1976b) Quantitative effects of climbing fibre deafferentation on the adult Purkinje cell dendritic tree. *Brain Res.,* 112: 133–140.

Bradley, P. and Berry, M. (1978a) The Purkinje cell dendritic tree in mutant mouse cerebellum. A quantitative Golgi study of weaver and staggerer mice. *Brain Res.,* 142: 135–141.

Bradley, P. and Berry, M. (1978b) Quantitative effects of methylazoxy-methanol acetate on Purkinje cell dendritic growth. *Brain Res.,* 143: 499–511.

Bradley, P. and Berry, M. (1979) Effects of thiophene on the Purkinje cell dendritic tree: a quantitative Golgi study. *Neuropath. appl. Neurobiol.,* 5: 9–16.

Cajal, S. Ramon y. (1911) *Histologie du Système Nerveux de l'Homme et des Vertebres,* Malione, Paris.

Cajal, S. Ramon y. (1960) *Studies on Vertebrate Neurogenesis* (translated by L. Guth), Charles C. Thomas, Springfield, Ill.

Calvet, M.C., Lepault, A.M. and Calvet, J. (1976) Procion yellow study of cultured Purkinje cells. *Brain Res.,* 111: 399–406.

Changeux, J.P. and Danchin, A. (1976) Selective stabilisation of developing synapses, a mechanism for the specification of neural networks. *Nature (Lond.),* 264: 705–712.

Chan-Palay, V. (1972) Arrested granule cells and their synapses with mossy fibres in the molecular layer of the cerebellar cortex. *Z. Anat. Entwickl.-Gesch.,* 139: 11–20.

Chan-Palay, V. (1975) Fine structure of labelled axons in the cerebellar cortex and nuclei of rodents and primates after intraventricular infusions with tritiated serotonin. *Anat. Embryol.,* 148: 235–265.

Chan-Palay, V. (1977) *Cerebellar Dentate Nucleus: Organisation, cytology and transmitters,* Springer-Verlag, Berlin.

Chan-Palay, V. and Palay, S.L. (1971a) Tendril and glomerular collaterals of climbing fibres in the granular layer of the rats' cerebellar cortex. *Z. Anat. Entwickl.-Gesch.,* 133: 247–273.

Chan-Palay, V. and Palay, S.L. (1971b) The synapse en marron between Golgi II neurons and mossy fibre in the rats' cerebellar cortex. *Z. Anat. Entwickl.-Gesch.,* 133: 274–289.

Chan-Palay, V., Plaitakis, A., Nicklas, W. and Berl, S. (1977) Autoradiographic demonstration of loss of labelled indoleamine axons of the cerebellum in chronic diet-induced thiamine deficiency. *Brain Res.,* 138: 380–384.

Crépel, F. (1971) Maturation of climbing fiber responses in the rat. *Brain Res.,* 35: 272–276.

Crépel, F., Delhaye-Bouchaud, N. and Legrand, J. (1976) Electrophysiological analysis of the circuitry and of the corticonuclear relationships in the agranular cerebellum of irradiated rats. *Arch. ital. Biol.,* 114: 49–74.

Crépel, F. and Mariani, J. (1976) Multiple innervation of Purkinje cells by climbing fibres in the cerebellum of the weaver mutant mouse. *J. Neurobiol.,* 7: 579–582.

Crépel, F. and Delhaye-Bouchaud, N. (1979) Distribution of climbing fibres on cerebellar Purkinje cells in X-irradiated rats. An electrophysiological study. *J. Physiol. (Lond.),* 290: 97–112.

Delhaye-Bouchaud, N., Mory, G. and Crépel, F. (1978) Differential role of granule cells in the specification of synapses between climbing fibres and cerebellar Purkinje cells in the rat. *Neurosci. Lett.,* 9: 51—58.

Descarries, L. and Saucier, G. (1972) Disappearance of the locus coeruleus in the rat after intraventricular 6-hydroxydopamine. *Brain Res.,* 37: 310—316.

Dreyfus, P.M. and Victor, M. (1961) Effects of thiamine deficiency in the central nervous system. *Amer. J. Clin. Nutr.,* 9: 414—425.

Ebels, E.J. (1972) Studies on ectopic granule cells in the cerebellar cortex with a hypothesis as to their aetiology and pathogenesis. *Acta neuropath. (Berl.),* 21: 117—129.

Eccles, J.C., Ito, M. and Szentagothai, J. (1967) *The Cerebellum as a Neural Machine,* Springer-Verlag, Berlin, Heidelberg, New York.

Garber, B.B. and Moscona, A.A. (1972) Reconstruction of brain tissue from cell suspensions. I. Aggregation patterns of cells dissociated from different regions of the developing brain. *Develop. Biol.,* 27: 235—247.

Hámori, J. (1969) Development of synaptic organisation in the partially agranular and in the trans-neuronally atrophied cerebellar cortex. In *Neurobiology of Cerebellar Evolution and Development,* Llinás, R. (Ed.), Amer. med. Ass., Chicago, Ill., pp. 845—858.

Hámori, J. (1973) The inductive role of presynaptic axons in the development of postsynaptic spines. *Brain Res.,* 62: 337—344.

Herndon, R.M. (1968) Thiophen induced granule cell necrosis in the rat cerebellum. An electron microscopic study. *Exp. Brain Res.,* 6: 49—68.

Hicks, S.P. and D'Amato, C.J. (1970) Motor-sensory and visual behaviour after hemispherectomy in newborn and mature rats. *Exp. Neurol.,* 29: 416—438.

Hoffer, B.J., Siggins, G.R. and Bloom, F.E. (1971) Studies on norepinephrine-containing afferents to Purkinje cells of rat cerebellum. II. Sensitivity of Purkinje cells to norepinephrine and related substances administered by microiontophoresis. *Brain Res.,* 25: 523—534.

Hollingworth, T. and Berry, M. (1975) Network analysis of dendritic fields of pyramidal cells in the neocortex and Purkinje cells in the cerebellum of the rat. *Phil. Trans. B,* 270: 227—262.

Hubel, D.H., Wiesel, T.N. and Le Vay, S. (1977) Plasticity of ocular dominance columns in monkey striate cortex. *Phil. Trans. B,* 278: 377—409.

Kasamatsu, T. and Pettigrew, J.D. (1976) Depletion of brain catecholamines: failure of ocular dominance shift after monocular occlusions in kittens. *Science,* 194: 206—209.

Kasamatsu, T. and Pettigrew, J.D. (1979) Preservation of binocularity after monocular deprivation in the striate cortex of kitten treated with 6-hydroxydopamine. *J. comp. Neurol.,* 185: 139—162.

Kasamatsu, T., Pettigrew, J.D. and Ary, M. (1979) Restoration of visual cortical plasticity by local microperfusion of norepinephrine. *J. comp. Neurol.,* 185: 163—182.

Kawaguchi, S., Yamamota, T., Luzimo, N. and Iwahori, N. (1975) The role of climbing fibres in the development of Purkinje cell dendrites. *Neurosci. Lett.,* 1: 301—304.

Kiernan, J. (1979) Regeneration in the central nervous system. *Biol. Rev.,* 54: 155—197.

Landis, S. (1971) Cerebellar cortical development in the staggerer mutant mouse. *J. Cell Biol.,* 51: 159a.

Landis, S.C. (1973) Granule cell heterotopia in normal and nervous mutant mice of the BALB/C strain. *Brain Res.,* 61: 175—189.

Lauder, J.M. and Krebs, H. (1976) Effects of *p*-chlorophenylalanine on time of neuronal origin during embryogenesis in the rat. *Brain Res.,* 107: 638—644.

Lewis, P.D., Patel, A.J., Bendek, G. and Balázs, R. (1977) Effect of reserpine on cell proliferation in the developing rat brain: a quantitative histological study. *Brain Res.,* 129: 299—308.

Lindvall, O. and Björklund, A. (1978) Organization of catecholamine neurons in the rat central nervous system. In *Handbook of Psychopharmacology, Vol. 9,* L.L. Iversen, S.D. Iversen and S.H. Snyder (Eds.), Plenum Press, Oxford.

Llinás, R., Hillman, D.E. and Precht, W. (1973) Neuronal circuit reorganisation in mammalian agranular cerebellar cortex. *J. Neurobiol.,* 4: 69—94.

Maeda, T., Tohyama, M. and Shimizu, N. (1974) Modification of postnatal development of neocortex in rat brain with experimental deprivation of locus coeruleus. *Brain Res.,* 70: 515—520.

Mallet, J., Huchet, M., Pongeois, R. and Changeux, J.P. (1976) Anatomical, physiological and biochemical studies on the cerebellum from mutant mice. III. Protein differences associated with the weaver, staggerer and nervous mutations. *Brain Res.,* 103: 291—312.

Mariani, J., Crépel, F., Mikoshiba, K., Changeux, J.P. and Sotelo, C. (1977) Anatomical, physiological and biochemical studies of the cerebellum from reeler mutant mouse. *Phil. Trans. B,* 281: 1—28.

McConnell, P. and Berry, M. (1978) The effect of refeeding after neonatal starvation on Purkinje cell dendritic growth in the rat. *J. comp. Neurol.,* 178: 759–772.

McConnell, P. and Berry, M. (1980) The effects of undernutrition on developing Purkinje cells in the cerebellum of the rat, *J. comp. Neurol.,* submitted.

McMahon, D. (1974) Chemical messengers in development: a hypothesis. *Science,* 185: 1012–1021.

Mettler, F.A. and Lubin, A.J. (1942) Termination of the branchium pontis. *J. comp. Neurol.,* 77: 391–397.

Mouren-Mathieu, A.-M. and Colonnier, M. (1969) The molecular layer of the adult cat cerebellar cortex after lesion of the parallel fibres. An optic and electron microscope study. *Brain Res.,* 16: 307–323.

Mugnaini, E. and Dahl, A.-L. (1975) Mode of distribution of aminergic fibres in the cerebellar cortex of the chicken. *J. comp. Neurol.,* 162: 417–432.

Olson, L. and Seiger, A. (1976) Locus coeruleus: fibre growth regulation in oculo. *Med. Biol.,* 54: 142–145.

Palay, S.L. and Chan-Palay, V. (1974) *Cerebellar Cortex. Cytology and Organisation,* Springer-Verlag. Berlin, Heidelberg and New York.

Patel, A.J., Bendek, G., Balázs, R. and Lewis, P.D. (1977) Effect of reserpine on cell proliferation in the developing rat brain: a biochemical study. *Brain Res.,* 129: 283–297.

Pettigrew, J.D. and Kasamatsu, T. (1978) Local perfusion of noradrenaline maintains visual cortical plasticity. *Nature (Lond.),* 271: 761–763.

Pfaffenroth, M.J. and Das, G.D. (1974) Heterotopic cell nests in the developing rat cerebellum. *Acta neuropath. (Berl.),* 30: 1–9.

Plaitakis, A., Nicklas, W.J. and Berl, S. (1977) Selective involvement of the cerebellar serotoninergic system in thiamine deficiency. *Neurology,* 27: 384–385.

Privat, A. (1975) Dendritic growth "in vitro". In *Physiology and Pathology of Dendrites, Advances in Neurology, Vol. 12.* G.W. Kreutzberg (Ed.), Raven Press, New York, pp. 201–216.

Privat, A., Drian, M.J. and Mandon, P. (1973) The outgrowth of rat cerebellum in organised culture. *Z. Zellforsch.,* 146: 45–67.

Privat, A., Drian, M.J. and Mandon, P. (1974) Synaptogenesis in the outgrowth of rat cerebellum in organized culture. *J. comp. Neurol.,* 153: 291–308.

Privat, A. and Drian, M.J. (1975) Specificity of the formation of the mossy fibre–granule cell synapse in the rat cerebellum. An "in vitro" study. *Brain Res.,* 88: 518–524.

Puro, D.G. and Woodward, D.J. (1977) The climbing fibre system in the Weaver mutant. *Brain Res.,* 129: 141–146.

Raisman, G. and Field, P.M. (1973) A quantitative investigation of the development of collateral reinnervation after partial deafferentation of the septal nuclei. *Brain Res.,* 50: 241–264.

Rakic, P. (1976) Synaptic specificity in the cerebellar cortex: study of anomalous circuits induced by single gene mutations in mice. *Cold Spr. Harb. Symp. quant. Biol.,* 40: 333–346.

Rakic, P. (1972) Extrinsic cytological determinants of basket and stellate cell dendritic pattern in the cerebellar molecular layer. *J. comp. Neurol.,* 146: 335–354.

Rakic, P. and Sidman, R.L. (1973a) Sequence of developmental abnormalities leading to granule cell deficit in cerebellar cortex of weaver mutant mice. *J. comp. Neurol.* 152: 103–132.

Rakic, P. and Sidman, R.L. (1973b) Organisation of cerebellar cortex secondary to deficit of granule cells in weaver mutant mice. *J. comp. Neurol.,* 152: 133–162.

Rezai, Z. and Yoon, C.H. (1972) Abnormal rate of granule cell migration in the cerebellum of "weaver" mutant mice. *Develop. Biol.,* 29: 17–26.

Rosenzweig, M.R., Krech, D., Bennett, E.L. and Diamond, M.C. (1962) Effects of environmental complexity and training on brain chemistry and anatomy. A replication and extension. *J. comp. physiol. Psychol.,* 55: 529–537.

Sachs, Ch. and Jonsson, G. (1975) Effects of 6-hydroxydopamine on central noradrenaline neurons during ontogeny. *Brain Res.,* 99: 277–291.

Schlumpf, M., Shoemaker, W.J. and Bloom, F.E. (1977) The development of catecholamine fibers in the prenatal cerebellar cortex of the rat. *Neurosci. Abstr.,* III: 361.

Schmidt, R.H. and Bhatnagar, R.K. (1979a) Distribution of hypertrophied locus coeruleus projections to adult cerebellum after neonatal 6-hydroxydopamine. *Brain Res.,* 172: 23–33.

Schmidt, R.H. and Bhatnagar, R.K. (1979b) Regional development of norepinephrine dopamine-β-hydroxylase and tyrosine hydroxylase in the rat brain subsequent to neonatal treatment with subcutaneous 6-hydroxydopamine. *Brain Res.,* 166: 293–308.

Schmidt, R.H., Hasik, S.A. and Bhatnagar, R.K. (1979) Regenerative critical periods for locus coeruleus in postnatal rat pups following intracisternal 6-hydroxydopamine: a model of noradrenergic development. *Brain Res.*, in press.

Seiger, A. and Olson, L. (1973) Late prenatal ontogeny of central monoamine neurons in the rat: fluorescence histochemical observations. *Z. Anat. Entwickl.-Gesch.*, 140: 281–318.

Seiger, A. and Olson, L. (1977) Reinitiation of directed nerve fibre growth in central monoamine neurons after intraocular maturation. *Exp. Brain Res.*, 29: 15–44.

Sidman, R.L. (1968) Development of interneuronal connections in brain of mutant mice. In *Physiological and Biochemical Aspects of Nervous Integration*, F.D. Carlson (Ed.), Prentice-Hall, Englewood Cliffs, N.J., pp. 163–193.

Sidman, R.L. (1972) Cell interactions in developing mammalian central nervous system. In *Proceedings of the 3rd Lepetit Colloquium*, L.G. Silvestri (Ed.), North-Holland, Amsterdam, pp. 1–13.

Sidman, R.L. (1974) Contact interaction among developing mammalian brain cells. In *The Cell Surface in Development*, A.A. Moscona (Ed.), J. Wiley, New York, pp. 221–253.

Sidman, R.L., Green, M.C. and Appel, S.H. (1965) *Catalog of the Neurological Mutants of the Mouse*, Harvard University Press, Cambridge.

Sievers, J., Klemm, H.P., Jenner, S., Baumgarten, H.G. and Berry, M. (1980a) Neuronal and extraneuronal effects of intracisternally administered 6-OHDA on the developing rat brain. *J. Neurochem.*, in press.

Sievers, R., Sievers, H. and Klemm, H.P. (1980b) Beitrage zur pranatalen Entwicklung des Locus coeruleus. *Verh. Anat. Ges.*, in press.

Siggins, G.R., Hoffer, B.J. and Bloom, F.E. (1971) Studies on norepinephrine-containing afferents to Purkinje cells of rat cerebellum. III. Evidence for mediation of norepinephrine effects by cyclic 3′,5′-adenosine monophosphate. *Brain Res.*, 25: 535–553.

Snider, R.S. (1936) Alterations which occur in mossy terminals of the cerebellum following transection of the branchium pontis. *J. comp. Neurol.*, 64: 417–435.

Sotelo, C. (1973) Permanence and fate of paramembranous synaptic specializations in "mutants" and experimental animals. *Brain Res.*, 62: 345–351.

Sotelo, C. (1975) Anatomical, physiological and biochemical studies of the cerebellum from mutant mice II. Morphological study of cerebellar cortical neurons and circuits in the Weaver mouse. *Brain Res.*, 94: 19–44.

Sotelo, C. and Arsenio-Nunes, L. (1976) Development of Purkinje cells in absence of climbing fibres. *Brain Res.*, 111: 389–395.

Sotelo, C. and Changeux, J.P. (1974) Transsynaptic degeneration "en cascade" in the cerebellar cortex of Staggerer mutant mice. *Brain Res.*, 67: 519–526.

Sotelo, C., Hillman, D.E., Zamora, A.J. and Llinás, R. (1975) Climbing fiber deafferentation: its action on Purkinje cell dendritic spines. *Brain Res.*, 98: 574–581.

Sosa, J.M., Palacios, E. and de Sosa, H.M. (1971) Heterotopic cerebellar granule cells inside the plexiform layer. *Acta anat.* 80: 91–98.

Špaček, J., Pařízek, J. and Lieberman, A.R. (1973) Golgi cells, granule cells and synaptic glomeruli in the molecular layer of the rabbit cerebellar cortex. *J. Neurocytol.*, 2: 407–428.

Stoughton, R.L., del Cerro, M., Walker, J.R. and Jeffrey, R. (1978) Presence of displaced neural elements within rat cerebellar fissures. *Brain Res.*, 148: 15–29.

Weiss, G.M. and Pysh, J.J. (1978) Evidence for loss of Purkinje cell dendrites during late development: a morphometric Golgi analysis in the mouse. *Brain Res.*, 154: 219–230.

Wendlandt, S., Crow, T.J. and Stirling, R.V. (1977) The involvement of the noradrenergic system arising from the locus coeruleus in the postnatal development of the cortex in rat brain. *Brain Res.*, 125: 1–9.

Woodward, D.J., Hoffer, B.J. and Altman, J. (1974) Physiological and pharmacological properties of Purkinje cells in rat cerebellum degranulated by postnatal X-irradiation. *J. Neurobiol.*, 5: 283–304.

Yoon, C.H. (1976) Pleiotropic effect of the Staggerer gene. *Brain Res.*, 109: 206–215.

Nutrition and Central Nervous System Development

MYRON WINICK

The Institute of Human Nutrition, Columbia University College of Physicians and Surgeons, New York, N.Y., U.S.A.

STRUCTURAL AND BIOCHEMICAL EFFECTS OF MALNUTRITION

During the past two decades evidence from a variety of sources has accumulated which demonstrates that severe early malnutrition can affect both brain structure and brain function. In the late 1950s, Widdowson and McCance demonstrated the importance of the time of the insult in determining subsequent outcome. They showed that rats malnourished from birth to weaning had smaller brains and that the size deficit persisted into adulthood no matter how they were re-fed. By contrast, animals malnourished after weaning showed smaller brains at the end of the period of malnutrition, but on re-feeding brain weight returned to normal (Widdowson and McCance, 1960). Subsequent studies have clarified the reason for the different responses. Brain growth is characterized by a series of cellular changes which take place in a sequential pattern. Early growth occurs primarily by repeated cell division as characterized by a linear increase in total organ DNA. Cell size as determined by weight/DNA ratio or protein/DNA ratio remains relatively constant (Enesco and LeBlond, 1962). The earliest growth in mammalian mrain is accompanied by proliferation of neurons. In the human this reaches a peak at about 26 weeks gestation (Dobbing and Sands, 1973). Later it is glial proliferation that predominates, reaching a peak around birth (Dobbing and Sands, 1973). The postnatal period in the human is characterized by a continuation in the proliferation of cells at a slower rate. Since net protein synthesis continues at the previous rate, the protein/DNA ratio (cell size) begins to increase. At about 18 months of age, cell division virtually stops in human brain (Winick, 1968), protein and lipids continue to be deposited and this results in growth which is entirely by increase in cell size. Thus 3 distinct periods can be described in the growing human brain: *hyperplasia* – during intrauterine life; *hyperplasia and hypertrophy* – birth to about 18 months; and *hypertrophy* – 18 months to beyond 3 years. These periods show considerable overlap and vary in their timing from one region to another.

In animals, malnutrition occurring during the period of rapid cell division (hyperplasia) results in a retardation in the overall rate of cell division, and hence ultimately results in fewer cells (Winick and Noble, 1966). This change is permanent. By contrast, malnutrition occurring during the period of hypertrophic growth results in curtailment of cell enlargement, a process which is reversible as soon as rehabilitation is instituted (Winick and Noble, 1966). Data from analysis of brains of children who died of malnutrition during the first year of life demonstrate a reduced number of cells (Winick and Rosso, 1969). Thus in the human, severe early undernutrition curtails cell division and results in fewer cells. From animal studies it must be inferred that this change is permanent.

In rats the hyperplastic phase is most pronounced in cerebellum postnatally and cell division stops earliest in this region. In cerebrum cell number increases more slowly but continues to increase for a longer period of time. In addition, whereas cerebral cellular increase is entirely glial, both glia and neurones are dividing postnatally in cerebellum (Winick, 1970). Malnutrition imposed at birth curtails the rate of cell division more profoundly in those areas exhibiting the most rapid rate of proliferation and impedes cell division in any type of cell that is dividing (Winick, 1970). Thus, because different cell types in different regions divide at different rates at any given time, early malnutrition may result in specific qualitative changes as well as general quantitative changes. These qualitative changes are the result of alterations in the neuronal/glial ratio in different regions.

In the human, regional patterns of cell division have not been worked out as precisely as in the rat and, because of the inability to employ radioautography, the types of cells dividing at any given time can only be inferred. However, from the data available, it appears that cell division virtually ceases in cerebrum, cerebellum and brain stem at about 18 months postnatally (Winick, Rosso and Waterlow, 1970). Malnutrition during the first year of life appears to reduce cell number in all 3 of these areas (Winick et al., 1970).

Malnutrition early in life has not only been shown to curtail cell division in brain but has also been shown to impede myelination (Davison and Dobbing, 1966). The deposition of lipids into myelin is slowed down and, since myelin turnover is relatively slow, the actual quantity of myelin in both rat (Chase, Dorsey and McKhann, 1967) and human (Rosso, Hormazabal and Winick, 1970) brain is reduced. In addition, the extent of dendritic arborization is found to be reduced in both rat and human brain and this reduction appears relatively greater than the reduction in either cell number or myelin content (Sima, 1974). Recent data demonstrate that the concentration of n-acetyl-neurominic acid (NANA) within the gangliosides is markedly reduced in rat cerebrum and cerebellum as a result of early malnutrition (Morgan and Winick, 1979).

Thus, reduction in protein-calorie intake during early brain growth will cause major structural and biochemical changes in the brain, many of which will persist into adult life.

While many studies have been done to examine general undernutrition, relatively few studies have attempted to document the changes induced by specific nutrient deficiencies. In recent years, because of the use of fat-free solutions for long-term parenteral nutrition in young infants, a number of investigators have examined the effect of essential fatty acid (EFA) deficiency on the developing brain. In rats, a fat-free diet from birth results in the deposition of myelin with an increased triene/tetraene ratio (Galli, 1973). In puppies, total parenteral nutrition from birth, using identical solutions to those generally employed in low birth weight infants, results in the deposition of a similarly abnormal myelin (Heird, personal communication). Moreover, this "abnormal" myelin is formed in large quantities only if caloric intake is adequate, suggesting that rapid growth must be maintained in order for the abnormality to manifest itself.

BEHAVIOURAL EFFECTS OF MALNUTRITION

At the same time that investigations like those described above, which were examining the effects of early malnutrition on brain structure were being conducted, other investigators were examining the effects of early undernutrition on brain function. By the early 1970s it became clear in both animals and children that, although malnutrition played an extremely important part in the complex of social deprivation leading to permanent changes in behaviour, it did not, *in itself,* induce severe permanent behavioural changes. Both the nutritional and the environmental components were important in determining outcome. These conclusions were reached only after a series of careful animal experiments indicated that even severely malnourished animals reared in a "stimulating" environment did not show behavioural abnormalities. Levitsky and Barnes in the United States (Levitsky and Barnes, 1972) and Frankova in Czechoslovakia (Frankova, 1974) demonstrated that environmental stimulation, either by repeated handling of the pups or by introducing a virgin female rat trained to care for rat pups into the cage with the mother and pups, could prevent the expected behavioural effects of early malnutrition. Moreover, these methods were at least partially effective even if the stimulation was introduced *after* the malnutrition had been going on for some time.

In humans, observations also suggested a complex relationship between early malnutrition, early environmental and subsequent mental development. While it was quite clear by the middle of the 1960's that children reared in poverty and malnutrition in developing countries showed retarded mental development, it was not clear to what extent the retardation could be attributed to malnutrition, and to what extent to environmental deprivation. In an important study carried out in Jamaica using, as controls, siblings who were not previously malnourished, Birch and his colleagues demonstrated that both early nutrition and early environment were important determinants of subsequent behaviour. In addition, they showed that not only were IQ and school performance affected by this complex but that social behaviour was also adversely affected (Hertzig, Birch, Richardson and Tizard, 1972).

In the early 1970s studies in children with cystic fibrosis who were severely malnourished during the first year of life but who were reared in an "enriched" environment revealed no evidence of retarded development by the time these children were 5 years old (Lloyd-Still, Wolff, Horwitz and Shwachman, 1975). These studies suggested that in the human, as in the rat, the expected effects of early malnutrition could be prevented if an "enriched" environment were supplied.

Two recent studies have demonstrated that such an "enriched" environment can prevent the behavioural changes that usually occur in malnourished children in developing countries. Korean orphans malnourished during the first year of life were compared with similar well-nourished orphans. All of the children were adopted into middle class U.S. families before they were 3 years old. The average IQ of the previously malnourished children, measured between ages 6 and 12, was 102. By contrast, the previously well-nourished children averaged 112, and the difference was statistically significant. Similar results were obtained when school performance was examined. The previously malnourished children performed at stanine 5 (equal to the U.S. norm) whereas the well-nourished children performed at about 6 (well above the U.S. norm) (Winick, Meyer and Harris, 1975). From these studies we have inferred that early environmental enrichment will increase IQ and school performance regardless of previous nutritional condition. However, the gap between previously malnourished and previously well-nourished children can be considerably narrowed by enriching the environment. Whether or not this gap will completely disappear with more time is not known. A second study, using the same experimental design but now examining children adopted between ages 3 and 5, revealed a drop in both IQ and school performance in both groups, with the difference between the previously malnourished and well-nourished children widening, and the malnourished children now doing significantly worse than the U.S. norms (Nguyzn, Meyer and Winick, 1977). Thus it would appear that the time of introduction of environmental stimulation is important in determining the extent of recovery. The earlier such intervention is introduced the more complete the recovery.

A recent study of black children from poor environments in the U.S. who were placed in foster care has suggested that an interaction between an "unstable" environment and early malnutrition may lead to retarded development, and that previously well-nourished children in an "unstable" environment or previously malnourished children in a stable environment do better than previously malnourished children in an "unstable" environment (Winick, Jaroslow and Winer, 1978).

Thus, the data from children both from developing and industrial countries suggest that early environment interacts with early nutrition and that it is the combination of poor environmental conditions and early malnutrition which leads to permanent behavioural changes. In addition, changing the environment even after a period of early nutritional deprivation can result in significant improvement.

BIOCHEMICAL MECHANISMS UNDERLYING BEHAVIOURAL CHANGES

Although just beginning, a final group of experiments deserve mention: these are studies aimed at defining the biochemical abnormalities responsible for the behavioural changes induced by malnutrition and early social deprivation.

As previously mentioned, a number of changes in brain chemistry occur with early malnutrition. Some of these changes also occur in animals subjected to early environmental deprivation, while others do not. One of the changes which occurs in both conditions is a reduced concentration of NANA. Moreover, the concentration of NANA in gangliosides increases when an enriched environment is supplied. In addition, environmental stimulation prevents the expected decrease in NANA concentration induced by early malnutrition. Finally, injection of NANA into malnourished animals results in incorporation of the injected NANA into brain gangliosides, and prevention of the subsequent abnormal behaviour (Morgan and Winick, 1979). Thus a specific substance (NANA) known to be reduced in the brains of both malnourished and environmentally deprived animals, can be increased by environmental enrichment or, if supplied exogenously to malnourished animals, can be incorporated into gangliosides and affect behaviour in a manner similar to environmental enrichment. These studies suggest for the first time a cause and effect relationship. Elucidation of the nature of this relationship may be one of the most exciting developments in the 1980s in the area of early malnutrition and brain development.

In summary, early malnutrition can retard structural and biochemical development of the brain. At least one biochemical change, reduced n-acetyl-neurominic acid (NANA) content of brain gangliosides, does not occur if an enriched environment is supplied concomitantly with early malnutrition. Behavioural changes are also prevented under these conditions. Simply supplying this compound exogenously, increases its incorporation into gangliosides and prevents the behavioural changes which usually accompany early malnutrition. We are suggesting the possibility of a cause and effect relationship between the concentration of ganglioside NANA and the behavioural abnormalities induced by both malnutrition and early environmental deprivation. We postulate that the final common pathway in both these conditions is a lowering of cerebral ganglioside NANA concentration. We further speculate that because of the similarity between the effects of early malnutrition and early environmental deprivation in the human infant and those in the infant rat, a similar final common pathway may exist.

REFERENCES

Chase, H.P., Dorsey, J. and McKhann, G.M. (1967) The effect of malnutrition on the synthesis of a myelin lipid. *Pediatrics,* 40: 551–559.

Davison, A.N. and Dobbing, J. (1966) Myelination as a vulnerable period in brain development. *Brit. Med. Bull.,* 22: 40–44.

Dobbing, J. and Sands, J. (1973) Quantitative growth and development of human brain. *Arch. Dis. Childh.,* 48: 757–767.

Enesco, M. and Le Blond, C.P. (1962) Increase in cell number as a factor in the growth of the organs of the young rat. *J. Embryol. exp. Morph.,* 10: 530–534.

Frankova, S. (1974) Interaction between early malnutrition and stimulation in animals. In *Symposia of the Swedish Nutrition Foundation XII, Early Malnutrition and Mental Development,* J. Cravioto, L. Hambraeus and B. Vahlquist (Eds.), Almqvist and Wiksell, Uppsala, pp. 202–210.

Galli, C. (1973) Dietary lipids in brain development. In *Dietary Lipids in Postnatal Development,* C. Galli, C. Jacini and Pecile, A. (Eds.), Raven Press, New York, pp. 191–202.

Hertzig, M.E., Birch, H.G., Richardson, S.A. and Tizard, J. (1972) Intellectual levels of school children severely malnourished during the first two years of life. *Pediatrics,* 49: 814–824.

Levitsky, D.A. and Barnes, R.H. (1972) Nutritional and environmental interactions in the behavioural development of the rat: long term effects. *Science,* 176: 68–71.

Lloyd-Still, J.D., Wolff, P.H., Horwitz, I. and Scwachman, H. (1975) Studies on intellectual development after severe malnutrition in infancy in cystic fibrosis and other intestinal lesions, *Proc. IX International Congress of Nutrition, Mexico, Vol. 2,* A. Chavez, H. Bourges and S. Basta (Eds.), S. Karger, Basel, p. 357.

Morgan, B. and Winick, M. (1979) A possible relationship between brain n-acetylneuraminic acid content and behavior. *Proc. Soc. exp. Biol. Med.,* 161: 534–537.

Nguyzn, M.L., Meyer, K.K. and Winick, M. (1977) Early malnutrition and "late" adoption: a study of their effects on the development of Korean orphans adopted into American families. *Amer. J. clin. Nutr.,* 30: 1734–1739.

Rosso, P., Hormazabal, J. and Winick, M. (1970) Changes in brain weight, cholesterol, phospholipid and DNA content in marasmic children. *Amer. J. clin. Nutr.,* 23: 1275–1279.

Sima, A. (1974) Studies on fibre size in developing sciatic nerve and spinal roots in normal, undernourished and rehabilitated rats. *Acta physiol. scand.* (Suppl.), 406: 1–55.

Widdowson, E.M. and McCance, R.A. (1960) Some effects of accelerating growth, I. General somatic development. *Proc. Roy. Soc. B,* 152: 88–206.

Winick, M. (1968) Changes in nucleic acid and protein content of human brain during growth. *Pediat. Res.* 2: 325–355.

Winick, M. (1970) Nutrition and nerve cell growth. *Fed. Proc.* 29: 1510–1515.

Winick, M., Jaroslow, A. and Winer, F. (1978) Foster placement, malnutrition and environment. *Growth,* 42: 391–397.

Winick, M., Meyer, K. and Harris, R. (1975) Malnutrition and environmental enrichment by early adoption. *Science,* 190: 1173–1175.

Winick, M. and Noble, A. (1966) Cellular response in rats during malnutrition at various ages. *J. Nutr.* 89: 300–304.

Winick, M. and Rosso, P. (1969) The effect of severe early malnutrition on cellular growth of human brain. *Pediat. Res.,* 3: 181–184.

Winick, M., Rosso, P. and Waterlow, J.C. (1970) Cellular growth of cerebrum, cerebellum and brain stem in normal and marasmic children. *Exp. Neurol.,* 26: 393–400.

Nutritional Effects on Non-Mitotic Aspects of Central Nervous System Development

P. McCONNELL

Netherlands Institute for Brain Research, IJdijk 28, 1095 KJ Amsterdam, The Netherlands

INTRODUCTION – VULNERABILITY TO UNDERNUTRITION

Of prime importance when considering the effects of nutritional deprivation on the development of the central nervous system (CNS) is the question of permanence. Are the sequelae of undernutrition immutable, or can they be reversed by subsequent nutritional rehabilitation?

In a series of articles, Dobbing and co-workers (Dobbing, 1968a and b; 1970a and b; 1971a and b; 1972; 1974a and b; Dobbing and Sands, 1971; Dobbing and Smart, 1973; 1974) have elaborated the hypothesis that there exists a finite period during the development of the brain when interference with its rate of growth produces a permanent deficit of growth attainment, resulting in structural distortions. They suggest that each individual event taking place during CNS development is most vulnerable when occurring at its maximum rate. Thus, the period of maximal vulnerability for the brain as a whole is thought to coincide with the so-called "brain growth spurt" (Dobbing, 1968b), the period when the majority of developmental events show their peak rate of change.

The proposition that a transient period of vulnerability exists during CNS development receives support from the results of Dobbing's own experiments (cited above) and from those of a large number of other studies of the long-term effects of undernutrition of rats during their neonatal "brain growth spurt" (review by Dodge, Prensky and Feigin, 1975; Shoemaker and Bloom, 1977, Balázs, Lewis and Patel, 1979). There is some controversy, however, as to the exact timing of the period of maximum vulnerability and, thus, some uncertainty as to which aspects of brain development are most likely to be permanently impaired. As stated above, Dobbing and his co-workers consider that the vulnerable period encompasses the whole of the "brain growth spurt", while a second hypothesis (Winick and Noble, 1966; Winick, this volume) proposes that it is solely the period of cell division, occupying the first half of the growth spurt, which is vulnerable. These latter workers studied the effects of undernutrition at various ages on the development of a variety of tissues in the rat, and concluded that permanent retardation of growth only ensues when cell number is reduced, since the latter cannot be restored unless nutritional supplementation is begun when cell division is still underway. Effects on cell size, on the other hand, can be reversed by re-feeding.

Whilst recognizing the value of Winick's hypothesis when applied to a wide range of body tissues, Dobbing and his colleagues have questioned its relevance to the impairment of brain development resulting from growth restriction (Dobbing, 1970a; 1971a; 1972; 1974;

Dobbing and Smart, 1973). They suggest that non-mitotic events, such as myelin synthesis, the growth of neuronal processes and the establishment of synaptic connections, which contribute to the hypertrophic phase of brain growth, may also be vulnerable.

Surprisingly, despite numerous suggestions that the impairment of non-mitotic events, particularly those involved in the establishment of connections between neurons, may have a direct bearing on the subsequent functioning of the brain (e.g. Cragg, 1972; Dobbing, 1972; 1973; Dobbing and Smart, 1973; Huttenlocher, 1974; 1975; Marin-Padilla, 1974; Jones, 1976), there is little evidence to either support or deny Dobbing's proposition. For example, whilst it is true that undernutrition during the "growth spurt" produces a permanent deficit in brain myelin (Dobbing, 1964; Culley and Lineberger, 1968; Dobbing, 1968b; Guthrie and Brown, 1968; Bass, Netsky and Young, 1970; Bass, 1971; Dobbing and Sands, 1971), a number of workers have suggested that such myelin deficits, both in the CNS (Bass et al., 1970; Dobbing, 1970a; Fox, Fishman, Dodge and Prensky, 1972) and in the peripheral nervous system (Hedley-Whyte and Meuser, 1971; Wood, 1973) may be attributable to a persistent numerical glial cell deficit, rather than to the impairment of myelin synthesis per se. Studies by Chase, Dorsey and McKhann (1967) and by Wiggins, Benjamins, Krigman and Morell (1974), however, have shown that the production of myelin-specific lipids and proteins is depressed during undernutrition, and that the resulting lipid deficit, at least, is irreversible (Chase et al., 1967). Lipid synthetic processes might, then, be permanently affected by undernutrition, although the data again refer to whole brain lipid content and it may be that the amount per glial cell remains normal.

DENDRITIC AND SYNAPTIC EFFECTS OF UNDERNUTRITION

The effects of undernutrition on the establishment of neuronal connections have been far less widely studied than effects on other non-mitotic developmental events. However, with recent advances in stereology (see for example, Underwood, 1970; Williams, 1977; Thomas, Bedi, Davies and Dobbing, 1979) and the advent of computer-aided methods of quantitative neuroanatomical analysis (e.g. Berry, Hollingworth, Anderson and Flinn, 1975; Berry and Bradley, 1976a; Lindsay, 1977; Overdijk, Uylings, Kuypers and Kamstra, 1978), it is now possible to obtain a precise assessment of the way in which dendritic and synaptic development is influenced by nutritional restriction. For example, it has recently been shown that undernutrition of both the rat (Griffin, Woodward and Chanda, 1977; McConnell and Berry, 1978a, 1979a) and the mouse (Pysh, Perkins and Singer-Beck, 1979) during the neonatal "brain growth spurt" produces marked abnormalities in the dendritic development of cerebellar Purkinje cells (PCs; Fig. 1). Rat pups, undernourished from birth until 30 days post-partum (dpp), showed alterations in the branching pattern of their dendritic trees and a deficit in overall length, resulting partly from a reduction in dendritic segment number and partly from a decrease in individual segment lengths, affecting the outermost segments of the tree (McConnell and Berry, 1978a). Similar results were obtained for a number of these parameters studied in 35-day-old, neonatally undernourished mice (Pysh et al., 1979).

With the exception of the alterations in topology, all of the dendritic alterations observed in undernourished rats followed a similar, age-related pattern of development, as illustrated in Fig. 2 (McConnell and Berry, 1979a). At 10 dpp there were no quantitative differences between control and undernourished cells, by 15 dpp small, though statistically insignificant, reductions in the various parameters were apparent, and these deficits increased so as to

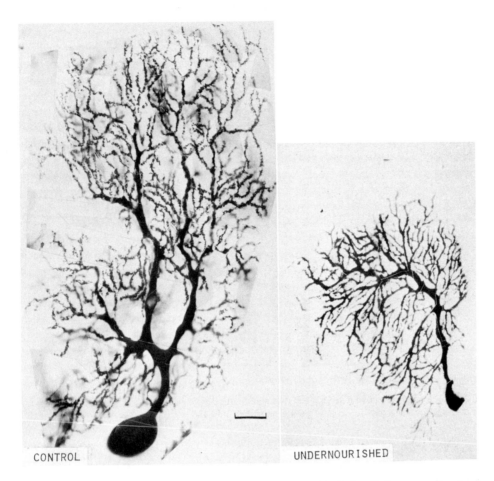

Fig. 1. Photomicrographs of representative Golgi–Cox impregnated Purkinje cells from control and under-nourished animals at 30 dpp. Magnification marker bar = 20 μm.

attain statistical significance in the 20- and 30-day animals.

This observation appears to support Dobbing's (1968a) suggestion that the individual processes occurring during brain development are most affected by nutritional insult when their rate of growth is maximal. The morphological abnormalities detected in under-nourished PCs by McConnell and Berry (1979a) showed their greatest increase in magnitude between 15 and 20 dpp, when the development of normal cells was most rapid (Fig. 2). Dobbing's further suggestion that such dendritic alterations would be irreversible, was investigated in a subsequent experiment.

Male rats, undernourished from birth until 30 dpp, were given ad libitum food supplies until 80 dpp (group R30) when their PCs were compared with those of 80-day animals given food ad libitum from birth (McConnell and Berry, 1978b). Qualitatively, there appeared to be little difference between the two groups of cells (Fig. 3). However, quantitative analysis revealed that, although some restoration of individual segment lengths occurred in the R30 group during the re-feeding period, there was no new segment production. The cells thus showed persistent deficits in total dendritic length and segment frequency, and the topology of the networks remained abnormal.

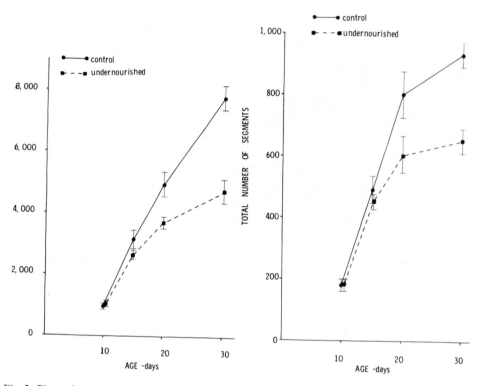

Fig. 2. Plots of total dendritic length and segment frequency (mean ± S.E.) against age for control and undernourished animals.

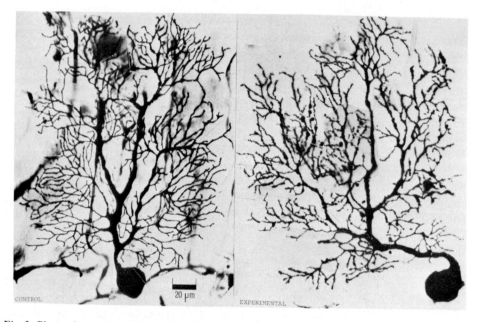

Fig. 3. Photomicrographs of Golgi–Cox impregnated Purkinje cells from an 80-day control animal and an 80-day animal re-fed after 30 days of neonatal undernutrition (= experimental; from McConnell and Berry, 1978b).

Superficially, then, the results appear to support Dobbing's hypothesis that the non-mitotic components of the brain growth spurt may be permanently impaired by under-nutrition. However, the observed dendritic abnormalities appear to be a manifestation of a number of interrelated changes. There is much evidence (Berry and Bradley, 1976b; Bradley and Berry, 1976; 1978a, b; Berry, Sievers and Baumgarten, this volume) that the extent of PC dendritic growth is influenced by the frequency of cerebellar parallel fibres (PFs) in the vicinity of the growing dendritic terminals. Indeed, in the normally developing cerebellum, a direct correlation has been observed between the deposition of PFs (as measured by cerebellar granule cell (GC) counts) and the formation of dendritic segments (McConnell and Berry, 1979a). This correlation was found to be maintained in undernourished animals. Thus, as several workers have suggested (Griffin et al., 1977; McConnell and Berry, 1978a; 1979a; Pysh et al., 1979), at least some of the PC dendritic field changes seen in under-nourished animals may be secondary to the deleterious effects of nutritional restriction on GC acquisition (Lewis, Balázs, Patel and Johnson, 1975; Lewis, 1975). Accordingly, the persistence of abnormal dendritic morphology in animals re-fed from 30 dpp may have been due, not to the absence of dendritic growth capabilities per se, but to the inability to restore this causative GC deficit in the absence of the external granular layer, which has dispersed by 30 dpp both in starved and in control animals (Rebière and Legrand, 1972; Lewis et al., 1975; Gopinath, Bijlani and Deo, 1976).

A study in which re-feeding was begun at various ages prior to the dispersion of the external granular layer supports this latter proposal (McConnell and Berry, 1979b). Eighty-day-old rats, re-fed after neonatal undernutrition to either 10 or 15 dpp, were found to be identical to controls both in dendritic length and segment frequency, and also in the number of GCs per PC. Thus, the deficits seen in these parameters in 15-day undernourished animals (McConnell and Berry, 1979a) could be fully restored by re-feeding from this age. Re-feeding after undernutrition to 20 dpp, on the other hand, failed to restore these parameters to normal. At 80 dpp, the latter animals showed deficits of 21.9% and 19.4% in dendritic length and segment frequency, respectively, together with a 21.1% reduction in the GC : PC ratio. These results, taken together with the observation that even animals re-fed from 30 dpp show a certain amount of dendritic growth during re-feeding, and the accumulating evidence of dendritic plasticity in the adult brain (see, for example, Rutledge, Wright and Duncan, 1974; McConnell and Berry, 1978b; Uylings, Kuypers and Veltman, 1978; Uylings, Kuypers, Diamond and Veltman, 1978; Weiss and Pysh, 1978; Greenough, Juraska and Volkmar, 1979), argue against the possibilities that the differing degrees of PC recovery recorded in the various re-fed groups are due to either: (i) a failure of re-feeding to restore metabolic damage caused by the longer periods of undernutrition: or (ii) the existence of a "once only" opportunity for dendritic growth. On the contrary, the results suggest that the restoration of PC dendritic morphology is related to the magnitude of PF replenishment achieved by re-feeding.

It is difficult to know, then, whether the observation that the growth of PC dendritic processes is apparently irreversibly impaired by undernutrition throughout the "growth spurt", can be extrapolated to other regions of the brain, as Dobbing's (1970a) hypothesis suggests. For example, whereas in the cerebellum, Purkinje cell dendritic growth coincides temporally with the production of granule cells, the production of the future afferent neurons to the cerebral cortex is completed prior to the occurrence of dendritic elaboration in this region (Eayrs and Goodhead, 1959; Altman and Das, 1966, Parnavelas, Bradford, Mounty and Lieberman, 1978). Thus, unless undernutrition causes the death of some of these already differentiated afferent neurons, any alterations in cerebral dendritic development are more likely to be due to metabolic lesions, affecting dendritic outgrowth either directly or as a result of disturbances in the afferent axon field. A priori, then, there seem to be more grounds for optimism that such growth deficiencies would be reversible.

Experimental studies of the effects of undernutrition on cortical dendrites have been concerned chiefly with the pyramidal neurons of frontal (Salas, Díaz and Nieto, 1973), occipital (Salas et al., 1974; Coredero, Díaz and Araya, 1976; West and Kemper, 1976) and somatosensory cortex (Angulo-Colmenares, Vaughan and Hinds, 1979). Deficits have been found in the number of basilar dendritic processes (Salas et al., 1974; Cordero et al., 1976), in dendritic thickness (Salas et al., 1974; West and Kemper, 1976; Angulo-Colmenares et al., 1979) and in the number of spines (Salas et al., 1974; West and Kemper, 1976). All of the studies which have been performed to date are incomplete, however, since there have been no systematic attempts to measure dendritic length and density, or to study the topology of the arborizations. Furthermore, only in the study by Angulo-Colmenares et al. (1979) was an attempt made to determine whether the deficits produced by undernutrition could be reversed by refeeding. In this experiment, deficits in basal dendritic thickness seen in mal-nourished rat pups at 20 dpp were restored by subsequent re-feeding to 40 dpp. Whether the cerebral dendritic trees of re-fed animals are normal in all other respects remains to be determined; such a study is at present underway in this laboratory.

Data concerning the permanence of nutritional effects on synaptic development are also scarce. Quantitative electron microscopic studies have detected deficits in the size (Gam-betti, Autilio-Gambetti, Rizzuto, Shafer and Pfaff, 1974) and numerical density (Gambetti et al., 1974; Dyson and Jones, 1976; Thomas et al., 1979) of presynaptic terminals in vari-ous regions of the cerebral cortex of undernourished rats, as well as deficits in mean number of synapses associated with each neuron (Cragg, 1972; Thomas et al., 1979). Only in two studies have the effects of subsequent nutrition rehabilitation been determined but, here again, the results indicate some "catch-up" of the various parameters during rehabilitation. For example, Dyson and Jones (1976) found that rehabilitation of undernourished rats from 35 dpp until 16 weeks eliminated the previously observed deficit in synaptic density and partially rectified the immaturity of undernourished synaptic junctions (Jones and Dyson, 1976), whilst Bedi (1979) found that the 37% deficit in synapse-to-neuron ratio seen in the frontal cortex of 30-day-old undernourished rats was completely restored if these animals were rehabilitated over a period of 5 months.

CONCLUSION

There have been relatively few attempts to determine whether or not the non-mitotic events contributing to the "brain growth spurt" are vulnerable to undernutrition. However, the available results suggest that the proposal that these events "may be vulnerable, simply because they are occurring rapidly at such a time" (Dobbing, 1970a) is perhaps too naïve an interpretation of the way in which the developing brain is influenced by undernutrition. Although the functional consequences of the recovery of dendritic and synaptic deficiencies in the cerebral cortices of previously undernourished animals remain unknown, from a morphological standpoint the hypothesis is untenable. On the other hand, Winick and Noble's (1966) general proposal that nutritional reduction of cell size can be reversed by re-feeding, also fails to account for the observed experimental results. Such recovery does not occur in the case of the PC dendritic tree. Indeed, Winick himself now appears to sup-port the concept that non-mitotic processes may also be vulnerable to undernutrition, since he suggests, in the preceding paper of this volume, that the apparently irreversible behavioural abnormalities associated with early undernutrition in the rat may be the result of alterations (presumably also permanent) in the concentration of the NANA (n-acetyl-neurominic acid) component of brain gangliosides.

Clearly much work remains to be done before a general conclusion can be reached concerning the nutritional vulnerability of the non-mitotic aspects of CNS development. Indeed, the conflicting nature of the preliminary results described above suggests that such a generalization may not be possible. In that case, attention could perhaps better be directed at defining the vulnerability of those developmental events which have the greatest significance for subsequent CNS performance.

ACKNOWLEDGEMENTS

I am grateful to Martin Berry, Michael Corner, John Dobbing and Harry Uylings for their comments on the manuscript.

REFERENCES

Altman, J. and Das, G.D. (1966) Autoradiographic and histological studies of postnatal neurogenesis 1. A longitudinal investigation of the kinetics, migration and transformation of cells incorporating tritiated thymidine in neonate rats, with special reference to postnatal neurogenesis in some brain regions. *J. comp. Neurol.,* 126: 337–390.

Angulo-Colmenares, A.G., Vaughan, D. and Hinds, J.W. (1979) Rehabilitation following early malnutrition in the rat: body weight, brain size and cerebral cortex development. *Brain Res.,* 169: 121–138.

Balázs, R., Lewis, P.D. and Patel, A.J. (1979) Nutritional deficiencies and brain development. In *Human Growth. 3. Neurobiology and Nutrition,* F. Falkner and J.M. Tanner (Eds.), Ballière Tindall, London, pp. 415–480.

Bass, N.H. (1971) Influence of neonatal undernutrition on the development of rat cerebral cortex: a microchemical study. In *Advances in Experimental Medicine and Biology, Vol. 13, Chemistry and Brain Development,* R. Paoletti and A.N. Davison (Eds.), pp. 413–424.

Bass, N.H., Netsky, M.G. and Young, E. (1970) Effects of neonatal malnutrition on developing cerebrum II. Microchemical and histological study of myelin formation in the rat. *Arch. Neurol.* 23: 303–313.

Bedi, K.S. (1979) Synapse-to-neuron ratios in previously undernourished rats. Poster presented at *11th International Summer School of Brain Research, "Adaptive capabilities of the Nervous System",* Amsterdam, August 13–14, 1979.

Berry, M. and Bradley, P. (1976a) The application of network analysis to the study of branching patterns of large dendritic fields. *Brain Res.,* 109: 111–132.

Berry, M. and Bradley, P. (1976b) The growth of the dendritic trees of Purkinje cells in irradiated agranular cerebellar cortex. *Brain Res.,* 116: 361–387.

Berry, M., Hollingworth, T., Anderson, E.M. and Flinn, R.M. (1975) Application of network analysis to the study of the branching patterns of dendritic fields. In *Advances in Neurology Vol. 12 Physiology and Pathology of Dendrites,* G.W. Kreutzberg (Ed.), Raven Press, New York, pp. 217–245.

Bradley, P. and Berry, M. (1976) The effects of reduced climbing and parallel fibre input on Purkinje cell dendritic growth. *Brain Res.,* 109: 133–151.

Bradley, P. and Berry, M. (1978a) The Purkinje cell dendritic tree in mutant mouse cerebellum. A quantitative Golgi study of weaver and staggerer mice. *Brain Res.,* 142: 135–141.

Bradley, P. and Berry, M. (1978b) Quantitative effects of methylazoxymethanol acetate on Purkinje cell dendritic growth. *Brain Res.,* 143: 499–511.

Chase, H.P., Dorsey, J. and McKhann, G.M. (1967) The effect of malnutrition on the synthesis of a myelin lipid. *Pediatrics,* 40: 551–559.

Cordero, M.E., Díaz, G. and Araya, J. (1976) Neocortex development during severe malnutrition in the rat. *Amer. J. clin. Nutr.*, 29: 358–365.

Cragg, B.G. (1972) The development of cortical synapses during starvation in the rat. *Brain*, 95: 143–150.

Culley, W.J. and Lineberger, R.O. (1968) Effects of undernutrition on the size and composition of the rat brain. *J. Nutr.*, 96: 375–381.

Dobbing, J. (1964) The influence of early nutrition on the development and myelination of the brain. *Proc. Roy. Soc. B.*, 159: 503–509.

Dobbing, J. (1968a) Vulnerable periods in developing brain. In *Applied Neurochemistry*, A.N. Davison and J. Dobbing (Eds.), Blackwell, Oxford, pp. 287–316.

Dobbing, J. (1968b) Effects of experimental undernutrition on development of the nervous system. In *Malnutrition, Learning and Behaviour*, N.S. Scrimshaw and J.E. Gordon (Eds.), M.I.T. Press, Cambridge, Mass. pp. 181–202.

Dobbing, J. (1970a) Undernutrition and the developing brain – the relevance of animal models to the human problem. *Amer. J. Dis. Childh.*, 120: 411–415.

Dobbing, J. (1970b) Undernutrition and the developing brain. In *Developmental Neurobiology*, W.A. Himwich (Ed.), Charles Thomas, Sprinfield, Ill., pp. 241–261.

Dobbing, J. (1971a) Undernutrition and the developing brain: the use of animal models to elucidate the human problem. In *Advances in Experimental Medicine and Biology Vol. 13, Chemistry and Brain Development.* R. Paoletti and A.N. Davidson (Eds.), Plenum Press, N.Y., pp. 399–412.

Dobbing, J. (1971b) Undernutrition and the developing brain: the use of animal models to elucidate the human problem. *Psychiat. Neurol. Neurochir.* 74: 433.

Dobbing, J. (1972) Lasting deficits and distortions of the adult brain following infantile undernutrition. *Pan. Amer. Health. Org.*, 251, Symposium on Nutrition, the Nervous System and Behaviour, pp. 15–23.

Dobbing, J. (1973) The developing brain: a plea for more critical interspecies extrapolation. *Nutr. Rep. Int.* 7: 401–406.

Dobbing, J. (1974a) The later growth of the brain and its vulnerability. *Pediatrics*, 53: 2–6.

Dobbing, J. (1974b) The later development of the brain and its vulnerability. In *Scientific Foundations of Paediatrics*, J.A. Davis and J. Dobbing (Eds.), William Heinemann Medical Books, London, pp. 565–577

Dobbing, J. (1974c) Prenatal nutrition and neurological development. In *Symposia of the Swedish Nutrition Foundation Vol. XII, Early Malnutrition and Mental Development*, J. Craviato, L. Hambraeus and B. Vahlquist (Eds.), Almqvist and Wiksell, Uppsala, pp. 96–110.

Dobbing, J. and Sands, J. (1971) Vulnerability of the developing brain. IX. The effect of nutritional growth retardation on the timing of the brain growth spurt. *Biol. Neonate* 19: 363–378.

Dobbing, J. and Smart, J.L. (1973) Early undernutrition, brain development and behaviour. In *Ethology and Development*, S.A. Barnett (Ed.), William Heinemann, London, pp. 16–36.

Dobbing, J. and Smart, J.L. (1974) Vulnerability of developing brain and behaviour. *Brit. Med. Bull.* 30: 164–168.

Dodge, P.R., Prensky, A.L. and Feigin, R.D. (1975) *Nutrition and the Developing Nervous System*, C.V. Mosby, St. Louis.

Dyson, S.E. and Jones, D.G. (1976) Some effects of undernutrition on synaptic development – a quantitative ultrastructural study. *Brain Res.*, 114: 365–378.

Eayrs, J.T. and Goodhead, B. (1959) Postnatal development of the cerebral cortex in the rat, *J. Anat.*, 93: 385–402.

Fox, J.H., Fishman, M.A., Dodge, P.R. and Prensky, A.L. (1972) The effect of malnutrition on human central nervous system myelin. *Neurology*, 22: 1213–1216.

Gambetti, P., Autilio-Gambetti, L., Rizzuto, N., Shafer, B. and Pfaff, L. (1974) Synapses and malnutrition: quantitative ultrastructural study of rat cerebral cortex. *Exp. Neurol.*, 43: 464–473.

Gopinath, G., Bijlani, V. and Deo, M.G. (1976) Undernutrition and the developing cerebellar cortex in the rat. *J. Neuropath. exp. Neurol.*, 35: 125–135.

Greenough, W.T., Juraska, J. and Volkmar, F.R. (1979) Maze training effects on dendritic branching in occipital cortex of adult rats. *Behav. neural Biol.*, 26: 287–297.

Griffin, W.S.T., Woodward, D.J. and Chanda, R. (1977) Malnutrition-induced alteration of developing Purkinje cells. *Exp. Neurol.* 56: 298–311.

Guthrie, H.A. and Brown, M.L. (1968) Effect of severe undernutrition in early life on growth, brain size and composition in adult rats. *J. Nutr.*, 94: 419–426.

Hedley-Whyte, E.T. and Meuser, C.S. (1971) The effect of undernutrition on myelination of rat sciatic nerve. *Lab. Invest.,* 24: 156–161.

Huttenlocher, P.R. (1974) Dendritic development in neocortex of children with mental defect and infantile spasms. *Neurology,* 24: 203–210.

Huttenlocher, P.R. (1975) Synaptic and dendritic development and mental defect. In *Brain Mechanisms in Mental Retardation,* N.A. Buchwald and M.A.B. Brazier (Eds.), Academic Press, New York, pp. 123–140.

Jones, D.G. (1976) The vulnerability of the brain to undernutrition. *Sci. Progr. (Oxford),* 63: 483–502.

Lewis, P.D. (1975) Cell death in the germinal layers of the postnatal rat brain. *Neuropath. appl. Neurobiol.,* 1: 21–29.

Lewis, P.D., Balázs, R., Patel, A.J. and Johnson, A.L. (1975) The effect of undernutrition in early life on cell generation in the rat brain. *Brain Res.,* 83: 235–247.

Lindsay, R.D. (1977) (Ed.) *Computer Analysis of Neuronal Structures,* Plenum Press, New York and London.

Marin-Padilla, M. (1974) Structural organization of the cerebral cortex (motor area) in human chromosomal aberrations. A Golgi study. ID$_1$ (13-15). Trisomy, Patau syndrome. *Brain Res.* 66: 375–391.

McConnell, P. and Berry, M. (1978a) Effects of undernutrition on Purkinje cell dendritic growth in the rat. *J. comp. Neurol.,* 177: 159–172.

McConnell, P. and Berry, M. (1978b) The effect of refeeding after neonatal starvation on Purkinje cell dendritic growth in the rat. *J. comp. Neurol.,* 178: 759–772.

McConnell, P. and Berry, M. (1979a) The effects of undernutrition on developing Purkinje cells in the cerebellum of the rat. *J. comp. Neurol.,* submitted for publication.

McConnell, P. and Berry, M. (1979b) The effect of refeeding after varying periods of neonatal undernutrition on the morphology of Purkinje cells in the cerebellum of the rat. *J. comp. Neurol.,* submitted for publication.

Overdijk, J., Uylings, H.B.M., Kuypers, K. and Kamstra, A.W. (1978) An economical, semi-automatic system for measuring cellular tree structures in three-dimensions, with special emphasis on Golgi-impregnated neurons. *J. Microsc.,* 114: 271–284.

Parnavelas, J.G., Bradford, R., Mounty, E.J. and Lieberman, A.R. (1978) The development of non-pyramidal neurons in the visual cortex of the rat. *Anat. Embryol.,* 155: 1–14.

Pysh, J.J., Perkins, R.E. and Singer Beck, L. (1979) The effect of postnatal undernutrition on the development of the mouse Purkinje cell dendritic trees. *Brain Res.* 163: 165–170.

Rebière, A. and Legrand, J. (1972) Effects comparés de la sous-alimentation, de l'hypothyroïdisme et de l'hyperthyroïdisme sur la maturation histologique de la zone moléculaire du cortex cérébelleux chez le jeune rat. *Arch. Anat. Microsc.,* 61: 105–126.

Rutledge, L.T., Wright, C. and Duncan, J. (1974) Morphological changes in pyramidal cells of mammalian neocortex associated with increased use. *Exp. Neurol.,* 44: 209–228.

Salas, M., Díaz, S. and Nieto, A. (1974) Effects of neonatal food deprivation on cortical spines and dendritic development of the rat. *Brain Res.,* 73: 139–144.

Shoemaker, W.J. and Bloom, F.E. (1977) Effect of undernutrition on brain morphology. In *Nutrition and the Brain, Vol. 2,* R.J. Wurtman and J.J. Wurtman (Eds.), Raven Press, New York, pp. 147–192.

Thomas, Y.M., Bedi, K.S., Davies, C.A. and Dobbing, J. (1979) A stereological analysis of the neuronal and synaptic content of the frontal and cerebellar cortex of weanling rats, undernourished from birth. *Early Human Develop.,* 3: 109–126.

Underwood, E.E. (1970) *Quantitative Stereology,* Addison-Wesley, Mass., Calif., London, Ontario.

Uylings, H.B.M., Kuypers, K., Diamond, M.C. and Veltman, W.A.M. (1978) Effects of differential environments on plasticity of dendrites of cortical pyramidal neurons in adult rats, *Exp. Neurol.,* 62, pp. 658–677.

Uylings, H.B.M., Kuypers, K. and Veltman, W.A.M. (1978) Environmental influences on the neocortex in later life. In *Maturation of the Nervous System, Progr. Brain Res., Vol. 48,* M.A. Corner, R.E. Baker, N.E. van de Pol, D.F. Swaab and H.B.M. Uylings (Eds.), Elsevier, Amsterdam, pp. 261–274.

Weiss, G.M. and Pysh, J.J. (1978) Evidence for loss of Purkinje cell dendrites during late development: a morphometric Golgi analysis in the mouse. *Brain Res.,* 154: 219–230.

West, C.D. and Kemper, T. (1976) The effect of a low protein diet on the anatomical development of the rat brain. *Brain Res.,* 107: 221–237.

108

Wiggins, R.C., Benjamins, J.A., Krigman, M.R. and Morell, P. (1974) Synthesis of myelin proteins during starvation. *Brain Res.,* 80: 345−349.

Williams, M.A. (1977) *Quantitative Methods in Biology,* North-Holland, Amsterdam, New York, Oxford.

Winick, M. and Noble, A. (1966) Cellular response in rats during malnutrition at various ages. *J. Nutr.,* 89: 300−306.

Wood, J.G. (1973) The effects of undernutrition on the proteins of optic and sciatic nerves during development. *J. Neurochem.,* 20: 423−429.

SECTION II

Peptide Hormones and Adaptive Mechanisms

(edited by G.J. Boer)

ACTH-Like Peptides, Pituitary–Adrenocortical Function and Avoidance Behavior

Central Research Division, Postgraduate Medical School, Budapest, Hungary

INTERACTIONS OF ALP, CHOLINOMIMETICS AND OPIATES ON CORTICOTROPIN-RELEASING HORMONE (CRH) SECRETORY ELEMENTS

Terenius (1975) showed that ACTH and its analogues have appreciable affinity for stereo-specific opiate receptors in synaptosomal membranes of brain tissue. Interestingly, α-melano-cyte stimulating hormone, vasopressin, substance P and thyroid releasing hormone proved to be inactive. These observations supported the view of Zimmerman and Krivoy (1973) that ACTH-like peptides (ALP) interfere with morphine in the central nervous system. In addition to this, the findings are in accordance with observations that ALP can antagonize the analgesic effects of opiates (see the review of Gispen et al., 1976).

Selye (1936) was the first to demonstrate the morphine-induced hyperactivity of the adrenal cortex. This finding was recently confirmed, among others, by Munson (1973) and by deWied and deJong (1974). Electrolytic lesions of the tubero-infundibular area prevented the morphine-induced rise of plasma corticosterone level (George and Leong Way, 1959), whereas local application of morphine into the basal and mid-hypothalamic nuclei increased the corticosterone production of the adrenal glands and elevated the plasma corticosterone level (van Ree et al., 1976). Local application of morphine into the dorsal and the caudal hypothalamic areas had no effect (Lotti et al., 1969). Cox et al. (1976) reported that hypothalamic sites where morphine elicits plasma corticosterone response are different from sites which are positive for temperature changes.

Recently, we studied the effects of intrahypothalamic administration of morphine into different parts of the hypothalamus in adult male rats. The drug or its vehicle was given bilaterally in 1 μl physiological saline through a chronically implanted cannula; the rats were killed 45 min following injection of 2 μg morphine, and the plasma corticosterone concentration was determined by the protein-binding technique. The cannulae were implanted 10 days prior to the experiments into different parts of the hypothalamus. Bilateral injections of 2 μg morphine into the arcuate nucleus and the suprachiasmatic area caused an increase in the plasma corticosterone level (Fig. 1). Other sites, such as the posterior hypothalamus and rostral preoptic area, proved to be ineffective. Simultaneous administration of 2 μg morphine together with 10 μg naloxone (a morphine antagonist) into the caudal suprachiasmatic region produced a significant decrease of the morphine-induced plasma corticosterone response level (Fig. 2). It is worth mentioning that naloxone alone did not modify the plasma corticosterone level and did not inhibit the daily rhythm of pituitary–adrenal axis when the drug was injected bilaterally into the preoptic or suprachiasmatic areas (unpublished observations).

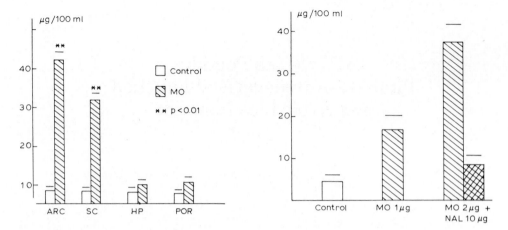

Fig. 1. Effect of bilateral microinjections of 2 μg morphine (MO) on the plasma corticosterone level in male rats. ARC, arcuate nucleus; SC, suprachiasmatic nucleus; HP, posterior hypothalamus; POR, preoptic region. Horizontal lines above bars give standard errors in this and the following figures.

Fig. 2. Effect of naloxone given simultaneously with morphine into the suprachiasmatic nuclei on plasma corticosterone level in rats. Control rats received physiological saline as vehicle. MO, morphine, NAL, naloxone.

Intrahypothalamic administration of drugs which inhibit the cholinesterase activity is followed by a significant rise of the plasma corticosterone level in rats. Thus, the microinjections of 20 μg physostigmine and 5 μg di-isopropyl-fluorophosphate (DFP) via chronically implanted cannulae into different parts of the hypothalamus revealed that the preoptic area is highly effective in inducing the activation of pituitary—adrenal axis. The hypothalamic sites where cholinomimetics cause the plasma corticosterone level to increase, do not overlap the sites where morphine activates the pituitary ACTH release (Fig. 3).

There is no causal relation between the inhibition of hypothalamic cholinesterase activity and the activation of pituitary ACTH release. Acetylcholinesterase activity was measured in

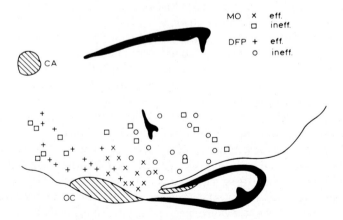

Fig. 3. Localization of effective and ineffective sites for DFP and morphine (MO) to induce elevation of plasma corticosterone level. CA, commissure anterior; OC, optic chiasma.

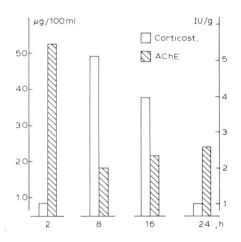 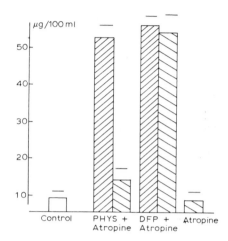

Fig. 4. Effect of 5 μg DFP injections into the preoptic area on the plasma corticosterone level and the acetylcholinesterase (AChE) activity of the hypothalamic tissue in rats. The enzyme activity was expressed in IU/g wet weight. The rats were killed at different time intervals following intrahypothalamic injections.

Fig. 5. Effect of atropine treatment (4 mg/kg body weight, subcutaneously) on the physostigmine- (PHYS) and DFP-induced increase of plasma corticosterone level in rats. Five μg DFP and 10 μg physostigmine were injected into the preoptic area and the rats were killed 45 min later.

those tissue pieces where the DFP was injected. Following administration of 5 μg DFP into the rostral preoptic area the elevation of plasma corticosterone level normalized within 24 h, although the enzyme activity was still suppressed by at least 50%, and returned to control values only 5–7 days later (Fig. 4).

Simultaneous administration of the anticholinergic drug, atropine, with physostigmine and/or DFP into the preoptic area or the suprachiasmatic nuclei, revealed that atropine can inhibit the physostigmine-induced increase of plasma corticosterone level, but it failed to suppress the effect of DFP (Fig. 5). These observations led us to assume that factors other than an excess of free acetylcholine at the synapses may be involved in DFP-induced activation of pituitary ACTH release. In higher doses, atropine blocks both muscarinic and nicotinergic receptors, and the local application of 10 μg atropine in our studies may be considered a large dosage.

OPIATE RECEPTORS AND CHOLINOMIMETICS

Combined injections of DFP with different doses of naloxone into the suprachiasmatic nuclei led to a dose-dependent decrease of the DFP-induced rise in plasma corticosterone level. Thus, 8–10 μg naloxone and 2 μg DFP resulted in at least 50% suppression of the presumed activation of the pituitary ACTH release (Fig. 6).

The experimental findings that naloxone can affect the DFP-induced acitvation of corticotrophin releasing hormone (CRH) neurosecretory elements supports the assumption that this organophosphorous substance acts at the opiate receptors, or else produces conformational changes of receptive sites. Irreversible inactivation of acetylcholinesterase by

114

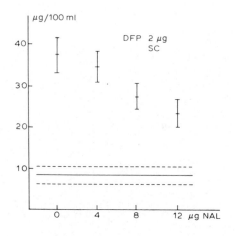 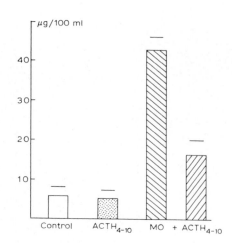

Fig. 6. Dose-dependent action of naloxone (NAL) on the DFP-induced increase of plasma corticosterone level in rats. The drugs were given simultaneously into the suprachiasmatic area (SC). Horizontal lines indicate the mean and standard deviations of resting plasma corticosterone concentration. Vertical lines indicate mean ± standard deviation of results.

Fig. 7. Inhibitory action of 4 µg ACTH 4–10 on the morphine- (MO) induced increase of plasma corticosterone level in male rats. The drugs were injected into the suprachiasmatic nuclei in single or combined microinjections.

DFP as a result of the phosphorylation of serine residues of the enzyme molecule is a known mechanism for inhibition of esterase activity. However, phosphorylation of membrane macromolecules possessing other receptive sites cannot be excluded.

Separate administration of naloxone into the arcuate nucleus and DFP into the preoptic area did not modify the DFP-induced activation of CRH neurosecretory elements. This observation led to the assumption that both drugs act upon the same pool of cells. However, it remains unclear whether these cells possess both cholinoreceptive and opiate receptor sites, or, whether they are separate elements.

Activation of pituitary ACTH release by microinjections of morphine into the suprachiasmatic nuclei was decreased by local application of ACTH 4–10. The ACTH analogue itself did not change the resting plasma corticosterone level. Intrahypothalamic injection of 4 µg ACTH 4–10 was performed simultaneously with 2 µg morphine through chronically implanted cannulae, the animals being killed 45 min later. ACTH 4–10 produced a significant decrease of the morphine-induced elevation of plasma corticosterone level (Fig. 7).

It is worth mentioning that combined injections of morphine plus atropine into the suprachiasmatic nuclei in different doses did not influence the morphine-induced increase of plasma corticosterone level. This finding indicates that opiate receptors are involved in the activation of CRH neurosecretory elements but the way in which neurotransmitters are involved is still unclear.

ACTH-INDUCED BEHAVIORAL REACTIONS AND BRAIN NOREPINEPHRINE NEURONAL SYSTEM

Considerable evidence suggests that brain catecholamines are involved in the organization of behavioral reactions, although the mechanisms behind these processes are still the subject of intensive investigation. In our earlier work in rats we studied the effect of ALP on brain norepinephrine (NE) turnover, and certain correlations were found between ACTH-induced behavioral reactions and NE-neuronal activity (see the review of Endröczi, 1976). Intraventricular administration of ACTH 1–24 and ACTH 4–10 produced an increase of brain NE turnover which could not be simulated by ACTH 11–24. Moreover, it was found that ALP produced a marked disappearance rate of [^{3}H]NE from the brain pool, which could not be prevented by blocking either the uptake or the biosynthesis (Endröczi et al., 1975). In studying the sites where ALP enhanced the activity of NE neuronal system we found that microinjections of ACTH 4–10 into the brain stem reticular formation at the level of the locus coeruleus were followed by a significant rise of NE turnover in the forebrain (Endröczi, 1976). Injections at other sites like septum, hippocampus, hypothalamus and neocortex were ineffective in this respect (Fig. 8).

In earlier investigations we found that the local application of ALP into the brain stem increased the resistance against extinction of avoidance responses. Rats were trained in a shuttlebox until a near 100% criterion level was attained. Naloxone (8 μg) and ACTH 4–10 (2 μg) were then injected, in 1 μl physiological saline, into the brain stem reticular formation at the locus coeruleus level, and the extinction of avoidance response was studied by presentations of non-reinforced trials. Fifteen trials were presented in each daily session, with the intracerebral injections given 30 min prior to the session. Fig. 9 shows that ACTH 4–10 retarded the extinction of avoidance response, but the combined injection with naloxone blocked the effect. Naloxone, injected alone into the brain stem in doses ranging between 4 and 12 μg, failed to influence the extinction rate.

With regard to the inhibitory action of naloxone upon the ACTH-induced behavioral reaction, we have tested the effect of ACTH plus simultaneous administration of naloxone upon brain NE turnover. Injections of 2 μg ACTH 4–10 and 8 μg naloxone bilaterally into

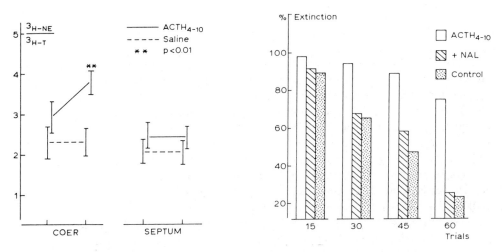

Fig. 8. Effect of 2 μg ACTH 4–10 on the forebrain NE turnover rates when given into the brain stem at the locus coeruleus (COER) level and into the septum. [^{3}H]NE/[^{3}H]tyrosine (T) ratio indicates the turnover rate. Time scale corresponds to 45 min. Vertical lines indicate mean ± standard deviation.

Fig. 9. Effect on the extinction of avoidance response in rats of 8 μg naloxone (NAL) given in combined injections with 2 μg ACTH 4–10. The drugs were administered into the brain stem reticular formation at the locus coeruleus level.

116

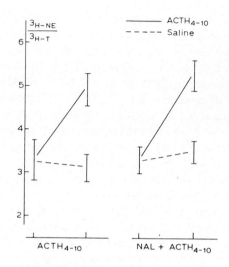

Fig. 10. Effect of naloxone (NAL) on the ACTH 4–10-induced increase of NE turnover of the forebrain in rats. The peptide (2 µg) and the drug (8 µg) were given into the brain stem reticular formation. Explanation of the symbols given in Fig. 8.

the brain stem reticular formation led to a marked increase in forebrain NE turnover. These observations indicate that ACTH-like peptides influence the NE neuronal system through a separate mechanism, and the blocking of opiate-receptors prevents the behavioral manifestations but not the activation of NE neurons ascending into the forebrain areas (Fig. 10).

EFFECTS OF DIBUTYRYL CYCLIC GMP ON THE CRH RELEASE

Recent findings suggest that analgesic effects of various drugs are mediated by more than one mechanism (Mayer and Price, 1976; Cohn et al., 1978). Enkephalins and morphine increase the cyclic GMP level in the brain (Minneman and Iversen, 1976; Racagni et al., 1976). Moreover, drugs affecting cholinergic transmission also altered the cyclic GMP content of the brain tissue (Ferrendelli et al., 1970). Centrally administered acetylcholine and cholinomimetics possess analgesic effects that are blocked by atropine (Pedigo et al., 1975).

Dibutyryl-cyclic guanosine 3'-monophosphate (dibutyryl-cGMP) administered directly into the central nervous system protects against noxious stimuli, without causing sedation or altering perception and locomotor activity. Unlike opiates, the analgesic properties of cyclic GMP (cGMP) are neither prevented nor reversed by naloxone (Cohn et al., 1978). It has not been established whether direct or indirect mechanisms are involved in morphine-induced elevation of cGMP content. For example, the cerebellar concentration of cGMP was altered by drugs affecting cholinergic transmission (Ferrendelli et al., 1970), and it is known that acetylcholine is the one of the transmitters implicated in the actions of both morphine and cGMP (Pert and Snyder, 1973; Ferrendelli et al., 1970). On the other hand, atropine does not antagonize the analgesic property of cGMP (Cohn et al., 1978), while iontophoretically applied atropine blocks the effect of acetylcholine but not of cGMP (Ferrendelli et al., 1970).

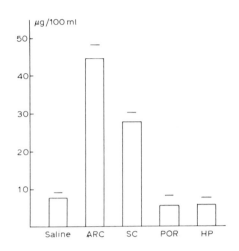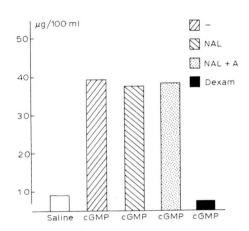

Fig. 11. Effect of bilateral dibutyryl-cGMP injections (250 nmol) on the plasma corticosterone level in male rats. The nucleotide was given into the arcuate nucleus (ARC), suprachiasmatic nucleus (SC), preoptic region (POR) and the posterior hypothalamus (HP).

Fig. 12. Effects on plasma corticosterone level of injections of cGMP, either in combination with atropine (A), naloxone (NAL), or following dexamethasone (Dexam) pretreatment. The nucleotide and the drugs were injected into the arcuate nucleus 30 min prior to sacrificing the rat.

Microinjections in conscious rats of 150–250 nmol dibutyryl-cGMP, in 1 μl physiological saline, produced a marked rise in plasma corticosterone level if the administration was performed into the arcuate nucleus. The plasma corticosterone concentration began to rise within 5–10 min, and had its peak about 25–40 min following the injections. Fig. 11 shows that injections of cGMP into the suprachiasmatic and preoptic nuclei or into the dorsal hippocampus did not increase the plasma corticosterone level which was measured 30 min later.

Simultaneous administration of atropine or naloxone with dibutyryl-cGMP into the arcuate nucleus did not modify the nucleotide-induced activation of the pituitary–adrenal axis (Fig. 12). Administration of 0.5 mg/kg dexamethasone 12 h prior to the intracerebral administration of nucleotide led to a complete inhibition of plasma corticosterone response.

EFFECTS OF cGMP ON BEHAVIORAL REACTIONS

Bilateral intraventricular administration of 250 nmol cGMP produced no remarkable changes in spontaneous behavior, with the rats showing normal orienting reactions and exploratory activity in a novel environment. The analgesic property of the nucleotide was not tested in these experiments although it was apparent, because the rats showed an increased resistance to the pain caused by penetration of the sharp points of the clamp to the tail.

The behavioral effect of cGMP was tested on the extinction of avoidance response in adult male rats. The animals were trained in a shuttle-box by presentations of buzzer sound with painful electric shocks (0.5 mA). Twenty associations were presented in each daily session until a near 100% criterion level was reached. The cGMP was then administered

118

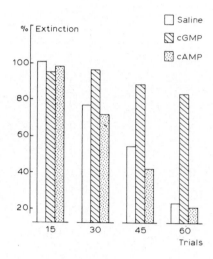

Fig. 13. Effect of cGMP and cAMP on the extinction of avoidance response in rats. The nucleotides were given bilaterally into the lateral ventricles (250 nmol in 5 μl physiological saline) and the extinction was performed by presentations of 15 trials per daily session. The administration of nucleotides was repeated each day 15 min prior to behavioral testing.

bilaterally via chronically implanted cannulae into the lateral ventricle 15 min prior to each behavioral test. Fifteen non-reinforced trials were presented in order to follow the extinction of avoidance response. The control rats received physiological saline, while another group of animals was treated with 250 nmol cyclic adenosine 5'-monophosphate (cAMP). Fig. 13 shows that intraventricular administration of 250 nmol cGMP resulted in a marked resistance to extinction of avoidance response. The cAMP treatment proved to be ineffective.

It is worthwhile mentioning that retardation of extinction by cGMP administration was more powerful than the effect observed after ALP treatment. Moreover, the systemic administration of cGMP in doses ranging between 500 and 1200 nmol/100 g body weight did not influence the extinction rate.

GENERAL CONCLUSIONS

More than 25 years ago Torda and Wolf (1952) reported that ACTH administration is followed by an increase of acetylcholine synthesis at the neuromuscular junction. It was demonstrated in other studies that ALP increase the NE turnover of the brain in both intact and adrenalectomized rats (Hökfelt and Fuxe, 1972; Versteeg, 1973; Endröczi et al., 1975; Endröczi, 1976). Correlation studies between the NE turnover rate and the extinction process of avoidance response postulated a direct role of the NE neuronal system in ACTH-induced behavioral changes (Endröczi, 1976). In the present investigations we have found that naloxone inhibits the behavioral action of ALP, although the effect of the peptide upon NE turnover remained unchanged. These observations indicate that ALP exert a multiple action on cells with different receptive sites, and that the activation of brain NE neuronal systems is not necessarily coupled to extinction of conditioned responses.

Terenius and Wahlström (1975) demonstrated the existence of an endogenous ligand of morphine receptors which was isolated from the cerebrospinal fluid. Terenius (1975) showed that ALP have an appreciable affinity for opiate binding sites, observations that are in accordance with the view of Zimmerman and Krivoy (1974) that ALP interfere with morphine in the central nervous system. Many studies indicate that brain tissue contains endogenous compounds which resemble opiates in their action. The most intensively investigated of these substances are peptides such as enkephalins and endorphins. However, there is another type of endogenous morphine-like compound which is not a peptide, but which binds to opiate receptors (Gintzler and Gershon, 1978). Immunocytochemical localization of such substances in various brain stem nuclei would imply their involvement with certain neuronal pathways associated with stimulus-produced analgesia. In connection with these findings, we must take into account that cGMP injections into the brain stem (e.g. periaqueductal gray matter and reticular formation) do not mimic the analgesic action of morphine, which suggests that opiates and nucleotides do not share a common mechanism of action.

Involvement of the brain NE neuronal system in controlling the behavioral reactions has been supported by a number of observations, although the recent investigations presented here, plus the fact that (D-Phe^7)-ACTH 4–10 is inactive in this respect are not in accordance with this view. Nevertheless, direct or indirect involvement of NE neurons in learning and memory processes is well-founded, although the mechanisms behind these events require further studies. Participation of cholinergic neurons in the central control of pituitary ACTH secretion has been supported by many observations. The present data are in accordance with the view that cholinergic transmission is involved in activation of CRH neurosecretory elements and the cholinoreceptive field located rostrally to the arcuate nucleus and the median eminence. These findings may help to interpret the observations of Makara and Stark (1976), who reported that deafferentation of the basal and medial hypothalamus prevents the activation of pituitary ACTH release after local application of cholinomimetics. The DFP-induced activation of pituitary–adrenocortical function was partially inhibited by naloxone, which supports the assumption that in addition to cholinoreceptive field the opiate receptors are involved in controlling the CRH-producing elements.

SUMMARY

The discovery of behavioral effects of adrenocorticotropin-like peptides (ALP) had a profound influence upon the study of endocrine control over adaptive behavior, and greatly contributed to the development of research into neuropeptides and peptidergic transmission in the brain (Mirsky et al., 1953; Murphy and Miller, 1955; Krivoy and Guillemin, 1961; deWied, 1965; Levine and Jones, 1965; Endröczi, 1972; Kastin et al., 1975). Considerable evidence suggests that ALP may act upon brain protein synthesis (Gispen et al., 1976) and catecholamine turnover (Endröczi et al., 1975), and that they bind to opiate receptors (Terenius, 1975). The experimental observations that ALP of extrapituitary origin are present in the brain led to the assumption that such neuropeptides are involved in neural transmission (Krieger et al., 1977; Pacold et al., 1978). The biologically active and immunoreactive ACTH content of the brain remained unchanged after either hypophysectomy or dexamethasone administration. These last observations indicate that other factors are involved in regulation of pituitary ACTH synthesis than that of the brain ALP. Whether the neuropeptides are directly involved in neural transmission or rather are playing a modulatory role, is still the subject of investigations.

REFERENCES

Cohn, M.L., Cohn, M. and Taylor, F.H. (1978) Guanosine 3',5'-monophosphate: a central nervous regulator of analgesia. *Science,* 199: 319–321.

Cox, B., Ary, M., Chesarek, W. and Lomax, P. (1976) Morphine hyperthermia in the rat: an action on the central thermostate. *Europ. J. Pharmacol.,* 36: 33–39.

Endröczi, E. (1972) *Limbic System, Learning and Pituitary–Adrenal Function,* Akadémiai Kiadó, Budapest.

Endröczi, E. (1976) Brain mechanisms involved in ACTH-induced changes of exploratory activity and conditioned avoidance behavior. In *Neuropeptides Influences on the Brain and Behavior,* L.H. Miller, C.A. Sandman and A.J. Kastin (Eds.), Raven Press, New York.

Endröczi, E., Hraschek, Á., Nyakas, Cs. and Szabó, G. (1975) Brain catecholamines and pituitary–adrenal function. In *Cellular and Molecular Bases of Neuroendocrine Processes,* Akadémiai Kiadó, Budapest, pp. 607–613.

Ferrendelli, J.A., Steiner, A. and Dougal, D.B. (1970) Effect of oxotremorine and atropine on cGMP and cAMP levels in mouse cerebral cortex and cerebellum. *Biochem. biophys. Res. Commun.,* 41: 1061–1067.

George, R. and Leong Way, E. (1959) The role of the hypothalamus in the pituitary–adrenal activation and antidiuresis by morphine. *J. Pharmacol. exp. Ther.,* 125: 111–125.

Gintzler, A.R. and Gershon, M.D. (1978) A nonpeptide morphine-like compound: immunocytochemical localization in the mouse brain. *Science,* 199: 447–448.

Gispen, W.H., Reith, M.E.A., Schotman, P., Wiegand, V.W., Zwiers, H. and deWied, D. (1976) CNS and ACTH-like peptides: neurochemical response and interactions with opiates. In *Neuropeptide Influences on the Brain and Behavior,* L.H. Miller, C.A. Sandman and A.J. Kastin (Eds.), Raven Press, New York, pp. 81–108.

Hökfelt, T. and Fuxe, K. (1972) On the morphology and neuroendocrine role of the hypothalamic catecholamine neurons. In *Brain–Endocrine Interactions, Median Eminence: Structure and Function,* K.M. Knigge, D.E. Scott and A. Weindl (Eds.), Karger, Basel, pp. 181–223.

Kastin, A.J., Plotnikoff, N.P., Hall, R. and Schally, A.V. (1975) Hypothalamic hormones and the central nervous system. In *Hypothalamic Hormones: Chemistry, Physiology, Pharmacology and Clinical Uses,* L. Martini (Ed.), Academic Press, New York, pp. 261–268.

Krieger, D.T., Liotta, A. and Brownstein, M.J. (1977) Presence of corticotropin in the brain of normal and hypophysectomized rats. *Proc. nat. Acad. Sci. (Wash.),* 74: 648–652.

Krivoy, W.A. and Guillemin, R. (1961) On a possible role of α-melanocyte stimulating hormone (α-MSH) in the central nervous system of the mammalia: an effect of α-MSH in the spinal cord of the cat. *Endocrinology,* 69: 170–175.

Levine, S. and Jones, L.E. (1965) Adrenocorticotropic hormone (ACTH) and passive avoidance behavior. *J. comp. physiol. Psychol.,* 59: 357–360.

Lotti, V.J., Kokka, N. and George, R. (1969) Pituitary–adrenal activation following intrahypothalamic microinjections of morphine. *Neuroendocrinology,* 4: 326–332.

Makara, G.B. and Stark, E. (1976) The effects of cholinomimetic drugs and atropine on ACTH release. *Neuroendocrinology,* 21: 31–39.

Mayer, D.J. and Price, D.D. (1976) Central nervous mechanisms of analgesia. *Pain,* 2: 379–404.

Minneman, K.P. and Iversen, I.L. (1976) Enkephalin and opiate narcotics increase cyclic GMP accumulation in slices of rat neostriatum. *Nature (Lond.),* 262: 313–314.

Mirsky, J., Miller, R. and Stein, M. (1953) Relation of adrenocortical activity and adaptive behavior. *Psychosom. Med.,* 15: 575–584.

Munson, P.L. (1973) Effects of morphine and related drugs on the corticotropin (ACTH)-stress reaction. In *Drug Effects on Neuroendrocine Regulation, Pro. Brain Res. Vol. 39,* D. DeWied (Ed.), Elsevier, Amsterdam, pp. 361–372.

Murphy, J.V. and Miller, R. (1965) The effect of adrenocorticotrophic hormone (ACTH) on avoidance learning in the rat. *J. comp. physiol. Psychol.,* 48: 48–49.

Pacold, S.T., Kristeins, L., Hojvat, S. and Lawrence, A.M. (1978) Biologically active pituitary hormones in the rat brain amygdaleoid nucleus. *Science,* 199: 804–805.

Pedigo, N.W., Dewey, W.L. and Harris, L.S. (1975) Determination and characterization of the antinociceptive activity of intraventricularly administered acetylcholine in mice. *J. Pharmacol. exp. Ther.,* 193: 845–852.

Pert, C.B. and Snyder, S.H. (1973) Opiate receptor: demonstration in nervous tissue. *Science,* 179: 1011–1014.

Racagni, G., Zsilla, G., Guidotti, A. and Costa, E. (1975) Accumulation of cGMP in striatum of rats injected with morphine analgesics: antagonism by naltrexone. *J. Pharm. Pharmacol.,* 28: 258–260.

Selye, H. (1936) The physiology and pathology of exposure to stress. *Acta Inc. (Montreal),* (1951).

Terenius, L. (1975) Effect of peptides and aminoacids on dihydromorphine binding to the opiate receptor. *J. Pharm. Pharmacol.,* 27: 450–452.

Terenius, L. and Wahlström, A. (1975) Morphine-like ligand for opiate receptors in human CSF. *Life Sci.,* 16: 1759–1764.

Torda, C. and Wolf, H.G. (1952) Effect of pituitary hormones, cortisone and adrenalectomy on some aspects of neuromuscular systems and acetylcholine synthesis. *Amer. J. Physiol.,* 169: 140–149.

Van Ree, J.M., Spaanen-Kok, W.B. and DeWied, D. (1976) Differential localization of pituitary–adrenal acitvation and temperature changes following intrahypothalamic microinjections of morphine in rats. *Neuroendocrinology,* 22: 318–324.

Versteeg, D.H.G. (1973) Effect of two ACTH analogues on noradrenaline metabolism in rat brain. *Brain Res.,* 49: 483–485.

deWied, D. (1965) The influence of the posterior and intermediate lobe of the pituitary and pituitary peptides on the maintenance of a conditional avoidance response in rats. *Int. J. Neuropharmacol.,* 4: 167–163.

deWied, D. and deJong, W. (1974) Drug effects and hypothalamic–anterior pituitary function. *Ann. Rev. Pharmacol.,* 14: 389–412.

Zimmerman, E. and Krivoy, W.A. (1973) Antagonism between the morphine and the polypeptides ACTH, ACTH 1-24 and α-MSH in the nervous system. In *Drug Effects on Neuroendocrine Regulation, Progress in Brain Research, Vol. 39,* D. De Wied (Ed.), Elsevier, Amsterdam, pp. 383–394.

The Interaction of Posterior Pituitary Neuropeptides with Monoaminergic Neurotransmission: Significance in Learning and Memory Processes

GÁBOR L. KOVÀCS, BÈLA BOHUS and DIRK H.G. VERSTEEG

Department of Pathophysiology, University Medical School, Szeged, Hungary and (B.B. and D.H.G. V.) Rudolf Magnus Institute for Pharmacology, University of Utrecht, The Netherlands

INTRODUCTION

Neuropeptides and neurotransmitters are integral constituents of the central nervous system. Certain neuropeptides (e.g. vasopressin, oxytocin, ACTH, MSH) affect the CNS processes underlying memory, motivation, behavioral adaptation and attention (for reviews, see De Wied et al., 1976, Endröczi, 1980, Sandman et al., 1976). Other neuropeptides (e.g. endorphin fragments) exert neuroleptic-like activity in animals (De Wied et al., 1978) and antipsychotic effects in psychiatric patients (Verhoeven et al., 1978, Van Praag and Verhoeven, 1980). Similar effects, however, have repeatedly been shown by classical neurotransmitter (norepinephrine, dopamine, serotonin, etc.) substances or by drugs acting on transmitter metabolism. Based on their CNS effects, neuropeptides have been classified as neuromodulators or as neurotransmitters (Barker and Smith, 1980). By either mechanism, however, neuropeptides may influence the production, secretion and actions of classical neurotransmitters.

This chapter is devoted to review the effects of monoaminergic neurotransmitters and posterior pituitary neuropeptides on learning and memory processes, with particular emphasis on the interactions between these biochemical messenger systems.

NEUROHUMORAL MECHANISMS IN LEARNING AND MEMORY

Role of monoaminergic neurotransmitters

There is a considerable body of evidence in support for a role of the monoamine neurotransmitters (norepinephrine, dopamine, serotonin, etc.) both in learning and in the processing of acquired information. Such evidence derives from studies in which the behavioral effects of centrally-acting drugs were either related to their actions on neurochemical processes, or were tested when specific brain sites or pathways were stimulated or lesioned. A third approach has been to search for correlations between alterations of behavioral processes and the activity of a particular neurotransmitter pathway in undisturbed animals.

Although no clear-cut evidence exists regarding a particular neurotransmitter as being the specific substrate of memory processes, there are many results which support the general view that catecholamines play an important role in modulating learning, memory storage and retrieval processes. Drugs which interfere with the synthesis of norepinephrine and dopamine disrupt conditioned avoidance responses during acquisition and extinction (Corrodi and

Hanson, 1966; McGaugh et al., 1975; Kovács and Telegdy, 1978). Administration of a dopamine-β-hydroxylase inhibitor shortly after training seriously impairs retention (McGaugh et al., 1975), indicating the possible role of noradrenaline in memory consolidation. Crow (1968), Kety (1970) and Anlezark et al. (1973) demonstrated that lesioning of the dorsal noradrenergic (coeruleotelencephalic) bundle (Dahlström and Fuxe, 1964; Jones and Moore, 1977) interferes with the animal's ability to acquire new information. More recently, this pathway has been suggested to be an anatomical substrate of attention and to play a role in the filtering out of irrelevant stimuli (Mason and Iversen, 1977; Mason and Fibiger, 1978). Correlational evidence also supports the role of catecholamines: Hraschek et al. (1977) have shown that good performance in a shuttle-box is associated with an increased [^{3}H]norepinephrine disappearance in the neocortex and dorsal hippocampus. In isolated brain nuclei, Kovács et al. (1980b) have demonstrated correlations between norepinephrine disappearance in the hippocampal dentate gyrus and the medial septal nucleus and the performance of a one-trial learning passive avoidance task. No correlation was found, on the other hand, between memory formation and the catecholamine levels of the whole brain (Pálfai et al., 1978), supporting the view that specific transmitter pathways rather than the overall metabolism of amines might be related to information processing.

Pharmacological manipulation of the cerebral dopaminergic activity (e.g. with amphetamine) also influences learning in a variety of behavioral situations (McGaugh, 1973; Haycock et al., 1977; Kovács and De Wied, 1978); however, the specific involvement of dopaminergic pathways in learning is not well understood. This is partly due to the fact that dopaminergic systems are closely involved in motor performance (Ranje and Ungerstedt, 1977).

It has been shown in a series of experiments (Essmann, 1971; 1973) that brain serotonin concentration and metabolism also influence memory consolidation. Since amnesia can be provoked in mice by the intracranial and intraventricular administration of 5-HT, it has been concluded that this indolamine mediates inhibitory events associated with, or leading to amnesia. The results from pharmacological manipulations of serotonin metabolism (Stevens, 1970; Knoll, 1973; Barchas and Usdin, 1973; Kovács and Telegdy, 1978; etc.) and also from lesion and stimulation of the ascending serotoninergic pathways (Kostowski et al., 1968; 1969; Lorens et al., 1971; Jacobs et al., 1974; Kovács and Telegdy, 1976; Knoll et al., 1976), support the view that the serotoninergic system has an inhibitory influence on neuronal processes associated with learning and memory.

Influence of posterior pituitary neuropeptides

It is now generally accepted that pituitary neuropeptides have an influence on various CNS functions. The pioneering work of De Wied (1964, 1969) has clearly demonstrated the importance of pituitary peptides in the acquisition and maintenance of learned behavior. While anterior pituitary neuropeptides (ACTH, MSH) primarily affect motivational and attentional processes (for refs. see Endröczi, 1972; De Wied, 1974; Miller et al., 1974; Bohus et al., 1975a), posterior pituitary neuropeptides (vasopressin and oxytocin) directly influence learning and memory. An extract of the posterior pituitary gland (Pitressin) caused long-lasting delay in the extinction of an active avoidance reaction (De Wied and Bohus, 1966). The same effects have been established with synthetic arginine[8]- and lysine[8]-vasopressin (De Wied, 1971; Ader and De Wied, 1972; Schulz et al., 1974). In accordance with these findings, avoidance latencies in various passive avoidance paradigms (step-through or step-down) are increased upon vasopressin challenge (Bohus et al., 1972; 1978a and b); Kovács et al., 1977). De Wied et al. (1976) concluded that vasopressin facilitates memory

TABLE I

OPPOSITE EFFECTS OF VASOPRESSIN AND OXYTOCIN ON CNS PROCESSES

Test method	Effect of vasopressin	Authors	Effect of oxytocin	Authors
Extinction of active avoidance reaction	delay	De Wied, 1971; Ader and De Wied, 1972; Schulz et al., 1974	facilitation	Schulz et al., 1974; 1976
One-trial learning passive avoidance	improvement	Bohus et al., 1972; 1978a and b, Kovàcs et al., 1977; 1978	attenuation	Kovàcs et al., 1978; Bohus et al., 1978a and b
Brain stimulation reward *	decrease	Schwarzberg et al., 1976	increase	Schwarzberg et al., 1976
Heroin self-administration *	decrease	Van Ree and De Wied, 1977	facilitation (slight)	Van Ree and De Wied, 1977
Hypothalamic neuronal activity	increase	Schulz et al., 1971	decrease	Schulz et al., 1971
Hippocampal theta rhythm *	shift to higher frequency	Bohus et al., 1978b	shift to lower frequency	Bohus et al., 1978b
Striatal dopamine disappearance	increase	Kovàcs et al., 1977; Tanaka et al., 1977b, Telegdy and Kovàcs, 1979a	decrease	Telegdy and Kovàcs, 1979a

* Test method indirectly related to learning and memory.

consolidation (the input stage of memory) as well as the retrieval of stored information (the output stage of memory). Studies involving retrograde amnesia also support the memory hypothesis: vasopressin and behaviorally-active peptide fragments protect against CO_2- and electroconvulsive shock-induced amnesia (Rigter et al., 1974; Rigter and Van Riezen, 1978), against pentylenetetrazol-induced amnesia (Bookin and Pfeifer, 1977) in rats, and against puromycin-induced amnesia in mice (Lande et al., 1972; Walter et al., 1975).

Vasopressin treatment affects the electrical activity of the cerebral cortex in humans (Timsit-Berthier et al., 1978). Treatment of volunteers with lysine[8]-vasopressin improves memory, as measured by visual retention, recognition and recall. Immediate memory and learning are also improved by the peptide (Legros et al., 1978). Vasopressin challenge improves memory in amnestic patients too (Oliveros et al., 1978).

Oxytocin, the other physiologically secreted neuropeptide of the posterior pituitary, affects CNS processes in a direction opposite to that of vasopressin (Table I). The two neuropeptides have opposite influences on the electrical activity of the hypothalamus (Schulz et al., 1971) and the rhythmic slow activity (theta rhythm) of the dorsal hippocampus during paradoxical sleep (Bohus et al., 1978b). Furthermore, behavioral processes are influenced in opposite ways by the two neuropeptides: in contrast to vasopressin, oxytocin facilitates the extinction of an active avoidance reaction (Schulz et al., 1974). This effect becomes more pronounced in water-deprived animals (endogenous vasopressin release?) (Schulz et al., 1976). Higher doses of peripherally administered oxytocin, however, mimic the effect of vasopressin on avoidance extinction (De Wied and Gispen, 1977). Both peripheral (Kovács et al., 1977; Telegdy and Kovács, 1979a) and intraventricular (Bohus et al., 1978b) administration of oxytocin attenuates passive avoidance behavior. It might thus be that oxytocin is a naturally occurring amnestic neuropeptide (Bohus et al., 1978a and b). Opposite effects of the two neuropeptides have been observed on other CNS processes as well, such as the brain stimulation reward (Schwarzberg et al., 1976) and self-administration of narcotic analgesics (Van Ree and De Wied, 1977; Van Ree et al., 1978b).

SITES OF ACTION OF POSTERIOR PITUITARY NEUROPEPTIDES IN THE BRAIN

Since both monoaminergic neurotransmitters and neuropeptides affect learning and memory, the question arose as to whether it might be that these two classes of neuro-humoral substances act in concert. The specific topographical distribution of transmitter pathways offers a means of approaching this question by testing the effects of peptides microinjected into discrete brain areas. As regards the noradrenergic systems in the brain implicated in learning and memory, noradrenergic cell bodies are concentrated in the A_6 catecholaminergic cell groups of the lower brain stem (locus coeruleus) and the ascending fibers innervate cortical, forebrain, limbic and brain stem structures (e.g. hippocampus, septum, etc.) (Dahlström and Fuxe, 1964; Loizou, 1969; Ungerstedt, 1971; Jones and Moore, 1977; Pasquier et al., 1977; Koda et al., 1978).

Wimersma Greidanus et al. (1975a) and Wimersma Greidanus and De Wied (1976) showed that lesions of the rostral septal region and the anterodorsal hippocampus completely prevented the effect of vasopressin on the extinction of one-way active avoidance behavior,

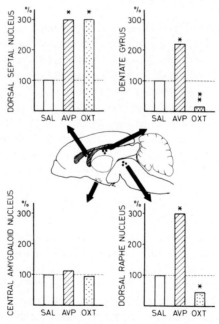

Fig. 1. Effects on passive avoidance behavior of microinjection of arginine[8]-vasopressin (AVP) and oxytocin (OXT). Metal microcannulae were implanted into various limbic-midbrain structures. Passive avoidance behavior was tested according to Ader et al. (1972) 10 days after surgery. The peptides were injected bilaterally (25 pg on each side) except in the dorsal raphe nucleus (50 pg). Treatment was given immediately after the single learning trial; passive avoidance latency was measured 24 h later. Avoidance latency is expressed as a percentage of the saline-treated controls. Asterisks indicate significant differences: * $P < 0.05$, ** $P < 0.01$. The schematic drawing in the middle depicts the sites of injection.

while lesion of the thalamic parafascicular area inhibited it only partially. Based on the combined results of these lesion studies, biochemical experiments to be discussed below and on the above described topographical distribution of the noradrenergic pathways, vasopressin and oxytocin have been microinjected into limbic-midbrain nuclei (dentate gyrus, dorsal septal nucleus, dorsal raphe nucleus, central amygdaloid nucleus), and their effects have been tested on the retention of a one-trial learning passive avoidance reaction (Ader et al., 1972). Local microinjection of small amounts of arginine[8]-vasopressin into the dorsal septal nucleus, hippocampal dentate area or the midbrain dorsal raphe nucleus was found to facilitate passive avoidance behavior (Fig. 1), while local microinjection of AVP into the central amygdaloid nucleus was without effect. Upon microinjection of oxytocin, two basically different kinds of behavioral effects were observed: the neuropeptide attenuated passive avoidance when injected into the dentate gyrus or the dorsal raphe nucleus, but when injected into the dorsal septal nucleus it facilitated passive avoidance behavior (Fig. 1).

Since it was found that 25–50 pg of the peptides is without any influence on behavioral processes when injected into the lateral cerebral ventricles (Bohus et al., 1978b), it was logical to conclude that certain limbic-midbrain areas are specifically sensitive for posterior pituitary neuropeptides and to suppose that these regions might mediate the effects of vasopressin and oxytocin on memory consolidation. It is of interest to note, however, that microinjection of the peptide into the central amygdaloid nucleus does not affect avoidance behavior, while lesions of the amygdala (Wimersma Greidanus et al., 1979) block the effect of vasopressin. One possible explanation for this apparent contradiction is that the lesion destroys more nuclei, whereas the microinjections are confined within the central nucleus. Such a restricted local sensitivity is observed in the hippocampus as well: vasopressin is highly effective in the dentate area, but is ineffective in the adjacent subiculum (Kovács et al., 1979b).

It is probably more than a coincidence that many brain regions with a specific sensitivity for vasopressin and oxytocin receive noradrenergic input via the dorsal noradrenergic bundle, and that extrahypothalamic vasopressinergic and oxytocinergic fibers enter these areas (Sterba, 1974; Buijs et al., 1978; Kozlowski et al., 1978) and form synaptic contacts there (Sofroniew and Weindl, 1978; Sterba et al., 1979; Buijs et al., 1980). This implies the possibility of an interaction presumably involving specific binding sites. However, specific binding or receptor sites for vasopressin or oxytocin have not been identified in the brain as yet, although morphological evidence suggests that these may exist (Castel, 1978).

INTERACTION OF NEUROPEPTIDES WITH MONOAMINERGIC BRAIN MECHANISMS

Influence of posterior pituitary neuropeptides on neurotransmitter metabolism

Although studies with whole brain have failed to reveal any effect of vasopressin on monoaminergic neurotransmission (Dunn et al., 1976), it is now known beyond any doubt that vasopressin does affect regional cerebral norepinephrine and dopamine metabolism. Peripheral administration of lysine[8]-vasopressin decreases the steady-state levels of dopamine in the hypothalamus septal region and striatum (Kovács et al., 1977). From studies of their effects on the disappearance of catecholamines following the inhibition of their synthesis by α-methyl-p-tyrosine, it has been concluded that both lysine[8]-vasopressin (Kovács et al., 1977) and arginine[8]-vasopressin (Tanaka et al., 1977a) influence the nerve impulse flow in catecholaminergic neurons. Vasopressin increases the α-MTP-induced disappearance in the hypothalamus (Kovács et al., 1977; Tanaka et al., 1977a), thalamus and medulla oblongata

(Tanaka et al., 1977a). Dopamine disappearance is facilitated in the septal area and striatum (Kovács et al., 1977) and also in the preoptic region (Tanaka et al., 1977a). The steady-state levels of serotonin (Telegdy and Kovács, 1979a) and the 5-HT accumulation (Kovács, Szabó and Telegdy, unpublished observation) are not affected by lysine[8]-vasopressin, although a correlation has been found between the anti-amnestic action of desglycinamide-vasopressin and the peptide-induced increase in 5-HT level of the dorsal hippocampus (Ramaekers et al., 1977).

A more specific regional distribution of vasopressin-induced changes has been described by Tanaka et al. (1977b). These authors studied the effect of arginine[8]-vasopressin on the disappearance of catecholamines in individual brain nuclei microdissected with a punch technique. Intraventricular administration of the peptide facilitated norepinephrine disappearance in 8 nuclei of limbic-midbrain and lower brain stem structures, but did not affect it in another 35 nuclei. Thus, limbic-midbrain and lower brain stem structures are rather selectively influenced by the neuropeptide. A facilitation of disappearance of dopamine in the caudate nucleus, median eminence and the dorsal raphe nucleus was also evident (Tanaka et al., 1977b).

Fewer data are available concerning the effects of oxytocin on cerebral neurotransmitter activity. Peripheral administration of oxytocin causes a decrease of norepinephrine levels in the hypothalamus, septum and striatum, whereas the dopamine levels are not altered. The 5-HT content of the hypothalamus increases, while the septal 5-HT decreases following oxytocin treatment (Telegdy and Kovács, 1979a). It is interesting to note that vasopressin and oxytocin exert opposite effects on striatal dopamine disappearance.

One obvious criticism of this type of approach is that the data do not indicate specifically the brain regions in which the effects of the neuropeptides on the brain monoamine metabolism are directly related to learning and memory processes. In a first attempt to overcome this problem, α-MTP-induced disappearance of catecholamines in individual brain nuclei was measured following the local microinjection of arginine[8]-vasopressin into those brain regions in which the peptide had been found to facilitate memory consolidation (Kovács et al., 1979b). Limbic-midbrain nuclei in which intraventricular administration of vasopressin had been found to affect catecholamine metabolism (Tanaka et al., 1977b) were selected for catecholamine assay.

Intracerebral injection of arginine[8]-vasopressin induced selective alterations of catecholamine metabolism (and facilitates memory consolidation, see above): bilateral microinjections of vasopressin into the dentate gyrus via chronically implanted cannulae facilitated norepinephrine disappearance in the dentate area itself, and increased the norepinephrine disappearance in the red nucleus of the midbrain (Fig. 2). Neither the norepinephrine nor the dopamine metabolism was changed in the other nuclei. Following septal injection of vasopressin, the norepinephrine disappearance was affected (inhibited) in the dorsal septal nucleus itself, and again facilitated in the red nucleus (Fig. 3). Intracerebral injection of vasopressin facilitates passive avoidance behavior and affects norepinephrine disappearance. Theoretically, the observed changes in catecholamine metabolism might be directly related to the ability of the peptide to influence norepinephrine metabolism. This mechanism would suggest that it is the changes in NE metabolism which mediate the action of vasopressin on memory consolidation. It is also possible, however, that the neuropeptide induces facilitation of memory consolidation by mechanisms other than via catecholamine metabolism, and that the changes in catecholaminergic neurotransmission merely reflect alterations in the motor performance of the animals. Such alterations in motor performance are the consequences of facilitated information processing. Since the red nucleus is a brain site which is

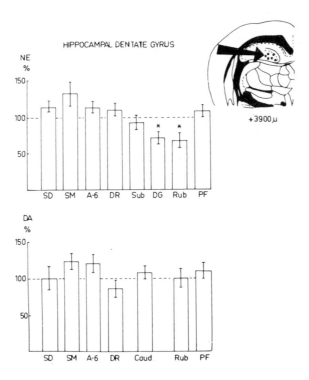

Fig. 2. Regional α-MPT-induced disappearance of catecholamines following intrahippocampal micro-injection of arginine[8]-vasopressin. α-Methyl-p-tyrosine was given i.p., followed by the intracerebral micro-injection of AVP 30 min later. After three hours, norepinephrine (NE) and dopamine (DA) were measured with the radioenzymatic method of Van der Gugten et al. (1976) in isolated brain nuclei (Palkovits, 1973). The results are expressed as percentages of the saline-treated controls; a lower catecholamine content, as it is the case for NE in the dentate gyrus of the hippocampus, indicates a facilitating effect of vasopressin on NE disappearance.

generally believed to be involved in the organization of motor patterns, this question was rather critical. In "naive" animals, which were not subjected to behavioral training, septal microinjection of vasopressin decreased rather than increased the NE turnover in the nucleus ruber (Kovács et al., 1979b). The same direction of change (i.e. a decrease) was observed in the nucleus ruber after intraventricular administration of vasopressin in naive animals (Tanaka et al., 1977b). These data suggest that the facilitated NE turnover in the red nucleus following intracerebral microinjection of vasopressin in trained animals might be a bio-chemical correlate of the altered motor performance (Kovács et al., 1979b). The in situ effect in the norepinephrine metabolism in limbic regions, on the other hand, was identical in trained and in naive animals. This led to the conclusion that peptide-induced effects on memory are quite likely coupled with in situ changes in limbic areas (Kovács et al., 1979b).

Posterior pituitary peptides have biological half-lives in the order of magnitude of minutes, but their effects on CNS processes, however, may persist for several days, or even longer (De Wied, 1971). Therefore, there was ample reason to test whether the changes in norepinephrine metabolism were short-term or long-term in nature. Vasopressin, given into the dorsal septal nucleus 3 h before decapitation, inhibited norepinephrine depletion at the injection site. When the injection was given 7 days prior to decapitation, however, the nore-pinephrine was unaltered on the day of sacrifice. The first injection did not potentiate the

130

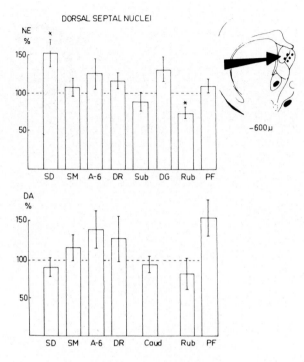

Fig. 3. Regional α-MPT-induced disappearance of catecholamines following intraseptal microinjection of arginine[8]-vasopressin. (For detailed legend see Fig. 2).

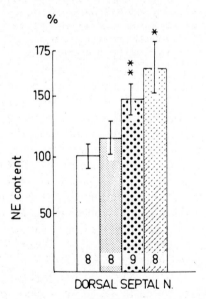

Fig. 4. Effects of repeated microinjections of arginine[8]-vasopressin on α-MPT-induced disappearance of norepinephrine. The peptide was microinjected bilaterally into the dorsal septal nucleus (25 pg on each side), and the NE disappearance of the injected area was determined as described above. First treatment 7 days, second one 3 h before decapitation. ▨, AVP + saline; ▨, saline + AVP; ▨, AVP + AVP; □, saline + saline.

effect of the second one (Fig. 4). Although additional studies are necessary to resolve this problem, it seems as if the effect of the neuropeptide outlasts the biological half-life, but does not persist nearly as long as the effects on avoidance behavior. It might be assumed, therefore, that the interaction with regional catecholamine neurotransmission represents an intermediate permissive step in the biochemical mediation of the effects of posterior pituitary neuropeptides on CNS functions.

Neurotransmitter pathways involved in CNS effects of vasopressin

Although the above data provide correlational evidence for the involvement of catecholaminergic mechanisms in some of the memory effects of vasopressin, this hypothesis needed further support. In fact, Kovács et al. (1977) reported that the inhibition of catecholamine biosynthesis by α-MPT prevented the effect of vasopressin on a passive avoidance reaction. A similar effect was found on the extinction of active avoidance behavior (Telegdy and Kovács,

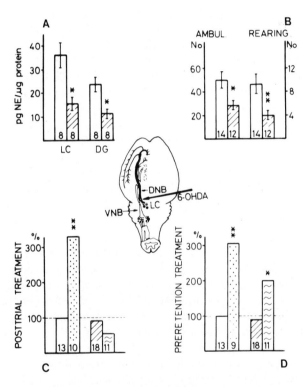

Fig. 5. Effects of arginine[8]-vasopressin on memory processes after lesioning of the dorsal noradrenergic bundle. Scheme represents the major noradrenergic pathways in the brain. DNB, dorsal noradrenergic bundle; VNB, ventral noradrenergic bundle; LC, locus coeruleus; arrow denotes the site of the lesion: microinjection of 6-OHDA (10 μg bilaterally). A: effects of lesion on the norepinephrine contents of the locus coeruleus (LC) and dentate gyrus (DG). □, sham-lesioned; ▨, lesioned. B: effects of lesion on the ambulation and rearing activities in an open field. Open-field behavior was measured in an open circular arena according to Weijnen and Slangen (1970) (Symbols: see A). C: effect of vasopressin on memory consolidation processes in DNB-lesioned animals. Arginine[8]-vasopressin (5 μg, s.c.) was injected immediately after a single learning trial and passive avoidance behavior was measured 24 h later. The data are expressed as percentages of the sham-operated saline treated controls. □, sham-operated + saline; ▧, sham-operated + AVP; ▨, 6-OHDA + saline; ▨, 6-OHDA + AVP. D: effect of vasopressin on memory retrieval in DNB-lesioned animals. Arginine[8]-vasopressin was injected 1 h before the retention trial (Symbols: see C).

1979a). However, the question as to whether noradrenergic or dopaminergic mechanisms (or both) are involved still remains open, nor can a role of the serotoninergic system be ruled out (Ramaekers et al., 1977).

The question has been approached by lesioning specific neurotransmitter pathways with neurotoxic drugs. Microinjection of 6-hydroxydopamine (6-OHDA) into the dorsal noradrenergic bundle causes degeneration of noradrenergic neurons, and results in a concomitant fall of forebrain and brain stem norepinephrine (Fig. 5A); (see also Roberts et al., 1976; Mason and Iversen, 1977; Kovács et al., 1979a). The lesion also decreases open-field ambulation and rearing (Fig. 5B). The effect of arginine[8]-vasopressin has been investigated in dorsal noradrenergic bundle-lesioned rats: a high amount (5 μg) of the peptide was injected s.c. either immediately after the single learning trial to test consolidation of memory (Fig. 5C), or 1 h prior to the retention to measure retrieval of memory (Fig. 5D). Post-trial AVP treatment did not facilitate passive avoidance reaction in DNB-lesioned animals, suggesting that the intact dorsal noradrenergic bundle is essential for a facilitating effect of vasopressin on memory consolidation. When the neuropeptide was administered shortly before the retention trial, its effect was present (although attenuated) in DNB-lesioned rats; thus, the retrieval effect of the neuropeptide was not abolished.

These results imply that consolidation and retrieval of newly-acquired information involve different neurotransmitter pathways (Kovács et al., 1979a) and that the dorsal noradrenergic bundle may play an essential role in mediating the influences of the neuropeptide on memory consolidation.

Bilateral destruction of the mesolimbic accumbens nucleus by 6-OHDA, or selective lesioning of the ascending serotoninergic system by 5,6-dihydroxytryptamine (5,6-DHT), did not interfere with the ability of vasopressin to induce facilitated memory consolidation, which shows that the role of the dorsal noradrenergic bundle seems to be rather selective (Kovács et al., 1979a). With regard to its effect on the retrieval processes, on the other hand, vasopressin has been suggested as acting via dopaminergic neurotransmission (Van Ree et al., 1978a, Telegdy and Kovács, 1979a).

Extrahypothalamic vasopressinergic and oxytocinergic fibers originating in the hypothalamic magnocellular nuclei project to limbic and midbrain areas (Sofroniew and Weindl, 1978; Buijs et al., 1978; Kozlowski et al., 1978; etc.). Therefore, the concept that neuropeptides may act as either neurotransmitters or neuromodulators (Barker and Gainer, 1974; Barker et al., 1978; Barker and Smith, 1980; Hökfelt et al., 1978) has gained anatomical support. As a neurotransmitter in the CNS, vasopressin should supposedly be released from presynaptic stores of the peptidergic neurons and interact with specific receptors on the postsynaptic membrane. As a neuromodulator, vasopressin could exert its effect presynaptically, by modifying synthesis and/or release of transmitters through axo-axonic synapses. Alternatively, it may affect the postsynaptic membranes, e.g. at the level of transmitter-sensitive receptors. It was of interest to study, therefore, whether the interaction of vasopressin with catecholaminergic neurotransmission takes place via regions containing the catecholamine cell bodies or via brain areas which contain the catecholaminergic terminals.

Microinjection of arginine[8]-vasopressin directly into the region which contains the cell bodies, the locus coeruleus, did not influence passive avoidance behavior (Kovács et al., 1979a), whereas the same amount of the peptide facilitated passive avoidance when injected into the regions which contain the terminals (septum, hippocampus, dorsal raphe). Thus, it might be tentatively concluded that the site of action of vasopressin is not located on noradrenergic cell bodies but rather in the terminal regions (Kovács et al., 1979a). Although this implies the possibility of a direct interaction via the terminals, it can not be excluded that the circuitry is more complex and that interneurons are transferring the information to the terminals. Using a different approach, Schulz et al. (1979) investigated the interaction of vasopressin and oxytocin with nigrostriatal dopaminergic neurons, and concluded that both peptides influence this system, independent of the cell bodies in the substantia nigra, most probably by eventually interacting with presynaptic dopaminergic terminals in the striatum.

Vasopressin facilitates memory consolidation when injected into the dorsal raphe nucleus. The synaptic organization of the raphe area has offered a model to investigate further the problem of terminals vs cell bodies. Serotoninergic cell bodies of the raphe nuclei give rise to fibers ascending in many forebrain regions (Anden et al., 1966; Daly et al., 1973; Fuxe and Jonsson, 1973). The serotoninergic cell bodies, on the other hand, receive noradrenergic afferents relayed from the locus coeruleus, and these noradrenergic terminals modulate the activity of the indolaminergic cells (Loizou, 1969; Jouvet, 1969; Kostowski et al., 1974; Roizen and Jacobowitz, 1976; Anderson et al., 1977; etc.). By means of local microinjection of selective neurotoxins into the raphe region, serotoninergic cell bodies (5,6-DHT) or catecholaminergic terminals (6-OHDA) can be destroyed independently of each other.

The results are depicted in Fig. 6. Local microinjection of arginine[8]-vasopressin into the dorsal raphe nucleus (given immediately after the learning trial) facilitated passive avoidance behavior 24 h after the learning trial. This effect was absent, however, when serotoninergic neurotoxin (5,6-DHT) or catecholaminergic neurotoxin (6-OHDA) was microinjected into the raphe area 10 days prior to the behavioral testing (Fig. 6). It might be supposed that the effects of vasopressin are primarily via the catecholaminergic nerve terminals directly, rather than via the serotoninergic cell bodies in the raphe area. This effect, however, results in secondary changes in the ascending indolaminergic system, as indicated by the observation that the serotoninergic neurotoxin also prevents the effect of the neuropeptide.

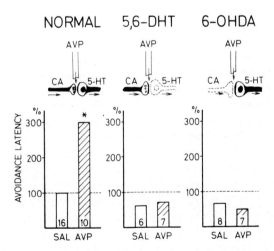

Fig. 6. Effect on memory consolidation of arginine[8]-vasopressin microinjected into the dorsal raphe nucleus: interference of locally-administered neurotoxic compounds. Normal: arginine[8]-vasopressin (50 pg) was microinjected into the dorsal raphe nucleus immediately after a single learning trial, and the passive avoidance behavior was tested 24 h later. Avoidance latency is expressed as a percentage of the saline-treated controls. 5,6-DHT: a serotoninergic neurotoxin (5,6-DHT, 10 μg) was injected into the raphe area 10 days prior to the behavioral testing. 6-OHDA: a catecholaminergic neurotoxin (6-OHDA, 10 μg) was injected into the raphe nucleus 10 days before the testing of passive avoidance.

In conclusion, the above data support the hypothesis that during the phase of memory consolidation, facilitated synaptic transmission in certain limbic-midbrain terminals of the dorsal noradrenergic bundle is presumably the initial event in the action of vasopressin on memory processes. This initial step then ultimately leads to changes in other neurotransmitter systems (e.g. serotoninergic neurotransmission), probably resulting in long-lasting biochemical changes. Blockade of the initial effect on neurotransmission by lesioning of the dorsal noradrenergic bundle prevents the subsequent steps which lead to facilitated consolidation of information. In contrast, facilitation of transmission, e.g. by local microinjection of the peptide into limbic-midbrain structures, favors the occurrence of consolidation.

NEUROPEPTIDE–NEUROTRANSMITTER INTERACTION: PHARMACOLOGICAL ARTIFACT OR PHYSIOLOGICAL REALITY?

De Wied et al. (1976) suggested that vasopressin might be involved in the normal, physiological regulation of learning and memory processes. This conclusion was based on experiments involving Brattleboro rats with hereditary hypothalamic diabetes insipidus (Valtin and Schroeder, 1964) as well as the effects of centrally administered anti-vasopressin serum. Both normal animals, following neutralization of centrally available vasopressin by specific antiserum (Wimersma-Greidanus et al., 1975b), and homozygous Brattleboro rats with diabetes insipidus (De Wied et al., 1975; Bohus et al., 1975b; Telegdy and Kovács, 1979b) exhibit a memory deficit. The inferior learning and memory is readily restored by the administration of vasopressin and vasopressin fragments (De Wied et al., 1975). The therapeutic value of vasopressin in amnestic patients (Oliveros et al., 1978) and its correlation with alterations of mood (Gold et al., 1978; Raskind et al., 1979) have also provided evidence that our understanding of behavioral and biochemical processes leading to CNS effects of posterior pituitary peptides is of significance.

In view of the likely physiological role of vasopressin (transported to cerebral target sites either by vascular or cerebrospinal circulation or by extrahypothalamic vasopressinergic fibers) on memory processes, it was logical to pose the question whether the effects of decreased amounts of neuropeptide in the brain would result in changes of "classical" neurotransmitter activities. If these changes were opposite to those found after increasing the intracerebral concentration of vasopressin, this would support the idea of a physiological modulating influence of the neuropeptide on these transmitter systems.

The biochemical and behavioral experiments done so far show that endogenous vasopressin in the central nervous system may indeed modulate monoaminergic neurotransmission. The catecholamine metabolism of homozygous Brattleboro rats with diabetes insipidus differs from those of homozygous non-diabetic (Versteeg et al., 1978) or heterozygous non-diabetic (Kovács et al., 1979c) littermates of the same strain. In various brain regions these differences are opposite to those which were observed in normal rats following vasopressin challenge (Versteeg et al., 1978; Telegdy and Kovács, 1979b). Furthermore, intraventricular administration of a vasopressin (Tanaka et al., 1977b) and of the antiserum against the neuropeptide influence the catecholamine turnover in opposite directions in some brain areas (Versteeg et al., 1979).

In recent experiments the effects of anti-vasopressin serum injected into the dorsal raphe nucleus was studied on the passive avoidance reaction of rats (Kovács et al., 1980a). It appeared that administration of the antiserum impairs passive avoidance behavior, as does the intraventricular administration of the serum (Wimersma-Greidanus et al., 1975b). This suggests that the normal, tonic influence of vasopressin in the raphe area is essential for the consolidation of memory. When, however, the antiserum was injected into animals in which the catecholaminergic terminals of the raphe region had been selectively destroyed by 6-OHDA, anti-vasopressin serum did not influence behavior. The results of these experiments also confirm the concept that the interaction of posterior pituitary peptides with neurotransmitters may well be a process that occurs physiologically in the brain.

Finally, it is of interest that McEntee and Mair (1978), in patients with Korsakoff's psychosis, described a decreased activity of the ascending noradrenergic pathway, which was likely to be related to the disturbances of memory processes. On the other hand, amnestic patients exhibiting this syndrome can be efficiently treated with vasopressin (Oliveros et al., 1978).

CONCLUDING REMARKS

Results of recent research have led to the concept that the interaction of posterior pituitary neuropeptides, vasopressin and oxytocin, with monoaminergic neurotransmitter mechanisms in the brain is of essential importance for the action of these peptides on memory processes. An increasing body of evidence, coming from behavioral, biochemical and from combined behavioral–biochemical studies favor the existence of a physiological, modulating influence of these neuropeptides on particular neurotransmitter systems. This neuropeptide–neurotransmitter interaction is presumably an essential permissive event in the mediation of neurohumoral influences on information processing. The involvement of neuropeptides in mental disease states has become a matter of major interest. The results of first human data concerning treatments with posterior pituitary neuropeptides are encouraging. It might be speculated that imbalances in neuropeptide–neurotransmitter interactions in the brain are contributing to certain human psychopathological disorders.

REFERENCES

Ader, R. and De Wied, D. (1972) Effects of lysine vasopressin on passive avoidance learning. *Psychon. Sci.*, 29: 46–48.

Ader, R., Weijnen, J.A.W.M. and Moleman, P. (1972) Retention of a passive avoidance response as a function of the intensity and duration of electric shock. *Psychon. Sci.*, 26: 125–129.

Andén, N.E., Dahlström, A., Fuxe, K., Larsson, K., Olsson, L., and Ungerstedt, U. (1966) Ascending monoamine neurons to the telencephalon and diencephalon. *Acta physiol. scand.*, 67: 313–326.

Anderson, C.D., Pasquier, D.A., Forbes, W.B. and Morgane, P.J. (1977) Locus coeruleus-to-dorsal raphe input examined by electrophysiological and morphological methods. *Brain Res. Bull.*, 2: 209–221.

Anlezark, G.M., Crow, T.J. and Greenway, A.P. (1973) Impaired learning and decreased cortical norepinephrine after bilateral locus coeruleus lesions. *Science*, 181: 682–684.

Barchas, J. and Usdin, E. (1973) *Serotonin and Behavior*, Academic Press, New York.

Barker, J.L. and Gainer, H. (1974) Peptide regulation of bursting pacemaker activity in a molluscan neurosecretory cell. *Science*, 184: 1371–1373.

Barker, J.L., Gruol, D.L., Huang, L.M., Neale, J.H. and Smith T.G. (1978) Enkephalin: pharmacological evidence for diverse functional roles in the nervous system using cultures of dissociated spinal neurons. In *Characteristics and Function of Opioids*, J.M. van Ree and L. Terenius (Eds.), Elsevier/North-Holland, Amsterdam, pp. 87–98.

Barker, J.L. and Smith, T.G. (1980) Three modes of intercellular neuronal communication. In *Adaptive Capabilities of the Nervous System, Progress in Brain Research, Vol. 53*, P. McConnell, G.J. Boer, H.J. Romijn, N. van de Poll and M.A. Corner (Eds.), Elsevier, Amsterdam, pp. 169–192.

136

Bohus, B., Ader, R. and De Wied, D. (1972) Effects of vasopressin on active and passive avoidance behavior. *Horm. Behav.*, 3: 191–197.

Bohus, B., Hendrickx, H.H.L., Van Kolfschoten, A.A. and Krediet, T.C. (1975a) Effect of $ACTH_{4-10}$ on copulatory and sexually motivated approach behavior in the male rat. In *Sexual Behavior: Pharmacology and Biochemistry*, M. Sandler and G.L. Gessa (Eds.), Raven Press, New York, pp. 269–275.

Bohus, B., Kovács, G.L. and De Wied, D. (1978a) Oxytocin, vasopressin and memory: opposite effects on consolidation and retrieval processes. *Brain Res.*, 157: 414–417.

Bohus, B., Urban, I., Wimersma-Greidanus, Tj.B. van and De Wied, D. (1978b) Opposite effects of oxytocin and vasopressin on avoidance behaviour and hippocampal theta rhythm in the rat. *Neuropharmacology*, 17: 239–247.

Bohus, B., Wimersma-Greidanus, Tj.B. van and De Wied, D. (1975b) Behavioral and endocrine responses of rats with hereditary hypothalamic diabetes insipidus (Brattleboro strain). *Physiol. Behav.*, 14: 609–615.

Bookin, H.B. and Pfeifer, W.D. (1977) Effect of lysine vasopressin on pentylenetetrazol-induced retrograde amnesia in rats. *Pharmacol. Biochem. Behav.*, 7: 51–54.

Buijs, R.M., Swaab, D.F., Dogterom, J. and Leeuwen, F.W. van (1978) Intra- and extrahypothalamic vasopressin and oxytocin pathways in the rat. *Cell. Tiss. Res.*, 186: 423–433.

Buijs, R.M., Velis, D. and Swaab, D.F. (1980) Extrahypothalamic vasopressin and oxytocin innervation of fetal and adult rat brain. In *Adaptive Capabilities of the Nervous System, Progress in Brain Research, Vol. 53*, P. McConnell, G.J. Boer, H.J. Romijn, N. van de Poll and M.A. Corner (Eds.), Elsevier, Amsterdam, pp. 159–167.

Castel, M. (1978) Immunocytochemical evidence for vasopressin receptors, *J. Histochem. Cytochem.*, 26: 581–592.

Corrodi, H. and Hanson, L.C.F. (1966) Central effects of an inhibitor of tyrosine hydroxylation. *Psychopharmacologia (Berl.)*, 10: 116–125.

Crow, T.J. (1968) Cortical synapses and reinforcement: a hypothesis, *Nature (Lond.)*, 219: 736–737.

Dahlström, A. and Fuxe, K. (1964) Evidence for the existence of monoamine neurons in the central nervous system. I. Demonstration of monoamines in the cell bodies of brain stem neurons. *Acta physiol. scand.*, 62: Suppl. 232, 1–55.

Daly, J., Fuxe, K. and Jonsson, G. (1973) Effects of intracerebral injections of 5,6-hydroxytryptamine on central monoamine neurons: evidence for selective degeneration of central 5-hydroxytryptamine neurons. *Brain Res.*, 49: 476–482.

De Wied, D. (1964) Influence of anterior pituitary on avoidance learning and escape behavior. *Amer. J. Physiol.*, 207: 255–259.

De Wied, D. (1969) Effects of peptide hormones on behaviour. In *Frontiers in Neuroendocrinology*, W.F. Ganong and L. Martini (Eds.), Oxford University Press, New York, pp. 97–140.

De Wied, D. (1971) Long term effect of vasopressin on the maintenance of a conditioned avoidance response in rats. *Nature (Lond.)*, 232: 58–60.

De Wied, D. (1974) Pituitary–adrenal system hormones and behavior. In *The Neurosciences, 3rd Study Program*, F.O. Schmitt and F.G. Worden (Eds.), MIT Press, Cambridge Mass., pp. 653–666.

De Wied, D. and Bohus, B. (1966) Long term and short term effects on retention of a conditioned avoidance response in rats by treatment with long acting Pitressin and α-MSH. *Nature (Lond.)*, 212: 1484–1486.

De Wied, D., Bohus, B. and Wimersma-Greidanus, Tj.B. van (1975) Memory deficit in rats with hereditary diabetes insipidus. *Brain Res.*, 85: 152–156.

De Wied, D. and Gispen, W.H. (1977) Behavioral effects of peptides. In *Peptides in Neurobiology*, H. Gainer (Ed.), Plenum Press, New York, pp. 391–442.

De Wied, D., Kovács, G.L., Bohus, B., van Ree, J.M. and Greven, H.M. (1978) Neuroleptic activity of the neuropeptide β-LPH_{62-77}/des-tyr^1-γ-endorphin/; DTγE. *Europ. J. Pharmacol.*, 49: 427–436.

De Wied, D., Wimersma-Greidanus, Tj.B. van, Bohus, B., Urban, I. and Gispen, W.H. (1976) Vasopressin and memory consolidation. In *Perspectives in Brain Research, Progr. Brain Res., Vol. 45*, M.A. Corner and D.F. Swaab (Eds.), Elsevier, Amsterdam, pp. 181–191.

Dunn, A.J., Iuvone, P.M. and Rees, H.D. (1976) Neurochemical responses of mice to ACTH and lysine vasopressin. *Pharmacol. Biochem. Behav.*, 5: Suppl. 1, 139–145.

Endröczi, E. (1972) *Limbic System, Learning and Pituitary-Adrenal Function*, Akadémiai Kiadó, Budapest.

Endröczi, E. (1980) ACTH-like peptides, pituitary–adrenocortical function and avoidance behavior. In *Adaptive Capabilities of the Nervous System, Progress in Brain Research, Vol. 53*, P. McConell, G.J. Boer, H.J. Romijn, N. van de Poll and M.A. Corner (Eds.), Elsevier, Amsterdam, pp. 111–121.

Essman, W.B. (1971) Drug effects on learning and memory processes. In *Advances in Pharmacology and Chemotherapy, Vol. 8*, S. Garattini, A. Goldin, F. Hawking and I.J. Kopin (Eds.), Academic Press, New York, pp. 241–330.

Essman, W.B. (1973) Pharmacological alteration of the retrograde amnestic effect of electroconvulsive shock: the modification of forebrain 5-hydroxytryptamine in mice. *Pharmacol. Res. Commun.*, 5: 295–302.

Fuxe, K. and Jonsson, G. (1973) Further mapping of central 5-hydroxytryptamine neurons: studies with the neurotoxic dihydroxytryptamines. In *Serotonin – New Vistas, Advances in Biochemical Psychopharmacology, Vol. 10*, E. Costa, G.L. Gessa and M. Sandler (Eds.), Raven Press, New York, pp. 1–12.

Gold, P., Goodwin, F.K. and Reus, V.I. (1978) Vasopressin in affective illness. *Lancet*, 1: 1233–1235.

Haycock, J.W., Van Buskirk, R. and Gold, P.E. (1977) Effects on retention of posttraining amphetamine injection in mice: interaction with pretraining experience. *Psychopharmacologia (Berl.)*, 54: 21–24.

Hökfelt, T., Elde, R., Johansson, O., Ljungdahl, A., Schultzberg, M., Fuxe, K., Goldstein, M., Nilsson, G., Pernow, B., Terenius, L., Ganten, D., Jeffcoate, S.L., Rehfeld, J. and Said, S. (1978) Distribution of peptide-containing neurons. In *Psychopharmacology: a Generation of Progress*, M.A. Lipton, A. DiMascio and K.F. Killam (Eds.), Raven Press, New York, pp. 39–66.

Hraschek, Á., Pavlik, A. and Endröczi, E. (1977) Brain catecholamine metabolism and avoidance conditioning in rats. *Acta physiol. Acad. Sci. hung.*, 49: 119–123.

Jacobs, B.L., Wise, W.D. and Taylor, K.M. (1974) Differential behavioral and neurochemical effects following lesions of the dorsal and median raphe nuclei in rats. *Brain Res.*, 79: 353–361.

Jones, B.E. and Moore, R.Y. (1977) Ascending projections of the locus coeruleus in the rat. II. Autoradiographic study. *Brain Res.*, 127: 23–53.

Jouvet, M. (1969) Biogenic amines and the states of sleep. *Science*, 163: 32–41.

Kety, S.S. (1970) The biogenic amines in the central nervous system: their possible roles in arousal, emotion and learning. In *The Neurosciences*, F.O. Schmitt (Ed.), Rockefeller University Press, New York, pp. 329–336.

Knoll, B., Timár, J., Jóna, G. and Knoll, J. (1976) Serotonin metabolism and learning. In *Symposium on Pharmacology of Catecholaminergic and Serotonergic Mechanisms*, K. Magyar (Ed.), Akadémiai Kiadó, Budapest, pp. 27–32.

Knoll, J. (1973) Modulations of learning and retention by amphetamines. In *Proceedings of the 5th International Congress of Pharmacology, Brain Nerves and Synapses, Vol. 4*, T.E. Bloom and G.H. Acheson (Eds.), Karger, Basel, pp. 55–68.

Koda, L.T., Wise, R.A. and Bloom, F.E. (1978) Light and electron microscopic changes in the rat dentate gyrus after lesions or stimulation of the ascending locus coeruleus pathway. *Brain Res.*, 144: 363–368.

Kostowski, W., Giacalone, E., Garattini, S. and Valzelli, L. (1968) Studies on behavioural and biochemical changes in rats after lesions of midbrain raphe. *Europ. J. Pharmacol.*, 4: 371–376.

Kostowski, W., Giacalone, E., Garattini, S. and Valzelli, L. (1969) Electrical stimulation of midbrain raphe: biochemical, behavioral and bioelectric effects. *Europ. J. Pharmacol.*, 7: 170–175.

Kostowski, W., Samanin, R., Bareggi, S.R., Marc, V., Garattini, S. and Valzelli, L. (1974) Biochemical aspects of the interaction between midbrain raphe and locus coeruleus in the rat. *Brain Res.*, 82: 178–182.

Kovács, G.L., Bohus, B. and Versteeg, D.H.G. (1979a) Facilitation of memory consolidation by vasopressin: mediation by terminals of the dorsal noradrenergic bundle?, *Brain Res.*, 172: 73–85.

Kovács, G.L., Bohus, B., Versteeg, D.H.G., De Kloet, E.R. and De Wied, D. (1979b) Effect of oxytocin and vasopressin on memory consolidation: sites of action and catecholaminergic correlates after local microinjection into limbic-midbrain structures. *Brain Res.*, 175: 303–314.

Kovács, G.L. and De Wied, D. (1978) Effects of amphetamine and haloperidol on avoidance behavior and exploratory activity. *Europ. J. Pharmacol.*, 53: 103–107.

Kovács, G.L., Szabó, G., Szontágh, L., Medve, L., Telegdy, G. and László, F. (1979c) Hereditary diabetes insipidus in rats: altered cerebral indolamine and catecholamine metabolism. *Neuroendocrinology*, in press.

Kovács, G.L. and Telegdy, C. (1976) Inhibitory effect of midbrain raphe stimulation on the maintenance of an active avoidance reflex. *Pharmacol. Biochem. Behav.*, 5: 709–711.

Kovács, G.L. and Telegdy, G. (1978) Indolamines and behaviour. The possible role of serotoninergic mechanisms in the pituitary–adrenocortical hormone-induced behavioural actions. In *Results in Neuroendocrinology, Neurochemistry and Sleep Research*, K. Lissák (Ed.), Akadémiai Kiadó, Budapest, pp. 31–97.

Kovács, G.L., Vécsei, L. and Telegdy, G. (1978) Opposite action of oxytocin to vasopressin in passive avoidance behaviour in rats. *Physiol. Behav.*, 20: 801–802.

Kovács, G.L., Vécsei, L., Medve, L. and Telegdy, G. (1980a) Effect of the endogenous vasopressin content of the brain on memory processes: the role of catecholaminergic mechanisms. *Exp. Brain Res.*, 38: 357–361.

Kovács, G.L., Vécsei, L., Szabó, G. and Telegdy, G. (1977) The involvement of catecholaminergic mechanisms in the behavioural action of vasopressin. *Neurosci. Lett.*, 5: 337–344.

Kovács, G.L., Versteeg, D.H.G., De Kloet, E.R. and Bohus, B. (1980b) Good and poor avoidance performance correlates with α-MPT-induced catecholamine disappearance in discrete rat brain regions, submitted.

Kozlowski, G.P., Brownfield, M.S. and Hostetter, G. (1978) Neurosecretory supply to extrahypothalamic structures: choroid plexus, circumventricular organs and limbic system. In *Neurosecretion and Neuroendocrine Activity. Evolution, Structure and Function*, W. Bargmann, A. Oksche, A.L. Polenow and B. Scharrer (Eds.), Springer, Berlin, pp. 217–227.

Lande, S., Flexner, J.B. and Flexner, L.B. (1972) Effect of corticotropin and desglycinamide-9-lysine vasopressin on suppression of memory by puromycin. *Proc. nat. Acad. Sci. (Wash.)*, 69: 558–560.

Legros, J.L., Gilot, P., Seron, X., Claessens, J., Adams, A., Moeglen, J.M., Audibert, A. and Berchier, P. (1978) Influence of vasopressin on learning and memory. *Lancet*, 1: 41–42.

Loizou, L.A. (1969) Projections of the nucleus locus coeruleus in the albino rat. *Brain Res.*, 15: 563–566.

Lorens, S.A., Sorenson, J.P. and Yunger, L.M. (1971) Behavioral and neurochemical effects of lesions in the raphe system of the rat. *J. comp. physiol. Psychol.*, 77: 48–52.

Mason, S.T. and Fibiger, H.C. (1978) Evidence for a role of brain noradrenaline in attention and stimulus sampling, *Brain Res.*, 159: 421–426.

Mason, S.T. and Iversen, S.D. (1977) Behavioural basis of the dorsal bundle extinction effect. *Pharmacol. Biochem. Behav.*, 7: 373–379.

McEntee, W.J. and Mair, R.G. (1978) Memory impairment in Korsakoff's psychosis: a correlation with brain noradrenergic activity. *Science*, 202: 905–907.

McGaugh, J.L. (1973) Drug facilitation of learning and memory. *Ann. Rev. Pharmacol.*, 13: 229–241.

McGaugh, J.L., Gold, P.E., Van Buskirk, R. and Haycock, J. (1975) Modulating influences of hormones and catecholamines on memory storage processes. In *Hormones, Homeostasis and the Brain*, W.H. Gispen, Tj.B. van Wimersma Greidanus, B. Bohus and D. De Wied (Eds.), Elsevier, Amsterdam, pp. 151–162.

Miller, L.H., Kastin, A.J., Sandman, C.A., Fink, M. and Van Veen, W.J. (1974) Polypeptide influences on attention, memory and anxiety in man. *Pharmacol. Biochem. Behav.*, 2: 663–668.

Oliveros, J.C., Jandali, M.K., Timsit-Berthier, M., Remy, R., Benghezal, A., Audibert, A. and Moeglen, J.M. (1978) Vasopressin in amnesia. *Lancet*, 1: 42.

Pálfai, T., Brown, O.M. and Walsh, T.J. (1978) Catecholamine levels in the whole brain and the probability of memory formation are not related. *Pharmacol. Biochem. Behav.*, 8: 717–721.

Palkovits, M. (1973) Isolated removal of hypothalamic or other brain nuclei of the rat. *Brain Res.*, 59: 449–450.

Pasquier, D.A., Kemper, T.L., Forbes, W.B. and Morgane, P.J. (1977) Dorsal raphe, substantia nigra and locus coeruleus: interconnections with each other and the neostriatum. *Brain Res. Bull.*, 2: 323–339.

Ramaekers, F., Rigter, H. and Leonard, B.E. (1977) Parallel changes in behaviour and hippocampal serotonin metabolism in rats following treatment with desglycinamide lysine vasopressin. *Brain Res.*, 120: 485–492.

Ranje, C. and Ungerstedt, U. (1977) High correlations between number of dopamine cells, dopamine levels and motor performance. *Brain Res.*, 134: 83–93.

Raskind, M., Orenstein, H. and Weitzman, R.E. (1979) Vasopressin in depression. *Lancet*, 1: 164.

Rigter, H., van Riezen, H. and De Wied, D. (1974) The effects of ACTH- and vasopressin-analogues on CO_2-induced retrograde amnesia in rats. *Physiol. Behav.*, 13, 120: 485–492.

Rigter, H. and van Riezen, H. (1978) Hormones and memory. In *Psychopharmacology: A Generation of Progress*, M.A. Lipton, A. DiMascio and K.F. Killam (Eds.), Raven Press, New York, pp. 677–689.

Roberts, D.C., Price, M.T.C. and Fibiger, H.C. (1976) The dorsal tegmental noradrenergic projection: an analysis of its role in maze learning. *J. comp. physiol. Psychol.*, 90: 363–372.

Roizen, M.F. and Jacobowitz, D.M. (1976) Studies on the origin of innervation of noradrenergic area bordering on the nucleus raphe dorsalis. *Brain Res.*, 101: 561–568.

Sandman, C.A., George, J., Walker, B.B., Nolan, J.D. and Kastin, A.J. (1976) Neuropeptide MSH/ACTH 4–10 enhances attention in the mentally retarded. *Pharmacol. Biochem. Behav.*, 5: Suppl. 1, 23–28.

Schulz, H., Kovács, G.L. and Telegdy, G. (1974) Effect of physiological doses of vasopressin and oxytocin on avoidance and exploratory behaviour in rats. *Acta physiol. Acad. Sci. hung.*, 45: 211–215.

Schulz, H., Kovács, G.L. and Telegdy, G. (1976) The effect of vasopressin and oxytocin on avoidance behaviour in rats. In *Cellular and Molecular Bases of Neuroendocrine Processes*, E. Endröczi (Ed.), Akadémiai Kiadó, Budapest, pp. 555–564.

Schulz, H., Kovács, G.L. and Telegdy, G. (1979) Action of posterior pituitary neuropeptides on the nigro-striatal dopaminergic system. *Europ. J. Pharmacol.*, 57: 185–190.

Schulz, H., Unger, H., Schwarzberg, H., Pommrich, G. and Stolze, R. (1971) Neuronenaktivität hypothalamischer Kerngebiete von Kaninchen nach intraventrikulärer Applikation von Vasopressin und Oxytocin. *Experientia (Basel)*, 27: 1482–1483.

Schwarzberg, H., Hartmann, G., Kovács, G.L. and Telegdy, G. (1976) Effect of intraventricular oxytocin and vasopressin on self-stimulation in rats. *Acta physiol. Acad. Sci. hung.*, 47: 127–131.

Sofroniew, M.V. and Weindl, A. (1978) Projections from the parvocellular vasopressin- and neurophysin-containing neurons of the suprachiasmatic nucleus. *Amer. J. Anat.*, 153: 391–430.

Sterba, G. (1974) Ascending neurosecretory pathway of the peptidergic type. In *Neurosecretion – The Final Neuroendocrine Pathway*, F. Knowles and L. Vollrath (Eds.), Springer, Berlin, pp. 38–47.

Sterba, G., Hoheisel, G., Wegelin, R., Naumann, W. and Schober, F. (1979) Peptide containing vesicles within neuro-neural synapses. *Brain Res.*, 169: 55–64.

Stevens, D.A. (1970) The effects of *p*-chlorophenylalanine on behavior: III. Facilitation of brightness discrimination in satiated rats. *Life Sci.*, 9: 1127–1134.

Tanaka, M., De Kloet, E.R., De Wied, D. and Versteeg, D.H.G. (1977b) Arginine[8]-vasopressin affects catecholamine metabolism in specific brain nuclei. *Life Sci.*, 20: 1799–1808.

Tanaka, M., Versteeg, D.H.G. and De Wied, D. (1977a) Regional effects of vasopressin on rat brain catecholamine metabolism. *Neurosci. Lett.*, 4: 321–325.

Telegdy, G. and Kovács, G.L. (1979a) Role of monoamines in mediating the action of hormones on learning and memory. In *Brain Mechanisms in Memory and Learning: from Single Neuron to Man, IBRO Monograph Series Vol. 4*, M.A.B. Brazier (Ed.), Raven Press, New York, pp. 249–268.

Telegdy, G. and Kovács, G.L. (1979b) Role of monoamines in mediating the action of ACTH, vasopressin and oxytocin. In *Central Nervous System Effects of Hypothalamic Hormones and Other Peptides*, R. Collu, A. Barbeau, J.R. Ducharme and J.G. Rochefort (Eds.), Raven Press, New York, pp. 189–205.

Timsit-Berthier, M., Audibert, A. and Moeglen, J.W. (1978) Influence de la lysine-vasopressine sur l'EEG chez l'homme. *Neuropsychobiology*, 4: 129–139.

Ungerstedt, U. (1971) Stereotaxic mapping of the monoamine pathway in the rat brain. *Acta physiol. scand.*, 367: 1–49.

Valtin, H. and Schroeder, H.A. (1964) Familial hypothalamic diabetes insipidus in rats (Brattleboro strain). *Amer. J. Physiol.*, 206: 424–430.

Van der Gugten, J., Palkovits, M., Wijnen, H.J.L.M. and Versteeg, D.H.G. (1976) Regional distribution of adrenaline in rat brain. *Brain Res.*, 107: 171–175.

Van Praag, H.M. and Verhoeven, W.M.A. (1980) Neuropeptides. A new dimension in biological psychiatry. In *Adaptive Capabilities of the Nervous System, Progress in Brain Research, Vol. 53*, P. McConnell, G.J. Boer, H.J. Romijn, N. van de Poll and M.A. Corner (Eds.), Elsevier, Amsterdam, pp. 229–252.

Van Ree, J.M., Bohus, B., Versteeg, D.H.G. and De Wied, D. (1978a) Neurohypophyseal principles and memory processes. *Biochem. Pharmacol.*, 28: 1793–1800.

Van Ree, J.M. and De Wied, D. (1977) Modulation of heroin self-administration by neurohypophyseal principles. *Europ. J. Pharmacol.*, 43: 199–202.

Van Ree, J.M., Dorsa, D.M. and Colpaert, F.C. (1978b) Neuropeptides and drug dependence. In *Characteristics and Function of Opioids,* J.M. van Ree and L. Terenius (Eds.), Elsevier, Amsterdam, pp. 1–12.

Verhoeven, W.M.A., Van Praag, H.M., Botter, P.A., Sunier, A., Van Ree, J.M. and De Wied, D. (1978) (Des-tyr[1])-γ-endorphin in schizophrenia. *Lancet,* 1: 1046.

Versteeg, D.H.G., De Kloet, E.R., Wimersma-Greidanus, Tj.B. van and De Wied, D. (1979) Vasopressin modulates the activity of catecholamine containing neurons in specific brain regions. *Neurosci. Lett.,* 11: 69–73.

Versteeg, D.H.G., Tanaka, M. and De Kloet, E.R. (1978) Catecholamine concentrations and turnover in discrete regions of the brain of homozygous Brattleboro rats deficient in vasopressin. *Endocrinology,* 103: 1654–1661.

Walter, R., Hoffman, P.L., Flexner, J.B. and Flexner, L.B. (1975) Neurohypophyseal hormones, analogs and fragments: their effect on puromycin-induced amnesia. *Proc. natl. Acad. Sci. (Wash).,* 72: 4180–4184.

Weijnen, J.A.W.M. and Slangen, J.L. (1970) Effects of ACTH-analogues on extinction of conditioned behavior. In *Pituitary, Adrenal and the Brain, Progr. Brain Res., Vol. 32,* D. De Wied and J.A.W.M. Weijnen (Eds.), Elsevier, Amsterdam, pp. 221–235.

Wimersma-Greidanus, Tj.B. van, Croiset, B.G., Bakker, E. and Bouman, H. (1979) Amygdaloid lesions block the effect of neuropeptides (vasopressin, $ACTH_{4-10}$) on avoidance behavior. *Physiol. Behav.,* 22: 291–295.

Wimersma-Greidanus, Tj.B. van, Bohus, B. and De Wied, D. (1975a) CNS sites of action of ACTH, MSH and vasopressin in relation to avoidance behavior. In *Anatomical Neuroendocrinology,* W.E. Stumpf and L.D. Grant (Eds.), Karger, Basel, pp. 284–289.

Wimersma-Greidanus, Tj.B. van and De Wied, D. (1976) Dorsal hippocampus: a site of action of neuropeptides on avoidance behavior? *Pharmacol. Biochem. Behav.,* 5: Suppl. 1, 29–33.

Wimersma-Greidanus, Tj.B. van, Dogterom, J. and De Wied, D. (1975b) Intraventricular administration of anti-vasopressin serum inhibits memory consolidation in rats. *Life Sci,* 16: 637–644.

Exohypothalamic Axons of the Classic Neurosecretory System and their Synapses[*]

GÜNTHER STERBA, WILFRIED NAUMANN and GEORG HOHEISEL

Department of Cell Biology and Regulation, Section of Biosciences, Karl-Marx University, Leipzig (G.D.R.)

INTRODUCTION

Bargmann (1949) discovered that the Gomori chrome—alum—hematoxylin stain clearly differentiates the hypothalamic neurosecretory system within the mammalian brain. Subsequently, the method was used by many investigators to demonstrate this system in other vertebrate classes and, already in 1953, at the first International Symposium on Neurosecretion in Naples, it could be stated that the hypothalamic neurosecretory system is organized in the same manner throughout the vertebrate phylum. In the following two decades interest became so strongly concentrated on the neurosecretory nuclei, the neurosecretory pathway and the neurohypophysis, that observations about exohypothalamic neurosecretory fibers were either neglected or considered to be artefacts. Especially Barry (1954, 1961) and the Legaits (1956, 1957, 1958) conducted a large number of tests to study extrahypothalamic neurosecretory structures. However, since the staining methods used gave insufficient assurance that the nerve fibers demonstrated outside the hypothalamus were indeed part of the hypothalamic system, no wider attention was paid to these studies.

During the same period, a variety of central actions of posterior lobe hormones, the chemical mediators of the hypothalamic neurosecretory system, were described. Faure et al. (1959, 1960) started with studies about the action of oxytocin and vasopressin on the EEG of rabbits. De Wied and his team discovered the action of posterior lobe hormones on memory processes (de Wied, 1965; for reviews see: van Wimersma-Greidanus et al., 1976; de Wied and Gispen, 1977; de Wied and Bohus, 1978). Unger and coworkers investigated different cerebral actions after peripheral or intraventricular application of vasopressin and oxytocin (for reviews see Unger, 1977; Sterba, 1977) while still other laboratories reported similar central effects upon nervous function. From these results we obtained the idea that posterior lobe hormones have intracerebral targets where they act either directly or in a modified form, and that the so-called hypothalamic neurosecretory system is not only restricted to the hypothalamus but also may have direct connections with other brain regions.

At the sixth International Symposium on Neurosecretion in London (1973) the concept could be enunciated that the hypothalamo—neurohypophysial complex represents only the descending part of a more differentiated system, which includes an ascending part as well. However, whereas most of the fibers of the descending part release their products within the

---

* Dedicated to Professor Dr. M. Gersch on the occasion of his 70th birthday.

142

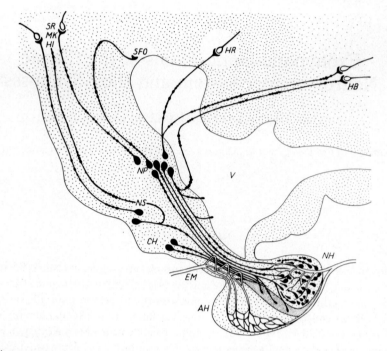

Fig. 1. Classic neurosecretory system of the mammal with its descending and ascending parts. AH, adeno-hypophysis; CH, chiasma; EM, median eminence; HB, hindbrain connection; HI, hippocampus connection; HR, habenular region; MK, amygdala nuclei; NH, neurohypophysis; NP, nucleus paraventricularis; NS, nucleus supraopticus; SFO, subfornical organ; SR, septal nuclei; V, third ventricle. The suprachiasmatic nucleus is involved in the ascending part too (Sofroniew and Weindl, 1978b; Buijs et al., 1978).

neurohypophysis directly into the blood circulation, most of the fibers of the ascending subsystem are not connected to capillaries but form true synapses with other neurons in different brain regions. The targets of the ascending fibers are mostly structures of the limbic

TABLE I

IMPORTANT TARGET REGIONS OF EXOHYPOTHALAMIC FIBRES IN THE VERTEBRATE CLASSES (BIBLIOGRAPHY AND OWN RESULTS)

1, rhinencephalic regions; 2, septal nuclei; 3, epithalamic nuclei and structures; 4, subfornical organ; 5, tectum opticum; 6, reticular formation of the midbrain; 7, somato-sensory and viscero-sensory areas of the caudal medulla. ○, proved by staining methods or by the pseudoisocyanine technique; ●, proved with immunocytochemical localization techniques as well.

	1	2	3	4	5	6	7
Cyclostomata	○	○	○		○	○	○
Chondrichthyes	○	○	○			○	○
Osteichthyes	○	○			○	●	●
Amphibia	●	●	●	●	○	○	○
Reptilia		○	○				
Aves	○	○	○	○	○	●	●
Mammalia	●	●	●	●	●	●	●

TABLE II

BRAIN AREAS OF THE RAT WHERE EXOHYPOTHALAMIC FIBRES OF THE CLASSIC NEURO-
SECRETORY SYSTEM COULD BE DEMONSTRATED. THE APPOSITE LITERATURE IS INDI-
CATED BY NUMBERS

NCH, suprachiasmatic nucleus; NP, paraventricular nucleus; NS, supraoptic nucleus.

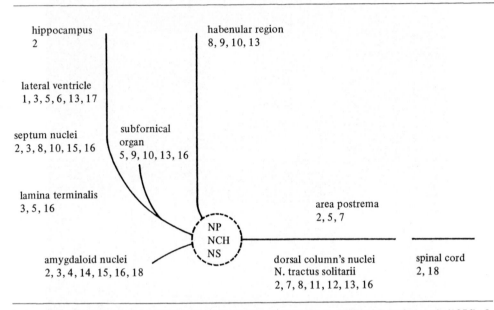

1, Brownfield and Kozlowski (1977); 2, Buijs (1978); 3, Buijs et al. (1978); 4, Burlet et al. (1976); 5,
Kozlowski et al. (1978); 6, Kozlowski et al. (1976); 7, Schober et al. (1977); 8, Sofroniew and Weindl
(1978a and b); 9, Sterba (1974b); 10, Sterba (1977); 11, Sterba (1978); 12, Sterba et al. (1979); 13,
Sterba und Schober (1979); 14, Swanson (1977); 15, Weindl and Sofroniew (1976); 16, Weindl and
Sofroniew (1978); 17, Weindl et al. (1976); 18, Wilkins et al. (1978).

system, but additional targets are situated both in the midbrain and hindbrain (Sterba,
1974a and b; Fig. 1, Tables I and II).

METHODS FOR DEMONSTRATING EXOHYPOTHALAMIC FIBERS OF THE CLASSIC
NEUROSECRETORY SYSTEM

Non-immunocytochemical techniques

As with the perikarya and fibers of the descending part of the system, the fibers of the
ascending part can be traced throughout their entire course by means of selective staining
with dyes. However, it has been established that not all relevant staining methods give
satisfactory results. In our own experience the best light microscopical visualization can be
obtained by the chrome–alum gallocyanine method according to Bock (1966). More sensitive, however, is the fluorescence microscopic method using pseudoisocyanine (Sterba,
1964). By this histochemical technique the disulfide groups of the neurophysin molecule are
oxidized to sulfonic acid groups, which in turn induce the association of the monomeric
pseudoisocyanine to polymeric aggregates. The polymeric pseudoisocyanine, but not the

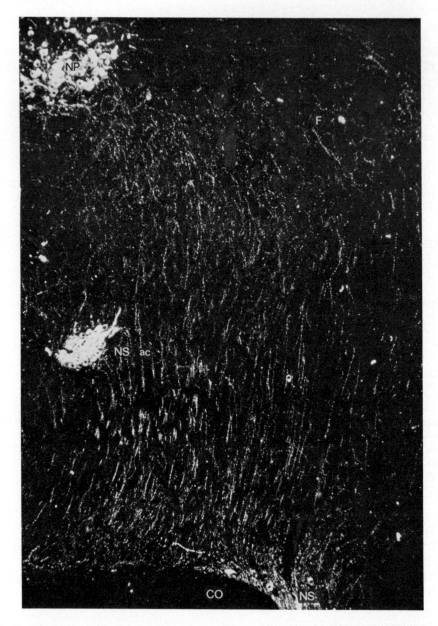

Fig. 2. Demonstration of the classic neurosecretory system of the rat with the pseudoisocyanine–fluorescence technique. CO, chiasma; F, fornix, NS, nucleus supraopticus; NS ac, nucleus supraopticus accessorius; NP, nucleus paraventricularis. ×170.

monomeric one, generates a strong yellow fluorescence when subjected to ultraviolet irradiation (Figs. 2 and 3). Most essential for understanding the specificity of this technique is the fact that the polymerization takes place only if the sulfonic acid groups are separated from each other by not more than 0.5 nm. Since, as far as is known, of all substances present within the vertebrate brain (with few exceptions) only the oxidized neurophysins and the secretory products in the subcommissural organ fulfill this condition, the technique can be conceived as a rather specific one.

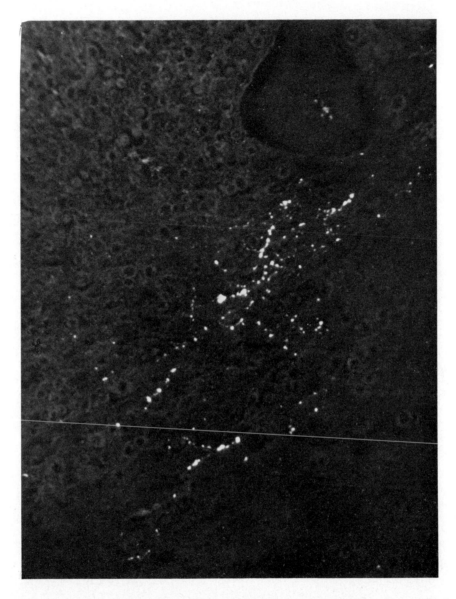

Fig. 3. Demonstration of very thin exohypothalamic fibers penetrating the tegmentum of the midbrain of a lamprey. Pseudoisocyanine—fluorescence technique. ×400.

The ascending fibers can of course also be demonstrated by means of the electron microscope. In the past few years we have demonstrated the presence of such fibers in the brains of several vertebrate species. As concerns the ultrastructure, the ascending fibers correspond to the well-known fibers of the hypothalamo—neurohypophysial tract but the caliber of the fibers is usually smaller, and the secretory vesicles more scattered throughout the entire course of the fibers (Hoheisel et al., 1978; Sterba et al., 1979a). The vesicles have the same size and the same shape as do the neurophysin-containing vesicles (NPV) of the posterior lobe. However, since ultrastructural similarities cannot be accepted as proof of identity, we

146

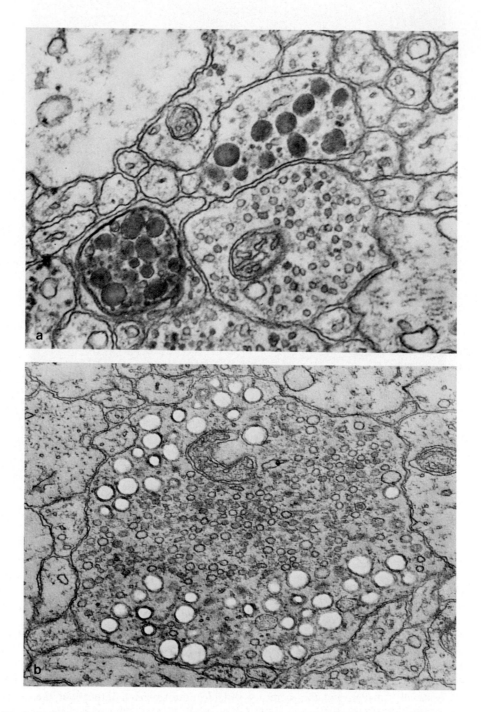

Fig. 4. Exohypothalamic fibers with neurophysin-containing vesicles within the rhombencephalic tegmen-tum motoricum of a lamprey. a: normal electron microscopic demonstration. b: ultrahistochemical demonstration. The electron-dense content of the vesicles is lacking. a and b ×70,000.

have tried to find a simple ultrahistochemical technique for the demonstration of NPV. This became possible after oxidation of the ultrathin sections, followed by contrasting with lead citrate (Naumann and Sterba, 1976). By this treatment the content of the NPV dissolves, while the vesicle membrane remains unaffected. Tangentially sectioned caps of the vesicles appear as spherical structures of high contrast. The procedure marks NPV in all structures of the classic neurosecretory system. Because monoamine vesicles, vesicles of the adenohypophysial cells and vesicles of unknown relation are all unaffected, the technique permits a well-defined identification and selective demonstration of NPV throughout the brain (Fig. 4).

Immunocytochemical techniques

The most up-to-date methods for demonstrating the peptide hormones in addition to their carrier proteins in the classic neurosecretory system are the immunocytochemical localization techniques (Fig. 5; for reviews see Sternberger, 1977). In the past 4 years these techniques have been employed for investigations concerning the ascending subsystem (Weindl et al., 1976, 1978; Brownfield and Kozlowski, 1977; Kozlowski et al., 1978; Sofroniew and Weindl, 1978a and b; Dogterom et al., 1978; Buijs, 1978; Buijs et al., 1978; Sterba, 1978; Sterba and Schober, 1979). Using these techniques, the results obtained with normal staining methods and with fluorescence microscopic techniques could not only be confirmed but also made more precise. The papers cited deal with exohypothalamic fibers in mammals which are oxytocinergic or vasopressinergic; furthermore they show that some targets of the brain are innervated both by oxytocinergic and by vasopressinergic fibers, whereas other targets receive one type only. Also the complementary neurophysins of both hormones can be demonstrated very specifically with these techniques.

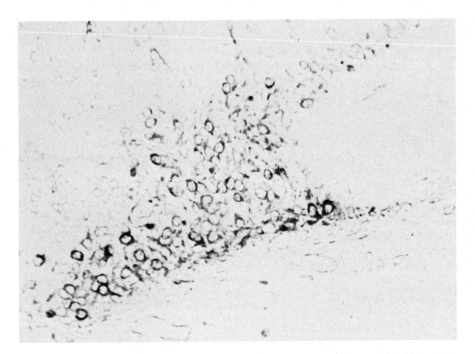

Fig. 5. Supraoptic nucleus of a 19-day fetal rat. Immunoperoxidase technique with rabbit anti-neurophysin antiserum. ×500.

Immunocytochemical methods have been recently used on the electron microscopic level too (Silverman and Zimmerman, 1975; Vossel et al., 1977; Krisch, 1977; Van Leeuwen, 1977; Van Leeuwen and Swaab, 1977), and in particular to identify ascending vaso-pressinergic fibers of the suprachiasmatic nucleus (Buijs et al., 1980).

The fundamental problem of the immunocytochemical localization technique is, of course, proof of the specificity (Swaab et al., 1975, 1977; Petrusz et al., 1976). Not all results obtained using antisera assumed to be monospecific in fact comply with all of the accepted criteria for specificity.

Retrograde labelling techniques

Exohypothalamic fibers can also be demonstrated by retrograde transport of horseradish peroxidase (HRP). Three to 4 days after HRP injections into the dorsal column's nuclei of medulla in rats, Schober (1978) observed labelled cells in the caudal part of the paraventricular nucleus, as well as some smaller ones in the lateral hypothalamic area. Proft (unpublished observations) used this technique to establish that neurosecretory fibers terminating within the subfornical organ of the rat originate from paraventricular neurons. In this connection, also the results of Saper et al. (1976) are of interest. They observed some labelled neurons in the hypothalamus after injections of HRP into the spinal cord of rats, cats and monkeys. Corresponding results were published by Hancock (1976), Ono et al. (1978) and Hosoya and Matsushita (1979).

THE SYNAPSES OF THE EXOHYPOTHALAMIC FIBERS

The concept of neurosecretion established at the first International Symposium on Neurosecretion in Naples (1953) started from the idea that the axons of neurosecretory neurons make no true synapses. It has been accepted for a long time that this feature is a very characteristic one (e.g. Knowles, 1974). The description of synapses connecting neurosecretory fibers of the classic neurosecretory system and glandular cells of the pars intermedia of cats (Bargmann et al., 1967; Bargmann, 1969), were regarded to be merely an

TABLE III

STRUCTURES OF THE VERTEBRATE BRAIN WHERE SYNAPSES OF EXOHYPOTHALAMIC FIBRES COULD BE DEMONSTRATED BY MEANS OF THE ELECTRON MICROSCOPE IN OUR LABORATORY.

Species	Brain structure
Lampetra planeri	reticular formation (1, 12)
Scardinius erythrophthalmus	tectum opticum (2)
Pleurodeles waltli	habenular nuclei (3); tectum opticum (3, 4, 12)
Rana esculenta (resp. temporaria)	subfornical organ (5); habenular nuclei (6)
Clemys caspica	lamina terminalis (7)
Columba livia	dorsal column's nuclei (8, 9, 12)
Wistar rat	nucleus tractus solitarii (8, 9, 10, 12); nucleus cuneatus medialis (8, 10); nucleus gracilis (10)

1, Hoheisel et al. (1978); 2, Weiss (not published); 3, Wegelin et al. (1975); 4, Sterba (1974a); 5, Wegelin and Sterba (1980); 6, Wegelin (not published); 7, Hoheisel (not published); 8, Schober et al. (1977); 9, Sterba (1978); 10, Sterba et al. (1979a); 11, Proft (not published); 12, Sterba et al. (1979b).

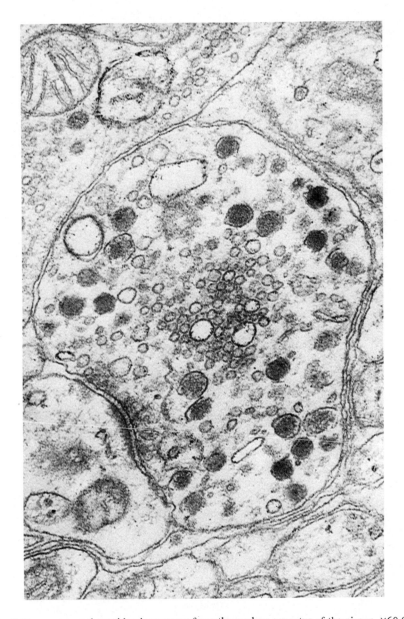

Fig. 6. Neuro-neuronal peptidergic synapses from the nucleus cuneatus of the pigeon. ×60,000.

exception to the above-mentioned generalization. At the sixth International Symposium on Neurosecretion in London (1973), Cross in fact postulated such synapses from the results of electrophysiologic recordings of recurrent inhibition in neurosecretory cells: "generation of the neurosecretory action potentials in the hypothalamus is facilitated by cholinergic (nicotinic receptors) mechanisms and inhibited by adrenergic (β-receptors) mechanisms but the morphological and neurotransmitter basis for the recurrent inhibition of neurosecretory cell discharges remains obscure" (Cross, 1974, p. 126).

At the same symposium the first results concerning neuro-neuronal synapses between

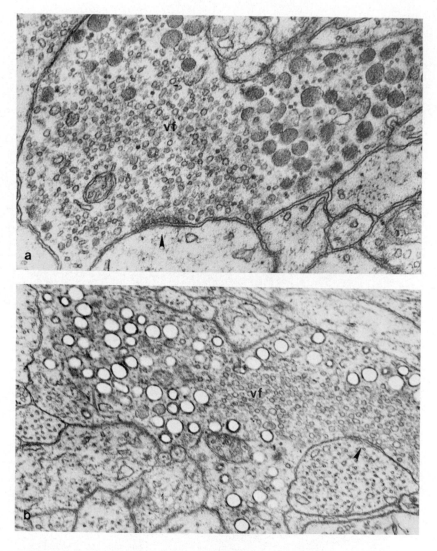

Fig. 7. Synaptic contacts (arrowheads) of vasotocinergic fibers (vf) with processes of other neurons from the rhombencephalic tegmentum of a lamprey. a: normal electron microscopic demonstration. b: ultra-histochemical demonstration. The electron dense material of the vesicles is lacking. a: ×60,000. b: ×52,000.

exohypothalamic fibers of the classic neurosecretory system and other neurons obtained by means of the electron microscope could be presented (Sterba, 1974a). Up to now we have been able to demonstrate such synapses in different brain regions from 6 vertebrate species (Table III). In all species investigated, the terminal portions of the exohypothalamic neurosecretory fibers make synaptic contacts with perikarya and nerve fibers of neurons not belonging to the classic neurosecretory system. Relatively frequently junctions "en passant" are found at small, spine-like protrusions of the contacted fibers. At the perikarya junctions "en passant" as well as junctions "termineaux" (Fig. 6) could be observed. The junctions "termineaux" examined in different brain areas are morphologically very similar throughout

151

the vertebrate phylum and meet the criteria of true synapses. The presynaptic boutons are bulb-like or disc-like and contain large vesicles (120–240 nm in diameter) in addition to small vesicles (40–50 nm in diameter), vacuoles and mitochondria. The large vesicles have a spherical, or slightly ovoid, shape and a homogeneously distributed, relatively electron-dense content which almost completely fills the vesicle lumen. Thus, they resemble the neurophysin-containing vesicles (NPV) in shape, appearance and size. The identity of the contents

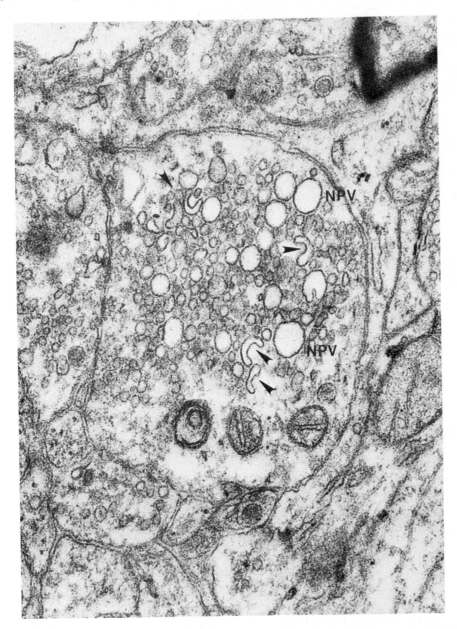

Fig. 8. Peptidergic synapses containing C-shaped vacuoles (arrowheads). As the slides were treated by the technique of Naumann and Sterba (1976), the neurophysin vesicles (NPV) appear empty. Wistar rat, dorsal column's nuclei. ×70,000.

152

with that of NPV could be demonstrated ultra-histochemically in all of the examined species (Fig. 7).

The small vesicles are clustered near the presynaptic axolemma, and resemble to a certain extent, the synaptic vesicles of cholinergic synapses. The synaptic cleft itself is a widened intercellular space, in some cases containing granulated intercleft material. Both presynaptic thickenings (dense projections) and postsynaptic densities could always be seen under the given conditions of preparation. Although we are not in the position to give proof of the mode of transmitter release from these synapses, a few remarks can be made. From the fiber terminals in the neurohypophysis it is known that the content of NPV is mainly released by exocytosis (Douglas, 1973; Dreifuss, 1975; Normann, 1976). The cytological process itself can be observed only rarely, even in the neurohypophysis. During exocytosis the NPV membrane fuses with the plasmalemma of the axon terminal, creating an opening by which the content of the vesicle is released into the extracellular space. It is generally assumed that the NPV membrane, which becomes incorporated into the plasmalemma for a short time, then subsequently is again internalized by endocytosis. The structures pinched off into the cytoplasm of the presynaptic bouton by a different mode of endocytosis are smooth microvesicles (Douglas et al., 1971) and larger vesicles or C-shaped vacuoles (Theodosis et al., 1976). The smooth microvesicles resemble morphologically the synaptic vesicles of cholinergic synapses (for review see Thorn, 1980).

Concerning the axon terminals of exohypothalamic neurosecretory fibers we have so far been unable to find any stage where the NPV membrane is fused with the plasmalemma. However, we occasionally find C-shaped vacuoles within the presynaptic bouton, of a size

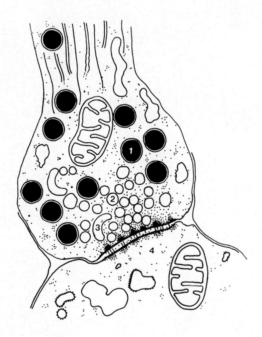

Fig. 9. Diagram of a peptidergic synapses. The presynaptic extremity of the exohypothalamic fiber is characterized morphologically by: (1) neurophysin-containing vesicles; and (2) empty microvesicles more or less massed together. Occasional C-shaped vacuoles (3) are present. (2) and (3) are thought to be related to the release of the content of the neurophysin-containing vesicles. The postsynaptic element (4) is formed by the receptive structures of another neuron.

comparable with or larger than that of the NPV (Fig. 8). We therefore assume that these structures as well as some larger microvesicles amongst the normal ones indicate that the exo-/endocytosis sequence takes place in the presynaptic endings of exohypothalamic fibers as well.

Fig. 9 includes all morphologic features of the described peptidergic synapses.

THE FUNCTIONAL SIGNIFICANCE OF THE ASCENDING SUBSYSTEM

The knowledge of the morphology of the descending and the ascending part include the possibility that the chemical mediators of the system are released from the neurohypophysis as well as from synaptically organized terminals in different brain regions. From the morphological point of view, different release sites suggest that a given chemical mediator might act both as a hormone and as a substance which affects other neurons directly. This last situation could be either by a short-term chemical mediation, in the sense of classical synaptic transmission, or by a more prolonged modulation of neuronal activities by changing the synaptic efficiency (Barker and Smith, 1980). This situation clearly points out that – as is well-known for monoamine mediators – protein mediators can serve different functions, and that the specificity of the function is always determined by the receptor sites.

The functional significance of the ascending subsystem is not clear. Most of the references concerning the function are purely speculative in character; two examples will be considered here. From the excellent work of De Wied and his coworkers, we are informed that vasopressin and oxytocin, their analogs and fragments thereof can affect learning processes after subcutaneous or cerebroventricular administration. Especially the acquisition and the resistance to extinction of active avoidance behaviour can be affected by the mentioned peptides. Furthermore, De Wied et al. determined the location of areas sensitive to some of these substances. The results point to an important role of structures of the limbic system, mainly the rostral region and the dorsal hippocampal region (for reviews see van Wimersma-Greidanus et al., 1976; De Wied and Gispen, 1977). These results underscore the problem of the physiological route involved in these effects, and we assume that the ascending part of the classic neurosecretory system participates in this process.

A direct action on brain structures might also be involved in our next example concerning functional significance. One of the most interesting exohypothalamic neurosecretory pathways is the hypothalamo–hindbrain connection (HHC). The axons belonging to the HHC originate from perikarya located in the caudal portion of the nucleus paraventricularis, and also from a small group of perikarya in the caudolateral hypothalamus. On their way to the hindbrain these fibers join fiber bundles from the mid- and hindbrain (for review see Sterba et al., 1979a). This pathway has been demonstrated by immunocytological localization techniques too (for review, see Buijs, 1978). In the hindbrain, most of the neurosecretory fibers terminate in the area of the nucleus tractus solitarii (NTS) and in the area of the dorsal column's nuclei (Fig. 10), and their axon terminals form synapses with other neurons. From the work of Korner (1971) and Chalmers (1975) we know that the NTS is a primary synaptic region for pressoreceptors. An increase in blood pressure recorded by these receptors leads to an activation of noradrenergic neurons of the NTS which are connected with sympathetic neurons in the vasomotor center by inhibitory synapses. The inhibition of the sympathetic component results in a decrease of the vascular tonus, a reduction of the minute output of the heart, and in a reduction of the noradrenaline level in the blood. The first suggestion that vasopressin might act on this system, was published by Tanaka et al. (1977).

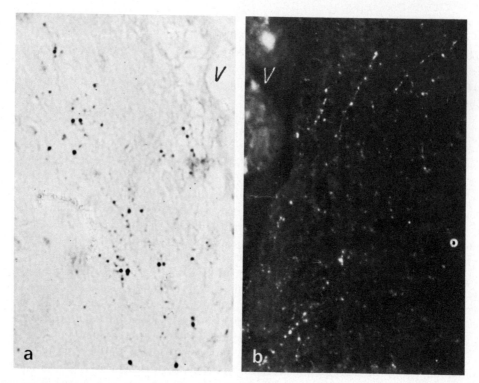

Fig. 10. Exohypothalamic neurosecretory fibers within the area of nucleus cuneatus medialis of the rat. V, fourth ventricle. a: immunoperoxidase technique with rabbit anti-neurophysin antiserum. b: contralateral brain-half of the same animal. Pseudoisocyanine–fluorescence technique. ×300.

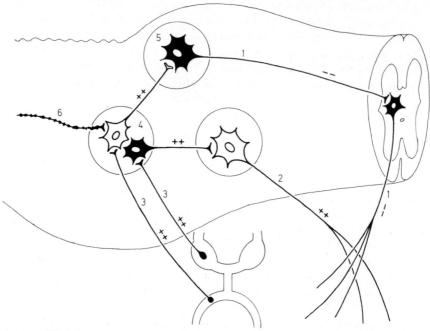

Fig. 11. Simplified diagram of connections serving blood pressure regulation, taking into consideration a possible participation of exohypothalamic fibers of the classic neurosecretory system. 1, orthosympathicus; 2, vagus (parasympaticus); 3, signal input from the baroreceptors; 4, nucleus tractus solitarii; 5, vasomotoric center; 6, neurosecretory fibers. Black: excitatory neurons. ++, increased impulse activity in the case of an increase in blood pressure; – –, decreased impulse activity in the case of an increase in blood pressure.

According to these authors, a very striking reduction of noradrenaline in the NTS can be observed in rats after intraventricular application of arginine-vasopressin. On the basis of this result, they suggested that this peptide may stimulate the release of noradrenaline from the neurons of the NTS and thus, bring about decrease in blood pressure. We assume that the demonstrated neurosecretory hypothalamo–hindbrain pathway terminating synaptically upon neurons of the NTS (Fig. 11) is the anatomical basis for the effects of posterior lobe mediators upon blood pressure (Sterba et al., 1979a).

SUMMARY

The classic neurosecretory system of the vertebrates is considerably more differentiated than has hitherto been supposed. Well-known is the descending part, that is: (a) the magnocellular nuclei which produce the peptides oxytocin, vasopressin, vasotocin, etc.; (b) the tractus hypothalamo-neurohypophyseus, by means of which the hormones are transported; and (c) the neural lobe, where the hormones are released into the blood circulation. But as yet we know little about the ascending part, through which the system is connected with different brain regions, e.g. the septal nuclei, the hippocampal and habenular structures, the reticular formation of the midbrain, and the areas of the dorsal column's nuclei of the hindbrain. All these connections formed by bundles of scattered fibers can be demonstrated by means of different techniques, e.g. fluorescence and electron microscopic methods, as well as by specific immunocytochemical and ultra-histochemical localization techniques.

Unlike the fibers of the descending part, the ascending fibers (exohypothalamic fibers) are not connected to capillaries, but rather make true synapses with other neurons. The most interesting feature of these peptidergic synapses is the presence of large vesicles containing neurophysins and nonapeptides. The existence of an ascending part makes it clear that the classic neurosecretory system cannot be viewed simply as a system involving signal transfer by neurohormone release and transfer of the mediators to the targets via the blood stream. Instead, we have to accept the view that the classic neurosecretory system also affects subsystems of the brain by direct neuronal intervention, and thus directly takes part in a variety of cerebral functions. Finally, the possibility is discussed that this system might be involved in such disparate processes as memory and the regulation of blood pressure.

REFERENCES

Bargmann, W. (1949) Über die neurosekretorische Verknüpfung von Hypothalamus und Neurohypophyse. Z. Zellforsch., 34: 610–634.

Bargmann, W. (1969) Das neurosekretorische Zwischenhirn-Hypophysensystem und seine synaptischen Verknüpfungen. J. Neuro-Visc. Rel., Suppl. 9: 64–77.

Bargmann, W., Lindner, E. und Andres, K.H. (1967) Über Synapsen an endokrinen Epithelzellen und die Definition sekretorischer Neurone. Untersuchungen am Zwischenlappen der Katzenhypophyse. Z. Zellforsch., 77: 282–298.

Barker, J.L. and Smith, T.G. (1980) Three modes of intercellular neuronal communication. In Adaptive Capabilities of the Nervous System, Progress in Brain Research, Vol. 53, P. McConnel, G.J. Boer, H.J. Romijn, N.E. van de Poll and M.A. Corner (Eds.), Elsevier, Amsterdam, pp. 169–192.

Barry, J. (1954) Neurocrinie et synapses "neurosecretoires". Arch. Anat. micr. Morph. exp., 43: 310–320.

Barry, J. (1961) Recherches morphologiques et expérimentales sur la glande diencéphalique et l'appareil hypothalamohypophysaire. Ann. Sci. Univ. Besancon, Zool. Physiol. Sér., 2: 3–133.

156

Bock, R. (1966) Über die Darstellbarkeit neurosekretorischer Substanz mit Chromalaun-Gallocyanin im supraoptico-hypophysären System beim Hund. *Histochemie,* 6: 362–369.

Brownfield, M.S. and Kozlowski, G.P. (1977) The hypothalamo-choroidal tract. I. Immunohistochemical demonstration of neurophysin pathways to telencephalic choroid plexuses and cerebrospinal fluid. *Cell Tiss. Res.,* 178: 111–127.

Buijs, R.M. (1978) Intra- and extrahypothalamic vasopressin and oxytocin pathways in the rat. Pathways to the limbic system, medulla oblongata and spinal cord. *Cell Tiss. Res.,* 192: 423–435.

Buijs, R.M., Swaab, D.F., Dogterom, J. and Leeuwen, F.W. van (1978) Intra- and extrahypothalamic vasopressin and oxytocin pathways in the rat. *Cell Tiss. Res.,* 186: 423–433.

Buijs, R.M., Velis, D. and Swaab, D.F. (1980) Extrahypothalamic vasopressin and oxytocin innervation of fetal and adult rat brain. In *Adaptive Capabilities of the Nervous System, Progress in Brain Research, Vol. 53,* P. McConnel, G.J. Boer, H.J. Romijn, N.E. van de Poll and M.A. Corner (Eds.), Elsevier, Amsterdam, pp. 159–167.

Burlet, A., Chateau, M. and Marchetti, J. (1976) Contributions of immunoenzymatic technique to the study of diencephalic localization of vasopressin, *First int. Symp. Immunoenzymatic techniques INSERM, Symp. No. 2,* G. Feldmann, P. Druet, J. Bignon, S. Avrameas (Eds.), Amsterdam, North-Holland, pp. 333–343.

Chalmers, J.P. (1975) Brain amines and models of experimental hypertension. *Circulat. Res.,* 36: 469–480.

Cross, B.A. (1974) The neurosecretory impulse. In *Neurosecretion – The Final Neuroendocrine Pathway,* F. Knowles and L. Vollrath (Eds.), Springer, Berlin–Heidelberg–New York, pp. 115–128.

Dogterom, J., Snijdewint, F.G.M. and Buijs, R.M. (1978) The distribution of vasopressin and oxytocin in the rat brain. *Neurosci. Lett.,* 9: 341–346.

Douglas, W.W. (1973) How do neurones secrete peptides? Exocytosis and its consequences, including "synaptic vesicle" formation, in the hypothalamo-neurohypophyseal system. In *Drug Effects on Neuroendocrine Regulation, Progress in Brain Research, Vol. 39,* E. Zimmerman, W.H. Gispen, B.H. Marks and D. De Wied (Eds.), Elsevier, Amsterdam, pp. 21–39.

Dreifuss, J.J. (1975) A review on neurosecretory granules: their contents and mechanisms of release. *Ann. N.Y. Acad. Sci.,* 248: 184–201.

Faure, J., Loiseau, P. et Friconneau, C. (1959) Influence de l'oxytocine sur l'électroencéphalogramme du lapin. *Rev. Neurol.,* 101: 302–308.

Faure, J., Loiseau, P. et Vincent, D. (1960) Influence de l'hormone antidiurétique (A.D.H.) sur l'électro-encéphalogramme du lapin éveillé et libre. *Rev. Neurol.,* 102: 333–338.

Hancock, M.B. (1976) Cells of origin of hypothalamo-spinal projections in the rat. *Neurosci. Lett.,* 3: 179–184.

Hoheisel, G., Rühle, H.-J. and Sterba, G. (1978) The reticular formation of lampreys (Petromyzonidae) – a target area for exohypothalamic vasotocinergic fibres. *Cell Tiss. Res.,* 189: 331–345.

Hosoya, Y. and Matsushita, M. (1979) Identification and distribution of the spinal and hypophyseal projection neurons in the paraventricular nucleus of the rat. A light and electron microscopic study with the horseradish peroxidase method. *Exp. Brain Res.,* 35: 315–331.

Knowles, F. (1974) Twenty years of neurosecretion. In *Neurosecretion – The Final Neuroendocrine Pathway,* F. Knowles and L. Vollrath (Eds.), Springer, Berlin–Heidelberg–New York, pp. 3–11.

Korner, P. (1971) Integrative neural cardiovascular control. *Physiol. Rev.,* 51: 312–367.

Kozlowski, G.P., Brownfield, M.S. and Hostetter, G. (1978) Neurosecretory supply to extrahypothalamic structures: choroid plexus, circumventricular organs, and limbic system. In *Neurosecretion and Neuroendocrine Activity, Evolution, Structure and Function,* W. Bargmann, A. Oksche, A. Polenov and B. Scharrer (Eds.), Springer, Berlin–Heidelberg, pp. 217–227.

Kozlowski, G.P., Brownfield, M.S. and Schultz, W.J. (1976) Neurosecretory pathways to the choroid plexus. *Int. Res. Commun. Sys.,* 4: 299.

Krisch, G. (1977) Electron microscopic immunocytochemical study on the vasopressin-containing neurons of the thirsting rat, *Cell Tiss. Res.,* 184: 237–247.

Leeuwen, F.W. van (1977) Immunoelectron microscopic visualization of neurohypophyseal hormones: evaluation of some tissue preparations and staining procedures, *J. Histochem. Cytochem.,* 11: 1213–1221.

Leeuwen, F.W. van and Swaab, D.F. (1977) Specific immunoelectronmicroscopic localization of vasopressin and oxytocin in the neurohypophysis of the rat. *Cell Tiss. Res.,* 177: 493–501.

Legait, H. (1958) Les voies extra-hypothalamo-neurohypophysaires de la neurosécrétion diencephalique dans la série des vertébrés. In *Zweites Internationales Symposium über Neurosekretion,* W. Bargmann, B. Hanström, B. and E. Scharrer (Eds.), Springer, Berlin–Göttingen–Heidelberg, pp. 42–51.

Legait, H. et Legait, E. (1956) Mise en évidence de voies neurosécrétoires extra-hypothalamo-hypophysaires chez quelques Batraciens et Reptiles. *C.R. Soc. Biol. (Paris)*, 150: 1429–1431.

Legait, H. et Legait, E. (1957) Relations entre les noyaux hypothalamiques neurosécrétoires et les régions septale et habénulaire chez quelques Oiseaux. *Acta neuroveg. (Wien)*, 17: 143–147.

Naumann, W. and Sterba, G. (1976) Ultrastructural studies on neurophysine-containing vesicles of the neurosecretory system of vertebrates. *Cell Tiss. Res.*, 165: 545–553.

Normann, T.Ch. (1976) Neurosecretion by exocytosis. *Int. Rev. Cytol.*, 46: 1–77.

Ono, T., Nishino, H., Sasaka, K., Muramoto, K., Yano, I. and Simpson, A. (1978) Paraventricular nucleus connections to spinal cord and pituitary. *Neurosci Lett.*, 10: 141–146.

Petrusz, P., Sar, M., Ordonneau, P. and Di Meo, P. (1976) Specificity in immunocytochemical staining, *J. Histochem. Cytochem.*, 24: 1110–1115.

Saper, C.B., Loewy, A.D., Swanson, L.W. and Cowan, W.M. (1976) Direct hypothalamo–autonomic connections. *Neurosci. Abstr.*, 2: 77.

Schober, F. (1978) Darstellung der neurosekretorischen hypothalamo-rhombencephalen Verbindung bei der Ratte durch retrograden axonalen Transport von Meerrettich-Peroxidase. *Acta biol. med. germ.*, 37: 165–167.

Schober, F., Trautmann, U., Naumann, W. und Sterba, G. (1977) Die oxytocinergen exohypothalamischen Verbindungen zur Medulla oblongata bei der Taube und der Ratte. *Acta biol. med. germ.*, 36: 1183–1186.

Silverman, A.J. and Zimmerman, E.A. (1975) Ultrastructural immunocytochemical localization of neurophysin and vasopressin in the median eminence and posterior pituitary of the guinea pig. *Cell Tiss. Res.*, 159: 291–301.

Sofroniew, M.V. and Weindl, A. (1978a) Extrahypothalamic neurophysin-containing perikarya, fiber pathways and fiber clusters in the rat brain. *Endocrinology*, 102: 334–337.

Sofroniew, M.V. and Weindl, A. (1978b) Projections from the vasopressin- and neurophysin-containing neurons of the suprachiasmatic nucleus. *Amer. J. Anat.*, 153: 391–429.

Sterba, G. (1964) Grundlagen des histochemischen und biochemischen Nachweises von Neurosekret (=Trägerprotein der Oxytozine) mit Pseudoisocyaninen. *Acta histochem.*, 17: 268–292.

Sterba, G. (1974a) Ascending neurosecretory pathways of the peptidergic type. In *Neurosecretion – The Final Neuroendocrine Pathway*, F. Knowles and L. Vollrath (Eds.), Springer, Berlin–Heidelberg–New York, pp. 38–47.

Sterba, G. (1974b) Das oxytocinerge neurosekretorische System der Wirbeltiere. Beitrag zu einem erweiterten Konzept. *Zool. Jb. Physiol.*, 78: 409–423.

Sterba, G. (1977) Morphologische Grundlagen der humoralen Informationsübermittlung durch Peptide bei Wirbeltieren. *Sitzungsberichte Akad. der Wissensch. DDR*, 5N: 40–61.

Sterba, G. (1978) Oxytocinergic extrahypothalamic neurosecretory system of the vertebrates and memory processes. In *Neurosecretion and Neuroendocrine Activity, Evolution, Structure and Function*, W. Bargmann, A. Oksche, A. Polenov and B. Scharrer (Eds.), Springer, Berlin–Heidelberg, pp. 293–299.

Sterba, G., Hoffmann, E., Solecki, R., Naumann, W., Hoheisel, G. and Schober, F. (1979a) The neurosecretory hypothalamo-hindbrain-pathway and its possible significance for the regulation of blood pressure and the milk-ejection reflex. *Cell Tiss. Res.*, 196: 321–336.

Sterba, G., Hoheisel, G., Wegelin, R., Naumann, W. and Schober, F. (1979b) Peptide-containing vesicles within neuro-neuronal synapses. *Brain Res.*, 169: 55–64.

Sterba, G. und Schober, F. (1979) *Topographie und Zytologie neurosekretorischer Systeme. Teil 1: Das klassische neurosekretorische System der Ratte*, VEB Gustav Fischer, Jena, pp. 1–119.

Sternberger, L.A. (1977) Immunocytochemistry of neuropeptides and their receptors. In *Peptides in Neurobiology*, H. Grainer (Ed.), Plenum Press, New York and London, pp. 61–97.

Swaab, D.F. and Pool, C.W. (1975) Specificity of oxytocin and vasopressin immunofluorescence. *J. Endocr.*, 66: 263–272.

Swaab, D.F., Pool, C.W. and Leeuwen, F.W. van (1977) Can specificity ever be proved in immunocytochemical staining. *J. Histochem. Cytochem.*, 25: 388–391.

Swanson, L.W. (1977) Immunohistochemical evidence for a neurophysin-containing autonomic pathway arising in the paraventricular nucleus of the hypothalamus. *Brain Res.*, 128: 346–353.

Tanaka, M., Kloet, R. De, Wied, D. De and Versteeg, D.H.G. (1977) Arginine[8]-vasopressin affects catecholamine metabolism in specific brain nuclei. *Life Sci.*, 20: 1799–1808.

158

Theodosis, D.T., Dreifuss, J.J., Harris, H.C. and Orci, L. (1976) Secretion-related uptake of horseradish peroxidase in neurohypophysial axons. *J. Cell Biol.* 70: 294–303.

Thorn, N.A. (1980) Biochemical mechanism of release of vasopressin, *Proc. IX Congress Hungarian Soc. of Endocrinology and Metabolism,* Akademia Kiodo, Budapest, in press.

Unger, H. (1977) Funktionelle Aspekte der Informationsübermittlung durch Vasopressin und Oxytocin bei Säugetieren, *Sitzungsber. Akad. Wiss. DDR,* 5N: 62–84.

Vossel, A. van, Vossel-Daeninck, J. van, Dierickx, K. and Vandesande, F. (1977) Electron microscopic immunocytochemical demonstration of separate mesotocinergic and vasotocinergic nerve fibres in the pars intermedia of the amphibian hypophysis. *Cell Tiss. Res.,* 178: 175–181.

Wegelin, R. and Sterba, G. (1980) Extrahypothalamic peptidergic neurosecretion. II. Neurosecretion in the subfornical organ of *Rana esculenta. Cell Tiss. Res.,* 205: 107–120.

Wegelin, R., Sterba, G. und Hoheisel, G. (1975) Licht- und elektronenmikroskopische Untersuchungen am exohypothalamischen oxytocinergen System von Pleurodeles waltli MICHAH. (Urodela). *Biol. Zbl.,* 94: 633–660.

Weindl, A. and Sofroniew, M.V. (1976) Demonstration of extrahypothalamic peptide secreting neurons. A morphological contribution to the investigation of psychotropic effects of neurohormones. *Pharmakopsychiatrie,* 5: 226–234.

Weindl, A. and Sofroniew, M.V. (1978) Neurohormones and circumventricular organs. In *Brain–Endocrine Interaction III. Neural Hormones and Reproduktion. 3rd Int. Symp. Würzburg 1977,* Karger, Basel, pp. 117–137.

Weindl, A., Sofroniew, M.V. und Schinko, I. (1976) Psychotrope Wirkungen hypothalamischer Hormone: Immunohistochemische Identifikation extrahypophysärer Verbindungen neuroendokriner Neurone. *Arzneim.-Forsch.,* 26: 1191–1194.

Weindl, A., Sofroniew, M.V. and Schinko, I. (1978) Distribution of vasopressin, oxytocin, neurophysin, somatostatin and luteinizing hormone releasing hormone-producing neurons. In *Neurosecretion and Neuroendocrine Activity, Evolution, Structure and Function,* W. Bargmann, A. Oksche, A. Polenov and B. Scharrer (Eds.), Springer, Berlin–Heidelberg, pp. 312–319.

Wied, D. De (1965) The influence of the posterior and intermediate lobe of the pituitary and pituitary peptides on the maintenance of a conditioned avoidance response in rats. *Int. J. Neuropharmacol.,* 4: 157–167.

Wied, D. De and Bohus, B. (1978) The modulation of memory processes by vasotocin, the evolutionarily oldest neurosecretory principle. In *Maturation of the Nervous System, Progress in Brain Research, Vol. 48,* M.A. Corner et al. (Eds.), Elsevier, Amsterdam, pp. 349–364.

Wied, D. De and Gispen, W.H. (1977) Behavioral effects of peptides. In *Peptides in Neurobiology,* H. Grainer (Ed.), Plenum Press, New York, pp. 397–448.

Wilkins, J., Michaels, J., Nilaver, G. and Zimmerman, E.A. (1978) Hypothalamic pathways to the lower brain stem containing neurophysins, oxytocin and vasopressin in the rat. *Endocr. Soc. Abstr.,* 60: 269.

Wimersma-Greidanus, Tj.B. van, Bohus, B. and Wied, D. De (1976) CNS sites of action of ACTH, MSH and vasopressin in relation to avoidance behaviour. In *Anatomical Neuroendocrinology.* W.E. Stumpf and L.D. Grant (Eds.), Karger, Basel, pp. 284–289.

Extrahypothalamic Vasopressin and Oxytocin Innervation of Fetal and Adult Rat Brain

R.M. BUIJS, D.N. VELIS and D.F. SWAAB

Netherlands Institute for Brain Research, IJdijk 28, 1095 KJ Amsterdam, The Netherlands

INTRODUCTION

After Ernst Scharrer (1951) demonstrated the existence of exohypothalamic pathways in the garter snake by means of the Gomori staining technique, Legait (1958) and Barry (1961), using the same method, convincingly demonstrated that this phenomenon holds true for many other species, ranging from fishes and amphibia to mammalians. Independently of each other, Barry et al. (1958) and Legait and Legait (1958) demonstrated, respectively, oxytocinergic activity in the area of the amygdala, and antidiuretic activity in the habenular region by means of bioassays. Twenty years later, Dogterom et al. (1978) were able to confirm and extend these studies using highly sensitive and specific radioimmunoassays for vasopressin (AVP) and oxytocin (OXT).

As early as 1954, Barry pointed to the possibility that these exohypothalamic fibres terminated by means of "de synapses neurosécrétoires" containing Gomori-positive material. However, the Gomori staining technique did not allow electron microscopic observation and identification of these structures.

In 1974 Sterba demonstrated the existence of such peptidergic synapses in the CNS of the salamander, using electron microscopy and an oxidation technique which was later described by Naumann and Sterba (1976). Due to the limitations of these techniques, particularly with regard to its specificity (Sterba et al., 1980), little or no attention was paid to these excellent studies. The demonstrated exohypothalamic fibres might represent the physiological route of transportation within the CNS for centrally effective vasopressin and oxytocin. An alternative route of transportation, the cerebrospinal fluid, was also proposed (De Wied and Gispen, 1977). We therefore decided to study the localization of vasopressin and oxytocin in the rat central nervous system using immunocytochemical techniques.

LOCALIZATION OF VASOPRESSIN AND OXYTOCIN IN THE RAT BRAIN

Antibodies against these two peptides were raised and purified using agarose beads coupled with the heterologous antigen (Swaab and Pool, 1975). Rat brains were perfused and fixed in 2.5% glutaraldehyde—1% paraformaldehyde in 0.1 M cacodylate buffer, after which the tissue was either embedded in paraffin for an immunolight microscopical procedure, or sectioned on a vibratome to be used both for immunolight- and immunoelectron microscopical observations. Immunolight- and immunoelectron microscopy were performed

160

using the unlabelled antibody enzyme method of Sternberger (1974). For further details about fixation, staining of the tissue and specificity controls see Buijs et al. (1978) and Buijs and Swaab (1979).

In the adult rat, vasopressin or oxytocin was demonstrated in cell bodies of the magnocellular nuclei and in fibres running towards the neurohypophysis, as well as in cell bodies scattered throughout the hypothalamus. From the paraventricular nucleus (PVN), vasopressin and oxytocin fibre pathways were found to run (Buijs, 1978; Buijs et al., 1978; Fig. 1): (a) via the ventral commissure of the fornix and subiculum, to reach the ventral hippocampus and entorhinal cortex (the ventral hippocampus is also reached by a ventral pathway via the amygdala); (b) via the stria terminalis to the nuclei of the amygdala; and (c) via the central grey and substantia nigra into the medulla oblongata and substantia gelatinosa of the spinal cord. The extent to which the SON contributes to the exohypothalamic system (EHS) is still unclear, but some of the fibres in the amygdala and ventral hippocampus might be derived from this nucleus. In rostal brain regions, including the hippocampus and "central grey", far more vasopressin than oxytocin fibres are present, while oxytocin fibres predominate more caudally. From the parvocellular suprachiasmatic nucleus (SCN), only vasopressin-containing fibres emerge, which run rostrally towards the organum vasculosum of the lamina terminalis and the lateral septum and dorsocaudally towards the lateral habenular nucleus (Buijs, 1978; Fig. 1).

Immunocytochemistry has enabled us to demonstrate vasopressin- and oxytocin-containing cells and/or fibres in the fetal rat hypothalamus as early as day 16. In contrast to the adult, OXT- and/or AVP-containing cells in the fetus come into direct contact with the ventricular system, with their somata lodged between the ependymal cells and their pro-

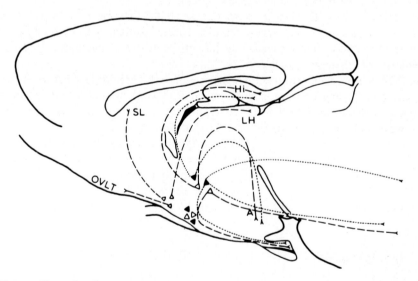

Fig. 1. Diagram illustrating pathways and sites of termination, originating from the suprachiasmatic nucleus (small triangles) and paraventricular nucleus (upper group of large triangles). The open triangles and broken lines indicate vasopressin-containing cell bodies and fibres while the closed triangles and dotted lines represent respectively, cell bodies and fibres containing oxytocin. From the suprachiasmatic nucleus, fibres run to the organum vasculosum lamina terminalis (OVLT), the lateral septum (SL) and the lateral habenular nucleus (LH). Paraventricular nucleus fibres run to the hippocampus (Hi) in which they terminate ventrally, the amygdala (A), and nuclei in the medulla oblongata and spinal cord.

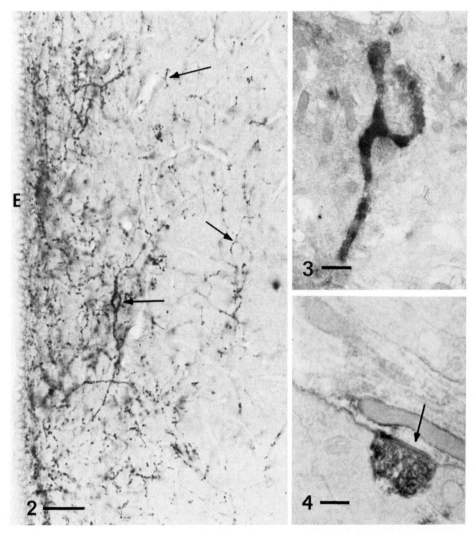

Fig. 2. Vasopressin-containing fibres in a transversal section of the lateral septum. Note the pericellular terminations, fibre branching (arrows) and the high concentration of fibres in the most lateral part of the septum. E, ependyma. Bar, 20 μm.

Fig. 3. Branching of a vasopressin-containing fibre in the lateral septum as seen by means of immunoelectronmicroscopy. Bar, 0.5 μm.

Fig. 4. Vasopressin-positive terminal forming a synapse (arrow) with an unlabelled dendrite in the lateral septum. Bar, 0.25 μm.

cesses pointing into the hypothalamus. The possibility of transport of neurohypophyseal hormones to other brain sites via the cerebrospinal fluid may thus be seriously considered for the developing brain (Boer et al., 1980). A ventromediorostral to dorsolaterocaudal gradient appeared to be present for the development of AVP- and OXT-containing cells, similar to the gradient reported for the general maturation of hypothalamic nuclei (Ifft, 1972; Anderson, 1978). In the fetal brain, large numbers of growth cones containing neurohypophyseal hormones seem to arise from the SON and PVN, and can be traced down into the central grey. Fibres of the EHS can be demonstrated in the nuclei of the amygdala from day 18. AVP in the parvocellular SCN can be demonstrated only from day 3 post-natally while innervation of the lateral septum is still absent (De Vries, unpublished results from The Netherlands Brain Research Institute).

THE PEPTIDERGIC SYNAPSE

Although no conclusive evidence for actual fibre termination in a given structure can be obtained by means of light microscopy, fibre density and branching and perineuronal structures indicate that this is the case in the lateral septum (Figs. 2 and 3), lateral habenular nucleus, ventral hippocampus, nuclei of the amygdala, nucleus tractus solitarius and nucleus ambiguus.

In order to verify these putative fibre terminations, immunoelectron microscopy was performed on the most densely innervated structures; i.e. the lateral septum and the lateral habenular nucleus as target areas of the SCN, and the nuclei of the amygdala for the PVN fibres. Using the pre-embedding staining technique, a very good correlation was found between the light microscopical results and electron microscopy (Buijs and Swaab, 1979).

In all 3 regions, synaptic structures containing vasopressin were frequently found to terminate mostly on dendrites (Figs. 4–7). These synapses contained clear vesicles and/or dense core vesicles, the latter with a diameter of approximately 100 nm were positively stained for vasopressin. A synaptic cleft with the presence of a postsynaptic density was also sometimes noted (Buijs and Swaab, 1979). These structures containing neurohypophyseal hormones were indistinguishable from classical neurotransmitter-containing synapses, as visualized by means of a similar pre-embeddding staining technique (e.g. Pickel et al., 1976). Infrequently, an oxytocin-containing synapse was seen in the nuclei of the amygdala. Most of these peptidergic synapses were found to terminate on dendrites, and not on the cell bodies as had been supposed on the basis of light microscopical results (Buijs et al., 1978; Sofroniew and Weindl, 1978). In the lateral septum, synapses "en passage" terminating both on a cell body and its dendrite were sometimes observed (Figs. 8 and 9). Since vaso-pressin-containing terminations were found on cell bodies (Fig. 7) and dendrites, and since monoamines are not reported to be present in cell bodies or dendrites in these parts of the limbic system, it is not plausible that the effect of vasopressin and oxytocin on the mono-amine metabolism in these regions (Kovacs et al., 1980) is a result of a direct action of these peptides. In order to enable a functional correlation between the finding of Kovacs et al. and ours, it seems necessary first to establish what type of transmitter the innervated cells produce and to what regions they project.

In the positively stained nerve fibres in the lateral septum and lateral habenular nucleus, vasopressin was present in granules of approximately 100 nm. This is in agreement with the observation that these fibres are derived from the SCN, where the same kind of vesicles are found (van Leeuwen et al., 1978). However, the presence of AVP and OXT in the amygdala and of OXT in the spinal cord, in granules of 100 nm, does not fit in with the observation that the PVN (where these fibres originate), contains granules of a larger size viz. 130 nm (Krisch, 1974). A comparable observation was reported by Dube et al. (1976) who demon-strated vasopressin-positive dense core vesicles, 90 nm in diameter, in fibres within the external zone of the median eminence, which are also thought to come from the PVN (Vandesande et al., 1977). Electrophysiological results suggest, moreover, that these fibres

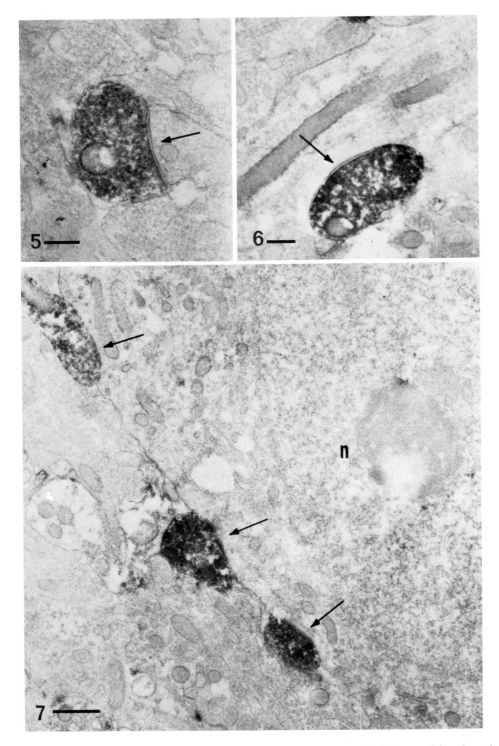

Fig. 5. Vasopressin-positive terminal forming a synapse (arrow) with a dendrite in the medial nucleus of the amygdala. Bar, 0.25 μm.

Fig. 6. Vasopressin-positive synapse (arrow) with an unlabelled dendrite in the lateral septum. Bar, 0.25 μm.

Fig. 7. Three vasopressin-positive synapses (arrows) with a cell body in the lateral septum. n, nucleus. Bar, 0.5 μm.

164

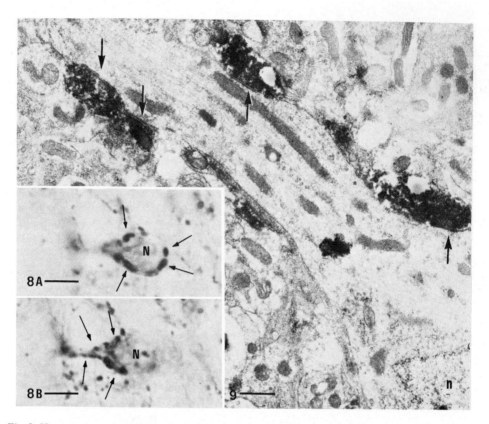

Fig. 8. Vasopressin-positive fibre (arrows) around a neuron (N) and its process, focused at two different levels (A, B) in a 20 μm thick section. Bar, 10 μm.

Fig. 9. Vasopressin-positive terminals (arrows) on a cell body (n, nucleus) and its dendrite, suggesting synapses "en passage". Contrasted with uranyl acetate and lead citrate. Bar, 0.5 μm.

in the external zone of the median eminence might be axon collaterals of PVN fibres that run towards the neurohypophysis (Pittman et al., 1978). Since in the neurohypophysis the granular size is approximately 150 nm (van Leeuwen and Swaab, 1977), this would point either to a selection mechanism for small granules in axon collaterals, or to a different release mechanism in central brain regions and the neurohypophysis. Vasopressin immuno-reactivity was frequently found at the surface of clear, vesicle-like structures. This might fit in with the idea that the smooth endoplasmic reticulum serves as an alternative vehicle for intra-axonal transport of non-granular neurosecretory material that gives rise to clear vesicles (Alonso and Assenmacher, 1978).

It is curious to note that neither the SCN nor its massive projections into the limbic system (Fig. 2) had been reported in the older studies by Barry, Legait or Sterba. Since the SCN has only once been reported to stain positively with such methods (Joussen, 1970), it is likely that its neurosecretory product is less readily stained than is that of the magnocel-lular system. In addition, the SCN fibres in general are thinner than those of the magno-cellular PVN or SON, which could make it impossible to detect these fibres, as has also been reported in the case of Sterba's pseudo-isocyanine technique (Sterba et al., 1979).

Since the limbic structures innervated by the SCN, are also found to be important for the AVP effects on avoidance behavior (van Wimersma-Greidanus et al., 1976), the SCN might be necessary in this respect. Another function in which the SCN might be involved is the central regulation of water balance. Thus lesions in the terminal field of the AVP fibres coming from the SCN, or lesions interrupting these fibres, caused a disturbed water balance in rats and goats (Johnson and Buggy, 1978; Andersson et al., 1975). This could mean that the SCN is involved in an indirect feed-back control mechanism upon the peripheral release of AVP. An indication in support of such a possibility is that septal stimulation inhibits PVN spike frequency (Negoro et al., 1973). In addition, direct connections exist between cells of the septum and the SON (Ellendorff et al., 1979).

CONCLUSION

It has been found both by immunocytochemistry and by radioimmunoassay (Dogterom et al., 1978) that AVP and OXT are present in a wide variety of regions in the central nervous system. In addition, it has now been demonstrated that these peptides are localized within synaptic structures which are morphologically indistinguishable from the classical neurotransmitter-containing synapses. It is therefore tempting to speculate that these peptides act as neurotransmitters within the central nervous system.

ACKNOWLEDGEMENTS

We wish to thank Ms. C. de Raay and Mr. P.S. Wolters for their expert technical assistance.

This study was supported by the Foundation for Fundamental Medical Research (FUNGO).

REFERENCES

Alonso, G. and Assenmacher, I. (1978) The smooth endoplasmic reticulum in neurosecretory axons of the rat neurohypophysis. *Biol. Cell.*, 32: 203–206.

Anderson, C.H. (1978) Time of neuron origin in the anterior hypothalamus of the rat. *Brain Res.*, 154: 119–122.

Andersson, B., Leksell, L.G. and Lishajko, F. (1975) Perturbation in fluid balance induced by medially placed forebrain lesions. *Brain Res.*, 99: 261–275.

Barry, J. (1954) Neurocrinie et synapses "neurosécrétoires". *Arch. Anat. Mikr.*, 43: 310–320.

Barry, J. (1961) Recherches morphologiques et expérimentales sur la glande diencephalique et l'appareil hypothalamo-hypophysaire. *Ann. Sci. Univ. Besancon Zool. Physiol.*, Ser. 2: 3–133.

Barry, J., Besson, S. and LaMarche, M. (1958) Recherches sur les activités post hypophysomimetiques des extraits de noyaux amygdaliens de cobayes. *Ann. Endocrinol. (Paris)*, 19: 1045.

Boer, G.J., Swaab, D.F., Uylings, H.B.N., Boer, K., Buijs, R.M. and Velis, D.N. (1980) Neuropeptides in rat brain development. In *Adaptive Capabilities of the Nervous System, Progress in Brain Research, Vol. 53*, P. McConnell, G.J. Boer, H.J. Romijn, N.E. van de Poll and M.A. Corner (Eds.), Elsevier, Amsterdam, pp. 207–227.

Buijs, R.M. (1978) Intra- and extrahypothalamic vasopressin and oxytocin pathways in the rat; pathways to the limbic system, medulla oblongata and spinal cord. *Cell Tiss. Res.*, 192: 423–435.

Buijs, R.M. and Swaab, D.F. (1980) Immuno-electron microscopical demonstration of vasopressin and oxytocin synapses in the limbic system of the rat. *Cell Tiss. Res.*, 204: 355–365.

Buijs, R.M., Swaab, D.F., Dogterom, J. and Leeuwen, F.W. van (1978) Intra- and extrahypothalamic vasopressin and oxytocin pathways in the rat. *Cell Tiss. Res.*, 186: 423–433.

Dogterom, J., Snijdewint, F.G.M. and Buijs, R.M. (1978) The distribution of vasopressin and oxytocin in the rat brain. *Neurosci. Lett.*, 9: 341–346.

Dube, D., Leclerc, R. and Pelletier, G. (1976) Electronmicroscopic immunohistochemical localization of vasopressin and neurophysin in the median eminence of normal and adrenalectomized rats. *Amer. J. Anat.*, 146: 103–108.

Ellendorff, F., Poulain, D.A. and Vincent, J.D. (1978) An electrophysiological study of septal input to oxytocin and vasopressin neurones in the supraoptic nucleus of the rat. *J. Physiol. (Lond)*, 284: 124P.

Ifft, J.D. (1972) An autoradiographic study of the time of final division of neurons in rat hypothalamic nuclei. *J. comp. Neurol.*, 144: 193–204.

Johnson, A.K. and Buggy, J. (1978) Periventricular preoptic hypothalamus is vital for thirst and normal water economy. *Amer. J. Physiol.*, 234: R122–R129.

Joussen, F. (1970) Zur morphologie des supraoptico-hypophysären systems beim Kaninchen. *Z. Zellforsch.*, 103: 544–558.

Kovács, G.L., Bohus, B. and Versteeg, D.H.G. (1980) The interaction of posterior pituitary neuropeptides with monoaminergic neurotransmission: significance in learning and memory processes. In *Adaptive Capabilities of the Nervous System. Progress in Brain Research, Vol. 53*, P. McConnell, G.J. Boer, H.J. Romijn, N.E. van de Poll and M.A. Corner (Eds.), Elsevier, Amsterdam, pp. 123–140.

Krisch (1974) Different populations of granules and their distribution in the hypothalamo-neurohypophysical tract of the rat under various experimental conditions. I. Neurohypophysis, nucleus supraopticus and nucleus paraventricularis. *Cell Tiss. Res.*, 151: 117–140.

Leeuwen, F.W. van, Swaab, D.F. and Raay, C. de (1978) Immunoelectronmicroscopic localization of vasopressin in the rat suprachiasmatic nucleus. *Cell Tiss. Res.*, 193: 1–10.

Leeuwen, F.W. van and Swaab, D.F. (1977) Specific immunoelectronmicroscopic localization of vasopressin and oxytocin in the neurohypohysis of the rat. *Cell Tiss. Res.*, 177: 493–501.

Legait, H. (1958) Les voies extra-hypothalamo-neurohypophysaires de la neurosécrétion diencéphalique dans la série des vertébrés. In *Zweites internationales symposium über neurosekretion*, W. Bargman, B. Hanström, B Scharrer and E. Scharrer (Eds.), Springer, Berlin, pp. 42–51.

Legait, H. and Legait, E. (1958) Présence d'une voie neurosécrétoire hypothalamo-habénulaire et mise en évidence d'une activité antidiurétique au niveau des ganglions de l'habénula chez la poule. *Comp. Rend. Soc. Biol.*, 152: 828–830.

Naumann, W. and Sterba, G. (1976) Ultrastructural studies on neurophysine-containing vesicles of the neurosecretory system of vertebrates. *Cell Tiss. Res.*, 165: 545–553.

Negoro, H., Visessuwan, S. and Holland, R.C. (1973) Inhibition and excitation of units in paraventricular nucleus after stimulation of septum amygdala and neurohypophysis. *Brain Res.*, 57: 479–483.

Pickel, V.M., Joh, T.H. and Reis, D.J. (1976) Monoamine synthesizing enzymes in central dopaminergic noradrenergic and serotonergic neurons. Immunocytochemical localization by light- and electronmicroscopy. *J. Histochem. Cytochem.*, 24: 792–806.

Pittman, Q.J., Blume, H.W. and Renaud, L.P. (1978) Electrophysiological indications that individual hypothalamic neurons innervate both median eminence and neurohypophysis. *Brain Res.*, 157: 364–368.

Scharrer, E. (1951) Neurosecretion X. A relationship between the paraphysis and the paraventricular nucleus in the garter snake (Thamnopsis sp.). *Biol. Bull.*, 101: 106–113.

Sofroniew, M.V. and Weindl, A. (1978) Projections from the parvocellular vasopressin and neurophysin containing neurons of the suprachiasmatic nucleus. *Amer. J. Anat.*, 153: 391–430.

Sterba, G. (1974) Ascending neurosecretory pathways of the peptidergic type. In *Neurosecretion – The Final Neuroendocrine Pathway*, F. Knowles, L. Vollrath (Eds.), Springer, Berlin, pp. 38–47.

Sterba, G., Hoffman, E., Solecki, R., Naumann, W., Hoheisel, G. and Schober, F. (1979) The neurosecretory hypothalamo-hindbrain pathway and its possible significance for the regulation of blood pressure and the milk ejection reflex. *Cell Tiss. Res.*, 196: 321–336.

Sterba, G., Naumann, W. and Hoheisel, G. (1980) Exohypothalamic axons of the classic neurosecretory system and their synapses. In *Adaptive Capabilities of the Nervous System, Progress in Brain Research, Vol. 53*, P. McConnell, G.J. Boer, H.J. Romijn, N.E. van de Poll and M.A. Corner (Eds.), Elsevier, Amsterdam, pp. 141–158.

Sternberger, L.A. (1974) *Immunocytochemistry,* New York, Prentice Hall, Englewood Cliffs.

Swaab, D.F. and Pool, C.W. (1975) Specificity of oxytocin and vasopressin immunofluorescence. *J. Endocr.,* 66: 263–272.

Vandesande, F., Dierickx, K. and Mey, J. de (1977) The origin of the vasopressinergic and oxytocinergic fibres of the external region of the median eminence of the rat hypophysis. *Cell Tiss. Res.,* 180: 443–452.

Wied, D. De and Gispen, W.H. (1977) Behavioral effects of peptides. In *Peptides in Neurobiology,* H. Gainer (Ed.), New York, Plenum Press, pp. 397–448.

Wimersma-Greidanus, Tj.B. van, Bohus, B. and Wied, D. De (1976) CNS sites of action of ACTH, MSH and vasopressin in relation to avoidance behavior. In *Anatomical Neuroendocrinology,* W.E. Stumpf and L.D. Grant (Eds.), Karger Basel, pp. 284–289.

Three Modes of
Intercellular Neuronal Communication

JEFFERY L. BARKER and THOMAS G. SMITH, Jr.

Laboratory of Neurophysiology, National Institute of Neurological and Communicativ Disorders and Stroke, National Institutes of Health, Bethesda, Md, 20205 (U.S.A.)

INTRODUCTION

Until rather recently, most neuroscientists held that intercellular communication between excitable cells was via specialized junctions called synapses and involved a process that is called neurotransmission. Such a conviction was eminently reasonable since that was the only form of communication known or for which there was any sound scientific evidence. In addition, many investigations have assumed that any naturally occurring neuroactive compound was, a priori, a neurotransmitter.

Lately, however, results have been found about the ways which cells may communicate that appear to be sufficiently different in their characteristics and mechanisms from neurotransmission via neurotransmitters to warrant different designations. We have classified these new modes of communication as neuromodulatory and neurohormonal communication (Barker and Smith, 1976, 1977, 1978, 1979a and 1979b); and, in this paper, we will compare and contrast them with neurotransmission and with each other. In addition, these modes of interneuronal communication will be illustrated by the use of peptides, particularly the opioid peptides, a relative new area of neuroscience.

It is instructive and therefore appropriate at a school such as this to enquire where and how the initial and/or the important findings were made that contributed significantly to our understanding of the basic membrane mechanisms of interneuronal communication. They were all made on simple preparations which provided for a maximum of experimental control. For the spike, which initiates synaptic transmission, it was, of course, the squid giant axon (Hodgkin, 1964; Cole, 1972); for the classical excitatory postsynaptic event, the end-plate potential, it was frog neuromuscular junction (Katz, 1966); for the initial inhibitory synaptic potential, the crayfish neuromuscular junction (Fatt and Katz, 1953); for electronic junctions, the giant neurons of the crayfish (Furshpan and Potter, 1959; Watanabe and Grundfest, 1961); for neurohormonal communication, the giant cells of molluscs (Barker and Gainer, 1974; Barker et al., 1975; Barker and Smith, 1976, 1977 and 1979b; Branton et al., 1978a and 1978b; Blankenship, 1979); and for neuromodulation, tissue-cultured spinal cord neurons (Barker et al., 1978a and 1978b; Barker et al., 1979a; Barker and Smith, 1979a). To repeat, for emphasis, *all* were simple preparations where the scientist had excellent experimental control of the input signals and high-precision measurement capabilities of the output signals. The intact vertebrate central nervous system (CNS) is just too complicated and cumbersome to allow the application of the technical procedures necessary to explore basic membrane mechanisms adequately and efficiently. While a lot has been learned about intercellular communication in the intact vertebrate CNS, virtually all of the information is conceptually and logically based on knowledge gained from simple preparations. For the young scientist, the lesson should be clear — if you want to work on basic membrane mechanisms, choose a simple preparation that allows for precise and efficient experimental control of the phenomena of interest.

The preparations that we have used are tissue-cultured mammalian spinal cord cells and molluscan neurons. The techniques we have employed involve intracellular recordings with one or two microelectrodes and include voltage clamping. With the latter technique, the tips of two microelectrodes are inserted into the cell, one for recording the membrane potential and the other for supplying the required current. The electrodes are connected to an electronic, negative-feedback circuit whose function is to control the membrane potential and to measure the membrane currents. From the data collected, one can calculate from Ohm's law the membrane conductances that are a measure of membrane ionic permeabilities (Cole, 1972; Smith et al., 1980). Neuroactive compounds of interest are applied to the external surface of the cell either locally with microelectrodes via iontophoresis or with pressure ejection or globally by bath perfusion. The results from all methods of application were the same.

NEUROTRANSMISSION

As is generally and well known, neurotransmission takes place between contiguous cells, where the axon terminal of the presynaptic neuron forms a specialized junction, called a synapse, with a patch of specialized somatic or dendritic membrane. Neurotransmission is initiated by the invasion of the axon terminal by an action potential. This usually leads to an increase in the terminal's intracellular calcium, which results in a synchronous release of packets or quanta of neurotransmitter molecules. These diffuse rapidly across the synaptic cleft and interact with stereospecific receptors on the external surface of the postsynaptic membrane. The successful interaction of transmitter molecules with individual receptors is the initial postsynaptic event in neurotransmission. This interaction leads to a momentary change, usually an increase, in the permeability or conductance of nearby transmembrane channels to particular ionic species. The conductance change results in a flow of ionic current through the membrane conductance and leads to a change in membrane potential. For a conductance increase, if the equilibrium potential to the ionic species is more positive or depolarized than the resting potential, the potential change will be positive-going and excitatory. Thus, if large enough to reach spike threshold, an excitatory postsynaptic potential (epsp) can lead to the initiation of a spike. Conversely, if the equilibrium potential is more negative than the resting potential, there will be a negative-going, inhibitory postsynaptic potential (ipsp), which can inhibit spike generation. For conductance decreases the potential changes will be the reverse of those just described.

The postsynaptic characteristics of neurotransmission can be demonstrated by locally applying a transmitter to the surface of the postsynaptic membrane. Fig. 1 shows the excitatory effect of iontophoresing the opiate peptide, leucine-enkephalin (ℓ-ENK), onto a tissue cultured mouse spinal cord neuron. A brief pulse of ℓ-ENK (at arrow) resulted in a transient depolarization (Fig. 1A_1, upper trace), which is due to an increase in membrane conductance. This is indicated by the fact that the repetitive, hyperpolarizing pulses, evoked by constant-current stimuli, decreased during the response (Fig. 1A_1, lower trace). The response is excitatory because, if large enough, it can lead to action potentials (Fig. 1A_2). The response amplitude varied linearly with membrane potential (Fig. 1B: squares), hence, by Ohm's law, the underlying conductance is independent of the membrane potential, a distinguishing characteristic of neurotransmission. The extrapolated reversal potential is around +15 mV, which is the potential reached by the sodium spike in this cell. Thus, one effect of enkephalin is to produce an increase in a voltage-dependent sodium conductance which can result in a neurotransmitter-like epsp. Although the conductance change is constant in neurotransmission, in some preparations the average duration of the elementary conductance change and the decay kinetics of the synaptic current does change with membrane potential (Dionne and Steven, 1975).

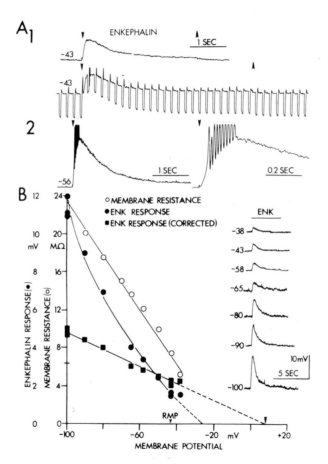

Fig. 1. Transmitter-like effects of enkephalin on cultured spinal neurons. Intracellular, KAc recordings from two different cells. A: depolarizing responses to iontophoresis of 50 nA leu-enkephalin (marked by arrowhead). At −56 mV the response is excitatory, eliciting a brief burst of spikes, while at −43 mV, with spikes inactivated, the response is simply depolarizing. The increase in membrane conductance, manifested by the decrease in voltage response to −0.8 nA−50 msec current stimuli, which is evident at the peak of the response, partly reflects the voltage-dependent nature of membrane conductance. B: effect of membrane potential on enkephalin response. Right: sample responses at membrane potentials indicated at beginning of trace. Left: plot of membrane resistance vs potential (open circles), recorded enkephalin response vs membrane potential (filled circles) and enkephalin response corrected for non-linear membrane resistance (filled squares). Extrapolated, corrected response (straight dotted line) indicates reversal potential of +15 mV (inverted arrowhead). In this and subsequent figures, all recordings are from intracellularly placed electrodes.

172

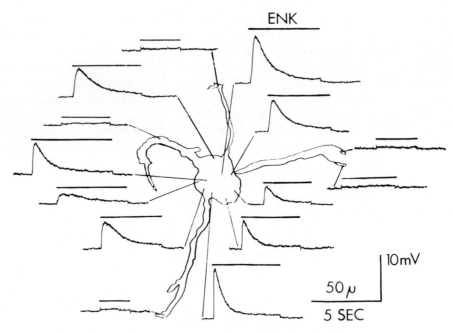

Fig. 2. Localization of sensitivity to enkephalin in evoking neurotransmitter-like response. Intracellular recordings from soma. Enkephalin applied from micropipette during times indicated by bar over response and at loci indicated by straight lines connecting response to outline drawing of spinal cord cell. See Text.

Two other distinguishing characteristics of neurotransmission are illustrated in Fig. 2. The first is called desensitization, so named because continued application of the putative transmitter results in a progressive decrease in receptor sensitivity to the transmitter and hence response amplitude (Fig. 2). The second is local sensitivity, in that sensitivity varies from site to site over the surface of the postsynaptic cell membrane. High sensitivity may represent the loci of synaptic junctions. In tissue-cultured neurons, large changes in sensitivity can occur over distances of only a few μm.

Another characteristic of neurotransmitters is that their activity can be blocked at the receptor site by stereospecific antagonists. In tissue-cultured spinal cord cells, the neurotransmitter-like action of ℓ-ENK is partially blocked by the specific opiate antagonist, naloxone (Fig. 3).

In summary, neurotransmission, defined both in terms of anatomical and physiological

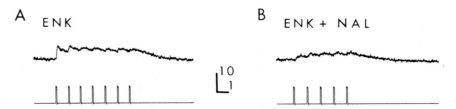

Fig. 3. Naloxone blocks enkephalin fast response. A: neurotransmitter-like fast response evoked by repetitive pressure application of enkephalin from tissue-cultured mouse spinal cord cell; lower traces monitor pressure. B: inhibition of enkephalin response by bath application of naloxone. Recovery of enkephalin response from naloxone (not shown) was complete.

properties involves a brief change of specific, voltage-independent, desensitizing conductances through the interaction of stereospecific receptors at specialized, local synaptic junctions (Katz, 1966; Eccles, 1964). Furthermore, these actions can be blocked by specific antagonists.

NEUROMODULATORS

We have observed another action of neuroactive substances that is distinctly different from neurotransmission, as just defined. This action has been seen with the peptides, substance P and leucine-enkephalin. It involves alteration of the magnitude and kinetics of the postsynaptic conductance responses to putative amino acid neurotransmitters, independent of any other membrane effects (Barker et al., 1978a and b; Vincent and Barker, 1979). We have labeled this action "neuromodulation" to distinguish it from neurotransmission. The peptide alteration in the neurotransmitter-evoked membrane response is dose-dependent, reversible and independent of membrane potential. The modulatory effect of the peptides may be either depression or enhancement or both.

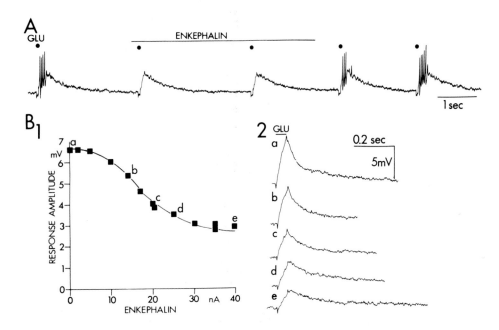

Fig. 4. Enkephalin depresses glutamate voltage responses on cultured spinal neurons. KAc recordings from two different cells. A: continuous trace of membrane potential showing depolarizing responses to 40 nA— 50 msec pulses of constant glutamate (black dots) which evoke spikes. Frequency responses of pen-writer attenuates spike amplitude. Iontophoresis of 20 nA ENK (marked by bar above trace) rapidly and reversibly blocks excitatory effect of constant glutamate without affecting resting membrane properties. Resting potential: −54 mV. B: ENK depression of depolarizing response to 25 nA−50 msec glutamate pulse is dose-dependent but incomplete with maximal depression being about 50%. Data plotted in B_1, specimen records in B_2. A slowing of the response time course is evident at higher ENK currents. Membrane potential: −80 mV. (From Barker et al., 1978b, reprinted with the permission of the *American Association for the Advancement of Science*, 1978.)

174

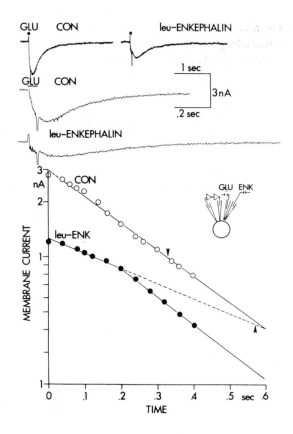

Fig. 5. Enkephalin alters amplitude and kinetics of glutamate response. Upper: voltage clamp currents of responses to short, constant pulses of glutamate (dots) before and during continuous co-application of enkephalin, on two different time scales. Lower: semi-log plots of falling phase of glutamate response vs time, before (CON: open circles) and during (leu-ENK: filled circles) application of leucine-enkephalin. Note lengthening of time constant (arrowhead) by enkephalin.

The experimental paradigm is to evoke repetitive responses with brief pulses of transmitter and, for a period during which responses were evoked, to apply a steady dose of ℓ-ENK. Both application of transmitter and ℓ-ENK are via iontophoresis or pressure ejection.

Fig. 4 illustrates the dose-dependent depressive effect of ℓ-ENK on the putative excitatory transmitter glutamate (Fig. 4A and B_2), without any direct effect on other membrane properties. If ℓ-ENK affected a glutamate response, it was always a reduction in amplitude; however, the suppression was never complete but ranged from 20 to 75% of control responses (Fig. 4B). In addition, ℓ-ENK changed the kinetics of the glutamate-induced response, viz. slowing down the time-to-peak and introducing an additional time constant (Fig. 5). Enkephalin depression of glutamate responses evoked in CNS neuron in vivo has been reported in the cat (Zieglgänsberger et al., 1976; Zieglgänsberger and Fry, 1978) and rat (Segal, 1977).

The mechanisms of action of these neuromodulatory effects are unknown. Fig. 6 illustrates that the reduction was not due to a change in the equilibrium potential of the glutamate response, since the equilibrium potential, i.e. the membrane potential at which the voltage clamp currents become zero (about −10 mV), was unchanged. Fig. 7 illustrates the

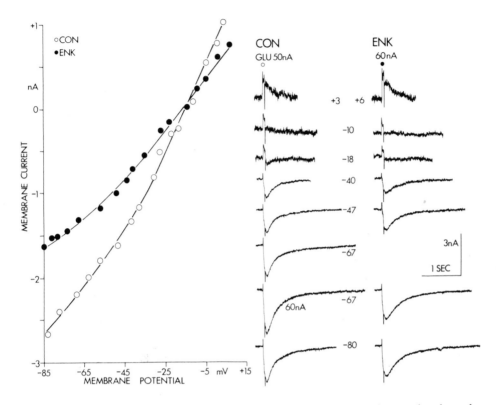

Fig. 6. Enkephalin does not alter reversal potential of glutamate response. Right: sample voltage clamp membrane currents evoked by brief constant-amplitude pulses of glutamate (GLU) as a function of membrane potential with and without the continuous application of enkephalin (ENK). Left: plot of glutamate-evoked membrane current vs membrane potential with (filled circles) and without (open circles) enkephalin.

dose–response curves of that effect of ℓ-ENK on the glutamate response (Fig. 7A). When this is plotted on a semi-logarithmic scale, the control and test curves are parallel with a slope of nearly one (Fig. 7C). The maximum, limiting slope of these Hill plots can be interpreted as indicative of the number of transmitter molecules required to activate the receptor-coupled conductance (Brooks and Werman, 1973). Since enkephalin produced no alteration in the Hill plot (Fig. 7C), the effect on the response was apparently not due to a change in the number of glutamate molecules needed to activate its receptor-coupled conductance.

The double-reciprocal plot of the dose–response curve, or Lineweaver-Burk plot, can give insight into the nature of the response reduction (Segel, 1975). Fig. 8, along with the non-parallel dose–response curve (Fig. 7A), indicate that the glutamate–ℓ-ENK interaction is non-competitive, suggesting that ℓ-ENK does not act at the glutamate receptor site. This leaves only two, at this point indistinguishable, possible mechanisms of action to account for the depression of ℓ-ENK on the glutamate-evoked response. The first mechanism is that ℓ-ENK acts on the conductance channel to which the glutamate receptor is connected. The second is that ℓ-ENK acts on another, non-glutamate, receptor that is coupled to the same conductance to which the glutamate receptor is connected.

Unlike the uniform results with the excitatory amino acid, glutamate, the action of ℓ-ENK on the putative inhibitory transmitter amino acids, α-aminobutyric acid (GABA) and

176

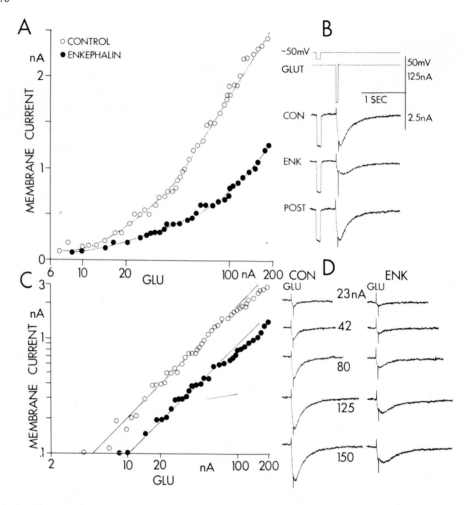

Fig. 7. Analysis of the enkephalin–glutamate interaction on cultured spinal neurons observed with the voltage clamp technique. The spinal neuron was impaled with two independent KCl micropipettes and the voltage was clamped to −50 mV. The experimental paradigm is illustrated in B. A 10 mV hyperpolarizing command followed by 100 msec-100 nA glutamate iontophoretic pulse before (CON) during (ENK), and after (POST) application of enkephalin (20 nA) at the same site. Depression and alteration in kinetics of glutamate-evoked inward membrane current during enkephalin application without change in current response to voltage command is evident. A: the dose–response curve of the membrane current as a function of the glutamate iontophoretic current in control and during enkephalin application. Specimen records are shown in D and a log–log plot is shown in C. Numbers in D refer to glutamate iontophoretic currents. See text. (From Barker et al., 1978b. Reprinted with the permission of the *American Association for the Advancement of Science*.)

glycine, are more complex. These effects will be illustrated with our glycine results. Fig. 9 shows that ℓ-ENK can have no effect on the glycine-induced response (Fig. 9A), a slight enhancement at low doses and depression at high doses of glycine (Fig. 9B) or marked enhancement at low doses and depression at high doses of glycine (Fig. 9C), while uniformly depressing glutamate responses at the same locations in the 3 cells illustrated.

Unlike the ℓ-ENK effect on the glutamate response, ℓ-ENK does not affect the kinetics of the inhibitory amino acid responses, either when enhanced (Fig. 10) or depressed. As with

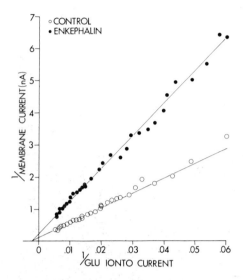

Fig. 8. Lineweaver-Burk plot of voltage clamp membrane current^{-1} vs glutamate current^{-1} with (ENKEPHALIN) and without (CONTROL) enkephalin. See text.

glutamate, there is no change in the reversal potential of the glycine or GABA responses (not illustrated) or in the Hill plots (Fig. 11, right). Also, as with glutamate, these modulations by ℓ-ENK of the inhibitory responses can be interpreted as neither affecting the equilibrium potential nor the number of amino acid molecules required to activate the receptor-coupled conductance.

The dose—response curve and the Lineweaver-Burk plot of the effects of ℓ-ENK on glycine are distinctly different from those on glutamate. With glycine, there is a roughly parallel shift in the dose—response curve (Fig. 11, left) and the lines in the Lineweaver-Burk plot intercept on the ordinate. Since ℓ-ENK has increased the glycine response-amplitude, the result is the inverse of competitive inhibition — a sort of "synergistic enhancement" by ℓ-ENK. In any event, the analysis suggests that glycine and ℓ-ENK are acting at a similar receptor site. However, while glycine can activate the receptor-coupled conductance, ℓ-ENK alone is without effect on the conductance.

Neuromodulation, defined electrophysiologically, involves the indirect alteration of post-synaptic neurotransmitter-activated membrane conductances independent of other effects on membrane properties. Neuromodulation, as defined here, has not yet been observed during the physiological elaboration of synaptic transmission nor has the anatomical rela-tionship between the neuromodulatory element and its target cells been described. A wide variety of clinically important drugs, including the opiates, benzodiazopenes and barbi-turates, can act on the postsynaptic membranes of CNS neurons to modulate transmitter-activated membrane conductance by altering either receptor affinity for neurotransmitter or the conductance activated by the neurotransmitter (Dostrovsky and Pomeranz, 1973; Zieglgänsberger and Bayerl, 1976; Segal, 1977; Choi et al., 1978; Barker and Ransom, 1978; Macdonald and Barker, 1978a and b). Thus, modulation of transmitter events at postsynap-tic sites by endogenous and exogenous substances may be an important aspect of both the normal physiological function of the CNS and the cellular mechanisms of action of clinically important CNS-active drugs. Alteration in synaptic transmission by clinically important

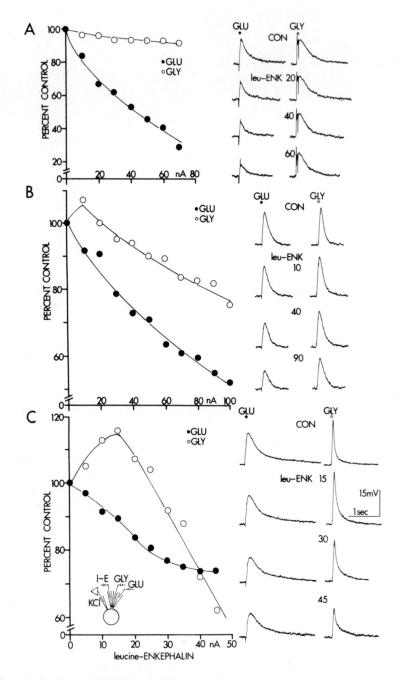

Fig. 9. Effect of enkephalin on glutamate- and glycine-evoked voltage responses. Records from 3 different cultured spinal cord cells. Right: sample records of responses evoked by constant pulses of glutamate (GLU) or glycine (GLY) without (CON) and different doses of enkephalin (leu-ENK; numbers indicate doses). Left: plots of effect of varying doses of enkephalin on responses evoked by constant glutamate (GLU: filled circles) and glycine (GLY: open circles). Enkephalin constantly attenuated glutamate responses (A, B and C), but variably affected glycine responses. Enkephalin either had no effect (A), slight enhancement at low and suppression at high doses (B) or marked enhancement at low and suppression at high doses (C) on glycine responses.

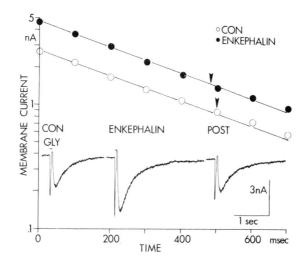

Fig. 10. Effect of enkephalin on voltage clamp membrane current evoked by brief pulses of glycine. Inset: enkephalin enhances glycine response (ENKEPHALIN) over control (CON, POST). Semi-log plot of decay of membrane current vs time shows no change in decay kinetics or time constant of decay (arrowheads).

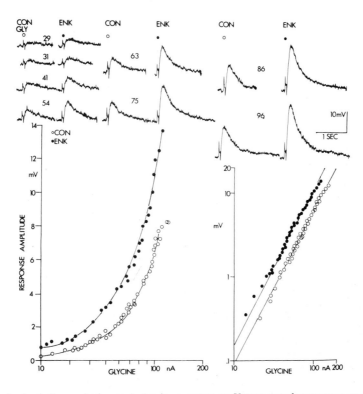

Fig. 11. Effect of enkephalin on glycine-evoked voltage responses. Upper: sample responses evoked by different amounts of glycine with (ENK) and without (CON) enkephalin. Lower: linear (left) and log–log (right) dose–response curves of glycine response vs glycine iontophoretic current, with (ENK) and without (CON) enkephalin. See text.

drugs acting at presynaptic sites in the CNS has also been reported (e.g. Weakly, 1969; Macdonald and Nelson, 1978), but the membrane mechanisms have yet to be elucidated.

NEUROHORMONAL COMMUNICATION

Another type of intercellular communication has recently been described in molluscan nervous systems, which we have termed "neurohormonal" communication. This communication in these invertebrates takes place between cells *not* in anatomical contiguity via synaptic or other contacts (Coggeshall, 1967; Frazier et al., 1967) and involves long-lasting changes in the activity of diverse and distant target cells following stimulation of specific peptidergic neurons called "bag cells" (Fig. 13) (Branton et al., 1978a; Stuart and Strumwasser, 1978). A peptide elaborated by the bag cells also induces egg-laying behavior (Kupfermann, 1970; Arch, 1972; Pinsker and Dudek, 1977; Blankenship, 1979). The effects of the peptide, vasopression, and of peptide extracts of both the bag cells (Barker and Smith, 1977) and other parts of the molluscan nervous system (Ifshin et al., 1975) on the excitability of several of the target neurons in the sea slug, *Aplysia californica,* and the land snail, *Otala lactea,* have previously been examined. In addition, a variety of peptides derived from the vertebrate nervous system have been applied to the same cells and found an action on membrane properties quite similar to those seen with the bag cell peptide (Barker and Gainer, 1974; Barker et al., 1975; Barker and Smith, 1976, 1977).

By way of background, the target cells of bag cell extract and the ones we have studied are the identified cells R15 in Aplysia (Frazier et al., 1967; Branton et al., 1978a and b; Blankenship, 1979) and its homologous identified cell in Otala, cell 11 (Gainer, 1972). These cells have a distinctive pattern of membrane potential behavior called bursting pacemaker potential activity (BPP). This activity is characterized by slow, endogenous membrane potential oscillations whose depolarizing phase is associated with a burst of spikes (Fig. 14B,

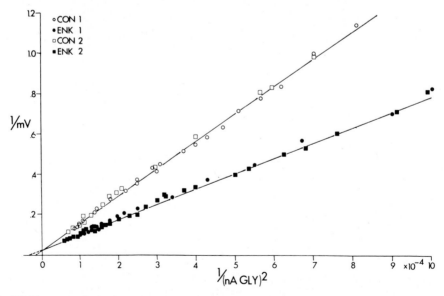

Fig. 12. Lineweaver-Burk plots of glycine-evoked response with (ENK; filled symbols) and without (CON; open symbols) enkephalin. See text.

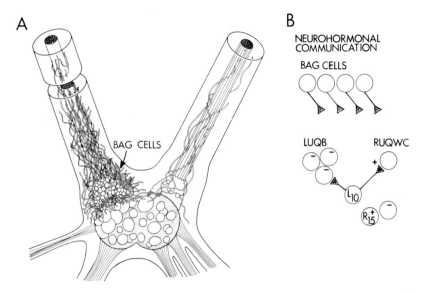

Fig. 13. Schema of bag cells and processes in the parietovisceral ganglion of Aplysia (ventral view). See text.

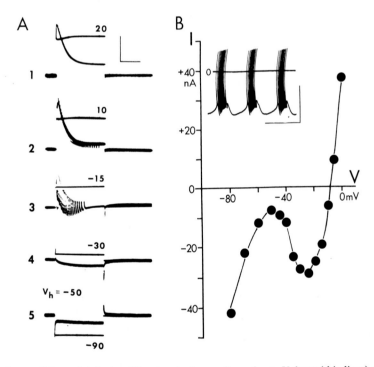

Fig. 14. Data from cell R_{15} of *Aplysia californica*. A: from voltage clamp. Voltage (thin lines) and current (thick lines) traces for 5 sec pulse commands from holding potential ($V_{holding}, V_h$) of 50 mV to potentials indicated by numbers adjacent to voltage trace. Traces begin with voltage and current traces superimposed. Positive-going potentials and (outward) currents are displayed upward. Calibration: 45 mV for voltage traces, 500 nA (trace 1); 200 nA (trace 2); 100 nA (trace 3); and 50 nA (traces 4 and 5) for current traces; 2.5 sec. B: quasi-steady-state I–V curve from voltage clamp data shown in A. Inset: spontaneous BPP oscillations in the unclamped cell. Calibrations: 50 mV, 25 sec. Zero membrane potential is indicated by a horizontal line marked 0. (Reproduced from Smith et al., 1975, with permission of *Nature*).

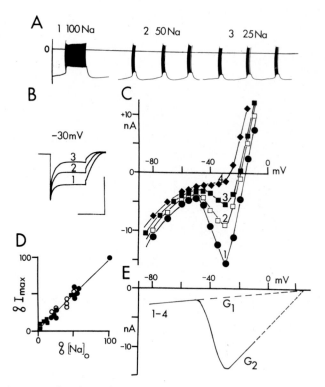

Fig. 15. Effects of altering $(Na^+)_0$ on membrane properties of BPP neurons. Data in A–C and E from cell 11 of *Otala lactea.* D: contains data from both cell 11 and cell R_{15}. Cs ions were iontophoresed intracellularly by means of a microelectrode in cell 11 before measurements. A–C: data labeled 1 (filled circles), 2 (open squares), and 3 (filled squares) were obtained when the $(Na^+)_0$ was, respectively, 100, 50, and 25 mM (Na^+ replaced with Tris). Other extracellular ions were kept constant (10 mM $SrCl_2$, 4 mM KCl). A: effect of reducing $(Na^+)_0$ on the BPP. B: line traces of voltage clamp currents recorded in pulsing the membrane from holding of −50 to −80 mV for 5 sec in different $(Na^+)_0$. C: plots of voltage clamp I–V curves. The curve linked by filled diamonds was taken in 25 mM NaCl, 80 mM $SrCl_2$, 4 mM KCl, and 5 mM Tris · Cl; V_h always −50 mV. D: clamp current, at −30 mV, as a percentage of current required to clamp the membrane at −30 mV in maximum $(Na^+)_0$ against the percentage of the maximum $(Na^+)_0$; $(Na^+)_0$ replacements were Li^+ (filled squares), $Tris^+$ (filled circles), and sucrose (open circles). E: curve 1 minus curve 4 of C. Solid parts of the curve are from data in C; dashed lines are straight-line extrapolations. Calibrations: 90 mV, 25 sec (A); 12.5 nA, 4sec (B). (Reproduced from Smith et al., 1975, with permission of *Nature*.)

inset), (Carpenter, 1973; Strumwasser, 1973). The basic membrane mechanisms underlying BPP activity involve sodium (Na_{pg}) and potassium (K_{pg}) pacemaker conductances (Smith et al., 1975; Barker and Smith, 1976, 1977, 1978, 1979b; Barker et al., 1978a).

The data indicating the existence of these conductances comes from electrophysiological studies employing the voltage clamp technique. The voltage-clamped pacemaker membrane current–voltage (I–V) curve has a region of negative slope and overall is N-shaped (Fig. 14B). In addition, there is no region in the range of the BPP where membrane current is zero, but there is a steady inward current (Fig. 14B); (Smith et al., 1975). The evidence that sodium ions (Na^+) are involved comes from studies where Na^+ in the Ringer's solution was replaced, in a step-wise manner, by a non-permanent solute. Reducing the Na^+ reduces the amplitude and duration of the BPP (Fig. 15A), the magnitude of the inward current (Fig. 15B and D) and the region of negative slope (Fig. 15C). When the I–V curve, obtained in the

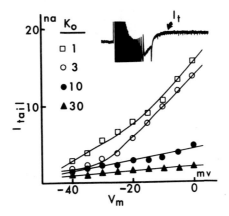

Fig. 16. Magnitude of outward tail currents as a function of membrane potential and $(K^+)_0$. Plot of magnitude of outward tail current (I_t in inset points to tail current) on ordinate as a function of potential to which membrane was clamped during a 5 sec depolarizing step. All currents recorded after the return of membrane to holding potential of -50 mV. Legend under "K_0" indicates symbols which correspond to each $(K^+)_0$. Graphs shows tail currents increase with increase in driving force of K^+ battery, i.e. as equilibrium potential of K^+, E_K, becomes more negative and -50 mV $-E_K$ increases. Results consistent with interpretation that tail currents are mainly K^+ currents.

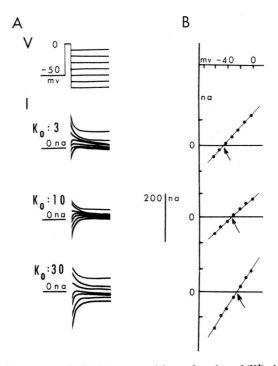

Fig. 17. Variations of tail currents and of driving potential as a function of $(K^+)_0$ in R_{15} of Aplysia. A_V shows experimental procedure: 5 sec steps from holding potential of -50 to 0 mV, followed by steps to different membrane potentials. A_I shows tail currents recorded at various potentials as a function of $(K^+)_0$ (3, 10, 30 mM KCl); all other ions constant 500 mM NaCl, 10 mM CaCl$_2$, 60 mM MgCl$_2$, 15 mM Tris, pH 7.8). B: plot of initial tail current as a function of membrane potential (shown at top) and of $(K^+)_0$ (to right of corresponding tail currents). Calibration: 200 nA applies to A_I and B. Equilibrium potential (arrow: membrane potential where I = 0), becomes less negative with increasing $(K^+)_0$ as expected if tail currents are K^+ currents. See text.

184

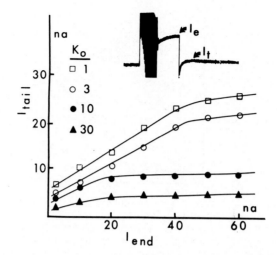

Fig. 18. Relationship between end-of-pulse currents and tail currents. Plot of magnitude of tail currents (I_t) vs the current recorded at the end (I_e) of a 5 sec depolarizing command. Legend under "K_0" indicates symbols which correspond to each $(K^+)_0$. Graph shows that I_t and I_e are directly related and hence consistent with slowly increasing I_e mainly a K^+ current.

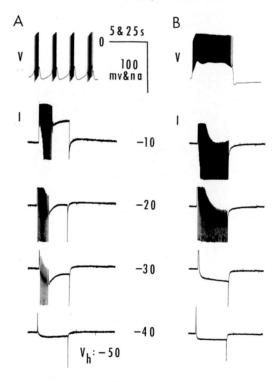

Fig. 19. Effect of $(Ca^{2+})_0$-free seawater on BPPs and voltage clamp currents in R_{15} of Aplysia. A: NaCl 500 mM; $CaCl_2$ 10 mM; $MgCl_2$ 60 mM; KCl 10 mM; Tris · Cl 15 mM; pH 7.8. B: Same solution as in A, except $CaCl_2$ 0 mM. Removal of $(CaCl_2)_0$ increases amplitude and duration of BPP and number of spikes per burst (compare A_V and B_V). In A_I and B_I, holding potential (V_h) −50 mV. Traces show voltage clamp currents evoked by 5 sec steps to potentials shown between A and B. $(Ca^{2+})_0$-free solution does not abolish persistent inward current (cf. −40 and −30 in A and B) but does remove most of late outward-going current during the step and the slow outward tail currents (cf. −10, −20 and −30 in A and B).
Calibrations: 5 sec and 100 nA for I-traces; 25 sec and 100 mV for V-traces.

absence of a negative slope (Fig. 15B, curve 4), is subtracted from the curve obtained in normal Na^+ (Fig. 15B, curve 1), the resultant curve (Fig. 15E) is the I–V curve for the Na_{pg}. This conductance has linear or voltage-independent (G_1) and non-linear or voltage-dependent (G_2) components, both of which extrapolate to the Na^+ equilibrium potential (+25 mV). (Smith et al., 1975; Barker and Smith, 1976, 1977, 1979b; Barker et al., 1978a.)

The potassium pacemaker conductance is less easily demonstrable, since there is no time or potential when only potassium (K_i) current is flowing – the K_i is always contaminated by other ionic currents. The best measure of K_i are the "tail" currents (I_t) (Cole, 1972). The I_t is that recorded upon change of the membrane potential to another value after a step change in membrane potential away from the holding potential (Fig. 16, I_t). These I_ts change in magnitude with changes in membrane potential and in extracellular K^+ as would be expected if they were potassium currents (Fig. 16).

Other data indicating that I_ts are mainly K^+ comes from the voltage-clamp, two-step paradigm (Smith et al., 1980). In the experiment illustrated in Fig. 17, the membrane potential was stepped from a holding potential of –50 mV to 0 mV for 5 sec and then changing to different membrane potential values on successive sweeps. The superimposed voltage sweeps are shown in Fig. 17A_V and the current sweeps are shown in Fig. 17A_I for different values of extracellular K^+ concentrations. When the earliest I_ts are plotted against the membrane potentials where the I_ts were recorded, the result is a straight line the slope of which is the tail conductance. Moreover, the potential at which the current is zero (Fig. 17B, arrows) is the tail equilibrium potential. The tail equilibrium potential becomes more positive as extracellular K^+ is increased (Fig. 17B; arrows), as would be expected for potassium-tail currents.

Another identified K_i is the current that develops slowly during long depolarizing steps in membrane potential, the "end" current, I_e (Fig. 18, inset I_e). The I_es vary with I_t and with changes in extracellular K^+ as expected for a K_i. These potassium I_es are present in normal sea water (Fig. 19A_I) but absent, as are the I_ts, in calcium- (Ca^{2+}) free sea water (Fig. 19B_I) or when no spikes occur (Fig. 19A, –40). It is known in these spikes that the spikes have both Na^+ and Ca^{2+} components (Carpenter, 1973) and that Ca^{2+} enters the cell in a pulsatile manner during the spikes (Stinnakre and Tauc, 1973; Gorman and Thomas, 1978). It is also known that entry of Ca^{2+} into the cell activates a voltage-dependent potassium conductance (Meech, 1972; Gorman and Thomas, 1978). Moreover, this potassium conductance can be blocked by barium ions (Barker and Smith, 1979b; Hermann and Gorman, 1979). Taken together, these data indicate that the K pacemaker conductance, whose activation by the entry of Ca^{2+} ions during spikes results in the K end and tail currents. This conclusion is supported by our finding that the magnitude of the tail current varies with the number of spikes evoked by depolarizing steps (Fig. 20).

The ways in which the Na, K and Ca conductances interact are illustrated in Fig. 21. In Fig. 21A are shown the unrestrained BPPs. In Fig. 21, recorded under voltage clamp, a sinewave was applied to the command amplifier, thus generating a sinusoid change in membrane potential (V) and the recorded current (I). At the beginning of the depolarizing (upward) phase there is a gradual decrease in the persistent inward sodium current. Early in the depolarization, the threshold for the voltage-dependent sodium conductance (Fig. 15E, G_2) is reached, which generates a further increase in inward Na_I, plus the spikes. The pulsatile increase in intracellular Ca^{2+}, which when large enough, activates the K pacemaker conductance. This activation leads to an outward-going K_i, which produces the hyperpolarizing phase of the BPP. This phase is terminated with the inactivation of the K pacemaker conductance and the persistent inward N_i^+ initiates the next cycle of the BPP.

In the estevating or hibernating land snail, *Otala lactea,* cell 11 does not spontaneously

186

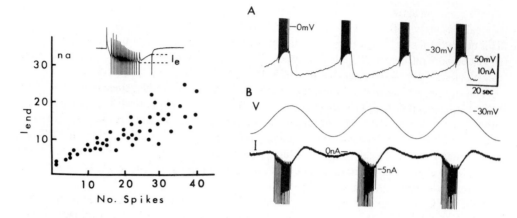

Fig. 20. Relationship between end-of-pulse current and number of spikes per burst. On the ordinate, the magnitude of the outward-going current at the end of a 5 sec depolarizing step (I_e shown in inset) to various membrane potentials (not indicated) is plotted vs the number of action current spikes during command. See text.

Fig. 21. Dynamics of net membrane currents during simulated BPP in Otala. A: recordings were made with CsCl microelectrodes from cell bathed in lysine-vasopressin (LVP) and 10 mM Sr^{2+}. Under unclamped conditions, pacemaker potential amplitude is about 40 mV, oscillating between −34 and −74 mV. B: after voltage clamping, a sinusoidal 50 mV command oscillating between −30 and −80 mV is imposed on the membrane (V), and the resulting net membrane current is recorded (I). On A: zero membrane curtain. At the beginning of the traces, voltage is −80 mV and net current is −2 nA. As membrane is depolarized, net current gradually becomes less negative until potential is about −40 mV, when net current becomes more negative, reaching −5 nA at peak of artificial pacemaker potential. While at peak of waveform, net current is rapidly reversed, momentarily becoming positive during the hyperpolarizing phase of oscillation. Current decays monophasically as potential is polarized to −80 mV. See text.

demonstrate BPPs. The cell is either electrically silent or firing spikes randomly (Fig. 22, inset: control) and its voltage clamp I–V curve has an all-positive slope (Fig. 22, open circles). The application of bag cell extract or nanomolar to micromolar amounts of the nonapeptide, vasopressin, to the bath perfusate initiates rigorous BPPs within minutes (Fig. 22, inset: vasopressin) and the I–V curve now shows a region of negative slope and has an N-shape (Fig. 22, filled circles). These BPPs persist for many minutes to hours following removal of the peptide from the perfusate (Barker and Gainer, 1974; Barker and Smith, 1976). Thus, these peptides are capable of producing prolonged activation of the Na and K pacemaker conductances in a peptidergic neuron that itself plays a role in water regulation (Kupferman and Weiss, 1976).

Thus, one group of cells, the bag cells, that have no anatomic connections with the pacemaker cell, secretes peptide substances, which travel via the circulatory system to engage receptors located on target pacemaker cells. This interaction activates the voltage-dependent Na and K pacemaker conductances, thereby altering the membrane potential behavior of the target cell, namely, by initiating or enhancing BPP activity. We have termed this form of interneuronal communication neurohormonal communication in obvious analogy with the well-known systemic hormonal communication (Barker and Smith, 1976, 1977, 1979a; 1979b; Barker et al., 1979).

There is another action of peptides on the membrane properties of cultured spinal

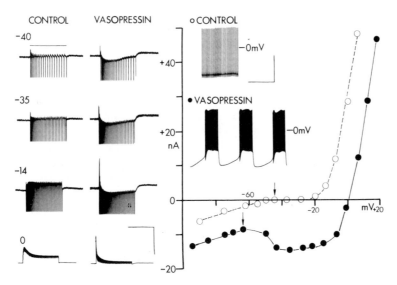

Fig. 22. Vasopressin initiates BPP and alters steady-state, voltage clamp, I–V curve. Recordings are from peptide-sensitive cell 11 from Otala before (CONTROL) and after (VASOPRESSIN) the bath application of 1 μM vasopressin. Membrane potential activity is illustrated in insets of I–V plot on right. Control trace shows random spiking activity. Vasopressin induces BPP. Zero membrane potential, "0 mV". Left: membrane of cell voltage clamped and 5 sec voltage steps imposed (during time indicated by bar above current trace marked −40). Currents are shown at different depolarizing voltage steps (to membrane potentials indicated by numbers above traces) under control conditions and in the presence of vasopressin. Rapid downward current events represent action potential currents. Presence of slow inward current that decreases during the command is apparent in the vasopressin-treated membrane. Right: I–V curve derived from quasi-steady-state currents using most negative or least positive current evoked after 1 sec during command. Current axis (nA), voltage axis (mV). Membrane of cell held at −45 mV in control and −65 mV in vasopressin (downward arrows). Calibrations: left − 10 nA (upper 3 traces) and 40 nA (lowermost traces), 5 sec; right (inset) − 50 mV, 20 sec. (From Barker and Smith (1976) with permission of *Brain Research*.)

neurons which is distinct from both conventional neurotransmitter actions and the aforementioned "neuromodulatory" effects. The action involves direct depression of excitability (Barker et al., 1978b) and consists of a dose-dependent, reversible elevation in threshold for spike generation either without any other detectable changes in membrane properties or independent of any other membrane effects (Barker et al., 1978b; Smith et al., 1978). The depression that had been observed with leucine-enkephalin, is evident within seconds of applying the peptide, does not desensitize during prolonged applications, and terminates within seconds of removal of the peptide. This action, though subtle, can effectively attenuate excitability. Since the anatomical relationship between enkephalin-containing nerve terminals and their target cells is not known, it is unclear whether this action on voltage-dependent spike conductance is mediated by peptides released at synapses, or whether it reflects an extra-synaptic or neurohormonal form of communication between cells.

Other examples of functional effects of putative "neurotransmitter" substances on voltage-dependent spike or pacemaker conductances have been reported (Tsein, 1974; Bolton, 1975; Kuba and Koketsu, 1975, 1976; Giles and Noble, 1976; Dunlop and Fischbach, 1978; Klein and Kandel, 1978). Moreover, some of these actions have been shown to occur on membranes apparently devoid of synapses (e.g. Dunlop and Fishbach, 1978) and

188

may be a vertebrate form of "neurohormonal communication". Thus, if these receptors, which are coupled to voltage-dependent conductances, are ever activated in vivo, the activating substances must arrive via a hormonal or circulatory route.

There is a teleological basis for the development and preservation of neurohormonal communication in the nervous system. It represents a class of operations whereby one species of communication molecule initiates and orchestrates the activities of diverse and distant target neurons whose concerted output may lead to an autonomic, endocrine and/or motor behavior of established survival value. In the invertebrate model system, the bag cell peptide causes egg-laying behavior, a clearly intricate and crucial pattern necessary for the survival of the species. In the vertebrate, central administration of angiotensin leads to elevation of blood pressure, release of antidiuretic hormone and drinking behavior. These complementary actions would serve to defend against salt-and-water imbalance. Whether these behaviors reflect a neurohormonal action of the peptide and whether the peptide mediates such events physiologically remain to be studied.

DISCUSSION

The recent development and extensive use of central and peripheral in vitro preparations, more complex than the neuromuscular junction, has generated a new wealth of physiological and pharmacological observations. Some of these findings appear to fall within classical definitions of neurotransmitter action, as defined in terms of carefully studied synaptic events at peripheral or invertebrate central synapses. However, a variety of observations have been reported which clearly do not fall within this definition, suggesting that there may be a variety of ways that cells communicate in the nervous system. Although much of the evidence to support the notion of multiple forms of intercellular communication has been obtained by pharmacological methods, there is reason to consider such data since some naturally occurring synaptic events can be closely mimicked by discrete pharmacological applications (e.g. Kuffler and Yoshikami, 1975). Such mimicry is possible in the case of synaptic potentials because they are brief and clearly detectable signals, properties which have led to the development of experimental techniques designed to mimic the natural membrane events. Since the physiological events occurring during "neurohormonal communication" can also be mimicked by pharmacological application of bag cell peptide, other membrane actions induced by pharmacological application of neuronal substances (e.g. peptide modulation of postsynaptic transmitter responses) might well reflect naturally occurring events.

From the foregoing it is reasonable to suggest that intercellular communication in the nervous system may not be restricted to "neurotransmission", occurring at specialized synaptic junctions between contiguous elements, but rather that intercellular communication in the nervous system may be more complex, utilizing a variety of signals and messengers to generate different patterns of excitability. The 3 types of intercellular signalling discussed here may be likened to several forms of modern electronic communication. For example, synaptic transmission is similar to a telephone conversation between two people in that the transmission is a form of single-cell-to-single-cell communication which requires contiguous neurons to be in contact with each other at specialized synaptic junctions. The signal generated during neurotransmission is brief and shaped by temporal, spatial, cooperative, desensitizing, diffusion and metabolic factors. Ostensibly, the signal functions to momentarily alter cell excitability, both by bringing membrane potential closer to, or further away from spike threshold, and by increasing or decreasing membrane resistance, thereby enhancing or attenuating the efficacy of other synaptically evoked events. Neuromodulation, as defined above, would be analogous to gain or volume control over telephone communication. Alteration in the time course of the synaptic conductance by peptides might be likened to a "tuning" of the transmitted signal. Whether neuromodulation requires immediate proximity of the controlling neuron with subsynaptic receptors remains to be known. Neurohormonal communication would be analogous to a radio broadcast which involves public transmission and private reception between remote elements. During this type of communication only those receivers properly tuned to the appropriate frequency will sense the signal. Thus, only those target cells with the proper receptors, possibly designed to engage different parts of the humorally conveyed molecule, will be activated. The neurohormone—receptor interaction, like the coupling of neurotransmitter receptors to functionally different conductances, may cause different effects in different target cells, leading to excitation in some and inhibition in others. Thus, the same signal may have a different meaning or consequence to different receivers. The neurohormonal mode of intercellular communication would allow one cell type to regulate the excitability of diverse and distant target neurons so as to produce concerted and complex patterns of autonomic, endocrine and motor behavior. This form of communication has not yet been demonstrated in the vertebrate CNS. The characteristics of 3 forms of communication are outlined in Table I.

TABLE I

	Neurotransmitters	Neurohormones	Neuromodulators
Avenue	Between contiguous cells at synaptic junctions	Between anatomically remote cells	Unknown
Means of distribution	By axonal connection	By extracellular space	Unknown
Release site	At synaptic terminals	At neurocirculatory terminals	Unknown
Effective concentration	Micro to millimolar	Nanomolar	Nanomolar?
Receptor localization	Subsynaptic localization	Extrasynaptic localization	Unknown
Operation	Change voltage-independent conductances	Change-voltage-dependent conductances	Modulates synaptic activity
Inactivation	Enzymatic; uptake?	Diffusion?	Enzymatic?
Desensitization	Yes	No	No
Antagonist	e.g. curare, bungarotoxin	Unknown	e.g. Naloxone
Kinetics	msec	sec—min—h	sec—min
Output	Simple, single cell activity: EPSPs and IPSPs	Complex and concerted activity of neuronal aggregates	Indirect regulation of neuronal activity
Examples	—ACh at neuromuscular junction —Amino acids in CNS —Catecholamine —Enkephalin on cultured CNS neurons	—Bag cell hormone and vasopressin in molluscs —Epinephrine and ACh on cardiac muscle —Norepinephrine and ACh in sympathetic neurons —Enkephalin modulation of spike threshold?	—Enkephlin on cultured CNS neurons

190

ACKNOWLEDGEMENTS

We thank the following colleagues for helpful discussion and for allowing us to use some previously unpublished data: Drs. Donna Gruol, Mae Huang, John MacDonald, and Jean-Didier Vincent. We thank Ann Huang and Lloyd LaGrange for unfailing technical assistance with the tissue cultures. We thank Dr. Phil Nelson for reviewing the manuscript and Mrs. Joan Kraft for typing the manuscript.

REFERENCES

Arch, S. (1972) Biosynthesis of egg-laying hormone (ELH) in bag cell neurons of *Aplysia californica, J. gen. Physiol.*, 60: 102–119.

Barker, J.L. and Gainer, H. (1974) Peptide regulation of bursting pacemaker activity in molluscan neurosecretory cell. *Science,* 184: 1371–1373.

Barker, J.L., Ifshin, M. and Gainer, H. (1975) Studies of bursting pacemaker potential activity in molluscan neurons. III. Effect of hormones. *Brain Res.,* 84: 501–513.

Barker, J.L. and Smith, T.G. (1976) Peptide regulation of neuronal membrane properties. *Brain Res.,* 103: 167–170.

Barker, J.L. and Smith, T.G. (1977) Peptides as neurohormones. In *Approaches to the Cell Biology of Neurons,* W.M. Cowan and J.A. Ferendelli (Eds.), Society for Neuroscience, Bethesda, pp. 340–373.

Barker, J.L. and Smith, T.G., Jr. (1978) Electrophysiological studies of molluscan neurons generating bursting pacemaker potential activity. In *Abnormal Neuronal Discharges,* N. Chalazonitis and M. Boisson (Eds.), Raven Press, New York, pp. 359–387.

Barker, J.L. and Ransom, B.R. (1978) Pentobarbitone pharmacology of mammalian central neurones grown in tissue culture. *J. Physiol. (Lond.),* 280: 355–372.

Barker, J.L., Neale, J.H., Smith, T.G., Jr. and Macdonald, R.L. (1978a) Opiate peptide modulation of amino acid responses suggests novel form of neuronal communication. *Science,* 199: 1451–1453.

Barker, J.L., Smith, T.G. and Neale, J.H. (1978b) Multiple membrane actions of enkephalin revealed using cultured spinal neurons. *Brain Res.,* 154: 153–158.

Barker, J.L. and Smith, T.G., Jr. (1979) Three modes of communication in the nervous system. In *Mediation, Modulation and Specifics in the Nervous System,* Y. Ehrlich (Ed.), Plenum Press, New York, in press.

Barker, J.L. and Smith, T.G., Jr. (1980) Bursting pacemaker potential activity in a peptidergic neuron. In *The Role of Peptides in Neuronal Function,* J.L. Barker and T.G. Smith, Jr. (Eds.), Marcel Dekker, New York, in press.

Barker, J.L., Gruol, D.L., Huang, A.L., Huang, L.M., MacDonald, J.F. and Smith, T.G. (1979) Peptide mediated modes of intercellular communication in the nervous system. In *The Role of Peptides in Neuronal Function,* J.L. Barker and T.G. Smith, Jr. (Eds.), Marcel Dekker, New York, in press.

Blankenship, J. (1980) Physiological properties of peptide-neuroendocrine cells in the marine mollusc Aplysia. In *The Role of Peptides in Neuronal Function,* J.L. Barker and T.G. Smith, Jr., (Eds), Marcel Dekker, New York, in press.

Bolton, T.B. (1975) Effects of stimulating the acetylcholine receptor on the current–voltage relationships of the smooth muscle membrane studied by voltage clamp of potential recorded by microelectrode. *J. Physiol. (Lond.),* 250: 175–202.

Branton, W.D., Mayeri, E., Brownell, P. and Simon, S.B. (1978a) Evidence for local hormonal communication between nervous hormonal communication between neurons in Aplysia. *Nature (Lond.),* 274: 78–79.

Branton, W.D., Arch, S., Smock, T. and Mayeri, E. (1978b) *Proc. Nat. Acad. Sci. (Wash.),* 75: 5732–5736.

Brooks, N. and Werman, R. (1973) The cooperativity of γ-aminobutyric acid on the membrane of locus muscle fibers. *Molec. Pharm.,* 9: 571–579.

Carpenter, D.O. (1973) Ionic mechanisms and models of endogenous discharge in Aplysia. In *Neurobiology of Invertebrates, Mechanisms of Rhythm Regulation,* T. Salanki (Ed.), Academiai Kiado, Budapest, pp. 35–38.

Choi, D.W., Farb, D.H. and Fishbach, G.D. (1978) Chlordiazepoxide selectivity augments GABA action in spinal cord cell cultures. *Nature (Lond.)*, 269: 342–343.

Coggeshall, R.E. (1967) A light and electron microscope study of the abdominal ganglion of *Aplysia californica, J. Neurophysiol.*, 30: 1263–1287.

Cole, K.S. (1972) *Membrane, Ions and Impulses*, University of California Press, Berkeley.

Dionne, V. and Stevens, C.F. (1975) Voltage dependence of agonists effectiveness at the frog neuro-muscular junction: resolution of a paradox. *J. Physiol. (Lond.)*, 251: 245–270.

Dostrovsky, J. and Pomeranz, B. (1973) Morphine blocks amino acid putative transmitters on cat spinal cord sensory interneurones. *Nature New Biol.*, 246: 222–224.

Dunlap, K. and Fischbach, G.D. (1978) Neurotransmitters decrease the calcium component of sensory neurone action potentials. *Nature (Lond.)*, 276: 837–839.

Eccles, J.C. (1964) *The Physiology of Synapses*, Springer, Heidelberg.

Fatt, P. and Katz, B. (1953) The effect of inhibitory nerve fibers on a crustacean muscle fiber. *J. Physiol. (Lond.)*, 121: 374–389.

Frazier, N.T., Kandel, E.R., Kupferman, I., Waziri, R. and Coggeshall, R.E. (1967) Morphological and functional properties of identified neurons in the abdominal ganglion on *Aplysia californica, J. Neurophysiol.*, 30: 1288–1351.

Furshpan, E.J. and Potter, D.D. (1959) Transmission at the giant motor synapse of the crayfish. *J. Physiol. (Lond.)*, 145: 289–325.

Gainer, H. (1972) Electrophysiological behavior of an endogenously active neurosecretory cell. *Brain Res.*, 39: 403–418.

Giles, W. and Noble, S.J. (1976) Changes in membrane currents in bullfrog atrium produced by acetyl-choline. *J. Physiol. (Lond.)*, 261: 103–123.

Gorman, A.L.F. and Thomas, M.V. (1978) Changes in intracellular concentration of free calcium ions in a pace-maker neurone, measured with a metallochromic indication dye arsenazo III. *J. Physiol. (Lond.)*, 275: 357–376.

Hermann, A. and Gorman, A.L.F. (1979) Blockage of voltage-dependent and Ca^{2+} dependent K^+ current components by Ba^{2+} in molluscan pacemaker neurons. *Experientia (Basel)*, 35: 229–231.

Hodgkin, A.L. (1964) *The Conduction of the Nerve Impulse*. Ch. Thomas, Springfield, Ill.

Ifshin, M., Gainer, H. and Barker, J.L. (1975) Peptide factor extracted from molluscan ganglia modulates bursting pacemaker activity. *Nature (Lond.)*, 254: 72–74.

Katz, B. (1966) *Nerve, Muscle and Synapse*, McGraw-Hill, New York.

Klein, M. and Kandel, E.R. (1978) Presynaptic modulation of voltage-dependent Ca^{2+} current: mecha-nism for behavioral sensitization in *Aplysia californica. Proc. Nat. Acad. Sci. (Wash.)*, 75: 3512–3516.

Kuba, K. and Koketsu, K. (1975) Direct control of action potentials by acetylcholine in bullfrog sym-pathetic ganglion cells. *Brain Res.*, 89: 166–169.

Kuba, K. and Koketsu, K. (1976) The muscarinic effects of acetylcholine on the action potential of bull-frog sympathetic ganglion cells. *Jap. J. Physiol.*, 26: 703–716.

Kuffler, S.W. and Yoshikami, D. (1975) The distribution of acetylcholine sensitivity at the post-synaptic membrane of vertebrate skeletal twitch muscles: iontophoretic mapping in the micron range. *J. Physiol. (Lond.)*, 244: 703–730.

Kupferman, I. (1970) Stimulation of egg laying by extracts of neuroendocrine cells (bag cells) of abdomi-nal ganglion of Aplysia. *J. Neurophysiol.*, 33: 877–881.

Kupferman, I. and Weiss, K.R. (1976) Water regulation by a presumptive hormone contained in identified neurosecretory cell R15 of Aplysia. *J. gen. Physiol.*, 67: 113–123.

Meech, R.W. (1972) Intracellular calcium injection causes increased potassium conductance in Aplysia nerve cells. *Comp. Biochem. Physiol.*, 42A: 493–499.

MacDonald, R.L. and Nelson, P.G. (1978) Specific opiate-induced depression of transmitter release from dorsal root ganglion cells in culture. *Science*, 199: 1449–1451.

MacDonald, R.L. and Barker, J.L. (1978a) Benzodiazepines specifically modulate GABA-mediated post-synaptic inhibition in cultured mammalian neurons. *Nature (Lond.)*, 271: 563–564.

MacDonald, R.L. and Barker, J.L. (1978b) Specific antagonism of GABA-mediated postsynaptic inhibi-tion in cultured mammalian spinal cord neurons: a common mode of convulsant action. *Neurol-ogy*, 28: 325–333.

Pinsker, H.M. and Dudek, F.E. (1977) Bag cell control of egg laying in freely behaving Aplysia. *Science*, 197: 490–493.

Segal, M. (1977) Morphine and enkephalin interactions with putative neurotransmitter in rat hippocampus. *Neuropharmacology,* 16: 587–592.

Segel, I.H. (1975) *Enzyme Kinetics,* John Wiley, New York.

Smith, T.G., Barker, J.L. and Gainer, H. (1975) Requirements for bursting pacemaker potential activity in molluscan neurons. *Nature (Lond.),* 253: 450–452.

Smith, T.G., Barker, T.L., Gruol, D.L., Huang, L.M. and Neale, J.H. (1978) Comparison of peptide and amino acid depression of excitability on cultured spinal neurons. *Neurosci. Abstr.,* 4: 415.

Smith, T.G., Barker, J.L., Smith, B.M. and Colburn, T.R. (1980) Voltage clamp techniques applied to cultured skeletal muscle and spinal neurons. In *Excitable Cells in Tissue Culture,* P.G. Nelson and M. Lieberman (Eds.), Plenum Press, New York, in press.

Stinnakre, J. and Tauc, L. (1973) Calcium influx in active Aplysia neurons detected by injected aquorin. *Nature (Lond.),* 242: 113–115.

Strumwasser, F. (1973) Neural and humoral factors in the temporal organization of behavior. *Physiologist,* 16: 9–42.

Stuart, D.G. and Strumwasser, F. (1978) Sites of action of the polypeptide egg-laying hormone (ELH) in the head ganglia of *Aplysia californica. Neurosci. Abstr.,* 4: 207.

Tsein, R.W. (1974) Effects of epinephrine on the pacemaker potassium current of cardiac purkinje fibers. *J. gen. Physiol.,* 64: 293–305.

Vincent, J.D. and Barker, J.L. (1979) Substance P: evidence for diverse roles in neuronal function using cultured mouse spinal neurons. *Science,* 205: 1409–1412.

Watanabe, A. and Grundfest, H. (1961) Impulse propagation at the septal and commissural junction of crayfish. *J. gen. Physiol.,* 45: 267–308.

Weakly, J.N. (1969) Effect of barbiturates on "quantal" synaptic transmission in spinal motoneurons. *J. Physiol. (Lond.),* 204: 63–77.

Zieglgänsberger, W. and Bayerl, H. (1976) The mechanism of inhibition of neuronal activity by opiates in the spinal cord of cat. *Brain Res.,* 115: 111–128.

Zieglgänsberger, W., Fry, J.P., Herz, A., Moroder, L. and Wursch, E. (1976) Enkephalin-induced inhibition of cortical neurons and the lack of this effect in morphine tolerant/dependent rats. *Brain Res.,* 115: 160–164.

Zieglgänsberger, W. and Fry, J.P. (1978) Actions of enkephalin on cortical and striatal neurons of naive and morphine tolerant/dependent rats. In *Opiates and Endogenous Opiate Peptides,* H.W. Kosterlitz (Ed.), North Holland, New York, pp. 231–238.

On the Neurochemical Mechanism of Action of ACTH[*]

W.H. GISPEN

Division of Molecular Neurobiology, Rudolf Magnus Institute for Pharmacology and Laboratory of Physiological Chemistry, Medical Faculty, Institute of Molecular Biology, University of Utrecht, The Netherlands

INTRODUCTION

For many years it has been known that pituitary peptides can modify behavior in animals and man. In 1969, de Wied formulated the hypothesis that the pituitary gland manufactures peptides, designated as neuropeptides, which are involved in learning, motivation and memory processes and which bring about their behavioral effect by a direct action on central nervous structures.

The importance of peptides for brain function is supported by a substantial body of reports in recent literature, describing the presence of a variety of peptides in brain cells and pathways. The discovery that some fragments of β-lipotropin (β-LPH) are naturally occurring brain-peptides with opiate-like activity (endorphins; Hughes et al., 1975; Guillemin et al., 1976; Bradbury et al., 1976), greatly enhanced the interest in neuropeptides. Such findings have led to speculation about the existence of a new type of neurotransmission, viz. peptidergic transmission.

As often happens in a rapidly expanding field, large amounts of data are collected and produced, the coherence of which in the beginning is poorly understood. Also, it would appear that there is sufficient imbalance between quantity and quality of the presently reported rapid communications on neuropeptides, making it a hazardous task to identify common principles in their reported effects which would allow the formulation of possible mechanisms of action.

In the present paper, I will attempt to outline the 3 most currently proposed neurochemical mechanisms by which peptides may affect brain function. First of all, neuropeptides may act transsynaptically in peptidergic synapses. Secondly, neuropeptides may exert their action by modulation of ongoing transmission in specific neuronal networks and, finally, they can be considered to act as effectors (neurohormones) in a classical endocrine view with the brain as the target tissue for circulating neurohormones. Emphasis will be given to the behaviorally active fragments of adrenocorticotropic hormone (ACTH) and their modulation of phosphorylation of synaptic membrane constituents (proteins, lipids), supporting the view that such peptides may act as neuromodulators. In view of the wide variety of behavioral, neurophysiological and neurochemical effects on record, one should reserve judgment regarding the unifying central mechanism of action of ACTH. Therefore, for the

---

[*] This manuscript is gratefully dedicated to my teacher and friend Prof. David de Wied.

moment, it seems appropriate to presume multiple sites and mechanisms of action of behaviorally active neuropeptides chemically related to ACTH.

ACTH AS NEUROHORMONE

In the periphery, peptide hormones are thought to interact with their respective target cells by binding with specific receptors at the outer membrane of these cells. In Sutherland's unifying concept (Sutherland, 1972) peptide hormones are regarded as effectors (*first messengers*) activating but not entering their target cell (Fig. 1). Peptide—receptor binding is thought to result in an allosteric activation of the membrane-bound adenylate cyclase which in turn amplifies the stimulus by the generation of free intracellular cyclic AMP (cAMP) from Mg-ATP. This cAMP (*second messenger*) binds to the regulatory subunit of a protein kinase complex which then releases the active catalytic protein kinase subunit (Rubin and Rosen, 1975). The cAMP-generating and protein kinase-activating system seems present in many cell types and can be found in both prokaryotic and eukaryotic cells. Thus, the activation of the cell constitutes a train of events which is identical in a variety of cell types irrespective of the nature of the first messenger. The specificity of the peptide—target cell interaction, giving a well-defined biological response, is ensured at two levels, i.e. extracellular peptide—receptor recognition and substrate specificity of the activated protein kinase. Additional regulatory influences on the free intracellular level of the second messenger cAMP can be envisaged to arise from the availability of Mg-ATP (ATPase) or the metabolism of cAMP (phosphodiesterase). Therefore, among the various criteria which are to be met before ascribing a mediating role of the cyclic nucleotide in hormone—cell interactions, it should be shown that cAMP alone can mimic the peptide-induced response, and that blockage of cAMP degradation leads to an enhancement of this response.

However, despite its generality in target tissue responses, the second messenger concept seems not to be the sole explanation for the metabolic response in the target cell (Goldfine, 1978). For instance, it is uncertain whether the trophic influence of a peptide on its target cell growth may be described solely in terms of cAMP activation. Increased blood circulation, and the concomitant enhanced supply of precursor substances, energy and oxygen, may by itself account for a number of metabolic changes seen in the target cell after expo-

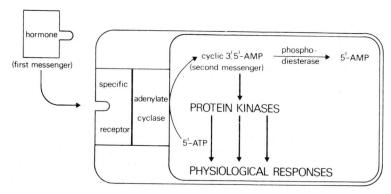

Fig. 1. Schematic representation of the second messenger concept. This scheme is a modified version of the concept as proposed by Sutherland (1972). (Figure taken from Wiegant, 1978.)

sure of the tissue to the first messenger. Furthermore, there is recent evidence to suggest that a peptide—membrane—receptor complex may be "internalized", and that in fact a certain amount of peptide will enter the cytosol. In this manner it would affect cell metabolism directly, by-passing cAMP mediation (Kolata, 1978).

In any event, characteristic of the neurohormonal mechanism is: (a) the production of the peptide at a specific place; (b) its humoral transport to the site of action; and (c) its binding to those cells which recognize the circulating peptide. For ACTH and congeners each of these points will be considered in more detail.

The *site of production* of a number of behaviorally active neuropeptides of this family is thought to be present in both the pituitary and the brain. The synthesis and release of β-endorphin, ACTH and melanocyte stimulating hormone (MSH) in pituitary cells is well documented, but neuro-immuno-cytochemical data also clearly revealed the presence of the pro-opiocortin precursor peptide for ACTH and endorphins suggestive of local production of these peptides in the brain (Akil et al., 1978). Such a notion is supported by experiments of Krieger c.s. indicating the substantial preservation of brain ACTH content even after long-term hypophysectomy (Krieger et al., 1977). Although these authors also showed that "brain"-immunoreactive ACTH-stimulated corticosteroid release in the adrenal cortex cell, structural identity of brain and pituitary ACTH is yet to be confirmed.

The location of the site of production (central vs pituitary) certainly co-determines by what mechanism the peptides are transported to their respective target cells and therefore a possible neurohormonal role. Peptides from the *blood stream* can enter the central nervous system (CNS), although not very efficiently. Recently, Conford et al. (1978) showed for a number of peptides a relatively low passage through the blood—brain barrier after intra-carotid administration. They concluded that the low brain uptake was in the same order of magnitude as that of other putative neurotransmitters. Verhoef and Witter (1976) also reported a low uptake for fragments of ACTH into brain tissue after systemic administration. Intact peptide concentrations of fresh brain tissue were in the order of $10^{-5}-10^{-4}$ times the administered dose for all 3 routes tested (orally, intravenously and subcutaneously). For pituitary ACTH, a special pituitary—brain transport mechanism has been described. Mezey et al. (1978) reported that following intra-pituitary injection of radioactively labelled peptide, an enhanced brain uptake of the peptide took place as compared to intravenous injection. There were clear regional differences with the highest uptake being into the hypothalamus. This transport is presumably partly vascular via the pituitary stalk. Transport to the other brain areas may have occurred via the cerebrospinal fluid but a neural route could not be excluded (Mezey et al., 1978).

The occurrence of ACTH in the *cerebrospinal fluid* (CSF) (Allen et al., 1974) and the behavioral and neuroendocrine effects known to occur after intracerebroventricular (i.c.v.) application of the peptide (De Wied and Gispen, 1977; Wiegant et al., 1979b), point to the importance of the CSF as a transport mechanism of behaviorally active neuropeptides. Intra-ventricular administration of an ACTH$_{4-9}$ analogue resulted in relatively high levels of intact peptide in brain tissue (Verhoef et al., 1977a). Furthermore, it was found that the highest uptake of the peptide occurred in the septal area, and that only in this area could the uptake be competitively displaced by pretreatment with peptides which were structurally and functionally related to ACTH (Verhoef et al., 1977b). Autoradiographic studies after i.c.v. administration revealed intracellular accumulation of the labelled ACTH$_{4-9}$ analogue in a morphologically distinct type of small neuron in the periventricular region, septum, caudate putamen, preoptic area, hypothalamus, thalamus, amygdala and hippocampus (Rees et al., 1980). Although the significance of the uptake of peptide hormones by target cells requires further research, several possible functions have been proposed, including the binding to intracellular receptors so as to exert long-term effects (Kolata, 1978; Schotman et al., 1980).

It remains to be seen whether or not the CSF is an efficient means of transport. Nonetheless, i.c.v. administration of ACTH can lead within minutes to the display of a characteristic behavior (excessive grooming) which has been demonstrated to depend upon dopaminergic projections from the substantia nigra to the neostriatum or the nucleus accumbens (Wiegant et al., 1977; Cools et al., 1978).

Although recognition by the *target cell* is essential in a neurohormonal concept, little if anything is known about specific ACTH—membrane binding sites (receptors) in the CNS. Recently, Witter (1980) reviewed the evidence for the presence of such ACTH receptors in the brain. Indeed, the clear structure—activity relationship for various CNS effects of ACTH (delay of extinction of conditioned avoidance behavior, induction of excessive grooming, counteraction of morphine analgesia; for review see Gispen et al., 1977b) point to the presence of multiple CNS binding sites for ACTH. However, the experiments showing displacement of dihydromorphin from its CNS membrane receptor by ACTH in vitro, are the only studies so far in which an interaction of the peptide with a binding site could conclusively be demonstrated (Terenius, 1975; Terenius et al., 1975). Because of the very low effective CNS concentrations of these peptides, Witter (1980) postulated that putative CNS receptors for ACTH are characterized by very high affinity and very low capacity. It might well be that this unfavourable situation is the main reason for the failure of such receptor sites to be demonstrated by currently available radioligand assays.

As discussed above, it is generally assumed that a peptide hormone will activate its target cell via a second messenger. The role of free *intracellular cAMP* as such a second messenger in ACTH—CNS interaction is unclear. Burkhard and Gey (1968) and Von Hungen and Roberts (1973) were unable to detect an effect of ACTH on adenylate cyclase in brain cell membrane preparations. Forn and Krishna (1971) did not observe an effect of ACTH on cAMP accumulation in rat brain cerebral cortex slices. On the other hand, indirect indications that peptides related to ACTH may affect brain cyclic nucleotide levels in vivo were presented by Rudman and coworker (Rudman and Isaacs, 1975; Rudman, 1976), who showed that intracisternal injection of ACTH or β-MSH in rabbits increased the cAMP but not the cGMP concentration in CSF. Furthermore, it was shown that in rabbit brain especially the circumventricular organs contain the ACTH-sensitive adenylate cyclase (Rudman, 1978). In a preliminary study it was reported that chronic treatment of rats with α-MSH ($[Ac-Ser^1]ACTH_{1-13}-NH_2$) increased the level of cAMP in the occipital cortex (Christensen et al., 1976), while the level of cGMP is unaltered by this treatment in all brain regions studied (Spirtes et al., 1978).

Recently, we have investigated the influence of N-terminal fragments of ACTH on the accumulation of cAMP in rat brain, using 3 different approaches: (a) broken cell preparations (adenylate cyclase activity); (b) slices from posterior thalamus and neostriatum; and (c) the intact brain (Wiegant and Gispen, 1975; Wiegant et al., 1979a).

$ACTH_{1-24}$ was found to have a biphasic effect on the activity of adenylate cyclase in broken cell preparations of rat brain subcortical tissue: concentrations below 25 μM stimulated, whereas higher concentrations inhibited adenylate cyclase activity. The magnitude of the observed stimulation was dependent upon the concentrations of ATP and Mg^{2+} in the incubation medium. Structure activity studies revealed that, at a concentration of 100 μM $ACTH_{1-16}-NH_2$ and $ACTH_{4-7}$ also inhibited the activity of adenylate cyclase, whereas $ACTH_{1-10}$, $ACTH_{4-10}$, $|D-Phe^7|ACTH_{1-10}$ and $|D-Phe^7|ACTH_{4-10}$ all were inactive in this respect (Fig. 2).

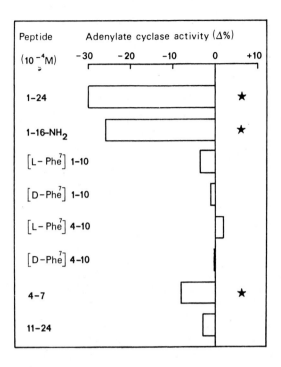

Fig. 2. Structure–activity relationship within ACTH$_{1-24}$ for the inhibitory effect on the adenylate cyclase activity in synaptosomal plasma membranes of rat brain subcortical tissue. The effect on the adenylate cyclase activity is expressed as percentage of the basal activity, and was determined at least in triplicate. Asterisks mean $P < 0.05$, Student t-test. (Figure taken from Wiegant et al., 1979.)

ACTH enhanced the accumulation of cAMP in slices from rat brain (posterior thalamus and neostriatum) in a dose-dependent manner. This effect was already maximal 7.5 min after the addition of the peptide, and was potentiated by isobutyl methylxanthine, a potent inhibitor of phosphodiesterase. Intraventricular injection of 1 μg ACTH$_{1-16}$-NH$_2$ in rats significantly elevated (+27%) the concentration of cAMP in the septal region 60 min after injection of the peptide. No effects were observed in the other brain regions studied (neocortex, hippocampus, basal ganglia, mesencephalon, substantia nigra, myelencephalon, cerebellum, Wiegant et al., 1979a). It was concluded therefore, that under certain circumstances ACTH and its congeners could serve as first messenger altering the intracellular cAMP levels in brain cells.

In a variety of tissues, effector–receptor binding is accompanied by a *calcium influx* into the cell. This calcium influx is also thought to serve as second messenger in the activation of target cell metabolism (Michell, 1975). In the membrane, concomitant with the calcium influx, an enhanced metabolism of (poly)phosphatidyl inositide(s) is observed (Michell, 1975). Especially in membranes from nervous tissue the *polyphosphoinositides* are present in considerable amounts and display an extremely rapid metabolism (Hawthorn and Pickard, 1979). It has been pointed out that these phospholipids are therefore likely candidates to play a role in the calcium influx into the nerve cell (Michell, 1975). Recently, we measured the effect of ACTH$_{1-24}$ on the metabolism of brain membrane phosphoinositides in vitro (Jolles et al., 1979). Preliminary data suggest a time- and dose-dependent acceleration of this phosphoinositide metabolism by the peptide. Further work is in progress, aimed at charac-

198

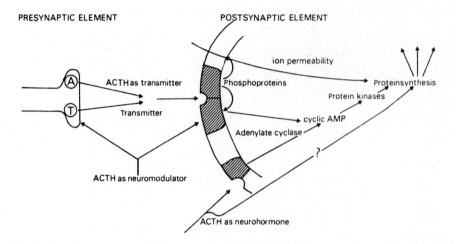

Fig. 3. Possible modes of action of ACTH in the central nervous system. A, ACTH; T, transmitter. *ACTH as neurohormone.* The brain is a target for circulating ACTH and brain cells with receptors for ACTH will recognize the peptide and may respond to ACTH–receptor binding with the intracellular production of a second messenger (cAMP). All subsequent events are then initiated by a cAMP-dependent protein kinase. *ACTH as neurotransmitter.* In peptidergic synapses, ACTH may serve as a transmitter itself and thus acting transsynaptically on the postsynaptic neuron. *ACTH as neuromodulator.* ACTH influences ongoing neurotransmission by altering either the release of transmitter from the presynaptic neuron or the excitability of the postsynaptic neuron. (Figure taken from Gispen et al., 1979.)

terizing this finding in more detail, and eventually correlating it with calcium uptake. Thus it is not unlikely that in some instances ACTH–brain membrane interactions involve phosphatidylinositide metabolism with calcium as a second messenger in ACTH-induced changes in rat brain metabolism.

The events following the influx of Ca^{2+} or the rise in intracellular cAMP are not well worked out (Fig. 3). There are numerous reports in the literature concerning effects of ACTH on brain RNA and protein metabolism, transmitter turnover, etc. (for reviews, see Schotman et al., 1976; Reith et al., 1977; Dunn and Gispen, 1977; Kovacs et al., 1980). It has been proposed that the effects on *protein metabolism* originate from actions of ACTH as a neurohormone, exerting a relatively long-lasting trophic influence upon CNS target cells (Dunn and Gispen, 1977; Schotman et al., 1980). It was argued that, by enhancement of protein synthesis, the nerve cell would acquire a larger adaptive capacity, e.g. new receptor molecules become incorporated into membranes or more enzymes are involved in the turn-over of neurotransmitters (Dunn and Gispen, 1977). Thus, such trophic influences could partly underlie the behavioral effects of ACTH. The peptide would in fact facilitate the brain's adaptation to a new environmental situation (Dunn, 1976). Indeed, peptides which enhanced the learning of an avoidance test by hypophysectomized rats, have been found to stimulate rat brain protein synthesis, whereas peptides which failed to enhance the learning behavior were without effect upon protein synthesis (Reith et al., 1977).

ACTH AS PUTATIVE NEUROTRANSMITTER

The suggestion that peptides could serve a role as neurotransmitter in peptidergic synapses (Fig. 3) is a fundamental one, and would place a number of reported findings in very different perspective. However, little evidence is presently on record to support the notion with respect to ACTH. Certainly, using immunocytochemical techniques, the existence of neuronal pathways containing ACTH-immunoreactive material is apparent (Krieger et al., 1977) as well as the presence of the precursor molecule of this peptide (Krieger et al., 1979; Akil et al., 1978). Furthermore, iontophoretic application of the peptide to nerve cells revealed the presence of ACTH-sensitive neurons (Segal, 1976; Steiner, 1970; Van Delft and Kitay, 1972). More work is needed, however, before a description in terms of putative ACTH transmission is possible. Further studies on release, production and breakdown, receptors, etc., may tackle this problem more precisely. Therefore, in this short survey on the neurochemical mechanisms of ACTH action, peptidergic neurotransmission has only been mentioned as a possible mode of action.

ACTH AS MODULATOR OF NEUROTRANSMISSION

Although current terminology does distinguish between "hormone" and "modulator", it is not entirely clear how much is semantics and how much this distinction can add to the understanding of how neuropeptides affect brain cells. The best defined terminology can be found in recent reviews by Barchas et al. (1978) and Barker and Smith (1979; 1980). In the context of this paper, neuromodulators are considered to be entities which alter interneuronal communication without serving as a transmitter of information themselves. Their effect should be of a rapid nature and is likely to take place at the membranes bordering the synaptic cleft (Fig. 3). Thus, per definition, their effects are different from the hormonal trophic responses as discussed above. Neuromodulators, like neurohormones, could either be transported by a general transport mechanism (for instance the CSF) or delivered via peptidergic neurons close to their site of action.

The process of neuromodulation could consist of altered transmitter release from the presynaptic terminal or of altered responsiveness of the postsynaptic element to incoming information (Fig. 3). Evidence is accumulating that phosphorylation of synaptic membrane proteins may affect the transmission of information between neurons, and thus could be an ideal target for putative neuromodulators. Early on, Heald speculated that the change in *protein phosphorylation* that occurred in response to electrical stimulation of respiring brain slices altered the conformation of neuronal membrane proteins, and that such changes might be involved in the regulation of ion movements through cell membranes (Heald, 1957; 1962). Trevor and Rodnight (1965) demonstrated that the protein-phosphoryl-serine groups that responded to electrical stimulation were indeed in the membrane fraction. Browning et al., (1977, 1979) reported that synaptic potentiation of the Schaeffer collaterals in rat hippocampal slices led to an altered Ca^{2+}-dependent phosphorylation of a specific protein band, associated with the synaptic plasma membrane fraction. Furthermore, phosphorylation of specific protein substrates seems to be involved in the release of neurotransmitters. Such a release is calcium-dependent and experiments were reported describing a calcium-dependent phosphorylation in relation to the exocytosis of neurotransmitters (Katz and Miledi, 1967; Douglas, 1973; DeLorenzo, 1976; Redburn et al., 1976; DeLorenzo and Freedman, 1977; Krueger et al., 1977; Herskowitz, 1978; Schulman and Greengard, 1978; Sieghart et al., 1978).

With respect to cAMP-sensitive brain membrane protein phosphorylation, it was hypothesized that enhanced phosphorylation of the substrate protein accounts for the membrane hyperpolarization (Greengard, 1976; Nathanson and Greengard, 1977). The involvement of protein phosphorylation in brain function is further evidenced by reports on correlative changes in membrane phosphoproteins with a variety of behavioral experiences (Glassman et al., 1973; Perumal et al., 1975, 1977; Ehrlich et al., 1977; Gispen et al., 1977a; Holmes et al., 1977).

We have been studying the endogenous phosphorylation of proteins from rat brain *synaptosomal plasma membranes* (SPM) in vitro with or without the behaviorally active peptide $ACTH_{1-24}$ in the incubation medium. Many factors may influence this in vitro process (Rodnight et al., 1975), and important determinants seem to be: the activity of ATPase(s) controlling the availability of the phosphate donor (ATP), the activity of the protein phosphatase(s) and, of course, that of the protein kinase(s). As was shown for total membrane protein (Rodnight et al., 1975), the phosphorylation of a given SPM protein band also depends very much on the ATP/SPM ratio used in the incubation system (Wiegant et al., 1978). Therefore, both a low and a high ATP/SPM ratio are routinely used in our experiments.

Incubation of SPM in the presence of $ACTH_{1-24}$ resulted in a decrease in phosphorylation of at least 5 SPM protein bands, as visualized by protein staining and by autoradiography after polyacrylamide slab gel electrophoresis (Zwiers et al., 1976). The decrease in phosphorylation showed a biphasic dose—response relationship. A marked reduction was observed at concentrations of $10^{-4}-10^{-5}$ M whereas at concentrations around $10^{-6}-10^{-7}$ M, hardly any effect could be detected. In freshly prepared preparations, a significant decrease was again observed consistently at concentrations around 10^{-8} M. The phosphoprotein bands affected by in vitro addition of $ACTH_{1-24}$ were of a smaller molecular weight than those affected by in vitro addition of cAMP. The peptide-sensitive bands ranged in mol. wt. from 15 000 to 48 000 daltons, whereas cAMP stimulated the endogenous phosphorylation of bands with molecular weights of 75 000, 57 000 and 54 000, respectively. The involvement of different protein bands, and the opposite direction of the peptide and cyclic nucleotide effects, make it highly unlikely that the peptide effect could have been mediated by cAMP (Zwiers et al., 1976).

Using the approach described by DeLorenzo and Greengard (1973), a first attempt was made to discriminate between a possible effect of $ACTH_{1-24}$ on phosphorylating and that on dephosphorylating activity in the SPM fraction. The data suggest that after the exhaustion of ATP, when there can be no net phosphorylation, $ACTH_{1-24}$ is ineffective in altering the amount of ^{32}P in SPM even over a long incubation period (dephosphorylation). If, however, new $[\gamma-^{32}P]ATP$ is added, and phosphorylation activity can thus again be monitored, a subsequent inhibition of ^{32}P incorporation by $ACTH_{1-24}$ is found (Zwiers et al., 1978). These data were therefore taken to mean that ACTH interacts with SPM protein kinase(s) and not with SPM protein phosphatase(s).

Further experiments were carried out to isolate, purify and partially characterize the *ACTH-sensitive protein kinase* from rat brain membranes and one of its endogenous substrates (B-50, mol. wt. 48 000, Zwiers et al., 1979). Treatment with 0.5% Triton X-100 in 75 mM KCl solubilized 15% of the total B-50 protein kinase activity and preserved the sensitivity of the enzyme to $ACTH_{1-24}$. Column chromatography of the solubilized material over DEAE-cellulose pointed to the presence of multiple protein kinase activities from rat brain SPM, one of which was the ACTH-sensitive *B-50 protein kinase* (Zwiers et al., 1979). The column fractions containing the B-50 protein kinase were subjected to ammonium sulphate precipitation and a protein fraction (55—80% ammonium sulphate) enriched in endogenous B-50 phosphorylating activity was obtained. The time course of the endogenous phosphorylation of B-50 in this fraction showed a linear incorporation with time for at least 10 min and a maximal incorporation of 0.65 mol P/mol B-50 was reached after 60 min. The inhibition by $ACTH_{1-24}$ of the B-50 protein kinase was dose-dependent; the half maximal effective concentration was 5×10^{-6} M, being 10–50 times lower as compared to intact SPM. cAMP, cGMP and various endorphins had no effect on the B-50 protein kinase. The B-50 protein kinase required both magnesium and calcium for optimal activity (Gispen et al., 1979; Zwiers et al., 1980).

After two-dimensional electrophoresis on polyacrylamide slab gels, the B-50 protein kinase and the B-50 protein could be further identified, purified and characterized. The isoelectric point (IEP) of the kinase is 5.5 and the apparent molecular weight 70 K dalton, whereas the IEP of the substrate protein B-50 is 4.5 and the apparent mol. wt. 48 K dalton. Amino acid analysis on µg quantities of purified kinase and B-50 protein revealed basic/acid amino acid ratios in agreement with the respective IEPs (Zwiers et al., 1980).

Structure–activity studies indicated that the interaction of ACTH with endogenous SPM phosphorylation is rather complex. It appeared that the capability of $ACTH_{1-24}$ to inhibit phosphorylation of the low molecular weight SPM bands (represented by B-50) is confined to the N-terminal part of the molecule. The shortest active sequence with the N-terminus intact is $ACTH_{1-13}$. The sequence $ACTH_{5-18}$ seems as active as $ACTH_{1-16}$, and it was therefore concluded that the active site is in the region $ACTH_{5-13}$. Possibly, C-terminal elongation of this sequence is necessary for expression of the activity since $ACTH_{5-16}$ was inactive and $ACTH_{5-18}$ active.

With respect to the effect of ACTH on avoidance behavior, there seems to exist an active site in $ACTH_{4-7}$ and a second site between the sequence $ACTH_{7-24}$ (Greven and de Wied, 1977). Also, the requirements necessary to displace dihydromorphine from its binding site in rat brain SPM and counteraction of morphine in vivo suggest a site in the sequence $ACTH_{4-10}$ along with that extra-active site (Gispen et al., 1976).

The ACTH-structure/CNS–activity relationships are not completely identical but the general principle of dormant activity and induction of such activity by chain elongation seems to apply. Apparently, information is encoded in a multiple form, making comparison among peptides, on the basis of primary structures alone, hazardous (de Wied and Gispen, 1977).

Interestingly, the effect of ACTH fragments on the phosphorylation of B-50 is very similar to that found for the induction of excessive grooming (Gispen et al., 1975). The ACTH sequences 1–24, 1–26, 1–13, 5–18 and, to some extent, 5–16 induce the display of excessive grooming in the rat after intraventricular administration, whereas 1–10, 4–10, 11–24, 7–16 and the combination of 1–10 plus 11–24 are ineffective.

It was of interest therefore, to see if in vivo intraventricular administration of a *behavioral active ACTH fragment* could result in subsequent changes in endogenous SPM phosphorylation in vitro. Administration of µg quantities of $ACTH_{1-24}$ in rat and subsequent preparation of SPM after 30 min resulted in an increased amount of in vitro incorporated ^{32}P into the same 5 phosphoprotein bands (Zwiers et al., 1977), which also responded after in vitro administration of ACTH. There appears to be a U-shaped dose–response curve of phosphate incorporation into SPM protein bands between 30 and 300 ng of injected $ACTH_{1-24}$. This effect of in vivo ACTH treatment on in vitro endogenous phosphorylation was also time-dependent, with maximal effect 30 min after the peptide injection (Zwiers et al., 1977). From a neurochemical point of view, one wonders what the meaning of the in vivo/in vitro approach is as used in these experiments and in those of others (Ehrlich et al., 1977; Holmes et al., 1977; Browning et al., 1979). A common feature of these studies is that the changes, induced under in vivo conditions, apparently are of long-lasting nature and are persistent in a

202

post hoc in vitro assay system. If ACTH also inhibits SPM protein kinase(s) in vivo, the resulting SPM preparation of an animal so treated, would have a higher percentage unphosphorylated amino acids in the ACTH-affected bands. Since the ACTH is washed out during the preparation of SPM (Zwiers, unpublished) the subsequent in vitro SPM phosphorylation assay will then result in higher phosphate incorporation in ACTH-sensitive bands than in the saline-treated controls (see Weller and Rodnight, 1973). In fact, this is exactly what we found.

We have elsewhere proposed that the direct effect of ACTH on a membrane-bound protein kinase may underlie its modulatory role in *neurotransmission* (Gispen et al., 1979). Since the membranes used in our studies will have been mainly of presynaptic origin, it may well be that this effect on membrane phosphorylation represents a presynaptic event. As the B-50 protein kinase is stimulated by magnesium and calcium, it may be the case that the function of the B-50 substrate protein resembles that described for other calcium-dependent phosphoproteins involved in the release of neurotransmitters. If, on the other hand, the B-50 protein kinase/substrate protein complex affected by ACTH primarily was postsynaptic in origin, the observed inhibition of phosphorylation could alter ion permeability, and hence

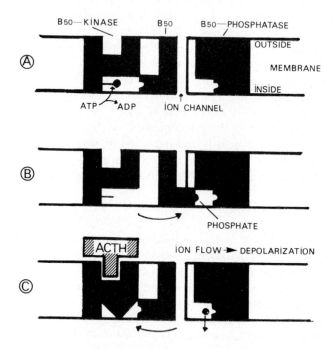

Fig. 4. Theoretical model explaining how ACTH could modulate neurotransmission. In panel A, the molecular components involved in protein phosphorylation occurring in the postsynaptic membrane are shown: the ACTH-sensitive B-50 protein kinase, its substrate protein B-50, bordering an ion channel, and the neighbouring B-50 protein phosphatase. In panel B, the result of phosphorylation of B-50 by B-50 protein kinase is shown. The transfer of a phosphate group (●) leads to an allosteric change in B-50 with the concomitant closure of the ion channel. Panel C represents the events occurring in the presence of ACTH. The peptide inhibits the B-50 protein kinase and subsequently the B-50 protein phosphatase dephosphorylates B-50 leading to the reopening of the ion channel. As a result, changes in ion permeability occur underlying presumably a reduced potential of the postsynaptic membrane. In such a way, the ACTH peptide could regulate the excitability of the postsynaptic neuron.

sensitivity to presynaptic input, as discussed earlier for the role of cAMP in neurotransmission (Fig. 4, Nathanson and Greengard, 1977).

ACKNOWLEDGEMENTS

The author acknowledges his collaboration with Drs. Zwiers, V.M. Wiegant, J. Jolles, K. Wirtz and P. Schotman in the experiments, summarized in this paper on the effect of neuropeptides on rat brain membrane phosphorylation. Furthermore he is grateful to Elly Looy and Greet Hoekstra for helping in the preparation of this manuscript.

REFERENCES

Akil, H., Watson, S.J., Levy, R.M. and Barchas, J.D. (1978) β-endorphin and other 31 K fragments: pituitary and brain systems. In *Characteristics and Functions of Opioids*, J. van Ree and L. Terenius (Eds.), Elsevier/North-Holland Biomedical Press, Amsterdam, pp. 123–134.

Allen, J.P., Kendall, J.W., McGilvra, R. and Vancura, C. (1974) Immunoreactive ACTH in cerebrospinal fluid. *J. clin. Endocr.*, 38: 586–593.

Barchas, J.D., Akil, H., Elliott, G.R., Holman, R.B. and Watson, S.J. (1978) Behavioral neurochemistry: Neuroregulators and behavioral states. *Science*, 200: 964–973.

Barker, J.L. and Smith, T.G., Jr. (1979) Three modes of communication in the nervous system. In *Modulators, Mediators, and Specifiers in Brain Function. Advances in Experimental Medicine and Biology, Vol. 116.* Y.H. Ehrlich, J. Volavka, L.G. Davis and E.G. Brunngraber (Eds.), Plenum Press, New York and London, pp. 3–25.

Barker, J.L. and Smith, T.G., Jr. (1980) Three modes of intercellular neuronal communication. In *Adaptive Capabilities of the Nervous System, Progress in Brain Research, Vol. 53,* P. McConnell, G.J. Boer, H.J. Romijn, N.E. van de Poll and M.A. Corner (Eds.), Elsevier, Amsterdam, pp. 169–192.

Bradbury, A.F., Smyth, D.G., Snell, C.R., Birdsall, N.J.M. and Hulme, E.C. (1976) The C-fragment of lipotropin: an endogenous peptide with high affinity for brain opiate receptors. *Nature (Lond.),* 260: 793–795.

Browning, M., Bennet, W. and Lynch, G. (1979) Phosphorylase kinase phosphorylates a brain protein which is influenced by repetitive synaptic activation. *Nature (Lond.),* 278: 273–275.

Browning, M., Dunwiddie, T., Gispen, W.H. and Lynch, G. (1977) Alterations in a specific membrane phosphoprotein following repetitive stimulation of the hippocampus. *Neurosci. Abstr.,* 3: 1341.

Burkhard, W.P. and Gey, K.F. (1968) Adenyl cyclase in rat brain. *Helv. physiol. pharmacol. acta,* 26: 197–198.

Christensen, C.W., Harston, C.T., Kastin, A.J., Kostrzewa, R.M. and Spirtes, M.A. (1976) Preliminary investigation on α-MSH and MIF I effects on cyclic AMP levels in rat brain. *Pharmacol. Biochem. Behav.,* 5, Suppl. 1: 117–120.

Cools, A.R., Wiegant, V.M. and Gispen, W.H. (1978) Distinct dopaminergic systems in ACTH-induced grooming. *Europ. J. Pharmacol.,* 50: 265–268.

Conford, E.M., Braun, L.D., Crane, P.D. and Oldendorf, W.H. (1978) Blood–brain barrier restriction of peptides and the low uptake of enkephalin. *Endocrinology,* 103: 1297–1303.

DeLorenzo, R.J. (1976) Calcium-dependent phosphorylation of specific synaptosomal fraction proteins: possible role of phosphoproteins in mediating neurotransmitter release. *Biochem. biophys. Res. Commun.,* 71: 590–597.

DeLorenzo, R.J. and Freedman, S.D. (1977) Calcium-dependent phosphorylation of synaptic vesicle proteins and its possible role in mediating neurotransmitter release and vesicle function. *Biochem. biophys. Res. Commun.,* 77: 1036–1043.

DeLorenzo, R.J. and Greengard, P. (1973) Activation by adenosine 3′,5′-monophosphate of a membrane-bound phosphoprotein phosphatase from toad bladder. *Proc. nat. Acad. Sci. (Wash.),* 70: 1831–1835.

De Wied, D. (1969) Effects of peptide hormones on behavior. In *Frontiers in Neuroendocrinology,* W.F. Ganong and L. Martini (Eds.), Oxford University Press, New York, pp. 97–140.

De Wied, D. and Gispen, W.H. (1977) Behavioral effects of peptides. In *Peptides in Neurobiology*, H. Gainer (Ed.), Plenum Press, New York, pp. 397–448.

Douglas, W.W. (1973) How do neurones secrete peptides? Exocytosis and its consequences, including "synaptic vesicle" formation, in the hypothalamo-neurohypophyseal system. In *Drug Effects on Neuroendocrine Regulation, Progress in Brain Research, Vol. 39*, E. Zimmermann, W.H. Gispen, B.H. Marks and D. de Wied (Eds.), Elsevier, Amsterdam, pp. 21–39.

Dunn, A.J. (1976) The chemistry of learning and the formation of memory. In *Molecular and Functional Neurobiology* W.H. Gispen (Ed.), Elsevier/North-Holland Biomedical Press, Amsterdam, pp. 347–387.

Dunn, A.J. and Gispen, W.H. (1977) How ACTH acts on the brain. *Biobehav. Rev.*, 1: 15–23.

Ehrlich, Y.H., Rabjohns, R.H. and Routtenberg, A. (1977) Experimental input alters the phosphorylation of specific proteins in brain membranes. *Pharmacol. Biochem. Behav.*, 6: 169–175.

Forn, J. and Krishna, G. (1971) Effect of norepinephrine, histamine and other drugs on cyclic 3',5'-AMP formation in brain slices of various animal species. *Pharmacology*, 5: 193–204.

Gispen, W.H., Buitelaar, J., Wiegant, V.M., Terenius, L. and De Wied, D. (1976) Interaction between ACTH fragments, brain opiate receptors and morphine induced analgesia. *Europ. J. Pharmacol.*, 39: 393–397.

Gispen, W.H., Perumal, R., Wilson, J.E. and Glassman, E. (1977a) Phosphorylation of proteins of synaptosome-enriched fractions of brain during short-term training experience: the effects of various behavioural treatments. *Behav. Biol.*, 21: 358–363.

Gispen, W.H., van Ree, J.M. and De Wied, D. (1977b) Lipotropin and the central nervous system. *Int. Rev. Neurobiol.*, 20: 209–250.

Gispen, W.H., Wiegant, V.M., Greven, H.M. and De Wied, D. (1975) The induction of excessive grooming in the rat by intraventricular application of peptides derived from ACTH: structure–activity studies. *Life Sci.*, 17: 645–652.

Gispen, W.H., Zwiers, H., Wiegant, V.M., Schotman, P. and Wilson, J.E. (1979) The behaviorally active neuropeptide ACTH as neurohormone and neuromodulator: the role of cyclic nucleotides and membrane phosphoproteins. In *Modulators, Mediators and Specifiers in Brain Function. Neuropeptides, Cyclic Nucleotides and Phosphoproteins. Advances in Experimental Medicine and Biology, Vol. 116*, Y.H. Ehrlich, J. Volavka, L.G. Davis and E.G. Brunngraber (Eds.), Plenum Press, New York and London, pp. 199–224.

Glassman, E., Gispen, W.H., Perumal, R., Machlus, B. and Wilson, J.E. (1973) The effect of short experiences on the incorporation of radioactive phosphate into synaptosomal and non-histone acid-extractable nuclear proteins from rat and mouse brain. In *Proc. 5th Int. Congress Pharmacology, San Francisco, 1972. Vol. 4*, pp. 14–17.

Goldfine, I.D. (1978) Insulin receptors and the site of action of insulin. *Life Sci.*, 23: 2639–2648.

Greengard, P. (1976) Possible role for cyclic nucleotides and phosphorylated membrane proteins in postsynaptic actions of neurotransmitters. *Nature (Lond.)*, 260: 101–108.

Greven, H.M. and De Wied, D. (1977) The influence of peptides structurally related to ACTH and MSH on active avoidance behaviour in rats. A structure–activity relationship study. In *Control, Chemistry and Effects of MSH*, F. Tilders, D. Swaab and Tj.B. van Wimersma-Greidanus (Eds.), Karger, Basel, pp. 140–152.

Guillemin, R., Ling, N. and Burgus, R. (1976) Endorphins. Hypothalamic and neurohypophyseal peptides with morphinomimetic activity. Isolation and primary structure of α-endorphin. *C.R. Acad. Sci. (Paris)*, 282: 783–785.

Hawthorne, J.N. and Pickard, M.R. (1979) Phospholipids in synaptic function. *J. Neurochem.*, 32: 5–14.

Heald, P.J. (1957) The incorporation of phosphate into cerebral phosphoprotein promoted by electrical impulses. *Biochem. J.*, 66: 659–663.

Heald, P.J. (1962) Phosphoprotein metabolism and ion transport in nervous tissue: a suggested connexion. *Nature (Lond.)*, 193: 451–454.

Hershkowitz, M. (1978) Influence of calcium on phosphorylation of a synaptosomal protein. *Biochim. biophys. acta (Amst.)*, 542: 274–283.

Holmes, H., Rodnight, R. and Kapoor, R. (1977) Effect of electroshock and drugs administered in vivo on protein kinase activity in rat. *Pharmacol. Biochem. Behav.*, 6: 415–420.

Hughes, J., Smith, T.W., Kosterlitz, H.W., Fothergill, L.A., Morgan, B.A. and Morris, H.R. (1975) Identification of two related pentapeptides from the brain with potent opiate agonist activity. *Nature (Lond.)*, 258: 577–579.

205

Jolles, J., Wirtz, K.W.A., Schotman, P. and Gispen, W.H. (1979) Pituitary hormones influence polyphosphoinositide metabolism in rat brain. *FEBS Lett.*, 105: 110–114.

Katz, B. and Miledi, R. (1967) A study of synaptic transmission in the absence of nerve impulses. *J. Physiol.*, 192: 407–436.

Kolata, G.B. (1978) Polypeptide hormones: what are they doing in cells? *Science*, 201: 895–897.

Kovacs, G.L., Bohus, B. and Versteeg, D.H.G. (1980) The interaction of posterior pituitary neuropeptides with monoaminergic neurotransmission: significance in learning and memory processes. In *Adaptive Capabilities of the Nervous System, Progress in Brain Research, Vol. 53*, P. McConnell, G.J. Boer, N.E. van de Poll, H.J. Romijn and M.A. Corner (Eds.), Elsevier, Amsterdam, pp. 123–140.

Krieger, D.T., Liotta, A. and Brownstein, M.J. (1977) Presence of corticotrophin in limbic system of normal and hypophysectomized rats. *Brain Res.*, 8: 575–579.

Krieger, D.T., Liotta, A.S., Nicholson, G. and Kizer, J.S. (1979) Brain ACTH and endorphin reduced in rats with monosodium glutamate induced arcuate nuclear lesions. *Nature (Lond.)*, 278: 562–563.

Krueger, B.K., Forn, J. and Greengard, P. (1977) Depolarization-induced phosphorylation of specific proteins, mediated by calcium ion influx, in rat brain synaptosomes. *J. biol. Chem.*, 252: 2764–2773.

Mezey, E., Palkovits, M., de Kloet, E.R., Verhoef, J. and De Wied, D. (1978) Evidence for pituitary–brain transport of a behaviorally potent ACTH analog. *Life Sci.*, 22: 831–838.

Michell, R.H. (1975) Inositol phospholipids and cell surface receptor function. *Biochim. biophys. acta (Amst.)*, 415: 81–148.

Nathanson, J.A. and Greengard, P. (1977) "Second messengers" in the brain. *Sci. American*, 237: 108–119.

Perumal, R., Gispen, W.H., Wilson, J.E. and Glassman, E. (1975) Phosphorylation of proteins from the brains of mice subjected to short-term behavioral experiences. In *Hormones, Homeostasis and the Brain, Progress in Brain Research. Vol. 42*, W.H. Gispen, Tj.B. van Wimersma-Greidanus, B. Bohus and D. de Wied (Eds.), Elsevier, Amsterdam, pp. 201–207.

Perumal, R., Gispen, W.H., Glassman, E. and Wilson, J.E. (1977) Phosphorylation of proteins of synaptosome-enriched fractions of brain during short-term training experiences: the effects of various behavioral treatment. *Behav. Biol.*, 21: 341–357.

Redburn, D.A., Shelton, D. and Cotman, C.W. (1976) Calcium-dependent release of exogenously loaded γ-amino-(U-^{14}C) butyrate from synaptosomes: time course of stimulation by potassium, veratridine, and the calcium ionophore A 23187. *J. Neurochem.*, 26: 297–303.

Rees, H.D., Verhoef, J., Witter, A., Gispen, W.H. and De Wied, D. (1980) Autoradiographic studies with a behaviorally potent ^{3}H-ACTH$_{4-9}$ analog in the brain after intraventricular injection in rats. *Brain Res. Bull.*, in press.

Reith, M.E.A., Schotman, P. and Gispen, W.H. (1977) Pituitary peptides and brain synthesis. In *Mechanisms, Regulation and Special Function of Protein Synthesis in the Brain*, S. Roberts, A. Lajtha and W.H. Gispen (Eds.), Elsevier/North-Holland Biomedical Press, Amsterdam, pp. 383–398.

Rodnight, R., Reddington, M. and Gordon, M. (1975) Methods for studying protein phosphorylation in cerebral tissues. In *Research Methods in Neurochemistry, Vol. 3*, N. Marks and R. Rodnight (Eds.), Plenum Press, New York, pp. 324–367.

Rubin, C.S. and Rosen, O.M. (1975) Protein phosphorylation. *Ann. Rev. Biochem.*, 44: 831–887.

Rudman, D. (1976) Injection of melatonin into cisterna magna increases concentrations of 3',5'-cyclic quanosine monophosphate in cerebrospinal fluid. *Neuroendocrinology*, 20: 235–242.

Rudman, D. (1978) Effect of melanotropic peptides on adenosine 3',5'-monophosphate accumulation by regions of rabbit brain. *Endocrinology*, 103: 1556–1561.

Rudman, D. and Isaacs, J.W. (1975) Effect of intrathecal injection of melanotropic-lipolytic peptides on the concentration of 3',5'-cyclic adenosine monophosphate in cerebrospinal fluid. *Endocrinology*, 97: 1476–1480.

Schotman, P., van Heuven-Nolson, D. and Gispen, W.H. (1980) Protein synthesis in a cell free system from rat brain sensitive to ACTH-like peptides. *J. Neurochem.*, in press.

Schotman, P., Reith, M.E.A., van Wimersma Greidanus, Tj.B., Gispen, W.H. and De Wied, D. (1976) Hypothalamic and pituitary peptide hormones and the central nervous system: with special reference to the neurochemical effects of ACTH. In *Molecular and Functional Neurobiology*, W.H. Gispen (Ed.), Elsevier, Amsterdam, pp. 309–344.

Schulman, H. and Greengard, P. (1978) Stimulation of brain membrane protein phosphorylation by calcium and an endogenous heat-stable protein. *Nature (Lond.)*, 271: 478–479.

Segal, M. (1976) Interactions of ACTH and norepinephrine on the activity of rat hippocampal cells. *Neuropharmacology*, 15: 329–333.

Sieghart, W., Theoharides, T.C., Alper, S.L., Douglas, W.W. and Greengard, P. (1978) Calcium-dependent protein phosphorylation during section by exocytosis in the mast cell. *Nature (Lond.)*, 279: 329–331.

Spirtes, M.A., Christensen, C.W., Hartston, C.T. and Kastin, A.J. (1978) a-MSH and MIF-I effects on cGMP levels in various rat brain regions. *Brain Res.*, 144: 189–193.

Steiner, F.A. (1970) Effects of ACTH and corticosteroids on single neurons in the hypothalamus. In *Pituitary, Adrenal and the Brain, Progress in Brain Res., Vol. 32.* D. de Wied and J.A.W.M. Weijnen (Eds.), Elsevier, Amsterdam, pp. 102–107.

Sutherland, E.W. (1972) Studies on the mechanism of hormone action. *Science*, 177: 401–408.

Terenius, L. (1975) Effect of peptides and amino acids on dihydromorphine binding to the opiate receptor. *J. Pharm. Pharmacol.*, 27: 450–452.

Terenius, L., Gispen, W.H. and De Wied, D. (1975) ACTH-like peptides and opiate receptors in the rat brain: structure–activity studies. *Europ. J. Pharmacol.*, 33: 395–399.

Trevor, A.J. and Rodnight, R. (1965) The subcellular localization of cerebral phosphoproteins sensitive to electrical stimulation. *Biochem. J.*, 95: 889–896.

Van Delft, A.M.L. and Kitay, J.I. (1972) Effect of ACTH on single unit activity in the diencephalon of intact and hypophysectomized rats. *Neuroendocrinology*, 9: 188–196.

Verhoef, J., Palkovits, M. and Witter, A. (1977a) Distribution of a behaviorally highly potent $ACTH_{4-9}$ analog in rat brain after intraventricular administration. *Brain Res.*, 126: 89–104.

Verhoef, J. and Witter, A. (1976) In vivo fate of a behaviorally active ACTH analog in rats after systemic administration. *Pharm. Biochem. Behav.*, 4: 583–590.

Verhoef, J., Witter, A, and De Wied, D. (1977b) Specific uptake of a behaviorally potent [^{3}H]$ACTH_{4-9}$ analog in the septal area after intraventricular injection in rats. *Brain Res.*, 131: 117–128.

Von Hungen, K. and Roberts, S. (1973) Adenylate cyclase receptors for adrenergic neurotransmitters in rat cerebral cortex. *Europ. J. Biochem.*, 36: 391–401.

Weller, M. and Rodnight, R. (1973) The state of phosphorylation in vivo of membrane-bound phosphoproteins in rat brain. *Biochem. J.*, 133: 387–389.

Wiegant, V.M. (1978) Cyclic nucleotides in nervous tissue. *Brain Res. Bull.*, 3: 611–622.

Wiegant, V.M., Cools, A.R. and Gispen, W.H. (1977) ACTH-induced excessive grooming involves brain dopamine. *Europ. J. Pharmacol.*, 41: 343–345.

Wiegant, V.M., Dunn, A.J., Schotman, P. and Gispen, W.H. (1979a) ACTH-like neurotropic peptides: possible regulators of rat brain cyclic AMP. *Brain Res.*, 168: 565–584.

Wiegant, V.M. and Gispen, W.H. (1975) Behaviorally active ACTH analogs and brain cyclic AMP. *Exp. Brain Res.*, 23: Suppl. 219.

Wiegant, V.M., Jolles, J., Colbern, D., Zimmermann, E. and Gispen, W.H. (1979b) Intracerebroventricular ACTH activates the pituitary–adrenal system: dissociation from a behavioral response. *Life Sci.*, 25: 1791–1796.

Wiegant, V.M., Zwiers, H., Schotman, P. and Gispen, W.H. (1978) Endogenous phosphorylation of rat brain synaptosomal plasma membranes in vitro: some methodological aspects. *Neurochem. Res.*, 3: 443–453.

Witter, A. (1980) On the presence of receptors for ACTH-neuropeptides in the brain. In *Proc. of the Colloquium on Receptors Neurotransmitters and Peptide Hormones, Capri, mei, 1979*, M. Kuhar, L. Enna and G.C. Pepeu (Eds.), Raven Press, in press.

Zwiers, H., Schotman, P. and Gispen, W.H. (1980) Purification and some characteristics of an ACTH-sensitive protein kinase and its substrate protein in rat brain membranes. *J. Neurochem.*, in press.

Zwiers, H., Tonnaer, J., Wiegant, V.M., Schotman, P. and Gispen, W.H. (1979) ACTH-sensitive protein kinase from rat brain membranes. *J. Neurochem.*, 33: 247–256.

Zwiers, H., Veldhuis, D., Schotman, P. and Gispen, W.H. (1976) ACTH, cyclic nucleotides and brain protein phosphorylation in vitro. *Neurochem. Res.*, 1: 669–677.

Zwiers, H., Wiegant, V.M., Schotman, P. and Gispen, W.H. (1977) Intraventricular administered ACTH and changes in rat brain protein phosphorylation: a preliminary report. In *Mechanism, Regulation and Special Functions of Protein Synthesis in the Brain.* S. Roberts, A. Lajtha and W.H. Gispen (Eds.), Elsevier/North-Holland Biomedical Press, Amsterdam, pp. 267–272.

Zwiers, H., Wiegant, V.M., Schotman, P. and Gispen, W.H. (1978) ACTH-induced inhibition of endogenous rat brain protein phosphorylation in vitro: structure–activity. *Neurochem. Res.*, 3: 455–463.

Neuropeptides in Rat Brain Development

G.J. BOER, D.F. SWAAB, H.B.M. UYLINGS, K. BOER, R.M. BUIJS and D.N. VELIS

Netherlands Institute for Brain Research, IJdijk 28, 1095 KJ Amsterdam, The Netherlands

INTRODUCTION

Normal development of the brain is the product of a complex interaction between genetics, environment, nutrition and circulating messengers. An imbalance in one of these factors during prenatal or early postnatal life can easily result in underdevelopment and malfunction of the central nervous system in later life. Apart from the influence of nutrition, the greatest advances in understanding the growth requirements of the brain have come from studies on the involvement of endocrine factors, e.g. thyroid hormones, corticosteroids and gonadal hormones. The same endocrine factors also influence adult brain function, especially during adaptive responses of the organism. The increasing knowledge of the involvement of neuropeptides in adaptation in a variety of behavioral situations (De Wied and Gispen, 1977), however, has so far not led to any systematic search for their possible involvement in brain development.

The present paper aims to give a train of thoughts from which it can be decided that neuropeptides play an important role in brain development. This idea will be illustrated by findings on the influence on brain development of peptides from the family of adreno-corticotropic hormone (ACTH) and by some recent observations on brain growth in the absence of vasopressin, i.e. in Brattleboro rats homozygous for diabetes insipidus.

NORMAL AND SUBNORMAL BRAIN DEVELOPMENT

Brain growth in mammals shows two peaks of extensive cell proliferation (Winick and Altman, 1969; Winick, 1971). In the rat, the first peak takes place intrauterine between days 13 and 17, and is almost completely determined by the birth of macroneurons (for review, see Altman, 1969). Information on factors influencing the growth of the brain in this period is almost completely lacking, in contrast to the second period of rapid cell formation which, for the rat, occurs postnatally between birth and day 20. Although predominantly glial cells are thought to be formed in this period, apparent sites of intensive neurogenesis can still be recognized: the subependymal layer of the lateral ventricles in the cerebrum, and the subpial zone of the cerebellar cortex, i.e. the external granular layer (EGL). These sites give rise to microneurons in the olfactory bulb, the dentate gyrus of the hippocampus and the cerebellum respectively (Altman and Das, 1965; Altman, 1966, 1969). Numerically, this second wave of cell proliferation is in fact the major process of neurogenesis in the cerebellum, during which 95% of the final number of cells is acquired (Fish and Winick, 1969).

Imbalances taking place in this postnatal cell acquisition period affect rat brain development with respect to both the number of cells formed and the functional organization of neuronal circuits. These conditions include changes in environmental conditions (Rosenzweig and Bennett, 1969; Diamond et al., 1972; Rosenzweig et al., 1972), undernutrition (e.g. Dobbing, 1970; Patel et al., 1973; Winick, 1976; Griffin et al., 1977; Balázs et al., 1979), abnormal endocrine state (Pasquini et al., 1967; Arai and Gorski, 1968; Howard, 1968; Balázs et al., 1971; Cotterrell et al., 1972; Balázs, 1974), and drug-induced changes in transmitter balance (Patel et al., 1977; Diaz and Schain, 1978; Wahlström and Nordberg, 1978) (Table I). For many of these influences, the developing brain has its "vulnerable period", in which a particular imbalance has its most prominent effect on later brain functional capacity. In the case of food deprivation, for instance, the periods of rapid cell formation appear to be the most sensitive, and lead to disturbances in learning behavior (see Dobbing, 1968). Abnormality of the thyroid state has its greatest influence in parts of the brain where postnatal neurogenesis is most extensive, for instance in the cerebellum (Balázs et al., 1971). Thyroid deficiency can lead to an impairment of adaptive behavior (Eayrs, 1968). Exposure to gonadal hormones during the first few days of life has a decisive influence upon later reproductive and sexual behavior in the rat (Arai and Gorski, 1968; Mullins and Levine, 1968). Although this effect has often been described as influencing mainly the "organization of neuroendocrine circuits" in the developing brain (Flerko, 1971; Dörner, 1978), it is apparent that DNA synthesis, i.e. cell proliferation, is involved in this process (Salaman, 1974). Monoamine neurotransmitters are probably acting as neurohumoral regulators of growth embryogenesis (Buznikow et al., 1970; Schlumpf et al., 1979) and seem also to influence later growth and differentiation of the developing brain (e.g. Patel et al., 1977). These and other observations concerning hormonal and neurotransmitter influences on the developing brain have led us to propose that those substances which influence central brain function in adult individuals, are also necessary for normal development of the brain, acting at certain critical periods during the prenatal and early postnatal life (e.g. Balázs, 1974; Dörner, 1978).

TABLE I

SURVEY OF FACTORS INFLUENCING THE POSTNATAL DEVELOPMENT OF THE RAT BRAIN AS MEASURED BIOCHEMICALLY *

Environment	
Nutrition	— malnutrition
	— undernutrition
Hormones	— growth hormone
	— thyroid hormones
	— gonadal hormones
	— corticosteroids
Neurotransmitters **	— reserpine
	— phenobarbital
	— 6-hydroxydopamine

* For refs. see text.
** Influences have almost always been determined by means of neurotransmission-affecting drugs.

NEUROPEPTIDES

The importance of hormone secretion by the brain for many fundamental processes of life is – 50 years after the first formulation of this concept by Scharrer (1928) – well established.

The classical neurosecretory cells in the mammalian brain, i.e. the cells of the supraoptic (SON) and paraventricular nuclei (PVN), which produce the peptide hormones, vasopressin and oxytocin, were already clearly distinguishable from "common" neurons by their size (Scharrer and Scharrer, 1954). More recently, however, hormones were also found in small neurons, e.g. vasopressin in the cells of suprachiasmatic nucleus (SCN) (Swaab et al., 1975; Vandesande et al., 1975), and the hypophysiotropic hormones in a number of hypothalamic neurons (e.g. Sétáló et al., 1978). Immunocytochemical observations have made it clear that the neurosecretory cells which produce vasopressin and oxytocin not only terminate on blood vessels in the hypophysis, the median eminence and the organum vasculosum laminae terminalis, but also send out fibres to extrahypothalamic areas as far away as the spinal cord (Sterba, 1974; Buijs, 1978). These exohypothalamic peptidergic fibres were found to terminate either as boutons or as perineural structures, especially in the limbic system (Buijs, 1978). Suprachiasmatic vasopressin fibres have projections to the lateral septum or the lateral habenular nucleus, while paraventricular fibres containing vasopressin and oxytocin innervate the amygdala, hippocampus, pineal gland, medulla oblongata and spinal cord. Immuno-electron microscopical visualization has revealed that these fibres indeed have synaptic endings in the limbic system (Buijs and Swaab, 1979; Buijs et al., 1980). The extensive innervation of limbic structures appeared, in addition, to be correlated (Buijs, 1978; Buijs and Swaab, 1979; Sterba et al., 1980) with the sites of effect of these hormones in behavioral studies (De Wied et al., 1976).

Many more centrally acting peptides are present in brain cells and fibres outside the originally described systems (Iversen, 1978; Swaab, 1980). This group of so-called neuropep-

TABLE II

NEUROPEPTIDES ARBITRARILY DIVIDED INTO (LEFT) SUBSTANCES ORIGINALLY DESCRIBED AS HORMONES OF THE HYPTHALAMO–HYPOPHYSIAL COMPLEX (HHC) AND (RIGHT) AS HORMONES OR PEPTIDES OUTSIDE THIS COMPLEX

Peptides HHC	Peptides outside HHC
Hypothalamic hormones	substance P
oxytocin	neurotensin
vasopressin	angiotensin
LH–RH	vasoactive intestinal peptide
TRH	bombesin
somatostatin	carnosine
Pituitary hormones	ameletin
ACTH	sleep promoting peptide
α-MSH	
endorphins	
enkephalin	
prolactin *	
growth hormone *	

* Because of its molecular weight this substance should be called a "neuroprotein" instead of a neuropeptide.

tides consists of: (1) all the known hypothalamic hormones (vasopressin, oxytocin, luteinizing hormone-releasing hormone or LHRH, thyrotropin-releasing hormone or TRH and growth hormone-release inhibiting hormone or somatostatin); (2) pituitary peptides of the ACTH/LPH (lipotropic hormone) family (ACTH, α-melanocyte stimulating or α-MSH, endorphins and enkephalins; cf. Miller, 1978) together with prolactin and growth hormone; and (3) a group of peptides which were originally not known to be hormones of the hypothalamo-hypophysial complex (Table II). By means of immunocytochemistry a number of these neuropeptides have also been demonstrated in nerve fibres and sometimes — using immuno-electron microscopy — like vasopressin and oxytocin also found in synaptic structures (enkephalin, Pickel et al., 1979; substance P, Chan Palay and Palay, 1977).

The presence of neuropeptides in nerve endings strongly supports the idea that they might act either as neurotransmitters or as neuromodulators (Barker and Smith, 1980) thus

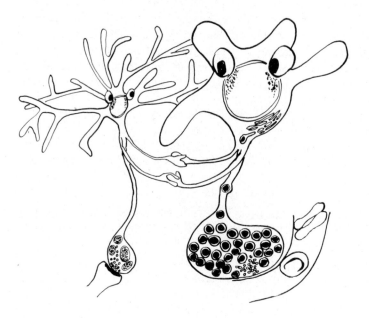

Fig. 1. Classical differences between neurotransmitter and neurosecretory neurons. Non-neurosecretory neurons are supposed to have a large dendritic tree and to both synthesize and release the transmitter substance present in small vesicles at the site of the synaptic cleft. Neurosecretory neurons would be magnocellular, have a less well-developed receptive field, and would synthesize and release hormone at separate sites (i.e. the Golgi apparatus in the perikaryon and the axonal swelling or ending on a capillary), with transport of hormone from the former to the latter by means of large neurosecretory vesicles. However, besides known common features for these cell types such as electric stimulus/secretion coupling and the exo-/endocytosis concept for release, it is now also known that: (1) a neurotransmitter can act as a neurohormone (e.g. dopamine); (2) the neurotransmitter-synthesizing enzyme rather than the neurotransmitter itself is synthesized in the cell body and is transported within vesicles to the axonal ending; (3) small neurosecretory cells and small secretory vesicles also exist; and (4) neurosecretory neurons can make synaptic contacts whereby the hormone might act as a true neurotransmitter. There thus seems to be no basis for making a fundamental distinction between these two classes of neurons.

being the anatomical substrate for the observed behavioral effects. Other arguments are derived from electrophysiological studies (Barker and Smith, 1980).

Thus, the classical neurosecretory cell which generates its secretion products into the circulatory system can also be characterized as a synaptic neuron. Since neurotransmitter-producing cells of the hypothalamus release their product, i.e. dopamine, also into the portal vessels of the hypothalamus–hypophysial complex (Neill et al., 1979), there no longer seems to be any fundamental distinction between neuroendocrine and neurotransmitter neurons (Fig. 1). A secretory substance of neuronal origin (peptides or amines) could therefore have either a distant (hormonal) or a local (neurotransmitter) effect, depending on the site of release. In this sense, neurotransmitters could be called "local hormones" (Dörner, 1978).

NEUROPEPTIDES IN DEVELOPING BRAIN

Only relatively little data are available concerning the presence of neuropeptides in the brain early in development. In the fetal rat at day 16, antiserum to neurophysin (part of the vasopressin or oxytocin precursor) stains the still immature SON (Wolff and Sterba, 1978), pointing to the presence of the neurohypophysial hormones. Positive staining in the second hypothalamic magnocellular nucleus (PVN) appears 3 days later, while the SCN content shows neurophysin immunoactivity only postnatally, from day 7 onwards. So far, using a combination of oxytocin and vasopressin antibodies, we have been able to demonstrate a positive reaction in the SON from fetal day 17 onwards, whereas radioimmunoassayable vasopressin and oxytocin have been found to be present in the fetal brain and pituitary at least as early as day 16. The total amount of hormones in brain and pituitary at prenatal day 16 as well as at the day of birth are moreover of the same ng order of magnitude, which is in sharp contrast to adults, where the amount in the pituitary is many times that of the brain (Table III). Similar data for α-MSH also point to an early prenatal appearance of this hormone in the brain (Table III). For α-MSH and oxytocin the concentration in the brain at very early stages of brain development is in fact close to the adult values, with lower concentrations being registered in between these two points (Table IV).

Immunocytochemistry for vasopressin and oxytocin in the brain outside the classical neurosecretory system clearly showed the existence of developing exohypothalamic pathways as early as day 17 (Fig. 2). This demonstrates that the radioimmunoassayable brain hormone content is indicative not only of the developing hypothalamo-neurohypophysial system, but also of the development of the exohypothalamic fibers (Fig. 3).

Other neuropeptides (see Table II) have also been found in developing brain using immunolocalization techniques and radioimmunoassays. LHRH appears in rat around birth (Araki et al., 1975; Daikoku et al., 1978) and somatostatin one day earlier (Ghirlanda et al., 1978).

In conclusion, the data, although scarce, clearly point to the early presence of neuropeptides in the developing brain, sometimes even in adult concentrations (α-MSH, oxytocin). All neuropeptides, so far assayed in development, appear to be present before the postnatal wave of brain cell generation. Vasopressin, oxytocin and α-MSH are, in addition, also present already at day 16, thus falling within the prenatal period of neurogenesis (days 13–17; the question of their possible presence still earlier has not yet been answered, because of difficulties in separately isolating the pituitary from the brain). Since these peptides are putative neurotransmitters or neuromodulators in the CNS, and given the probability that neurotransmitters serve as neurohumoral regulators affecting cell growth and development, one

TABLE III

RADIOIMMUNOASSAYABLE VASOPRESSIN, OXYTOCIN AND α-MSH CONTENTS OF PITUITARY AND TOTAL BRAIN OF THE DEVELOPING WISTAR RAT *,**

	Vasopressin (ng)		Oxytocin (ng)		α-MSH (ng)	
	Pituitary	Brain	Pituitary	Brain	Pituitary	Brain
Prenatal day 16	0.12 ± 0.06	0.09 ± 0.04	0.023 ± 0.002	0.13 ± 0.05	0.22 ± 0.09	0.27 ± 0.08
Birth	5.0 ± 0.7	3.6 ± 0.8	0.29 ± 0.03	0.11 ± 0.01	7.7 ± 0.6	0.26 ± 0.2
Adult	650 ± 150	14 ± 7.6	460 ± 110	5.2 ± 1.4	2620 ± 840	12.3 ± 2.1

* No distinction is made between males and females, except for adults, where males were used.
** Data are mean values ± S.E.M. of 15 animals for young stages and 5 animals in adulthood.

TABLE IV

CONCENTRATION OF VASOPRESSIN, OXYTOCIN AND α-MSH IN WISTER RAT BRAIN DURING DEVELOPMENT (ng/g w/w)

	Vasopressin	Oxytocin	α-MSH
Prenatal day 16	1.5 ± 0.7 *	2.2 ± 0.8	4.7 ± 1.3
Birth	15 ± 3	0.45 ± 0.06	1.06 ± 0.09
Adult	6.9 ± 3.9	2.5 ± 0.7	5.7 ± 0.9

* Data are mean ± S.E.M. values and calculated with the data of Table III.

may expect neuropeptides to play a role in the growth and differentiation of the brain in particular. However, only for peptides of the ACTH/LPH family are some indications for such a role known, while we are currently investigating the possible involvement of vaso-pressin.

PEPTIDES OF THE ACTH/LPH FAMILY

The peptides of the ACTH/LPH family originally were described as being synthesized in the pituitary gland, but since these peptides remained demonstrable in the brain even after hypophysectomy (e.g. Rudman et al., 1974; Krieger et al., 1977), the nervous system seems to be a second site of production (Krieger and Liotta, 1979). This is all the more likely since at least one of them (enkephalin) is present even in cultured neurons (Neale et al., 1978). A single large precursor molecule for all these peptides has recently been proposed to exist (Nakanishi et al., 1979), making it plausible that the presence of one family member could, in some cases, implicate the presence of others as well.

A single subcutaneous injection of long-acting ACTH in newborn female (but not male) rats accelerated the time of eye-opening, which is commonly considered to be a reliable marker for the degree of brain maturation. Of the 39 amino acids in the ACTH molecule, at least the first 16 appeared necessary for this effect (Van der Helm-Hylkema, 1973; Van der Helm-Hylkema and De Wied, 1976). Other ACTH fragments, including α-MSH, as well as endogenous corticosteroids had no effect upon the time of eye-opening, the last observation being indicative that the adrenal gland is not involved in this effect. Such single ACTH injec-tions, also of α-MSH, in neonatal rat life were also found to accelerate the development of motor behavior (Van der Helm-Hylkema, 1973). Other behavioral changes were found by Nyakas (1973), who treated young animals (days 3—5) with ACTH and found an increase in passive avoidance behavior 3 weeks later, without any concomitant change in the adrenocor-tical response level. In addition, neonatal α-MSH treatment resulted in changes in later behavior as observed in open-field body contact and in learning and memory tasks (Beckwith et al., 1977a and b). These results all point to an "organizing" effect of ACTH and α-MSH on the developing brain.

During normal intra-uterine growth of rats, a sudden acceleration can be seen at day 19. This growth spurt disappears completely when the brain and pituitary are removed, resulting in a difference in "brain-corrected" body weight of about 50% (Swaab and Honnebier, 1973). The only factor of hypothalamo-hypophysial origin which was found, after a single dose, to restore this defect to a certain degree (50%) was α-MSH (Swaab and Honnebier, 1974; Honnebier and Swaab, 1974). To verify that endogenous α-MSH really was involved

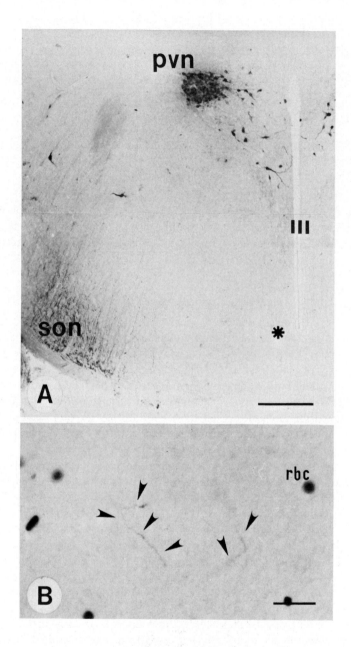

Fig. 2. Neurohypophysial hormone immuno-staining of the fetal Wistar rat brain. The staining procedure is described previously by Buijs et al. (1978) and, in short, comprises the incubation of 100 μm transversal vibratome sections of glutar-/formaldehyde-fixed tissue, using an antivasopressin serum and the 3-step peroxidase-anti-peroxidase (PAP) technique, while diaminobenzidine was used for developing the sites of antibody coupling. A: positive reaction in both the supraoptic (SON) and paraventricular nucleus (PVN) of the hypothalamus of a day 20 fetal rat. Note the absence of staining at the site (asterisk) of the postnatally vasopressin-positive suprachiasmatic nucleus. III, third ventricle. Bar = 200 μm. B: a few hormone-containing fibers (arrowheads) in the amygdala of a day-18 fetal rat. The density of these extrahypothalamic fibers at that stage, however, is very low. rbc, red blood cell, stained aspecifically. Bar = 20 μm.

(The photographs as well as those of Figs. 3 and 6 were taken by A.T. Potjer.)

in intra-uterine growth, Swaab et al. (1976) injected purified anti-α-MSH subcutaneously into the rat fetus on day 19, and found that the growth acceleration could indeed be partially inhibited. By a similar experimental approach with anti-α-MSH, also the prenatal brain maturation was found to be inhibited (Swaab et al., 1978). On prenatal day 21, i.e. two days after the administration of the antiserum, a 4% decrease was observed in brain weight and its protein and total lipid content. Since the DNA content did not differ from control values, endogenous α-MSH in prenatal life seems primarily to be involved in individual cell growth rather than cell proliferation. On the other hand, however, the DNA is assayed in a period in which cell generation is normally reduced (Winick, 1971), so that differences in brain cell content will not be easy to show up in such an experiment.

Daily subcutaneous injections with α-MSH and anti-α-MSH had no effect on body weight development in neonatal rats (Swaab et al., 1978). Likewise, after intracerebroventricular injections of anti-α-MSH on day 10, 12 and 14, both the body growth and the brain size at day 16 appeared normal (Boer and Swaab, unpublished observations). The cerebellum, the growth of which is most sensitive to internal and external influences during the second and third week of postnatal life, develops normally as well. If anti-α-MSH were also effective in neutralizing endogenous α-MSH in neonatal life, this would mean that α-MSH probably has no influence on cell multiplication and maturation after birth. Since, on the contrary, prenatal α-MSH seems just necessary for maturation of brain cells, it appears as if this neuropeptide, while keeping its organizing effect loses, around the time of birth, its trophic influence on further development of the brain. Growth hormone does not seem to be involved in in utero body and brain growth in the rat (Croskerry et al., 1973; Swaab and Honnebier, 1974), but may take over in the neonatal period, where it is necessary for normal postnatal growth (Duquesnoy and Good, 1970).

VASOPRESSIN AND BRAIN DEVELOPMENT

From the discovery of the genetically recessive vasopressin-deficient Brattleboro rat, the retarded body growth of the homozygous (HOM) form has been recognized (Valtin and Schroeder, 1964). In a later study, in which adult animals (which suffer from diabetes insipidus with a diuresis of up to 80% of their body weight per day) were daily injected subcutaneously with Pitressin tannate (a long-acting vasopressin preparation in oil) for one month, no increase in body weight approaching heterozygous (HET) control levels could be observed (Sokol and Sise, 1973). Wright and Kutscher (1977), using vasopressin in oil, also observed no improvement in the first month of life, and both groups concluded that the absence of vasopressin in HOM-DI Brattleboros could not be the origin of the stunted body growth. In both cases, however, a dose just sufficient to normalize water metabolism was given. The putative growth requirement for vasopressin perhaps demands a still higher level or else the replenishment of this hormone in the brain itself. In other words, the absence of hypothalamic innervation delivering vasopressin in the brain of these animals might not be compensated by vasopressin given peripherally, more so since it does not pass the blood—brain barrier very well (Willumsen and Bie, 1969). Moreover, lysine[8]-vasopressin (Wright and Kutscher, 1977), or a mixture of this with (absent in Brattleboros) arginine[8]-vasopressin (Pitressin tannate; Sokol and Sise, 1973), was used in these studies, and it could well be that lysine[8]-vasopressin has an antidiuretic action, but does not affect body growth.

216

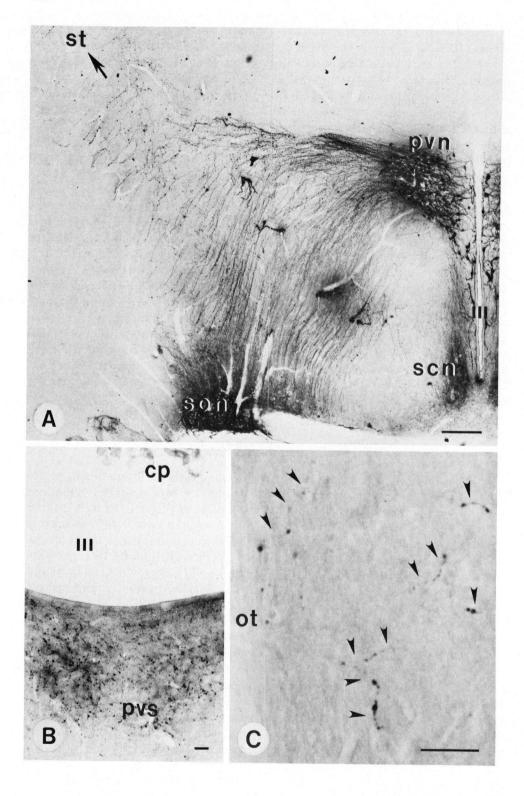

Body growth

In previous reports on body growth in Brattleboros (Arimura et al., 1968; Sokol and Sise, 1973; Wright and Kutscher, 1977; Dlouhá et al., 1977), the extent to which postnatal growth can be seriously affected by early environmental factors, e.g. prenatal condition, fostering, litter size (e.g. Winick, 1976), cage conditions (Rosenzweig and Bennett, 1969), etc., has never sufficiently been taken into consideration. Using homozygous normal (HOM-N) Brattleboros, which were bred and selected from HET- and HOM-DI animals by our animal supplier (TNO, Zeist, The Netherlands) and a large stock of HOM-DI male and females, a breeding program has been set up in order to investigate postnatal body development in homogeneous HOM- or HET-DI litters with the same type of mother (HOM-DI). Maternal care of pups during weaning is then presumed to be the same and possible influences of intra-litter competition are excluded as well. This last is of importance, since HOM-DI newborns are lighter in weight than HET-DI controls and, normally, heavier animals in a nest of constant size keep this lead throughout life (Dobbing, 1970; Bührdel et al., 1978).

Nevertheless, even with this breeding scheme and great care in keeping the constantly urinating mothers with their litters on dry embedding material and providing ready accessibility for the young to the water bottles, a retardation in body growth for HOM-DI pups was quickly apparent (Fig. 4). Although the mean litter size for HET- and HOM-DI nests was not different (cf. Boer et al., 1980), a lower body weight for the HOM pups was already present at birth (HET-DI: 6.42 ± 0.03 g; HOM-DI: 6.29 ± 0.03 g), showing that the growth-affecting factors probably start working already during intra-uterine development. When litter size was kept constant at 7—8 pups, an increasing retardation of growth became apparent in the HOM-DI pups, amounting up to almost 20% in the 5th—6th week of life. After a small recovery in the second month of life, a difference with HET-values of about 12% finally stabilizes in both sexes and throughout the period studied (up to 150 days).

Since higher body growth impairments (up to 43%) had been found in an earlier study (Boer et al., 1978, 1979) in which HOM-DI pups, delivered and weaned by a HOM-DI mother, were compared with the 75% non-HOM-DI pups from litters raised in a HET-DI mother, which had been interbred with a HET-DI male (50% HET-DI and 25% HOM-N), there might be an additional detrimental factor which must be attributed to the HOM-DI mother.

An interesting observation moreover, is that in the present controlled study the opening of the eyes occurs one day earlier in HOM-DI pups than in HET-DI pups (12.6 ± 0.2 (14) against 13.4 ± 0.4 (7); Boer et al., unpublished observation), indicating that brain development might be influenced too.

Brain development

In the first breeding experiment (Boer et al., 1978, 1979), postnatal brain development

---

Fig. 3. Neurophysial hormone immuno-staining of the brain of a 14-day-old Wistar rat. The staining procedure is given at Fig. 2. A: hypothalamic vibratome section with positive cell bodies in supraoptic (SON), paraventricular (PVN) and suprachiasmatic (SCN) nuclei, showing not only the rather extensive fiber tract from the PVN towards the neurohypophysis (via the SON) but in addition, an exohypothalamic fiber tract going dorsolaterally in the direction of the stria terminalis (→st). Compare with Fig. 2A. III, third ventricle, Bar = 200 μm. B: exohypothalamic fiber tract originating from the SCN and traversing the periventricular nucleus (PVS) along the third ventricle (III) near to the choroid plexus (cp). Bar = 20 μm. C: exohypothalamic fibers (arrowheads) in the amygdala near the optic tract (ot). Bar = 20 μm. (Photographs taken from preparations of G.J. de Vries.)

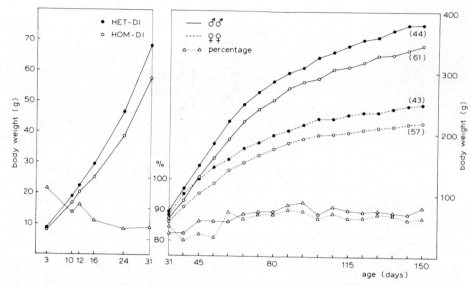

Fig. 4. Body weight development of HOM- and HET-DI Brattleboro rats under constant conditions. Pups were all born from HOM-DI mothers and in litters of a constant number of genetic homogeneous litter mates (7 or 8). Mother and pups were kept under standard conditions in small cages with sawdust until day 21, and thereafter up to day 31 in a larger one. The litters were then sexed, and males and females were kept in groups of 10 on grids in large metal boxes. n = number of animals.

of Brattleboro rats has been assessed on the basis of measurements made on days 12, 16, 24 and 180 of postnatal life. A reduced brain weight was observed during the postnatal brain growth spurt as well as in adulthood. The stunted growth of the brain in neonatal life (10–15%) did not show up very much in the cerebral cortex (0–7%), in comparison with the remaining part of the brain (17–31%). In adulthood, a cerebral cortex deficit becomes somewhat more apparent (8%), while the rest of the brain has recovered to a great extent (8–14% weight deficit) – perhaps in the same period as the partial recovery in body weight (cf. Fig. 4).

In the 180-day-old animals, the cerebellum and medulla oblongata appeared to be the brain parts that were permanently affected the most (Table V). The DNA content gave a similar but even more pronounced picture (Fig. 5; Table V). An almost normal development

TABLE V

WEIGHT AND DNA CONTENT IN BRAIN AREAS OF HOMOZYGOUS BRATTLEBORO MALE RATS AS PERCENTAGE OF NON-HOMOZYGOUS VALUES (180 DAYS) *,**

	Cerebral cortex	Sub-cortex	Cerebellum	Medulla oblongata
Wet weight	93 ± 3 ***	97 ± 7	84 ± 7 ***	90 ± 9
Dry weight	93 ± 4	94 ± 7	85 ± 7 ***	88 ± 10
DNA	88 ± 3 ***	87 ± 9	80 ± 7 ***	78 ± 5 ***

* Number of non-HOM-/HOM-DI animals: 18/13 for cerebral cortex, 12/6 for other areas.
** Data given are means ± S.E.M.
*** Difference statistically significant at $P \leqslant 0.05$ according to the Student's t-test.

in the cerebral cortex was found in the first 3 weeks of life for the HOM-DI pups, still leading to an about 14% lower cell content at 180 days. Cell proliferation appeared to be more seriously affected in the rest of the brain: 30% fewer cells at day 24, which becomes 13–22% in the adults. This again demonstrates the existence of a partial catch-up after the period of rapid brain growth.

The cerebellum is the most active site of cell proliferation in the second and third weeks of rat life (40% of the final total brain DNA is synthesized in this period; cf. Fish and Winick, 1969). However, our preliminary morphological study of the cerebellum in HOM-DI pups has shown no EGL later than day 21 (Uylings and Boer, unpublished observations). So, the recovery in number of cells therefore does not seem to be related to a prolonged period of EGL cell proliferation and might perhaps be due to a glial response.

Comparison with other types of disturbed brain development

The results described above do not prove, of course, that vasopressin is directly involved in normal brain development. Other (endocrine or non-endocrine) systems of the Brattleboro rats might be affected as well. Comparison of the Brattleboro data with other known factors affecting brain development seems, however, to exclude a number of such possible disturbances (Table VI). For instance, although *undernutrition* shows similarities in reduction of the final number of brain cells, in lack of effect on the period of postnatal neurogenesis and in final cell size, the opposite shift in the day of eye opening — later in undernutrition and earlier in the absence of vasopressin — clearly differentiates the two conditions. In contrast, the difference with *thyriod deficiency* is that postnatal cell acquisition in the EGL of the cerebellum is extended by more than a week (Lewis et al., 1976), resulting in a normal (but less mature) final cell number (Legrand, 1967; Balázs et al., 1968). *Hyper-*

TABLE VI

COMPARISON OF BRAIN DEVELOPMENTAL DATA FOR HOM-DI BRATTLEBORO RATS WITH OTHER BIOCHEMICALLY STUDIED FACTORS REPORTED TO AFFECT "BRAINOGENESIS".

	Under-nutrition [a]	Hypo-thyroidism [b]	Hyper-thyroidism [b]	Cortico-steroids [c]	HOM-DI Brattleboro [d]
Final effects on:					
body weight	↓ [e]	↓	↓	↓	↓
brain weight	↓	↓	↓	↓	↓
brain cell number	↓	=	↓	↓	↓
cell size	=	↓	=	=	=
Effects in postnatal germinal zones:					
period of cell formation	=	↑	↓	=	=?
mitotic activity	↓	↓ → ↑	= → ↓	↓	
cell loss	↑	↑	=	=	
cell cycle length	↑	=			
Day of eye opening[5]	↓	↓	↑	= or ↑	↑

[a] Lewis et al. (1975); Smart and Dobbing (1971); Neville and Chase (1971); Patel et al. (1973); Winick (1976).
[b] Balázs et al. (1968, 1971); Bakke et al. (1972, 1976); Balázs (1974); Lewis et al. (1976).
[c] Howard (1968); Cotterrell et al. (1972); Howard and Benjamins (1975); Van der Helm-Hylkema and De Wied (1976).
[d] Boer et al. (1978) and present data.
[e] ↓ delayed; ↑ accelerated.

thyroidism, on the other hand, produces effects on brain development which look quite similar to the defects found in HOM-DI Brattleboro rats. However, in contrast to the Brattleboros, the cerebral cortex of thyroid-treated neonatal normal rats is also affected during the first 3 weeks of life in thyroid-treated rats (Balázs et al., 1971). Furthermore, thyroid function in HOM-DI rats has been described as being normal (Galton et al., 1966), so that thyroid involvement in the abnormalities of Brattleboro brain development seems unlikely. Brain developmental parameters of *corticosteroid*-treated animals too, are similar to that of Brattleboros, but while the adrenocortical capacity does seem to be enhanced (Arimura et al., 1968; Kenyon et al., 1978), corticosteroid serum levels in adult HOM-DI animals are actually lower than in HET-DI controls (Möhring et al., 1978). Therefore, although no analogous data for young stages are available, the involvement of endogenous corticosteroids on Brattleboro growth retardation also seems doubtful. Additional data on mitotic activity, cell loss and cell cycle length during brain development in HOM-DI rats should be more conclusive in this respect (cf. Table VI).

It has been suggested by Arimura et al. (1968) that reduced body weight in the Brattleboro is caused by an impairment of *growth hormone* (GH) production. This was concluded from: (a) the normal GH-releasing activity in hypothalamic tissue; (b) the much lower levels of GH in the pituitary; and (c) the observation that chronic treatment with large amounts of GH increases the body weight of adult HOM-DI animals more than that of HET-DI animals (while in contrast Pitressin tannate treatment did not affect body growth or only slightly for the males; Sokol and Sise, 1973). In themselves, however, neither pituitary GH levels nor GH-hypophysiotropic activity of the hypothalamus say anything about their rate of synthesis and release. In addition, neither growth hormone treatment (Croskerry et al., 1973; Swaab and Honnebier, 1974) nor inhibition of GH release by somatostatin (cf. Sara et al., 1979) was found to affect early brain development in normal Wistar rat; GH only starts to express its influence around the 10th postnatal day (Duquesnoy and Good, 1970; Winick, 1971). Already by this time, severe growth retardation of body and brain was seen in the HOM-DI Brattleboros, thus arguing against an influence of GH.

Taking all the above data together, a number of factors can be safely excluded as contributing to the underdevelopment of the Brattleboro brain. At present, therefore, the absence of vasopressin in the Brattleboro rat seems to have its own expression in brain development.

Vasopressin supplementation

Chronic treatment with Pitressin tannate, given subcutaneously in a dose normalizing the diuresis, slightly increases the body weight of adult HOM-DI males, but not the females (Sokol and Sise, 1973; Table VII), but the brain weight is not influenced in either sex (Table VII). Since only a small percentage of vasopressin given peripherally reaches the brain (Willumsen and Bie, 1969), we have investigated the effect of intraventricular administered vasopressin. Via a permanent cannula placed into the lateral ventricule of 150-day-old HOM-DI Brattleboros, 50 ng of arginine[8]-vasopressin was given daily for one month either with or without subcutaneous Pitressin tannate administration. No effect on the total brain weight was found (Table VII). Water content of the male brain does not change following the central application of vasopressin, but in females the ventricular injection by itself increases water content — especially of the forebrain (unpublished result) — accounting for the higher brain weight observed (Table VII). Thus, if vasopressing indeed has a direct influence on brain size, its presence seems necessary in early development rather than in later life. In the study of Wright and Kutscher (1978) mentioned before, daily subcutane-

TABLE VII

BODY AND BRAIN WEIGHT OF HET- AND HOM-DI BRATTLEBORO RATS AT 180 DAYS OF AGE
AND UNDER DIFFERENT REGIMES OF VASOPRESSIN SUBSTITUTION (g)

Condition		Males			Females		
		n	Body	Brain	n	Body	Brain
HOM-DI	oil [b]	5	347 ± 24 [a]	1.92 ± 0.04	7	233 ± 5	1.76 ± 0.03
	P [b]	6	403 ± 28 [d]	1.92 ± 0.03	7	246 ± 9	1.74 ± 0.02
HOM-DI	oil [b] + VP [c]	5	359 ± 12	2.09 ± 0.05	7	215 ± 5	1.92 ± 0.06
	P [b] + saline [c]	4	345 ± 18	1.96 ± 0.04	8	242 ± 12	2.03 ± 0.05
	P [b] + VP [c]	7	363 ± 13	1.94 ± 0.04	2	243 ± 20	1.90 ± 0.03

[a] Mean ± S.E.M.

[b] 0.1 ml/100 g body weight daily of oil and Pitressin tannate (P) respectively starting at day 150.

[c] Daily injection starting at day 150 via polyethylene cannula implanted in the right lateral ventricle of 2 μl saline or 50 ng vasopressin (VP) in 2 μl saline. Vasopressin derived from Sigma (type VIII, 360 IU/mg, lot 28C-0287).

[d] Difference with oil-treated animals statistically significant at $P \leqslant 0.05$ for weight increment between day 150 and 180.

ous injections of lysine[8]-vasopressin did not improve postnatal body growth. This study, however, needs to be repeated with the actual missing arginine[8]-vasopressin and, preferably, applied directly into the developing brain.

HOM-DI Brattleboros have an elevated oxytocin blood level (Dogterom et al., 1977), perhaps as a consequence of their increased blood osmolality (by which both vasopressin- and oxytocin-producing cells are activated; Valtin et al., 1968; Swaab et al., 1973). Vaso-

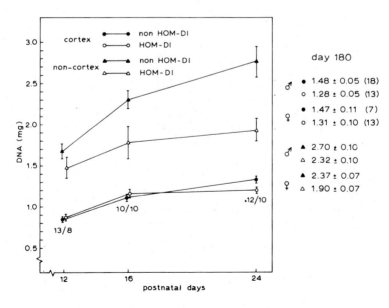

Fig. 5. DNA content in the developing Brattleboro brain and in adulthood (180 days). The cerebral cortex and the remaining brain tissue (non-cortex) have been separately assayed. Adult values are given in mg (From Boer et al., 1978.)

222

pressin supplementation in amounts sufficient to normalize diuresis, as in the studies of
Wright and Kutscher (1978), will most probably have lowered the oxytocin levels as indicated by the restoration of pituitary stores (Sunde and Sokol, 1975). This argues against the
idea that high circulating oxytocin levels are responsible for the stunted postnatal growth in
HOM-DI pups.

Mode of action

An intriguing question is how vasopressin might act on the developing brain and, especially on the cerebellum. Exohypothalamic neurosecretory vasopressin pathways do not reach

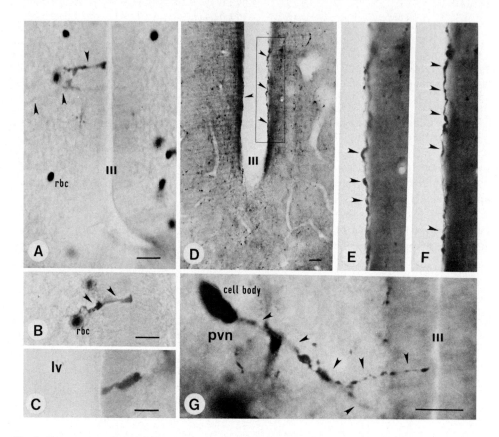

Fig. 6. Immunocytochemical images of neurohypophyseal hormone-containing fibres contacting the
cerebrospinal fluid pre- (A–C) and early postnatally (D–G) in the rat. For immunocytochemical procedure see legends to Fig. 2. Bars = 20 μm. In prenatal stages positive-stained fibres (arrowheads) were
frequently seen to cross the ependymal cell layer of the third ventricle (III) (fetal day 20–21: A–B).
The few red blood cells (rbc) show pseudo-peroxidase staining. Typical formed positive-stained cells were
seen in between the ependymal cells of the ventricles in late gestation, thereby contacting the CSF too.
C: shows such a cell at the lateral ventricle (LV) of a fetus of day 19. These images, however, have disappeared two weeks after birth. Postnatally at least up to day 16, the lateral wall of the third ventricle is
layered with a few vasopressin fibres (postnatal day 16: D–F) which mainly run from dorsal to ventral.
Because of the thickness of the vibratome section one fibre has been magnified further and photographed
on two levels of focusing (E–F), thereby manifesting its full length and appearance. Besides these intraventricular fibres, some vasopressin cells of the PVN were seen to send their fibres directly in between the
ependymal cells and into the third ventricle (postnatal day 4: G). Both images have not been noticed in
adults. (Photographs D–G were taken from preparations of G.J. de Vries.)

this structure in the adult (Buijs, unpublished result). Although this could be different for the developing cerebellum, a direct endocrine or indirect influence might be involved in this case. This last indirect possibility is thought to be executed, e.g. via catecholaminergic transmitter systems, which are known in vivo to be under the influence of vasopressin (Kovács et al., 1980). However, although the exohypothalamic fibres reach the medulla oblongata and most probably innervate catecholaminergic nuclei (nucleus ambiguus and nucleus tractus solitarius; Buijs, 1978), no vasopressinergic innervation of the locus coeruleus — which is the main source of noradrenergic fibres projecting to the cerebellum — had been noticed (Buijs, 1978).

The existence of neurosecretory neuron processes, shown immunocytochemically and which penetrate the ependymal cell layer of the third ventricle, making a direct contact with the cerebrospinal fluid (CSF) in the rat between day 18 prenatally and day 16 postnatally (Fig. 6), might be indicative of a direct release of vasopressin into the CSF of the developing brain and so, a pathway for direct hormonal action of vasopressin in other brain areas, e.g. the developing cerebellum. A considerable amount of vasopressin (and oxytocin) is present in the adult CSF (Dogterom et al., 1977), although by that time vasopressin containing fibers ending in the CSF have disappeared (Buijs, unpublished result). It is therefore most probable that in adults the hormone is released within extrahypothalamic areas, and subsequently is removed by the CSF.

A direct hormonal action of vasopressin on cell proliferation is also suggested by the work of Rozengurt et al. (1979). In their cultured mice fibroblasts, mitotic activity under suboptimal serum concentrations could be enhanced by low concentrations of vasopressin, which is a thousand-fold more potent than oxytocin in this respect. Also, the higher body weight in mice suffering from a hereditary nephrogenic defect in urinary concentration (Naik and Valtin, 1969; Naik, 1972) seems to point in the same direction. In complete contrast to HOM-DI Brattleboros, these animals are supposed to have a high circulating level of vasopressin throughout life (Naik and Kobayashi, 1971).

SUMMARY

Peptides that are present in the CNS and have central actions are called neuropeptides. These neuropeptides can be divided, on historical grounds, into 3 groups: the hypothalamic hormones, the pituitary hormones and those peptides, which were originally described as hormones or substances from outside the hypothalamo—hypophysial complex. Their central actions are likely to be explained by the existence of peptidergic synapses in the brain areas involved.

Other centrally acting substances, such as gonadal and thyroid hormones and aminergic neurotransmitters, are each indispensable for the normal development of the rat brain. Because the neuropeptides are putative neurotransmitters and are present in the brain early in the prenatal period, the hypothesis is put forward that these peptides play a role in brain development as well.

Observations on the influence of α-MSH upon prenatal brain development have given evidence for a growth-promoting role of this peptide. Vasopressin-deficient Brattleboro rats manifest a stunted body and brain growth, both pre- and postnatally. Brain weight and tissue parameters, so far, point to a different etiology for this syndrome than in the case of other nutritional and hormonal factors, which have been studied so far.

These data are certainly not inconsistent with the idea that neuropeptides obey the rule that factors which are of importance for adult brain function are also involved in brain development (Swaab, 1980).

ACKNOWLEDGEMENTS

The authors wish to thank Ms. E.M. Verbraak for breeding the Brattleboro rats so carefully, Mrs. C.M.F. van Rheenen-Verberg and B. Fisser for their technical assistance and Ms. J. van de Velde and Mrs. W. Chen-Pelt for typing the manuscript.

REFERENCES

Altman, J. (1966) Autoradiographic and histological studies of postnatal neurogenesis. II. A longitudinal investigation of the kinetics, migration and transformation of cells incorporating tritiated thymidine in infant rats, with special reference to neurogenesis in some brain regions. *J. comp. Neurol.,* 128: 431–473.

Altman, J. (1969) DNA metabolism and cell proliferation. In *Structural Neurochemistry, Handbook of Neurochemistry, Vol. II,* A. Lajtha (Ed.), pp. 137–182.

Altman, J. and Das, G.D. (1965) Postnatal origin of microneurons in the rat brain. *Nature (Lond.),* 207: 953–956.

Arai, Y. and Gorski, R.A. (1968) Critical exposure time for androgenization of the developing hypothalamus in the female rat. *Endocrinology,* 82: 1010–1014.

Araki, S., Toran-Allerand, C.D., Ferin, M. and Van de Wiele, R.L. (1975) Immunoreactive gonadotropin-releasing hormone (Gn-RH) during maturation in the rat: ontogeny of regional hypothalamic differences. *Endocrinology,* 97: 693–697.

Arimura, A., Saito, T., Bowers, C.Y. and Schally, A.V. (1968) Pituitary–adrenal activation in rats with hereditary hypothalamic diabetes insipidus. *Acta Endocrinol.,* 54: 155–165.

Balázs, R. (1974) Hormonal influence on brain development. *Biochem. Soc. Spec. Publ.,* 1: 39–57.

Balázs, R., Cocks, W.A., Eayrs, J.T. and Kovács, S. (1971) Biochemical effects of thyroid hormones on the developing brain. In *Hormones in Development,* N. Hamburg and E.J.W. Barrington (Eds.), Appleton-Century-Crofts, New York, pp. 357–379.

Balázs, R., Kovács, S., Cocks, W.A., Johnson, A.L. and Eayrs, J.T. (1971) Effect of thyroid hormone on the biochemical maturation of rat brain: postnatal cell formation. *Brain Res.,* 25: 555–570.

Balázs, R., Lewis, P.D. Patel, A.J. (1979) Nutritional deficiencies and brain development. In *Human Growth, Vol. 3,* F. Faulkner and J.M. Tanner (Eds.), Plenum Press, London, pp. 415–480.

Beckwith, B.E., O'Quin, R.K., Petro, M.S., Kastin, A.J. and Sandman, C.A. (1977a) The effects of neonatal injections of α-MSH on the open-field behavior of juvenile and adult rats. *Physiol. Psychol.,* 5: 295–299.

Beckwith, B.E., Sandman, C.A., Hothersall, D. and Kastin, A.J. (1977b) Influence of neonatal injections of α-MSH on learning, memory and attention in rats. *Physiol. Behav.,* 18: 63–71.

Boer, G.J., Uylings, H.B.M., Rheenen-Verberg, C.M.F. van and Fisser, B. (1978) Postnatal brain development in rats which hereditary diabetes insipidus (Brattleboro strain). In *Hormones and Brain Development.* G. Dörner and M. Kawakami, Elsevier, Amsterdam, pp. 253–258.

Boer, G.J., Van Rheenen-Verberg, C., Uylings, H.B.M. and Fisser, B. (1979) Postnatal brain development in the absence of vasopressin. *J. Endocr.,* 80: 64P–65P.

Boer, K., Boer, G.J. and Swaab, D.F. (1980) Reproduction in the Brattleboro diabetes insipidus rat. Submitted for publication.

Bührdel, P., Willgerodt, H., Keller, E. and Theile, H. (1978) Postnatal development of rats born preterm and postterm. I. Body weight. *Biol. Neonate,* 33: 184–188.

Buijs, R.M. (1978) Intra- and extrahypothalamic vasopressin and oxytocin pathways in the rat. Pathways to the limbic system, medulla oblongata and spinal cord. *Cell Tiss. Res.,* 192: 423–435.

Buijs, R.M. and Swaab, D.F. (1979) Immunoelectronmicroscopical demonstration of vasopressin and oxytocin synapses in the rat limbic system. *Cell Tiss. Res.,* 204: 355–365.

Buijs, R.M., Velis, D.N. and Swaab, D.F. (1980) Immunocytochemical demonstration of vasopressin and oxytocin in the rat central nervous system by light- and electronmicroscopy. In *Adaptive Capabilities of the Nervous System, Progress in Brain Research Vol. 53*, P. McConnel, G.J. Boer, N.E. van de Poll, H.J. Romijn and M.A. Corner (Eds.), Elsevier, Amsterdam, pp. 159–167.

Buznikow, G.A., Kost, A.N., Kucherova, N.F., Mndzhoyan, A.L., Suvorov, N.N. and Berdysheva, L.V. (1970) The role of neurohumours in early embryogenesis. III. Pharmacological analysis of the role of neurohumours in cleavage divisions. *J. Embryol. exp. Morph.*, 23: 549–569.

Chan-Palay, V. and Palay, S.L. (1977) Ultrastructural identification of substance P cells and their processes in rat sensory glia ganglia and their terminals in the spinal cord immunocytochemistry. *Proc. nat. Acad. Sci. (Wash.)*, 74: 4050–4054.

Cotterrell, M., Balázs, R. and Johnson, A.L. (1972) Effects of corticosteroids on the biochemical maturation of rat brain: postnatal cell formation. *J. Neurochem.*, 19: 2151–2167.

Croskerry, P.G., Smith, G.K., Shepard, B.J. and Freeman, K.B. (1973) Perinatal brain DNA in the normal and growth hormone-treated rat. *Brain Res.*, 52: 413–418.

Daikohn, S., Kawano, H., Matsumura, H. and Saito, S. (1978) In vivo and in vitro studies on the appearance of LHRH neurons in the hypothalamus of perinatal rats. *Cell Tiss. Res.*, 194: 433–445.

Diamond, M.C., Rosenzweig, M.R., Bennett, E.L., Lindner, B. and Lyon, C. (1972) Effects of environmental enrichment and impoverishment on rat cerebral cortex. *J. Neurobiol.*, 3: 47–64.

Diaz, J. and Schain, R.J. (1978) Phenobarbital: effects of long-term administration on behavior and brain of artificially reared rats. *Science*, 199: 90–91.

Dobbing, J. (1968) Vulnerable periods in developing brain. In *Applied Neurochemistry*, A.N. Davison and J. Dobbing (Eds.), Blackwell, Oxford, pp. 287–316.

Dobbing, J. (1970) Undernutrition and the developing brain. In *Developmental Neurobiology*, W.A. Himwich (Ed.), Charles C. Thomas, Springfield, Ill., pp. 241–261.

Dogterom, J., Wimersma-Greidanus, Tj.B. van and Swaab, D.F. (1977) Evidence for the release of vasopressin and oxytocin into cerebrospinal fluid: measurements in plasma and CSF of intact and hypophysectomized rats. *Neuroendocrinology*, 24: 108–118.

Dörner, G. (1978) Hormones, brain development and fundamental processes of life. In *Hormones and Brain Development*, G. Dörner and M. Kawakami (Eds.), Elsevier, Amsterdam, pp. 13–25.

DuQuesnoy, R.J. and Good, R.A. (1970) Growth inhibition of newborn rats by plasma of monkeys immunized against rat growth hormones. *J. Endocr.*, 48: 465–466.

Eayrs, J.T. (1968) Developmental relationships between brain and thyroid. In *Endocrinology and Human Behavior*, R.P. Michael (Ed.), Oxford University Press, London, pp. 239–255.

Fish, I. and Winick, M. (1969) Cellular growth in various regions of the developing rat brain. *Pediat Res.*, 3: 407–412.

Flerkó, B. (1971) Steroid hormones and the differentiation of the central nervous system. In *Current Topics in Experimental Endocrinology, Vol. I*, L. Martini and V.H.T. James (Eds.), Academic Press, New York, pp. 41–80.

Ghirlanda, G., Bataille, D., DuBois, M.P. and Rosselin, G. (1978) Variations of the somatostatin content of gut, pancreas and brain in the developing rat. *Metabolism*, 27 Suppl. 1: 1167–1170.

Griffin, W.S.T., Woodward, D.J. and Chanda, R. (1977) Malnutrition and brain development: cerebellar weight, DNA, RNA, protein and histological correlations. *J. Neurochem.*, 28: 1269–1279.

Helm-Hylkema, H. van der (1973) *Effecten van Vroeg Neonatal Toegediend ACTH en aan ACTH Verwante Peptiden op de Somatische en Gedragsontwikkeling van de Rat*, Thesis, University of Utrecht, The Netherlands.

Helm-Hylkema, H. van der and Wied, de, D. (1976) Effect of neonatally injected ACTH and ACTH analogues on eye-opening of the rat. *Life Sci.*, 18: 1099–1104.

Honnebier, W.J. and Swaab, D.F. (1974) Influence of α-melanocyte-stimulating hormone (α-MSH), growth hormone (GH) and fetal brain extracts on intrauterine growth of fetus and placenta in the rat. *J. Obstet. Gynaecol.*, 81: 439–447.

Howard, E. (1968) Reduction in size and total DNA of cerebrum and cerebellum in adult mice after corticosterone treatment in infancy. *Exp. Neurol.*, 22: 191–208.

Iversen, L.L. (1978) Chemical messengers in the brain. *Trends Neurosci.*, 1: 15–16.

Kenyon, G.J., Hargreaves, G. and Henderson, I.W. (1978) Adrenocortical function in rats with inherited hypothalamic diabetes insipidus (Brattleboro strain). *J. Steroid Biochem.*, 9: 345–348.

Kovács, G.L., Bohus, B. and Versteeg, D.H.G. (1980) The interaction of posterior pituitary neuropeptides with monoaminergic neurotransmission: significance in learning and memory processes. In *Adap-

226

tive Capabilities in the Nervous System, Progress in Brain Research Vol. 53, P. McConnell, G.J. Boer, H.J. Romijn, N.E. van de Poll and M.A. Corner (Eds.), Elsevier, Amsterdam, pp. 123–140.

Krieger, D.T. and Liotta, A.S. (1979) Pituitary hormones in brain: where, how, and why? Science, 205: 366–372.

Krieger, D.T., Liotta, A. and Brownstein, M.J. (1977) Presence of corticotropin in brain of normal and hypophysectomized rats. Proc. nat. Acad. Sci. (Wash.), 74: 648–652.

Lewis, P.D., Balázs, R., Patel, A.J. and Johnson, A.L. (1975) The effect of undernutrition in early life on cell generation in the rat brain. Brain Res., 83: 235–247.

Miller, R.J. (1978) Enkephalin: a peptide with morphine-like properties. Trends Neurosci., 1: 2931–31.

Möhring, J., Kohrs, G., Möhring, B., Petri, M., Homsy, E. and Haack, D. (1978) Effects of prolonged vasopressin treatment in Brattleboro rats with diabetes insipidus. Amer. J. Physiol., 234: F106–F111.

Mullins, R.F. and Levine, S. (1968) Hormonal determinants during infancy of adult sexual behavior in the female rat. Physiol. Behav., 3: 333–338.

Naik, D.V. (1972) Salt and water metabolism and neurohypophyseal vasopressor activity in mice with hereditary nephrogenic diabetes insipidus. Acta endocrinol., 69: 434–444.

Naik, D.V. and Kobayashi, H. (1971) Neurohypophyseal hormones in the pars nervosa of the mouse with hereditary nephrogenic diabetes insipidus. Neuroendocrinology, 7: 322–328.

Naik, D.V. and Valtin, H. (1969) Hereditary vasopressin resistant urinary concentrating defects in mice. Amer. J. Physiol., 217: 1183–1190.

Nakanishi, S., Inone, A., Kita, T., Nakamura, M., Chang, A.C.Y., Cohen, S.N. and Numa, S. (1979) Nucleotide sequence of cloned cDNA for bovine corticotropin-β-lipotropin precursor. Nature (Lond.), 278: 423–427.

Neale, J.H., Barker, J.C., Uhl, G.R. and Snijder, S.H. (1978) Enkephalin-containing neurons visualized in spinal cord cell cultures. Science, 201: 467–469.

Neill, J.D., Plotsky, P.M. and Greef, W.J. de (1979) Catecholamines, the hypothalamus and neuroendocrinology – applications of electrochemical methods. Trends Neurosci., 2: 60–63.

Neville, H.E. and Chase, H.P. (1971) Undernutrition and cerebellar development. Exp. Neurol., 33: 485–497.

Nyakas, Cs. (1973) Influence of corticosterone and ACTH on the postnatal development of learning and memory functions. In Hormones and Brain Function, K. Lissak (Ed.), Plenum Press, New York, pp. 83–89.

Patel, A.J., Balázs, R. and Johnson, A.L. (1973) Effect of undernutrition on cell formation in the rat brain. J. Neurochem., 20: 1151–1165.

Patel, A.J., Beridek, G., Balázs, R. and Lewis, P.D. (1977) Effect of reserpine on cell proliferation in the developing rat brain: a biochemical study. Brain Res., 129: 283–297.

Pasquini, J.M., Kaplún, B., García Argiz, C.A. and Gómez, G.J. (1967) Hormonal regulation of brain development I. The effect of neonatal thyroidectomy upon nucleic acid, protein and two enzymes in developing cerebral cortex and cerebellum of the rat. Brain Res., 6: 621–634.

Pickel, V.M., Joh, T.H., Reis, D.J., Leeman, S.E. and Miller, R.J. (1979) Electron microscopic localization of substance P and enkephalin in axon terminals related to dendrites of catecholaminergic neurons. Brain Res., 160: 387–400.

Rozengurt, E., Legg, A. and Pettican, P. (1979) Vasopressin stimulation of mouse 3T3 cell growth. Proc. nat. Acad. Sci. (Wash.), 76: 1284–1287.

Rosenzweig, M.R. and Bennett, E.L. (1969) Effects of differential environments on brain weights and enzyme activities in gerbils, rats and mice. Develop. Psychobiol., 2: 87–95.

Rosenzweig, M.R., Bennett, E.L. and Diamond, M.C. (1970) Anatomical plasticity of brain: replications and extensions. In Macromolecules and Behavior, J. Gaito (Ed.), Appleton-Century-Crofts, New York, pp. 205–277.

Rudman, D., Scott, J.W., Del Rio, A.E., Honser, D.H. and Sheen, S. (1974) Melanotropic activity in regions of rodent brain. Amer. J. Physiol., 226: 682–686.

Salaman, D.F. (1974) The role of DNA, RNA and protein synthesis in sexual differentiation of the brain. In Integrative Hypothalamic Activity, Progress in Brain Research, Vol. 41, D.F. Swaab and J.P. Schadé (Eds.), Elsevier, Amsterdam, pp. 349–362.

Sara, V.R., Rutherford, R. and Smythe, G.A. (1979) The influence of maternal somatostatin administration on fetal brain cell proliferation and its relationship to serum growth hormone and brain trophin activity. Horm. Metab. Res., 11: 147–149.

Scharrer, E. (1928) Die Lichtempfindlichkeit blinder Elritzen. (Untersuchungen über das Zwischenhirn der Fische I.). Z. Vergl. Physiol., 7: 1–38.

Scharrer, E. and Scharrer, B. (1954) Hormones produced by neurosecretory cells. In *Recent Progress in Hormone Research, Vol. X,* pp. 183–240.

Schlumf, M., Lichtensteiger, W., Shoemaker, W.J. and Bloom, F.E. (1979) Catecholamines in early development. In *Catecholamines: Basic and Clinical Frontiers,* H. Usdin, H. Kopin and H. Bancla (Eds.), Pergamon Press, New York, pp. 806–808.

Sétáló, G., Flerkó, B., Arimura, A. and Schally, A.V. (1978) Brain cells as producers of releasing and inhibiting hormones. *Int. Rev. Cytol.,* Suppl. 7: 1–52.

Sokol, H.W. and Sise, J. (1973) The effect of exogenous vasopressin and growth hormone on the growth of rats with hereditary hypothalamic diabetes insipidus. *Growth,* 37: 127–142.

Sterba, G. (1974) Ascending neurosecretory pathways of the peptidergic type. In *Neurosecretion – the Final Neuroendocrine Pathway,* F. Knowles and L. Vollrath (Eds.), Springer, Berlin, pp. 38–47.

Sterba, G., Naumann, W. and Hoheisel, G. (1980) Exohypothalamic axons of the classic neurosecretory system and their synapses. In *Adaptive Capabilities in Nervous System, Progress in Brain Research, Vol. 53,* P. McConnell, G.J. Boer, H.J. Romijn, N.E. van de Poll and M.A. Corner (Eds.), Elsevier, Amsterdam, pp. 141–158.

Sunde, D.A. and Sokol, H.W. (1975) Quantification of rat neurophysins by polyacrylamide gel electrophoresis (PAGE): application to the rat with hereditary hypothalamic diabetes insipidus. *Ann. N.Y. Acad. Sci.,* 248: 345–364.

Swaab, D.F. (1980) Neuropeptides and brain development – a working hypothesis. In *A Multidisciplinary Approach to Brain Development,* C. Di Benedetta, R. Balázs and G. Gombos (Eds.), Elsevier, Amsterdam, in press.

Swaab, D.F., Boer, G.J. and Nolten, J.W.L. (1973) The hypothalamo–neurohypophysial system (HNS) of the Brattleboro rat. *Acta endocrinol.,* Suppl. 177: 80.

Swaab, D.F., Boer, G.J. and Visser, M. (1978) The fetal brain and intrauterine growth. In *Paediatrics and Growth,* D. Barltrop (Ed.), Fellowship of postgraduate Medicine, London, pp. 63–69.

Swaab, D.F. and Honnebier, W.J. (1973) The influence of removal of the fetal rat brain upon intrauterine growth of the fetus and the placenta and on gestation length. *J. Obstet. Gynaecol.,* 80: 589–597.

Swaab, D.F. and Honnebier, W.J. (1974) The role of the fetal hypothalamus in development of the fetoplacental unit and in parturition. In *Integrative Hypothalamic Activity, Progress in Brain Research, Vol. 41,* D.F. Swaab and J.P. Schadé (Eds.), Elsevier, Amsterdam, pp. 255–280.

Swaab, D.F., Pool, C.W. and Nijveldt, F. (1975) Immunofluorescence of vasopressin and oxytocin in rat hypothalamo–neurohypophyseal system. *J. neural Transm.,* 36: 195–215.

Swaab, D.F., Visser, M. and Tilders, F.J.H. (1976) Stimulation of intra-uterine growth in rat by α-melanocyte-stimulating hormone. *J. Endocr.,* 70: 445–455.

Valtin, H. and Schroeder, H.A. (1964) Familial hypothalamic diabetes insipidus in rats (Brattleboro strain). *Amer. J. Physiol.,* 206: 425–430.

Vandesande, F., Dierickx, K. and De Mey, J. (1975) Identification of the vasopressin–neurophysin producing neurons of the rat suprachiasmatic nuclei. *Cell Tiss. Res.,* 156: 377–380.

Wahlström, G. and Nordberg, A. (1978) Decreased brain weights in rats after long-term barbital treatments. *Life Sci.,* 23: 1583–1590.

Wied, D. de, Wimersma-Greidanus, Tj.B. van, Bohus, B., Urban, I. and Gispen, W.H. (1976) Vasopressin and memory consolidation. In *Perspective in Brain Research, Progress in Brain Research,* M.A. Corner and D.F. Swaab (Eds.), Elsevier, Amsterdam, pp. 181–194.

Wied, D. de and Gispen, W.H. (1977) Behavioral effects of peptides. In *Peptides in Neurobiology,* H. Gainer (Ed.), Plenum Press, New York, pp. 397–448.

Wikumsen, N.B.S. and Bie, P. (1969) Tissue to plasma ratios of radioactivity in the rat hypothalamo–hypophyseal system after intravenous injection of ^{3}H-lysine^8-vasopressin and ^{3}H-mannitol. *Acta endocr.,* 60: 389–400.

Winick, M. (1971) Cellular changes during placental and fetal growth. *Amer. J. Obstet. Gynecol.,* 109: 166–176.

Winick, M. (1976) *Malnutrition and Brain Development,* Oxford University Press, London.

Winick, M. and Noble, A. (1965) Quantitative changes in DNA, RNA and protein during prenatal and postnatal growth in the rat. *Develop. Biol.,* 12: 451–466.

Wolf, G. and Sterba, G. (1978) Development of the hypothalamic–neurohypophysial system in rats. In *Hormones and Brain Development.* G. Dörner and M. Kawakami (Eds.), Elsevier, Amsterdam, pp. 217–222.

Wright, W.A. and Kutscher, C.L. (1977) Vasopressin administration in the first month of life: effects on growth and water metabolism in hypothalamic diabetes insipidus rats. *Pharm. Biochem. Behav.,* 6: 505–509.

Neuropeptides.
A New Dimension in Biological Psychiatry

H.M. van PRAAG and W.M.A. VERHOEVEN

Department of Psychiatry, University of Utrecht, (The Netherlands)

INTRODUCTION

In the past 20 years, research into biochemical determinants of disturbed behavior has focused mainly on the central monoamines (MA) (Van Praag, 1978). There were sound reasons for this: (1) effective methods were evolved for determination of MA metabolites in cerebrospinal fluid (CSF) and peripheral body fluids; (2) the so-called probenecid technique enhanced the instructive value of determining these compounds in the CSF; (3) the degradation of MA is a "linear" process. MA metabolites are degradation products and have no precursor function in MA synthesis. The level of MA metabolites therefore reflects to some extent the rate of degradation of the mother substances in a given region; and (4) several enzymes involved in MA metabolism are measurable in peripheral blood (monoamine oxidase, catechol-O-methyltransferase and dopamine-β-hydroxylase).

Other central transmitters either did not fulfil these criteria, or did so only to a partial extent. An example is acetylcholine. Choline is both precursor and metabolite of acetylcholine. Moreover, choline is not utilized exclusively for central acetylcholine synthesis. Finally, determination of these compounds in CSF has until recently been difficult and cumbersome. We were in fact able to demonstrate that determination of choline in CSF warrants no reliable conclusion about the acetylcholine turnover in the central nervous system (CNS) (Klaver et al., 1979).

The discovery of the neuropeptides was of importance to biological psychiatry for two reasons. The first is a general reason: neuropeptides represent a new principle in neurobiology, that of hormone-like compounds produced in the brain, whose target is the brain. The second is a specific biological psychiatric reason: the neuropeptides have added a new dimension to human brain and behaviour research, supplementary to the MA dimension. This new dimension as such seems amply to merit investigation, but in addition raises the question whether (and, if so, how) neuropeptide and MA systems are related. The first question is discussed in this paper. On the second question there are (as yet) no adequate (human) data.

NEUROPEPTIDES

Neuropeptides are peptides which are produced by and are active in the CNS. Some neuropeptides also show peripheral endocrine activity but their effect on the CNS is independent of this. This direct effect on the CNS can give rise to specific behavior changes. It is with these neuropeptides that this paper is concerned. It does not claim comprehensiveness but confines itself to those peptides that: (1) influence behaviour via a direct effect on the CNS; and (2) have already been tested in human subjects.

Discovery of the neuropeptides

Three independent lines of research have led to the discovery of behaviorally-active peptides (De Wied, 1977b; Schally, 1978; Guillemin, 1978; Hughes, 1979; Nemeroff and Prange, 1978).

Pituitary hormones. Certain pituitary hormones — specifically adrenocorticotropic hormone (ACTH), melanocyte-stimulating hormone (MSH), vasopressin and oxytocin — exert an influence on amnestic and motivational processes. Since derivatives which lack peripheral endocrine activity retain their effects on behavior, it seemed plausible that these effects are based upon a direct effect on the CNS.

Releasing and inhibiting factors. These hormones are produced in the hypothalamus and control the release of anterior pituitary hormones. Research into thyrotropin-releasing hormone (TRH) in depressions (Prange et al., 1972) revealed that peptides of this group can cause effects on behaviour. Behaviour research has since been carried out, not only with TRH but also with some other hypothalamic hormones such as luteinizing hormone-releasing hormone (LH-RH) and the growth hormone release-inhibiting factor (somatostatin).

Endorphins (and enkephalins). The discovery of these peptides followed that of the so-called opiate receptors in the brain. The existence of these receptors prompted the question of the nature of the physiological candidates for these receptors. This led, first to the discovery of two pentapeptides, methionine-enkephalin and leucine-enkephalin, mainly localized in the brain, followed by the discovery of a few larger peptides, called endorphins. There are 3 known endorphins which, in order of diminishing size, are known as β-, γ- and α-endorphin. They are localized mainly in the pituitary gland; far less are found in the brain.

PITUITARY HORMONES; VASOPRESSIN AND OXYTOCIN

Vasopressin and oxytocin are mainly produced in the cell bodies of two hypothalamic nuclei, the supraoptic and the paraventricular nucleus. They are stored in so-called neurosecretory granules, which are transported along the axons of these neurons to, and stored in the axonal endings of the posterior pituitary. Oxytocin influences lactation and uterine contractions. Vasopressin inhibits renal water excretion and, in larger doses, increases blood pressure. Vasopressin is released, not only into the peripheral circulation but also into the hypothalamic–pituitary vascular system. This suggests that it may influence the function of the anterior pituitary gland.

Vasopressin is also found in the median eminence, but the function of this pool is still obscure, nor is it known how vasopressin reaches this site. Vasopressin is released, not only into the systemic and local circulation but also into the CSF, via which it could reach various brain structures. An alternative possibility is that it is transported via axons of the neurosecretory cells in the paraventricular and the supraoptic nucleus.

Data from animal experiments: memory research

De Wied et al. (1976a) demonstrated that resection of the posterior pituitary lobe (including the intermediate lobe) in rats leads to disturbances in avoidance learning, specifically in the capacity to fix the new behavioral patterns in memory (consolidation). The rate at which behavior is learned (acquisition), on the other hand, is not affected. In other words, rats deprived of the neurohypophysis learn normally but the extinction of what they have learned is accelerated: they "forget" more quickly. There are indications, moreover, that the retrieval of stored information is also disturbed in these animals. These phenomena can be reversed with the aid of vasopressin, and with vasopressin derivatives which lack peripheral endocrine activity, e.g. desglycinamide-lysine vasopressin.

Vasopressin has a comparable effect in intact rats: it inhibits the extinction of conditioned behaviour — a long-term effect which may persist for several days after a single injection. The first hours after the learning trial are critical for the effect of vasopressin, the effect being most marked within the first hour, and disappearing within 6 h. When retrograde amnesia is provoked in rats with an intact brain, e.g. with the aid of electroshocks or by carbon dioxide inhalation, restoration of memory can be facilitated with vasopressin.

The physiological involvement of vasopressin in memory and learning processes is clinched by the following two experiments. Intracerebrally administered anti-vasopressin serum induces in normal rats the above-described consolidation defects. Peripherally administered antiserum does not produce this effect. This suggests furthermore that the effect of vasopressin on memory is based on a direct influence within the CNS (Van Wimersma Greidanus and De Wied, 1976). The second experiment was carried out on rats of the Brattleboro strain by De Wied et al. (1975b). These rats have a genetic defect in vasopressin production and consequently suffer from diabetes insipius. In addition, they were found to show marked memory disorders which could be reversed with the aid of vasopressin.

The effect of the second posterior pituitary hormone (oxytocin) on the learning of avoidance behavior is the opposite of that of vasopressin (Van Ree et al., 1978a). Oxytocin administration leads to diminished consolidation and retrieval, rendering the animals amnesic, so to speak, for the aversive experience. Conversely, intraventricular injection of oxytocin antiserum facilitates the learning of avoidance behaviour. Posterior pituitary hormones are thus proven to be closely involved both in the acquisition of new types of behavior, and in the extinction of established ones. It therefore seems likely that their activity plays a role in the individual's ability to maintain himself in his life environment.

Data from animal experiments: addiction research

Apart from the effects of vasopressin in learning processes, there are reports on a second series of behavior effects of this peptide in animals which may have medical significance: effects on opiate addiction behaviour (Van Ree et al., 1978b). Des-glycinamide[9]-arginine[8]-vasopressin (DG-AVP) reduces i.v. self-administration of heroin in rats, both when subcutaneously and when intraventricularly injected. Anti-vasopressin antibodies, which neutralize the effect of endogenous vasopressin, have the opposite effect. The effectiveness of the vasopressin analog appears to be long-lasting, so that the specific rewarding effect of heroin in animals appears to be counteracted by vasopressin.

Another effect of vasopressin upon addiction behavior is the acceleration of habituation to the effects of morphine and related compounds (Krivoy et al., 1974; Van Ree et al., 1978b; Hoffman et al., 1978). In the absence of vasopressin (rats with diabetes insipidus or normal rats treated with vasopressin antiserum), on the other hand, the development of tolerance is delayed. Since the development of tolerance has been compared with a learning process, this vasopressin effect may come under the same denominator as the above described facilitation of consolidation and inhibition of extinction of conditioned behavior. The former effect seems to hold promise for the treatment of addicts, but the latter effect would be therapeutically undesirable.

Oxytocin exerts no significant influence on heroin self-administration. Its effect on the development of tolerance is similar to that of DG-AVP: it facilitates it. In this respect, oxytocin was found to be 5 times as potent as DG-AVP (Van Ree et al., 1978b).

Human studies

In a few recent human studies the effect of vasopressin (about 14 IU/day) on learning and memory processes was studied by means of psychometric tests (Table I). On the basis of a controlled study of 23 volunteers (aged 60–65 years), Legros et al. (1978) reached the conclusion that vasopressin (administered as nasal spray) improved attention, concentration, learning and memory. Oliveros et al. (1978), Blake et al. (1978) and La Boeuf et al. (1978) described the effect of vasopressin in a total of 8 patients with an amnesic syndrome. Oliveros et al. (1978) observed a favorable effect on memory functions in patients with post-traumatic amnesia. Blake et al. (1978) observed no effect in patients with disturbed memory functions as a result of alcoholism. La Boeuf et al. (1978) observed marked improvement of memory functions in two patients with a Korsakoff syndrome. Further investigations will be needed to establish whether or not vasopressin treatment is of clinical significance in amnesia and other memory disorders with an anatomically intact cerebral substrate. To avoid side effects, moreover, it would be advisable to use a vasopressin analog which lacks peripheral endocrine effects.

So far, only one study has focused on the effect of vasopressin in heroin addicts. In the vasopressin group, the number of heroin administrations was significantly smaller than that in the placebo group (Van Ree, personal communication). Follow-up studies will be needed to see if there are also influences on tolerance development, which might cause the gain made on the one hand to be lost on the other.

TABLE I

BEHAVIORAL STUDIES WITH VASOPRESSIN IN HUMAN BEINGS

Study	Diagnosis	n	Design	Dosage	Result
Blake et al., 1978	Korsakoff syndrome	2	open	16 IU daily 15 or 21 days	No effect
LeBoeuf et al., 1978	Korsakoff syndrome	2	double-blind	22,5 IU daily 14 days	Improvement of memory and concentration
Legros et al., 1978	Volunteers with memory disorders, age: 50–65 years	12	double-blind	16 IU daily 3 days	Improvement of memory, concentration and attention
Oliveros et al., 1978	Post-traumatic amnesia	3	double-blind	11–15 IU daily	Improvement of memory and mood
	Alcoholic amnesia	1		7–21 days	
Total		20			+ = 18

Patients with acute psychoses and a high degree of anxiety were found to have increased plasma vasopressin concentrations as compared both with non-psychotic patients having a high degree of anxiety, and with normal controls (Raskind et al., 1978). Anxiety is therefore probably not the cause of this phenomenon, the significance of which remains obscure. There have been speculations on the possible involvement of vasopressin in the pathogenesis of depressions (Gold et al., 1978), but no experimental data have yet been reported.

As pointed out earlier, the effect of oxytocin on conditioned behavior is the opposite of the effect of vasopressin. The latter facilitates consolidation of new information, whereas the former facilitates its extinction. We considered the fact that there are categories of psychiatric patients with memory traces that lead to entirely dysfunctional, repetitive behaviour. Typical examples are patients with obsessive-compulsive disorders, in whom extinction of the memory traces in question might produce a therapeutically desirable effect. We are now studying the effect of oxytocin on compulsive behavior and our preliminary results indicate that compulsive activities are indeed less frequent during oxytocin medication than during placebo administration (Kraaimaat, Verhoeven, Van Praag, De Wied and Van Ree, unpublished results).

PITUITARY HORMONES; ADRENOCORTICOTROPIC HORMONE

ACTH is produced by the basophilic cells in the anterior pituitary lobe and is released directly into the blood stream. It stimulates the adrenal cortex to increased hormone release, especially of glucocorticosteroids. ACTH release in turn is stimulated by the corticotropin-releasing factor (CRF) from the hypothalamus. The structure of CRF is still unknown. In rats, ACTH is found also in the basal hypothalamus and the median eminence.

ACTH consists of 39 amino acids. The amino acid sequence of this molecule is in part found also in β-lipotropin (β-LPH). β-LPH has been known for some time as a pituitary hormone involved in fat mobilization in the periphery (Li, 1964), and is probably the precursor substance of the endorphins and met-enkephalin. It has recently been established that β-LPH and ACTH originate from a common precursor molecule (Nakanishi et al., 1979). The first 13 amino acids of ACTH (ACTH 1–13) are identical to those in α-melanocyte-stimulating hormone (α-MSH) (Fig. 1).

Data from animal experiments

Rats deprived of the anterior pituitary lobe learn conditioned behaviour less readily and also forget more quickly what they have learned (De Wied et al., 1975a). This disorder can-

	1	8 9 10	11 12 13 14 15 16 17	18 19 20 21 22	
β-MSH	Ala.....	Pro-Tyr-Arg	-Met-Glu-His-Phe-Arg-Try-Gly	-Ser-Pro-Pro-Lys-Asp	
		1 2 3	4 5 6 7 8 9 10	11 12 13	
α-MSH		Ser-Tyr-Ser	-Met-Glu-His-Phe-Arg-Try-Gly	-Lys-Pro-Val	-NH_2
		1 2 3	4 5 6 7 8 9 10	11 12 13	39
ACTH		Ser-Tyr-Ser	-Met-Glu-His-Phe-Arg-Try-Gly	-Lys-Pro-Val	..........Phe

Fig. 1. Common amino acid sequences in corticotropin-related peptides. (From Prange et al., 1978.) ACTH 4–10 = α-MSH 4–10 = β-MSH 11–17. ACTH 1–13 = α-MSH 1–13.

not be reversed with corticosteroids but can be effectively treated with ACTH or ACTH fragments without corticotropic activity, e.g. ACTH 4–10. The amino acid sequence ACTH 4–7 is the smallest behaviourally-active ACTH fragment.

When given to intact rats, ACTH and its behaviourally-active fragments exert little influence on the acquisition of conditioned behavior, but they do delay its extinction. This applies to conditioned avoidance behavior, but in equal measure to sexual and food-rewarded behavior. The effect of these compound is brief (hours) as compared with that of vasopressin (days) (De Wied, 1977a).

Other behavioural effects of ACTH observed in rats were increased arousal, increased attentive ability and increased "motivational value" of external clues (Donovan, 1978). These effects presumably enable animals treated with ACTH peptides to retain new information more easily.

Intrathecal and intraventricular (not intravenous) administration of ACTH leads to frequent yawning and stretching in test animals (Bertolini et al., 1975). The significance of this syndrome is not clear, but it is conceivable that it suppresses sleep and therefore relates to the positive effects of ACTH on attention. Moreover, animals thus treated show frequently repeated erections, ejaculations and copulation movements without seeking contacts with females.

Human studies

Only ACTH 4–10 has so far been studied in normal volunteers and in aged patients with memory disorders (Table II). In the former category, there were indications of a general arousal effect and improved concentration of attention. The fragment reduces performance deficits during serial reaction time tasks, delays the development of electroencephalographic

TABLE II

BEHAVIORAL STUDIES WITH ACTH 4–10 IN HUMAN BEINGS

Study	Diagnosis	n	Dosage (single dose)	Results
Galliard and Sanders 1975	Volunteers 21–29 years	18	30 mg s.c.	Improvement of general motivation and activation
Dornbusch and Nikolevski, 1976	Volunteers 63–70 years	9	15–60 mg s.c.	Improvement of visual reaction time
Sannita et al., 1976	Volunteers 19–29 years	12	60 mg i.v.	Improvement of level of attention
Miller et al., 1977	Volunteers 21–35 years	20	30 mg s.c.	No effect
Sandman et al., 1977	Volunteers 21–23 years	11	15 mg i.v. during 2 h	Improvement of level of attention
Rapoport et al., 1976	Children with learning difficulties	20	30 mg i.v.	No effect
Will et al., 1978	Geriatric volunteers complaining of memory loss, 65–80 years	22	15 mg s.c.	No effect
Branconnier et al., 1979	Organic brain syndrome >60 years	18	30 mg s.c.	Improvement of affective state and retrieval from memory
Total	Volunteers	70		+ = 50
	Organic brain syndrome	60		+ = 18

signs of habituation, increases the arousal level, and improves short-term memory (Van Riezen et al., 1977; Miller et al., 1974; Gaillard and Sanders, 1975; Dornbush and Nikolovski, 1976; Kastin et al., 1975).

It can be concluded from two controlled studies that ACTH may be valuable also in aged patients suffering from slight deterioration based on organic cerebral lesions. Ferris et al. (1976) reported improvement of cognitive functions, while Branconnier et al. (1979) placed more emphasis on motor and affective effects than on cognitive effects. Subjects experienced a reduction of depression and confusion along with increased vigor. This evidence of increased vigor was supported behaviorally by a delay in the onset of increased latency in reaction time. The findings also indicated that retrieval from memory stores may be enhanced by ACTH 4–10. Although significant, these effects were not very pronounced. Further investigation will be needed to show whether ACTH 4–10 has any true therapeutic significance.

According to Small et al. (1977), ACTH 4–10 has no effect on memory disorders caused by electroshock therapy (EST). The strength of this compound may after all be more that it increases the level of arousal — resulting in improved mood level, motivation and selective attention — than that it improves memory functions per se. If so, then the compound would in fact much more useful in the treatment of patients with mild senile organic brain syndromes than in "pure" memory disorders such as those observed after EST or after head injuries.

PITUITARY HORMONES; MELANOCYTE-STIMULATING HORMONE

The pituitary gland contains two melanocyte-stimulating hormones: α-MSH which consists of 13 amino acids, and β-MSH which consists of 22 amino acids. The first 13 amino acids of ACTH are identical to the α-MSH molecule (Fig. 1). The minimal chain which still shows MSH activity consists of the amino acids 4–10 of the α-MSH molecule. Both α-MSH and β-MSH are found in the pars intermedia of the pituitary gland, as well as in the hypothalamus.

MSH plays no role in the mammalian pigment metabolism, its function being in fact unknown. It is remarkable, moreover, that the hypothalamus contains a MSH release-inhibiting factor (MSH-RIF), but that no blood vessels which could transport this product from hypothalamus to pars intermedia of the pituitary gland have been identified.

Data from animal experiments

Like ACTH and its fragment ACTH 4–10, α-MSH and β-MSH are able to reverse memory and learning disorders resulting from extirpation of the anterior pituitary lobe. When given intrathecally or intracerebrally, they too provoke the previously mentioned yawning and stretching syndrome (Van Wimersma Greidanus, 1977).

Human studies

Cotzias et al. (1967) reported that MSH aggrevates the symptoms of Parkinson's disease. It therefore seemed plausible that a substance which inhibits MSH release, e.g. MSH-RIF, might have a therapeutic effect on this disease. It was also observed that MSH-RIF vigorously potentiates dopamine (DA) effects (Donovan, 1978). For these two reasons MSH-RIF

was given to Parkinson patients (Fischer et al., 1974) and was indeed found to be therapeutically effective. The same was observed in depressions (Ehrensing and Kastin, 1974), but
the latter experiments have not yet been repeated and confirmed. Nor is it known whether
these MSH-RIF effects are produced via MSH release or whether they are based on a direct
influence on the CNS.

HYPOPHYSIOTROPIC HORMONES; THYROTROPIN-RELEASING HORMONE

Thyrotropin-releasing hormone (TRH) was the first pituitary-regulating hormone whose
chemical structure was identified. It is a tripeptide which was named TRH in view of its
ability to enhance the release of thyroid-stimulating hormone (TSH, thyrotropin) by the
anterior pituitary lobe. It was later found that TRH can also increase prolactin release, but
it is still uncertain whether this is a physiological effect.

This hormone is found, not only in the median eminence but also in other parts of the
hypothalamus and outside it, e.g. in the cerebral cortex, cerebellum brain stem and CSF.
The hypothalamus contains in fact no more than 20% of the total amount of TRH in the
brain. The TRH concentration is relatively high in brain parts which are also rich in monoamines.

Motives for behaviour research with TRH

Interest in a possible effect of TRH on certain types of disturbed behavior was aroused
by the following observations. Prange and his groups had demonstrated (Prange et al., 1969)
that the thyroid hormone T_3 potentiates the therapeutic effect of the tricyclic antidepressant imipramine (Tofranil). The pituitary thyroid-stimulating hormone TSH produced
a similar potentiating effect (Prange et al., 1970). This prompted the question of the possible
effect of TRH in depressions. The urgency of this question was further increased by a
number of observations made in animal experiments.

When given to rats and mice treated with the monoamine oxidase (MAO) inhibitor
pargyline, L-DOPA has a central stimulating effect (hyperactivity, increased aggressiveness
and irritability). Antidepressants potentiate this DOPA effect. This phenomenon is used in
screening potential antidepressants. TRH proved to behave like an antidepressant in this test,
even in animals deprived of pituitary gland or thyroid (Plotnikoff et al., 1972). The effect is
therefore independent of the pituitary-thyroid axis, and is probably based on a direct
influence of TRH on the brain.

Moreover, TRH antagonizes the sedative and hypothermal effects of various central
depressants such as barbiturates, chloral hydrate, chlorpromazine (Largactil) and diazepam
(Valium). This effect, too, persists in animals deprived of the pituitary gland. Thyroid
hormones lack this potency. TRH analogs which lack the ability to enhance TSH release, do
antagonize sedatives (Prange et al., 1978). This warrants the conclusion that the analeptic
potency of TRH is independent of its endocrine effects.

Finally, it was found that TRH potentiates the behavioural effects resulting from an
excess of serotonin in the brain (Green and Grahame-Smith, 1974). In addition, indications
were found that TRH increases the release of noradrenaline from the presynaptic nerve
terminals (Horst and Spirt, 1974). In view of the monoamine (MA) hypothesis on the
pathogenesis of depressions, serotonin and/or noradrenaline-potentiating compound can be
expected to have an antidepressant effect.

TRH in depression

Two publications which appeared in 1972 (Prange et al.; Kastin et al.) presented promising data on the use of TRH in depression. In a double-blind cross-over design, the former authors treated 10 women with unipolar depressions with a single dose of 0.6 mg TRH and reported a favorable effect within a few hours. The depression scores diminished by about 50%, and this (partial) therapeutic effect persisted for an appreciable time (about a week). Kastin et al. (1972), using the same design, treated 4 women and 1 man with manic-depressive illness (depressed type) and involutional depression. After being given 500 μg TRH by i.v. injection for 3 consecutive days, 4 showed pronounced improvement, while the fifth improved moderately. In 3 of these patients the favorable effect persisted for several days.

A fairly large series of studies has since been devoted to the effect of TRH in depression. However, they show a marked diversity of design, dosage scheme, measuring methods, type of patients, etc. This material is therefore too heterogeneous to allow for any definite conclusion, so that we have to confine ourselves to a few general, more tentative conclusions (Prange et al., 1978; Nemeroff et al., 1979).

(1) The results obtained with orally given TRH are disappointing. Perhaps the effective blood concentration was never attained, for TRH is degraded fairly rapidly in the blood, the half-time value being about 2 min. Should absorption of TRH from the intestine be gradual, then the rate of degradation is possibly higher than the rate of absorption.

(2) The majority of authors have observed that TRH had a psychopharmacological effect if given by rapid i.v. injection. However, the effect is described not so much as antidepressant but rather in such terms as: decrease in tension, increase in energy, enhanced capacity to cope with feelings, etc. In terms of effect, therefore, TRH seems to resemble a central stimulant more than a traditional antidepressant.

(3) The conclusion given in the preceding point is supported by findings in normal test subjects, in whom TRH induces relaxation, mild euphoria and a sense of increased energy. This effect develops also if TRH administration is preceded by administration of thyroid hormone in order to block the TSH response of the pituitary gland. The behaviour effects, therefore, are probably based upon the activity of TRH per se.

(4) The TRH effect in cases of depression is brief and of little significance therapeutically.

(5) Hardly any research has been done into the question of whether or not there exists a "TRH-susceptible" subgroup of depressions which can be distinguished in biochemical or psychopathological terms from "TRH-insusceptible" patients. Such research would be of interest, however, for most authors intimate that, if TRH has any effect, only certain of the depressive patients notice it. MA research in depressions has revealed the concept of the biochemical and endocrinological classifiability of depressions. These variables should be taken into account in analyzing the results of antidepressant medications, particularly if they involve compounds with an effect on central MA metabolism.

(6) TRH fails in any way to potentiate the effect of the tricyclic antidepressant amitriptyline. This shows that the thyroid-stimulating effect of TRH plays no role in its psychopharmacological effect, for the thyroid hormone T3 does potentiate the effect of this antidepressant.

TRH in schizophrenic psychoses

An endogenous substance is not likely to have a specific therapeutic effect in a given syndrome, unless this involves a deficiency. There are no indications of TRH deficiency in depression. This is why TRH has also been used in other psychiatric disorders, and more specifically in schizophrenic psychoses (Prange et al., 1978).

The number of available studies is too small, and their design not sufficiently perfect, to warrant any firm conclusions as yet. The impression gained from the available data is that TRH can have a favorable effect on autistic, inert and reticent patients. In this category of patients, too, there is evidently a mild stimulating and euphorizing effect. As in the case of depression, this effect has been reported to persist often for days after discontinuation of the medication.

TRH in Parkinson's disease

The compound has proved ineffective against neurological symptoms (Lakke et al., 1974), but a shift toward optimism and a sense of well-being has been repeatedly reported (Chase et al., 1974).

Conclusions

In normal test subjects and in several categories of psychiatric patients, TRH has a mild stimulating and activating effect. It is neither a specific nor an effective antidepressant.

HYPOPHYSIOTROPIC HORMONES; LUTEINIZING HORMONE-RELEASING HORMONE

Luteinizing hormone-releasing hormone (LH-RH) stimulates both the release of LH and that of follicle-stimulating hormone (FSH) from the anterior pituitary lobe. We do not know whether a separate FSH-releasing hormone also exists. LH-RH is localized chiefly in the hypothalamus but small amounts are found also in periventricular tissue.

In animal experiments this releasing factor has been demonstrated to have 3 major behavioral effects: activation of sexual behavior (Moss et al., 1975), antagonism of barbiturate effects such as sedation and hypothermia (Bisette et al., 1976), and inhibition of the extinction of active avoidance behavior (De Wied et al., 1975a). Female rats show their sexual willingness by assuming a lordotic posture and lifting the hindquarters. Small amounts of LH-RH (s.c.) provoke this behavior, even in animals without pituitary gland or ovaries (Donovan, 1978), evidently via an extra-pituitary mechanism. Human studies have been scanty. In a recent controlled study (McAdoo et al., 1978), 12 healthy male volunteers were given 500 μg LH-RH by continuous infusion. Psychological tests yielded indications of a slight increase in both reaction speed and level of attention for a few hours after administration. A decrease in anxiety and fatigue was likewise observed. Doering et al. (1977), however, observed no effect of LH-RH on mood and behavior in a study of human volunteers. Nor did it have any therapeutic effect in cases of depression and in impotence (Benkert, 1975).

HYPOPHYSIOTROPIC HORMONES; SOMATOSTATIN

Growth hormone release-inhibiting factor, somatostatin, inhibits not only the release of growth hormone (GH) by the anterior pituitary lobe but also the TRH-induced release of

TSH. It is localized, not only in the hypothalamus but also in other brain areas (e.g. mid-brain, brain stem, cerebral cortex) and also outside the CNS (e.g. stomach, pancreas and intestine). Over 60% of the somatostatin in the brain is localized outside the hypothalamus. GH secretion diminishes to immeasurable values after sectioning of the hypophyseal stalk. It is therefore unlikely that somatostatin inhibits GH secretion tonically, i.e. continuously.

Test animals treated by somatostatin infusion show less motor activity and an increased sensitivity to the sedative, sleep-inducing effect of barbiturates. This effect is observed also in hypophysectomized animals. Direct application of somatostatin to hippocampus or cerebral cortex induces a complex pattern of motor symptoms such as tremors, stereotyped movements and ataxia. Behavioral effects in human subjects have not yet been studied (Kastin et al., 1978).

HYPOPHYSIOTROPIC HORMONES; MSH RELEASE-INHIBITING FACTOR

The tripeptide Pro-Leu-Gly (PLG) inhibits the release of MSH from the pituitary gland. Apart from PLG, a tetrapeptide (Pro-His-Arg-Gly) has been isolated from hypothalamic tissue which shows about 20% of the effect of PLG on MSH release. PLG is therefore some-times referred to as MIF-I, while the tetrapeptide is called MIF-II. PLG is believed to be enzymatically split off from oxytocin in the hypothalamus. PLG is effective in the pargy-line/DOPA model (see section on motives for behavior research with TRH), even in hypo-physectomized animals. It increases the rate of synthesis of central dopamine but not that of noradrenaline or serotonin. This dopamine effect, however, requires the presence of the pituitary gland (Prange et al., 1978).

Human studies have already been briefly mentioned in the subsections dealing with pituitary hormones. The results can be summarized in the statement that PLG seems to have a mild antidepressant effect, and also exerts a favorable influence on the motor pathology in Parkinson patients. However, the available data are limited, and have not always been the result of methodologically well-designed research.

ENDORPHINS

The discovery of the endorphins resulted from the following observations: (1) the mammalian CNS proved to contain receptors with a high affinity for morphine and related compounds, which were insensitive to any of the known neurotransmitters (Pert and Snyder, 1973; Simon et al., 1973; Terenius, 1975), and (2) pain can be alleviated in test animals by electrical stimulation of certain brain areas. This stimulation-induced analgesia can be antagonized with a morphine antagonist such as naloxone (Mayer et al., 1971; Akil et al., 1976). These observations seemed to suggest the existence of an endogenous ligand for these so-called opiate receptors. Within a remarkably short time, two such compounds were isolated from the brain and identified (Hughes, 1975; Terenius, 1975). They were pentapep-tides and named enkephalins: methionine-enkephalin (met-enkephalin) and leucine-enkephalin (leu-enkephalin).

After the discovery of the enkephalins, the search for other morphomimetic peptides was further intensified by the fact that the amino acid sequence of met-enkephalin proved to be present in the 91 amino acid pituitary hormone β-LPH. This research led to the discovery of β-endorphin (β-LPH 61-91) (Li and Chung, 1976), γ-endorphin (β-LPH 61-77) and α-endorphin (β-LPH 61-76) (Fig. 2).

240

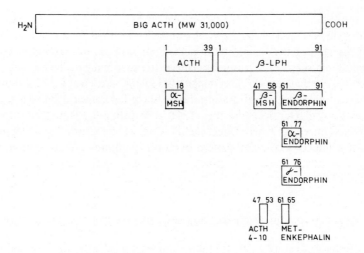

Fig. 2. Precursor relationships of corticotropins and pituitary endorphins. The 31,000 molecular weight peptide "big ACTH" contains within its sequence the entire ACTH and β-lipotropin (β-LPH) molecules, which appear to be located next to each other. Within the ACTH molecule lies the sequence of α-MSH, while the sequence of β-MSH, as well as the sequence of β-endorphin, is contained within the structure of β-LPH. The sequence ACTH 4–10 is also present within the β-LPH sequence, so that this portion of the ACTH molecule is repeated twice within the big ACTH precursor. The sequence of γ-endorphin, α-endorphin and met-enkephalin is contained within that of β-endorphin. Supposedly α- and γ-endorphin are formed from β-endorphin. There is no evidence that β-endorphin is the precursor of met-enkephalin in the brain. (From Snyder and Childers, 1979.)

All endorphins and enkephalins except leu-enkephalin, therefore, are incorporated in the β-LPH molecule. The endorphins, i.e. the larger β-LPH fragments, are chiefly found in the pituitary gland, like β-LPH itself. The enkephalins on the other hand are found almost exclusively in the brain. Neurons and pituitary cells with β-endorphin, also contain β-LPH and ACTH. The brain contains neurons with β-endorphin as well as with enkephalin. There are sound reasons to assume that, in these cells, they play a role in impulse transmission (Snyder and Childers, 1979). In the following, I shall use the term endorphins as a collective term both for endorphins in the strict sense, and for enkephalins.

Interest in endorphins in psychiatry

Endorphins have attracted psychiatric attention from the start. The following factors have contributed to this: (1) high endorphin concentrations are found in brain areas involved in pain conduction, motor activity and, probably, regulation of mood and affects (Snyder and Childers, 1979); (2) opiates have a distinct effect on pain threshold, mood and level of psychological integration. A similar effect could be expected of the "endogenous morphines"; (3) patients whose periventricular grey matter was electrically stimulated in order to alleviate chronic pain, showed increased enkephalin-like activity in the CSF (Akil et al., 1978a); (4) stress increases the release of ACTH as well as β-endorphin by the pituitary gland (Guillemin et al., 1977; Watson et al., 1979); and (5) β-endorphin exerts an unmistakable influence on animal behavior. In large doses, it gives rise to a catatonia-like condition with motor retardation (Jacquet and Marks, 1976; Bloom et al., 1976; Snyder, 1978).

Clinical endorphin research has so far fanned out in the following directions: (1) measurement of the endorphin concentration in body fluids (specially, CSF and dialysate after haemodialysis); and (2) the effects of morphine (and endorphin) antagonists and of endorphin or endorphin derivatives in psychiatric patients.

Endorphin research in psychiatric patients

Endorphins in human cerebrospinal fluid. Terenius and Wåhlström (1975a,b) isolated two opiate-like fractions from human CSF. Neither of these fractions is identical to any of the endorphins now known. The concentrations of these fractions were determined in 13 patients with schizophrenic and 7 with manic-depressive psychoses (Terenius et al., 1976, 1977; Lindström et al., 1978). Abnormally high "fraction I" endorphin concentration was found in the schizophrenic patients, which was normalized by neuroleptic medication resulting in reduction of psychotic symptoms. In the manic patients, an increased fraction I endorphin fraction was found during the manic phase. A correlation between "fraction II" endorphin and clinical symptoms was not demonstrated.

The β-endorphin concentration in the CSF was found to be markedly increased in patients with acute schizophrenic psychoses, whereas in chronic psychotic patients it varied from normal to slightly decreased (Domschke et al., 1979). Loeber et al. (1979) demonstrated the presence of α- and γ-endorphin in human CSF. Whether their concentrations can show changes in psychiatric patients has yet to be established.

Endorphins in dialysate

Opiate antagonists. The two pure opiate antagonists, naloxone and naltrexone (with a slightly more prolonged effect and, unlike naloxone, orally administrable), have been used in human studies. Naltrexone has a dysphoric effect in normal test subjects (Mendelson et al., 1979). In psychiatric patients, these compounds have been studied mostly in schizophrenic and manic syndromes (Table III).

In 3 double-blind cross-over studies (Emrich et al., 1977; Watson et al., 1978; Akil et al., 1978b), 20, 11 and 8 patients respectively, with schizophrenic psychoses were given naloxone intravenously. In 26 patients the psychotic symptoms (specifically the acoustic hallucinations) showed a transient reduction 2–7 h after the injection. In a single-blind study (Gunne et al., 1977), a similar effect was observed in 4 out of 6 patients. In two uncontrolled studies involving 5 and 3 schizophrenic patients, respectively (Mielke and Gallant, 1977; Gitlin and Rosenblatt, 1978), no effect was observed after oral administration of 250 mg and 50–100 mg naltrexone per day. In 4 controlled studies involving 14, 7, 8 and 20 patients with schizophrenic psychoses (Davis et al., 1977; Volavka et al., 1977; Janowsky et al., 1977; Hertz et al., 1978), no clinically demonstrable effect of naloxone was found.

Reduction of manic symptoms was demonstrated in 16 out of a total of 24 patients involved in two double-blind controlled studies (Janowsky et al., 1978; Judd et al., 1978). In both, 20 mg naloxone was given by continuous drip within 20 min: the maximum effect developed 15–30 min after the drip and lasted 1–2 h. A pilot study of 5 patients with vital depressions (Terenius et al., 1977) revealed no effect of naloxone on the depressive symptoms.

In a recent study we focused on the effect of naloxone on acoustic hallucinations and manic symptoms (Verhoeven et al., 1979b). In a double-blind placebo-controlled design, 10 patients were given a single injection of 20 mg naloxone s.c. Five patients had verifiable acoustic hallucinations in the context of a schizophrenic psychosis, and the other 5 showed

TABLE III

EFFECTS OF NALOXONE IN SCHIZOPHRENIC AND MANIC SYNDROMES

Study	Diagnosis	n	Neuroleptic medication	Design	Dosage naloxone *	Result	Duration	Attenuation of symptoms
Emrich et al., 1977	Schizophrenia	20	– = 2, + = 18	Double-blind Cross-over	4.0 mg i.v.	+12	2 – 7 h	Auditory hallicunations
Watson et al., 1978	Schizophrenia	11	– = 6, + = 5	Double-blind Cross-over: 9 Single-blind: 2	10 mg i.v.	+6	3 – 6 h = 4, 48 h = 2	Auditory hallicunations
Akil et al., 1978	Schizophrenia	8	– = 4, + = 4	Double-blind Cross-over	10 mg i.v.	+8	75 –90 min	Auditory hallicunations
Gunne et al., 1977	Schizophrenia	6	+ = 6	Single-blind	0.4 mg i.v.	+4	1 – 6 h	Auditory hallicunations
Kurland et al., 1977	Schizophrenia	12	+ = 12	Double-blind	0.4–1.2 mg i.v. naltrexone 250 mg, 9 days	–		
Mielke and Gallant, 1977	Schizophrenia	5	– = 5	Open		–		
Gitlin and Rosenblatt, 1978	Schizophrenia	3	– = 1, + = 2	Single-blind	naltrexone 50–100 mg, 14 days	–		
Davis et al., 1977	Schizophrenia	14	– = 9, + = 5	Double-blind	0.4–10 mg i.v.	–		
Volavka et al., 1977	Schizophrenia	7	+ = 7	Double-blind	0.4 mg i.v.	–		
Janowsky et al., 1977	Schizophrenia	8	+ = 8	Double-blind Cross-over	1.2 mg i.v.	–		
Hertz et al., 1978	Schizophrenia	20	– = 20	Double-blind Cross-over	4.0 mg i.v.	–		
Janowsky et al., 1978	Manic syndrome	12	– = 3, + = 9	Double-blind Cross-over	20 mg i.v. (infusion)	+12	30 –90 min	Manic symptoms
Judd et al., 1978	Manic syndrome	12	– = 12	Double-blind Cross-over	20 mg i.v. (infusion)	+4	0.5– 2 h	Manic symptoms
Verhoeven et al., 1979a,b	Schizophrenia Manic syndrome	5 5	+ = 10	Double-blind Cross-over	20 mg s.c.	–		
Total	Schizophrenia	119				+30	2 – 7 h	Auditory hallucinations
	Manic syndrome	29				+16	0.5– 2 h	Manic symptoms

* So far only single administration studies have been carried out.

manic symptoms in the context of either a bipolar depression or a (schizophrenic) psychosis. All had already received neuroleptic medication without complete therapeutic success; the neuroleptic maintenance therapy was continued during the naloxone treatment. The symptoms of the manic patients were scored with the aid of the Brief Psychiatric Rating Scale and the Biegel–Murphy Mania Rating Scale, while those of the schizophrenic patients were scored with the aid of the Brief Psychiatric Rating Scale and a Hallucination Scale. In all cases, moreover, a checklist of individual symptoms was completed on the basis of a complete Present State Examination Interview. This controlled study disclosed no demonstrable influence of naloxone on any of the psychopathological symptoms scored: in particular no influence on acoustic hallucinations and/or manic symptoms was found.

To conclude, in only 3 out of 8 controlled clinical trials (Emrich et al., 1977; Watson et al., 1978; Akil et al., 1978b) was a favourable effect of naloxone reported consisting of transient reduction or disappearance of acoustic hallucinations. Some 30% of the 107 patients so far treated with naloxone responded to this medication. Unlike neuroleptics, naloxone has no effect on serum prolactin (Lal et al., 1979). Dopamine receptors in the tubero-infundibular system are therefore not blocked. There are sound reasons to assume that the therapeutic effect of neuroleptics depends upon their ability to block dopamine receptors (Van Praag, 1977, 1980). Therefore, in so far as naloxone has any antipsychotic properties, they must be mediated via another mechanism. The two controlled clinical studies of Janowsky et al. (1978) and Judd et al. (1978) reported a transient reduction of manic symptoms in 16 out of 24 patients (Table III). One controlled study (Verhoeven et al., 1979) produced negative results. We conclude tentatively from these data either that there could exist a subgroup of psychotic patients or that psychotic symptoms exist which are susceptible to opiate antagonists. However, further definition of this range of indications is not yet possible.

Dialysate studies. In 1977 Wagemaker and Cade described a favorable effect of long-term haemodialysis in chronic schizophrenic patients. Several centers are now conducting studies in which dialysis and sham-dialysis are being compared. A conclusion concerning the therapeutic validity of this method in schizophrenic patients would be highly premature.

Palmour et al. (1977) isolated a hitherto unknown peptide from the dialysate of schizophrenic patients. It is believed to be β-endorphin in which the methionine in the 5-position has been replaced by leucine (β-leu^5-endorphin), a sensational statement which implies the possibility of a correlation between disorders of endorphin metabolism and schizophrenic psychoses. However, Lewis et al. (1979) recently reported that they had been unable to isolate a peptide of the above-mentioned structure from the haemodialysate of two schizophrenic patients.

Therapeutic applications of endorphins and endorphin derivatives

β-Endorphin. In an open study without a clearly defined protocol, Kline et al. (1977) have injected i.v. a total dose of 9 mg β-endorphin – distributed over 4 days – injected in 5 patients with schizophrenic psychoses and in 2 with depression (unipolar and bipolar, respectively). The following psychotropic effects were observed: (1) the injection was followed within a few min by an activating, anxiolytic and antidepressant effect which persisted for 2–3 h; (2) a degree of drowsiness developed 2–4 h after injection; and (3) about 12 h after injection of β-endorphin, a therapeutic effect was observed which was characterized by reduction of the psychotic or depressive symptoms lasting 1–10 days.

Des-tyrosine-γ-endorphin (DTγE). Most endorphins (β-endorphin, α-endorphin, met-enkephalin and leu-enkephalin) are able to delay the extinction of conditioned behavior (e.g. conditioned active or passive avoidance behavior). This effect must be independent of the opiate receptors, for it persists after blockade of these receptors by means of naloxone.

One endorphin deviates from this general pattern: γ-endorphin (De Wied et al., 1978). It does have morphinomimetic properties but it facilitates extinction instead of consolidation of new information. In this respect it behaves like the traditional neuroleptics of, say, the phenothiazine and butyrophenone series. If the terminal tyrosine molecule is split off (thus producing DTγE) then the molecule loses its morphinomimetic characteristics, and its facilitating effect on the extinction of conditioned behavior is intensified.

Apart from its suppressive effect on conditioned behavior, DTγE has other properties in common with traditional neuroleptics, e.g. a positive grip test. In other ways, however, its profile differs from that of traditional neuroleptics. For example, DTγE has no effect on gross behavior in an open field, nor does it antagonize the effects of apomorphine and amphetamine — compounds with a dopamine-potentiating capacity.

In biochemical terms too, there is a similarity between neuroleptics and DTγE. Both compounds increase the dopamine turnover in certain brain areas. With the neuroleptics, this effect is probably secondary to blockade of postsynaptic dopamine receptors. Exactly how DTγE increases the dopamine turnover remains to be established (Versteeg et al., 1979). In view of the similarities between DTγE and the traditional neuroleptics we decided to study this peptide in patients with schizophrenic psychoses.

DTγE has so far been used in clinical research in one single-blind and one controlled study, involving a total of 14 patients (Verhoeven et al., 1978, 1979b) with recurrent schizophrenic and schizo-affective psychoses. Twelve had been hospitalized for at least 6 months when the study started, and were still psychotic despite medication with adequate doses of neuroleptics. The remaining two were treated with DTγE for acute schizophrenic psychosis immediately after admission. They had had no neuroleptics prior to admission. In the past, they had been repeatedly hospitalized with an acute psychotic episode.

In the first single-blind study, 6 patients were given a single i.m. dose of 1 mg DTγE per day for 7 days. In the second study (a double-blind cross-over design), 6 patients received 1 mg DTγE by i.m. injection per day for 8 days. In the first study, neuroleptics were discontinued one week before DTγE injections were started, while in the second study, neuroleptic maintenance was continued. The 6 patients in the first study all showed marked exacerbation of the psychotic symptoms after discontinuation of neuroleptics. From the fourth day of DTγE medication onwards, 3 of these patients showed a reduction in psychotic symptoms; these symptoms were entirely absent from the sixth day through the third week after discontinuation of DTγE. Two of the 3 patients showed a recurrence of psychotic symptoms after the third week (the follow-up on the third patient had to be discontinued when she was transferred to another hospital). The remaining 3 patients showed reduction of psychotic symptoms on days 3 and 4 of the medication, but from the fifth day onwards became psychotic again with severe agitation and aggressiveness. DTγE was then discontinued and neuroleptic medication reinstituted.

In the second study, progressive reduction of psychotic symptoms was observed from the first day of DTγE medication (Fig. 3). Four of the six patients became psychotic again 4–10 days after discontinuation of treatment, but their symptoms seemed less severe than those prior to DTγE medication. The remaining 2 patients remained free from psychotic symptoms. The same double-blind cross-over design was used for two acutely psychotic drug-free patients treated with DTγE immediately after admission. Both showed reduction of psychotic symptoms from the third day of medication and, from the sixth day on, both

245

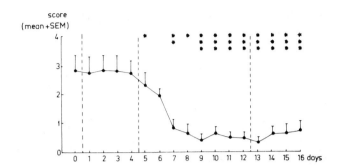

Fig. 3. Influence of (des-Tyr')-γ-endorphin on the score of 6 schizophrenic patients. Days 1–4 refer to days preceding (des-Tyr')-γ-endorphin treatment (days 5–12), followed by placebo treatment (days 13–16). Student's paired *t*-test was used to compare individual values on a given day to those obtained on day 4. * indicates $P < 0.05$; ** $P < 0.01$; *** $P < 0.005$. (From Verhoeven et al., 1979.)

remained free from psychotic symptoms for some considerable time (a few months). All patients treated with DTγE seemed to show improved emotional responsiveness. No extrapyramidal, cardiovascular or gastrointestinal side effects were observed.

Interpretation of clinical DTγE data. It is important to note that, like γ-endorphin, DTγE has recently been demonstrated in human CSF (Loeber et al., 1979). It therefore seems plausible that this compound is normally formed in the brain, probably from γ-endorphin itself which (like α-endorphin) is a fragment of β-endorphin (Fig. 4). It is conceivable that DTγE has antipsychotic properties because the patients involved are suffering from a DTγE deficiency (De Wied, 1978). Such a deficiency could in principle develop either by a deficient formation of DTγE from β-endorphin or by an accelerated conversion to α-endorphin. This hypothesis is now being investigated in our endorphin research. If evidence to support the deficiency theory were found, it would mean that a disturbed endorphin metabolism plays a role in the pathogenesis of (some types of) schizophrenic psychoses, and also that treatment with DTγE could be regarded as a form of substitution therapy.

A similar development, i.e. treatment of a psychiatric syndrome with endogenous substances in which the brain is probably deficient, has occurred in the field of depression (Van Praag, 1980). The use of the serotonin precursor 5-hydroxytryptophan in the treatment and prevention of certain types of vital depression can probably be so regarded. In 3 patients in our first (i.e. open) study, initial improvement was followed by marked psychotic exacerbation with intensive agitation and aggressiveness. In principle, there are two possible expla-

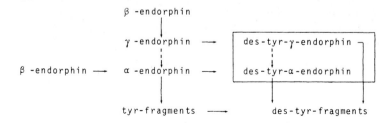

Fig. 4. Schematic representation of the fragmentation of β-endorphin. (De Wied, 1978.)

nations. To begin with, the exacarbation could have resulted from discontinuation of neuro-leptics. Secondly, it may have been due to the DTγE medication itself. In the context of the latter possibility the following hypothesis might be advanced: the exogenous (administered DTγE is unusually quickly converted to DTαE, and the latter is responsible for the exacer-bation. This seems a plausible hypothesis since De Wied (personal communication) has found that in rats, DTαE has amphetamine-like properties; and central stimulants are known for their ability to induce psychoses or exacerbate existing psychoses. That this complication did not develop in the second experiment could have been due to the fact that neuroleptic maintenance therapy was continued during the DTγE study in these patients. Testing of this hypothesis has to be postponed until reliable methods are evolved to determine DTγE and its metabolites in body fluids.

FK 33-824: a synthetic met-enkephalin. FK 33-824 is a met-enkephalin derivative syn-thesized by Sandoz, with the amino acid sequence: Tyr-D-Ala-Gly-Mephe-Met(O)-ol (met-enkephalin: Tyr-Gly-Gly-Phe-Meth). FK 33-824 thus differs from met-enkephalin in: (a) replacement of glycine by D-alanine; (b) N-methylation of phenylalanine; (c) alteration of methionine by oxidizing its sulphur to sulphoxide; and (d) conversion of the carboxyl to a carbinol group.

Jørgensen et al. (1979) used FK 33-824 in 9 patients with chronic psychoses: 8 of them chronic schizophrenics and the other patient with alcohol hallucinosis. The patients had been hospitalized for 7–15 years. Their medication was continued, but in addition they received, in a single-blind design, i.m. injections of 1, 2 and 3 mg of this peptide on 3 con-secutive days. An unmistakable therapeutic effect was observed in 6 patients. Four of them showed a striking decrease in hallucinations ("voices") and an increased sense of well-being: "they felt better than they had for years". In two patients there was no effect on the hal-lucinations but they became more open and spontaneous, speaking more freely than usual, and euphoric. The effect persisted for 4–7 days after the last injection.

A rebound effect was observed (as in the case of DTγE) in 3 patients. Initial improvement in these patients was followed by exacerbation of the psychotic symptoms, which in turn was followed by renewed improvement. The DTγE patients who showed exacerbation were given neuroleptics in order to control it, and consequently it was not established whether their rebound effect would have been transient. Unlike DTγE, FK 33-824 has retained its terminal tyrosine molecule and therefore possesses morphinomimetic properties. It is there-fore uncertain whether its therapeutic effect is based upon these properties or upon a "genuine", opiate receptor-independent antipsychotic action.

CONCLUSIONS

Until recently it was thought that pituitary hormones occurred only in the pituitary gland and had a peripheral endocrine function solely. It has been established, however, that several pituitary hormones and their fragments are also found outside the pituitary and also exert a direct influence on the CNS, as manifested by their effects on certain types of behavior. Neuropeptides derived from ACTH, vasopressin and oxytocin prove able to influ-ence motivation, learning and memory processes in animals. ACTH fragments have a short-term effect and probably play a role in attention and motivation, whereas vasopressin deriva-tives have a long-term effect, specifically on memory processes. This is expressed in improved consolidation and retrieval of information. Oxytocin has the opposite effect and could therefore be regarded as an amnestic peptide. Vasopressin derivatives also tend to reduce addictive behavior to heroin in rats. The clinical significance of these ACTH- and vasopressin-derived neuropeptides could therefore lie on the one hand in the treatment of cerebral disorders accompanied by disturbed memory function (which may in part be due to a diminished function of these hormonal systems), and on the other hand in the control of addiction to heroin and other morphine-like substances. Clinical research has so far been scanty, but preliminary results are sufficiently encouraging to suggest that conclusions based on animal experiments may also have some validity for human individuals.

Of the releasing and inhibiting factors, the same can be said as of the pituitary hormones. They were at first believed to occur exclusively in the hypothalamus and to have solely a regulating function with regard to hormone release by the anterior pituitary lobe. It has recently been found, however, that they also occur in the CNS outside the hypothalamus, and can exert a direct influence on the CNS, resulting in behavioural changes. It is to be noted that even modest therapeutic effects have been demonstrated only with TRH and PLG: TRH has a brief, slight central stimulant effect, while PLG slightly alleviates the symptoms in Parkinson's disease and depression. The clinical effects of the peptides of this group have so far been disappointing, perhaps because the proper indications have not yet been defined.

Since 1975, the identification of the endorphins, which can perhaps be justifiably regarded as neurotransmitters or neuromodulators, has given the field of psychoneuroendocrinology a new dimension. Animal experiments have shown that, in addition to a morphinomimetic effect, the endorphins exert an unmistakable influence on behavior which may or may not be mediated by opiate receptors. Therapeutic effects have so far been obtained with β-endorphin, DTγE (a split product of γ-endorphin) and FK 33-824 (a synthetic met-enkephalin derivative). However, the clinical data available are still far too limited to warrant any definite conclusion. So far, observations on DTγE have been the most interesting in scientific terms. This is an endogenous, natural peptide in the brain, with certain properties also found in the pharmacological action profile of "true" neuroleptics. It is therefore conceivable that DTγE, or a compound closely related to it, is an endogenous "antipsychotic" agent and that a DTγE deficiency based on disturbed endorphin metabolism contributes to the pathogenesis of (certain types of) schizophrenia. The heuristic value of this theory is quite substantial, for it generates a number of hypotheses that can be clinically tested, always provided that reliable methods can be developed for separating and measuring endorphins in the body fluids.

REFERENCES

Akil, H., Mayer, D.J. and Liebeskind, J.C. (1976) Antagonism of stimulation produced analgesia by naloxone, a narcotic antagonist. *Science,* 191: 961–962.

Akil, H., Richardson, D.E., Hughes, J. and Barchas, J.D. (1978a) Enkephalin-like material elevated in ventricular cerebrospinal fluid of pain patients after analgetic focal stimulation. *Science,* 201: 463–465.

Akil, H., Watson, S.J., Berger, Ph.A. and Barchas, J.D. (1978b). Endorphins, β-LPH, and ACTH: biochemical, pharmacological and anatomical studies. In *Advances in Biochemical Psychopharmacology, Vol. 18,* E. Costa and M. Trabucchi (Eds.), New York, pp. 125–137.

Benkert, O. (1975) Effects of hypothalamic releasing hormones in depression and sexual impotence. *Excerpta Medica International Congress Series,* 359: 663–671.

Bertolini, A., Gessa, G.L. and Ferrari, W. (1975) Penile erection and ejaculation: a central effect of ACTH-like peptides in mammals. In *Sexual Behavior: Pharmacology and Biochemistry,* M. Sandler and G.L. Gessa (Eds.), Raven Press, New York, 247–257.

248

Bisette, G., Nemerhoff, C.B., Loosen, P.T., Prange, A.J., Jr., Breese, G.R. and Lipton, M.A. (1976) Comparison of the potency of TRH, ACTH 4—10 and related peptides to reverse pentobarbital-induced narcosis and hypothermia. In *Hypothalamus and Endocrine Function*, F. Labrie, J. Meites and G. Pelletier (Eds.), Proceedings of the International Symposium on Hypothalamus and Endocrine Functions, Quebec City, Canada, September 1975, Plenum Press, New York, pp. 478—479.

Blake, D.R., Dodd, M.J. and Grimley Evans, J. (1978) Vasopressin in amnesia. *Lancet*, I: 608.

Bloom, F., Segal, D., Ling, N. and Guillemin, R. (1976) Endorphins: profound behavioral effects in rats suggest new etiological factors in mental illness. *Science*, 194: 630—632.

Branconnier, R.J., Cole, J.O. and Gardos, G. (1979) ACTH 4—10 in the amelioration of neuropsychological symptomatology associated with senile organic brain syndrome. *Psychopharmacology*, 61: 161—165.

Chase, T.N., Woods, A.C., Lipton, M.A. and Morris, C.E. (1974) Hypothalamic releasing factors and Parkinson disease. *Arch. Neurol.*, 31, 55—56.

Cotzias, G.C., Woert, M.H. van and Schiffer, L.M. (1967) Aromatic amino acids and modification of Parkinsonism. *New Engl. J. Med.*, 276: 374—379.

Davis, G.C., Bunney, W.E., Jr., DeFraites, E.G., Kleinman, J.E., Van Kammen, D.P., Post, R.M. and Wyatt, R.J. (1977) Intravenous naloxone administration in schizophrenia and affective illness. *Science*, 197: 74—76.

Doering, G.H., McAdoo, B.C., Kraemer, H.C., Brodie, H.K.H., Dessert, N.J. and Hamburg, D.A. (1977) Psychological effects of gonadotropin-releasing hormone in the adult male. In *Neuroregulators and Psychiatric Disorders*, E. Usdin, L.D.A. Hamburg and J.D. Barchas (Eds.), Oxford University Press, New York, pp. 267—275.

Domschke, W., Dickschas, A. and Mitznegg, P. (1979) CSF β-endorphin in schizophrenia. *Lancet*, I: 1029.

Donovan, D.T. (1978) The behavioural actions of hypothalamic peptides: a review. *Psychol. Med.*, 8: 305—316.

Dorbusch, R.L. and Nikolovski, O. (1976). ACTH 4—10 and short-term memory. In *The Neuropeptides — Pharmacology, Biochemistry and Behavior, Vol. 5*, C.A. Sandman, L.H. Miller and A.J. Kastin (Eds.), Phoenix, New York, Ankho, pp. 69—72.

Ehrensing, R.H. and Kastin, A.J. (1974) Melanocyte-stimulating hormone-release inhibiting hormone as an antidepressant. *Arch. gen. Psychiat.*, 30: 63—65.

Emrich, H.M., Cording, C. Piree, S., Kölling, A., Zerssen, D. von and Herz, A. (1977) Indication of an antipsychotic action of the opiate antagonist naloxone. *Pharmakopsychiatrie*, 10: 265—270.

Ferris, S.H., Sathananthan, G., Gershon, S., Clark, C. and Moshinsky, J. (1976) Cognitive effects of ACTH 4—10 in the elderly. In *The Neuropeptides — Pharmacology, Biochemistry and Behavior, Vol. 5*, C.A. Sandman, L.H. Miller and A.J. Kastin (Eds.), Phoenix, New York, Ankho, 73—78.

Fischer, P.A., Schneider, E., Jacobi, P. and Maxion, H. (1974) Effect of melanocyte-stimulating hormone-release inhibiting factor (MIF) in Parkinson's syndrome. *Europ. Neurol.*, 12: 360—368.

Gaillard, A.W.K. and Sanders, A.F. (1975) Some effects of ACTH 4—10 on performance during a serial reaction task. *Psychopharmacologia (Berl.)*, 42: 201—208.

Gitlin, M. and Rosenblatt, M. (1978) Possible withdrawal from endogenous opiates in schizophrenics. *Amer. J. Psychiat.*, 135: 377—378.

Gold, Ph.W., Goodwin, F.K. and Rens, V.I. (1978) Vasopressin in affective illness. *Lancet*, II: 1233—1235.

Green, A.R. and Grahame-Smith, D.G. (1974) TRH potentiates behavioral changes following increased brain 5-hydroxytryptamine accumulation in rats. *Nature (Lond.)*, 251: 524—526.

Guillemin, R., Vargo, T., Rossier, J., Minick, I., Ling, N., Rivier, C., Vale, W. and Bloom, F. (1977) β-Endorphin and adrenocorticotropin are secreted by the pituitary gland. *Science*, 197: 1367—1369.

Guillemin, R. (1978) Peptides in the brain: the new endocrinology of the neuron. *Science*, 202: 390—402.

Gunne, L.-M., Lindström, L. and Terenius, L. (1977) Naloxone-induced reversal of schizophrenic hallucinations. *J. neural. Transm.*, 40: 13—19.

Hertz, A., Bläsig, J., Emrich, H.M., Cording, C., Pirée, S., Kölling, A. and Zerssen, D. von (1978) Is there some indication from behavioral effects of endorphins for their involvement in psychiatric disorders? *Advances in Biochemical Psychopharmacology, Vol. 18*, E. Costa and M. Trabucchi (Eds.), Raven Press, New York, pp. 333—339.

Hoffman, P., Ritzmann, R.F., Walter, R. and Tabakoff, B. (1978) Arginine vasopressin maintains ethanol tolerance. *Nature (Lond.)*, 276: 614–616.

Horst, W.D. and Spirt, N. (1974) A possible mechanism for the anti-depressant activity of thyrotropin-releasing hormone. *Life Sci.*, 15: 1073–1082.

Hughes, J. (1975) Isolation of an endogenous compound from the brain with pharmacological properties similar to morphine. *Brain Res.*, 88: 295–308.

Hughes, J. (1979) Opioid peptides and their relatives. *Nature (Lond.)*, 278: 394–395.

Jacquet, Y.F. and Marks, N. (1976) The C-fragment of β-lipotropin: an endogenous neuroleptic or antipsychotogen. *Science*, 194: 632–635.

Janowsky, D.S., Segal, D.S., Bloom, F., Abrams, A. and Guillemin, R. (1977) Lack of effect of naloxone on schizophrenic symptoms. *Amer. J. Psychiat.*, 134: 926–927.

Janowsky, D.S., Judd, L.L., Huey, L., Roitman, N., Parker, D. and Segal, D. (1978) Naloxone effects on manic symptoms and growth-hormone levels. *Lancet*, II: 320.

Jørgensen, A., Fog, R. and Veilis, B. (1979) Synthetic enkephalin analogue in treatment of schizophrenia. *Lancet*, I: 935.

Judd, L.L., Janowsky, D.S., Segal, D.S., Leighton, Ph.D. and Huey, L. (1978) Naloxone related attenuation of manic symptoms in certain bipolar depressives. In *Characteristics and Function of Opioids, Vol. 4*, J.M. van Ree and L. Terenius (Eds.), Elsevier/North-Holland, Amsterdam, pp. 173–175.

Kastin, A.J., Ehrensing, R.H., Schalch, D.S. and Anderson, M.S. (1972) Improvement in mental depression with decreased thyrotropin response after administration of thyrotropin-releasing hormone. *Lancet*, II: 740–742.

Kastin, A.J., Sandman, C.A., Stratton, L.O., Goldman, H., Schally, A.V. and Miller, L.H. (1975) Influences of MSH on behavioral and electrographic correlates of attention, memory and anxiety in rat and man. In *Hormones, Homeostasis and the Brain, Progress in Brain Research, Vol. 42*, W.H. Gispen, Tj.B. van Wimersma Greidanus, B. Bohus and D. de Wied (Eds.), Elsevier, Amsterdam, 143–150.

Kastin, A.J., Cov, D.H., Jacquet, J., Schally, A.V. and Plotnikoff, N.P. (1978) CNS effect of somatostatin. *Metabolism*, 27 (Suppl. 1): 1247–1252.

Klaver, M.M., Flentge, F., Nienhuis-Kuiper, H.E. and Praag, H.M. van (1979) The origin of CSF choline and its relation to acetylcholine metabolism in brain. *Life Sci.*, 24: 231–236.

Kline, N.S., Li, C.H., Lehmann, H.E., Lajtha, A., Laski, E. and Cooper, T. (1977) β-Endorphin-induced changes in schizophrenic and depressed patients. *Arch. gen. Psychiat.*, 34: 1111–1113.

Krivoy, W.A., Zimmerman, E. and Lande, S. (1974) Facilitation of development of resistance to morphine analgesia by desglycinamide[9]-lysine vasopressin. *Proc. nat. Acad. Sci. (Wash.)*, 71: 1852–1856.

Kurland, A.A., McCabe, A.L., Haulon, Th. and Silivan, D. (1977) The treatment of perceptuate disturbances in schizophrenia with naloxone hydrochloride. *Am. J. Psychiat.*, 134: 1408–1410.

LeBoeuf, A., Lodge, J. and Eames, P.G. (1978) Vasopressin and memory in Korsakoff syndrome. *Lancet*, II: 1370.

Lakke, J.P.W.F., Praag, H.M. van, Twisk, R. van, Doorenbos, H. and Witt, F.G.J. (1974) Effects of administration of thyrotropin releasing hormone in Parkinsonism. *Clin. Neurol. Neurosurg.*, 3/4: 1–5.

Lal, S., Nair, N.P.V., Cervantes, P., Pulman, J. and Snyder, H. (1979) Effects of naloxone or levallorphan on serum prolactin concentrations and apomorphine induced growth hormone secretion. *Acta psychiat. scand.*, 59: 173–179.

Legros, J.J., Gilot, P., Seron, X., Claessens, J., Adam, A., Moeglen, J.W., Audibert, A. and Berchier, P. (1978) Influence of vasopressin on learning and memory. *Lancet*, I: 41.

Lewis, R.V., Gerber, L.D., Stein, S., Stephen, R.L., Grosser, B.I., Velick, S.F. and Udenfriend, S. (1979) On β[H]-Leu[5]-endorphin and schizophrenia. *Arch. gen. Psychiat.*, 36: 237–239.

Li, C.H. (1964) Lipotropin, a new active peptide from pituitary glands. *Nature (Lond.)*, 201: 924.

Li, C.H. and Chung, D. (1976) Isolation and structure of an untriakontapeptide with opiate activity from camel pituitary glands. *Proc. nat. Acad. Sci. (Wash.)*, 73: 1145–1148.

Lindström, L.H., Widerlöv, E., Gunne, L.-M., Wahlström, A. and Terenius, L. (1978) Endorphins in human cerebrospinal fluid: clinical correlations to some psychotic states. *Acta psychiat. scand.*, 57: 153–164.

Loeber, J., Verhoef, J., Burbach, J.P.H. and Ree, J.M. van (1979) Endorphins and related peptides in human cerebrospinal fluid. *Abstract Acta Endocrinologica Congress*, Munich.

Mayer, D.J., Wolfe, T.L., Akil, H., Cardner, B. and Liebeskind, J.C. (1971) Analgesia from electrical stimulation in the brain-stem of the rat. *Science*, 174: 1351–1354.

McAdoo, B.C., Doering, C.H., Kraemer, H.C., Dessert, N., Brodie, H.K.H. and Hamburg, D.A. (1978) A study of the effects of gonadotropin-releasing hormone on human mood and behavior. *Psychosomat. Med.*, 40: 199–209.

Mendelson, J.H., Ellingboe, J., Keuhule, J.C. and Mello, N.K. (1979) Effects of naltrexone on mood and neuroendocrine function in normal adult males. *Psychoneuroendocrinology*, 3: 231–236.

Mielke, D.H. and Gallant, D.M. (1977) An oral opiate antagonist in chronic schizophrenia: a pilot study. *Amer. J. Psychiat.*, 134: 1430–1431.

Miller, L.H., Fiswer, S.C., Groves, G.A., Rudrauff, M.E. and Kastin, A.J. (1977) MSH/ACTH$_{4-10}$. Influences on the CAR in human subjects: a negative finding. *Pharmacol. Biochem. Behav.*, 7: 417–419.

Miller, L.H., Kastin, A.J., Sandman, C.A., Fink, M. and Veen, W.J. van (1974) Polypeptide influences on attention, memory and anxiety in man. *Pharmacol. Biochem. Behav.*, 2: 663–668.

Moss, R.L., McCann, S.M. and Dudley, C.A. (1975) Releasing factors and sexual behavior. In *Hormones, Homeostasis and the Brain. Progress in Brain Research, Vol. 42*, W.H. Gispen, Tj.B. van Wimersma Greidanus, B. Bohus and D. de Wied (Eds.), Elsevier, Amsterdam, pp. 37–46.

Nakanishi, S., Inone, A., Kita, T., Nakamura, M., Chang, A.C.J., Cohen, S.N. and Numa, S. (1979) Nucleotide sequence of cloned cDNA for bovine corticotropin β-lipotropin precursor. *Nature (Lond.)*, 278: 423–427.

Nemeroff, Ch.B. and Prange, A.J. (1978) Peptides and psychoneuroendocrinology. *Arch. gen. Psychiat.*, 35: 999–1010.

Nemeroff, Ch.B., Loosen, P.T., Bisette, G., Manberg, P.J., Wilson, I.C., Lipton, M.A. and Prange, A.J. (1979) Pharmaco-behavioral effects of hypothalamic peptides in animals and man: focus on thyrotropin-releasing hormone and neurotensine. *Psychoneuroendocrinology*, 3: 279–310.

Oliveros, J.C., Jandali, M.K., Timsit-Berthier, M., Remy, R., Benghezal, A., Audibert, A. and Moeglen, J.M. (1978) Vasopressin in amnesia. *Lancet*, I, 42.

Palmour, R.M., Ervin, F.R. and Wagemaker, H. (1977) Characterization of a peptide derived from the serum of psychiatric patients. *Neurosci. Abstr.*, 7: 32.

Pert, C.B. and Snyder, S.H. (Johns Hopkins) (1973) Opiate receptor: demonstration in nervous tissue. *Science*, 179: 1011–1014.

Plotnikoff, N.P., Prange, A.J., Jr., Breese, G.R., Anderson, M.S. and Wilson, I.C. (1972) Thyrotropin releasing hormone: enhancement of DOPA activity by a hypothalamic hormone. *Science*, 178: 417–418.

Praag, H.M. van (1977) The significance of dopamine for the mode of action of neuroleptics and the pathogenesis of schizophrenia. *Brit. J. Psychiat.*, 130: 463–474.

Praag, H.M. van (1978) Amine hypotheses of affective disorders In: *Handbook of Psychopharmacology. Biology of Mood and Anti-Anxiety Drugs, Vol. 13*. L.L. Iversen, S.D. Iversen and S.H. Snyder (Eds.), Plenum Press, New York, Amsterdam.

Praag, H.M. van (1980) Central monoamine metabolism in depressions. I. Serotonin and related compounds. *Compr. Psyhiatr.*, 21: 30–43.

Prange, A.J., Wilson, I.C., Rabon, A.M. and Lipton, M.A. (1969) Enhancement of imipramine antidepressant activity by thyroid hormone. *Amer. J. Psychiat.*, 126: 457–469.

Prange, A.J., Wilson, I.C., Knox, A., McClane, T.K. and Lipton, M.A. (1970) Enhancement of imipramine by thyroid stimulating hormone: clinical and theoretical implications. *Amer. J. Psychiat.*, 127: 191–199.

Prange, A.J., Jr., Lara, P.P., Wilson, I.C., Alltop, L.B. and Breese, G.R. (1972) Effects of thyrotropin-releasing hormone in depression. *Lancet*, I: 999–1002.

Prange, A.J., Nemeroff, Ch.B., Lipton, M.A., Breese, J.R. and Wilson, I.C. (1978) Pentides and the central nervous system. In *Handbook of Psychopharmacology, Vol. 13*, pp. 1–107.

Rapoport, J.L., Quina, P.O., Copeland, A.P. and Burg, C. (1976) ACTH 4–10: cognitive and behavioral effects in hyperactive learning – disabled children. *Neuropsychobiology*, 2: 283–290.

Raskind, M.A., Weitzman, R.E., Orenstein, H., Fischer, D.A. and Courtney, N. (1978) Is antidiuretic hormone elevated in psychosis? *Biol. Psychiat.*, 13: 385–390.

Ree, J.M. van, Bohus, B., Versteeg, D.H.G. and Wied, D. de (1978a) Neurohypophyseal principles and memory processes. *Biochem. Pharmacol.*, 27: 1793–1800.

Ree, J.M. van, Dorsa, D.M. and Colpaert, F.C. (1978b) Neuropeptides and drug dependence. In *Characteristics and Function of Opioids, Vol. 4*, J.M. van Ree and L. Terenius, Elsevier/North-Holland, Amsterdam, pp. 1–13.

Riezen, H. van, Rigter, H. and Wied, D. de (1977) Possible significance of ACTH fragments for human mental performance. *Behav. Biol.*, 20: 311–324.

Sandman, C.A., George, J., McCann, T.R., Nolan, J.D., Kaswan, J. and Kastin, A.J. (1977) MSH/ACTH 4–10; influence on behavioral and physiological measures of attention. *J. clin. Endocr. Metab.*, 44: 884–891.

Sannita, W.G., Irwin, P. and Fink, M. (1976) EEG and task performance after ACTH 4–10 in man. *Neuropsychobiology*, 2: 283–290.

Schally, A.V. (1978) Aspects of hypothalamic regulation of the pituitary gland. *Science*, 202: 18–28.

Simon, E., Hiller, J.M. and Edelman, I. (1973) Stereospecific binding of the potent narcotic analgesic (^{3}H) etorphine to rat brain homogenate. *Proc. nat. Acad. Sci. (Wash.)*, 70: 1947–1949.

Small, J.G., Small, I.F., Milstein, V. and Dian, D.A. (1977) Effects of ACTH 4–10 on ECT-induced memory dysfunctions. *Acta psychiat. scand.*, 55: 241–250.

Snyder, S.H. (1978) The opiate receptor and morphine-like peptides in the brain. *Amer. J. Psychiat.*, 135: 645–652.

Snyder, S.H. and Childers, S.R. (1979) Opiate receptors and opioids peptides. *Ann. Rev. Neurosci.*, 2: 35–64.

Terenius, L. (1975) Characteristics of the "receptor" for narcotic analgesics in synaptic plasma membrane fraction from rat brain. *Acta pharmacol. toxicol.*, 33: 377–384.

Terenius, L. and Wahlström, A. (1975a) Search for an endogenous ligand for the opiate receptor. *Acta physiol. scand.*, 94: 74–81.

Terenius, L. and Wahlström, A. (1975b) Morphine-like ligand for opiate receptors in human CSF. *Life Sci.*, 16: 1759–1764.

Terenius, L., Wahlström, A., Lindström, L. and Widerlöv, E. (1976) Increased CSF levels of endorphins in chronic psychosis. *Neurosci. Lett.*, 3: 157–162.

Terenius, L., Wahlström, A. and Agren, H. (1977) Naloxone (Narcan®) treatment in depression: clinical observations and effects on CSF endorphins and monoamine metabolites. *Psychopharmacologia (Berl.)*, 54: 31–33.

Verhoeven, W.M.A., Praag, H.M. van, Botter, P.A., Sunier, A., Ree, J.M. van and Wied, D. de (1978) (des-tyr[1])-γ-endorphin in schizophrenia. *Lancet*, I: 1046–1047.

Verhoeven, W.M.A., Praag, H.M. van, Ree, J.M. van and Wied, D. de (1979a) Improvement of schizophrenic patients by treatment with (des-tyr[1])-γ-endorphin (DTγE). *Arch. gen. Psychiat.*, 36: 294–298.

Verhoeven, W.M.A., Jong, J.T.V.M. de and Praag, H.M. van (1979b) The effects of naloxone on psychotic symptoms. In *Proceedings of the 20th Dutch Federation Meeting*, p. 435.

Versteeg, D.H.G., Kloet, E.R. de and Wied, D. de (1979) Effects of α-endorphine, β-endorphin and (des-tyr[1])-γ-endorphin on α-MPT-induced catecholamine disappearance in discrete regions of the rat brain. *Brain Res.*, 179: 85–92.

Volavka, J., Mallya, A., Baig, S. and Perez-Cruet, J. (1977) Naloxone in chronic schizophrenia. *Science*, 196: 1227–1228.

Wagemaker, H. and Cade, R. (1977) The use of hemodialysis in chronic schizophrenia. *Amer. J. Psychiat.*, 134: 684–685.

Watson, S.J., Berger, Ph.A., Akil, H., Mills, M.J. and Barchas, J.D. (1978) Effects of naloxone on schizophrenia: reduction in hallucinations in a subpopulation of subjects. *Science*, 201: 73–76.

Watson, S., Akil, H., Berger, Ph.A. and Barchas, J.D. (1979) Some observations on the opiate peptides and schizophrenia. *Arch. gen. Psychiat.*, 36: 35–41.

Wied, D. de (1977a) Behavioral effects of neuropeptides related to ACTH, MSH, and β-LPH. *Ann. N.Y. Acad. Sci.*, 297: 263–274.

Wied, D. de (1977b) Peptides and behavior. *Life Sci.*, 20: 195–204.

Wied, D. de (1978) Psychopathology as a neuropeptide dysfunction. In *Characteristics and Function of Opioids, Vol. 4*, J.M. van Ree and L. Terenius (Eds.), Elsevier/North-Holland, Amsterdam, pp. 113–123.

Wied, D. de, Witter, A. and Greven, H.M. (1975a) Behaviourally active ACTH analogues. *Biochem. Pharmacol.*, 24: 1463–1468.

Wied, D. de, Bohus, B. and Wimersma Greidanus, Tj.D. van (1975b) Memory deficit in rats with hereditary diabetes insipidus. *Brain Res.*, 85: 152–156.

Wied, D. de, Wimersma Greidanus, Tj.B. van, Bohus, B., Urban, I. and Gispen, W.H. (1976a) Vasopressin and memory consolidation. In *Perspectives in Brain Research. Progress in Brain Research, Vol. 4,*

252

M.A. Corner and D.F. Swaab (Eds.), Elsevier/North-Holland Biomedical Press: Amsterdam, pp. 181–194.

Wied, D. de, Kovacs, G., Bohus, B., Ree, J.M. van and Greven, H.M. (1978) Neuroleptic activity of the neuropeptide β-LPH 62-77 ([des-tyr[1]]γ-endorphin; DTγE). *Europ. J. Pharmacol.*, 49: 427–436.

Will, J.C., Abuzzahab, F.S. and Zimmermann, R.L. (1978) The effects of ACTH 4–10 versus placebo in the memory of symptomatic geriatric volunteers. *Psychopharmacol. Bull.*, 14: 25–26.

Wimersma Greidanus, Tj.B. van (1977) Effects of MSH and related peptides on avoidance behavior in rats. *Frontiers Horm. Res.*, 4: 129–139.

Wimersma Greidanus, Tj.B. van and Wied, D. de (1976) Modulation of passive-avoidance behavior of rats by intracerebroventricular administration of antivasopressin serum. *Behav. Biol.*, 18: 325–333.

SECTION III

Sleep and Dreams: their Origin and Significance

(edited by H.J. Romijn)

Sleep as an Adaptation for Energy Conservation Functionally Related to Hibernation and Shallow Torpor

JAMES M. WALKER and RALPH J. BERGER

Thimann Laboratories, University of California, Santa Cruz, Santa Cruz, Calif. 95064 (U.S.A.)

INTRODUCTION

A vast amount of research on sleep has been generated during the past two decades and much has been learned about its phenomenology and underlying physiological and biochemical mechanisms. Yet the biological function of sleep remains enigmatic.

A recent approach that might shed light on this question is to study sleep in relationship to behaviorally similar states, states whose biological function is obvious. Hibernation and shallow torpor are two such states. Although the mechanism underlying hibernation and torpor are not completely understood, there can be little doubt that their biological function is that of energy conservation. We propose that sleep constitutes another, albeit less well recognized, variation on the theme of mammalian dormancy that is functionally related to hibernation and torpor.

We shall review here the behavioral and physiological characteristics of sleep, shallow torpor, and hibernation in mammals and birds and propose that they are functionally homologous processes. In addition, we shall describe phylogenetic and ontogenetic correlations between sleep and endothermy, and sleep-dependent thermoregulatory adjustments associated with decreased metabolism consistent with an energy conserving role for sleep. Electrophysiological studies demonstrate physiological continuities between sleep, shallow torpor and hibernation, such that thermoregulatory changes initiated during sleep are extended during shallow torpor and hibernation. Finally, data demonstrating circannual rhythms of sleep with maximum amounts coinciding with winter hibernation in alpine ground squirrels will be presented. These findings lead us to speculate that the other states of dormancy mentioned above evolved through a gradual extension of thermoregulatory adjustments initiated in all mammals during sleep.

DORMANCY IN MAMMALS AND BIRDS

Sleep

It is now well-established that sleep as a form of dormancy is characterized by thermoregulatory adjustments resulting in a slight decline ($2°C$) of body temperature (T_b) (Heller and Glotzbach, 1977).

The behavioral characteristics of sleep are fairly obvious and have changed little from those originally proposed by Pieron (1913). He described sleep as comprising behavioral quiescence and an increased threshold of arousal to sensory stimulation. Sleep could be differentiated from other inactive states such as coma or hibernation on the basis of the ability to become aroused rapidly in response to sufficiently strong sensory stimulation. A criterion customarily added to Pieron's description of sleep is the requirement of a stereotypic, species-specific posture during sleep.

The discovery of the electroencephalogram (EEG) by Berger (1929) and its subsequent measurement during sleep (Davis et al., 1937, 1938; Loomis et al., 1937) added a new dimension to the categorization of sleep and wakefulness. Because of their utility, electrophysiological criteria of sleep gained importance and became dominant in the definition of sleep. Although correlations between physiological and behavioral measures of sleep may be weak or non-existent in ectotherms (Walker and Berger, 1973) both measures are highly concordant in endotherms.

Sleep is ubiquitous in mammals and birds and consists of two distinct phases of physiological activity whose characterization stems from the discovery of Aserinsky and Kleitman (1953) of recurrent phases of rapid-eye-movement (REM) sleep (for a review see Berger, 1969) alternating with phases of non-rapid-eye-movement (NREM) sleep (Dement and Kleitman, 1957). NREM sleep, which comprises from 70–95% of sleep time, is also called slow wave sleep (SWS) because of its predominant slow wave EEG activity, and this term will be used throughout this paper.

Shallow torpor

Shallow torpor is a form of dormancy present in some birds and many small mammals which is characterized by a decrease of about $5-20°C$ in T_b, an immobile stereotyped posture and decreased responsiveness. Reversibility to wakefulness occurs in response to strong environmental stimuli, but is diminished in comparison to sleep because of the decreased T_b. Shallow torpor usually occurs with a circadian rhythm (also called daily torpor) during the normal major sleep period but may be extended to encompass multiday periods. Shallow torpor which occurs seasonally in the hotter, drier portions of the year has also been termed estivation.

Hibernation (or deep torpor)

Hibernation is a less frequent phenomenon than shallow torpor and occurs in only a few small species within one-third of the mammalian orders. It is defined by profound decreases in T_b, amounting to $15-35°C$, occurs seasonally and is manifested in multiday bouts separated by periodic arousals. Similar to sleep and shallow torpor, hibernation is characterized by immobility, decreased responsiveness, and a stereotypic posture. However, because of the low T_b, there is a greatly diminished capacity for arousal to strong stimulation, the length of time for an animal to arouse being inversely correlated with body weight.

SLEEP AS AN ADAPTATION FOR ENERGY CONSERVATION

Mammals and birds are endothermic. They generate heat through high rates of metabolism (8–10 times greater than reptiles of similar size and at the same T_b) and maintain relatively constant T_bs ranging from $36-40°C$ (euthermia). Hibernation and shallow torpor represent physiological adaptations to this costly energetic process, whereby endotherms cope with limited energy supplies through periodic reductions of T_b and metabolism. The magnitude of the decrease in T_b and temporal patterns of dormancy are acutely tuned to the specific energy balance (either immediate or projected) of each particular species displaying this adaptation. Thus, pocket mice and hummingbirds exhibit daily torpor in instances of acute food shortages or low ambient temperatures (T_a) whereas some squirrels and marmots hibernate in preparation for a recurrent energy shortage occurring during a seasonally harsh portion of the year. Species survival depends not only upon effective reproduction and parental care but also upon the effective utilization of energy resources. Endotherms are generally specialized to forage during either the light or the dark portion of the day and are inactive during the other portion. During periods of inactivity, when the search for and ingestion of food is not possible, any reduction in basal metabolism is energetically adaptive, given the finite amount of energy available at each trophic level in an ecosystem (Berger, 1975; Berger et al., 1973).

Derived in part from earlier suggestions by Snyder (1966) and Allison and Van Twyver (1970), the hypothesis of this paper is that SWS constitutes a state of reduced metabolism during periods of obligate inactivity, that evolved to partially offset the increased energy requirements of endothermy, while retaining a sufficiently high T_b for critical reactivity. SWS is considered as a variation on the theme of dormancy, functionally lying on a continuum of arousal and energy conservation processes. This continuum extends from waking behavioral inactivity, with immediate capabilities for rapid arousal, through sleep to shallow torpor and hibernation with their greatly diminished capabilities for arousal.

SWS is unique to endotherms

If the foregoing hypothesis is valid, then slow wave sleep (SWS) should be confined to endotherms, which are subject to severe energy constraints by virtue of their high metabolism.

All mammals in which electrophysiological characteristics of sleep have been extensively recorded have exhibited unequivocal SWS (Snyder, 1969). Birds studied thus far, including the pigeon (Tradardi, 1966; Van Twyver and Allison, 1972; Walker and Berger, 1972), owl (Berger and Walker, 1972), hawk and falcon (Rojas-Ramirez and Tauber, 1970), and chicken (Ookawa, 1972; Ookawa and Gotoh, 1965) have also exhibited unmistakable SWS similar to that observed in mammals. By contrast, amphibians studied to data, viz. the bull frog (Hobson, 1967), toad (Segura, 1966), and salamander (Lucas et al., 1969), did not exhibit any signs of SWS.

The status of sleep in reptiles to this data remains unclear and continues to be a controversial issue. Tauber et al. (1968) attributed sleep to the lizard on the basis of a reduction in EEG amplitude associated with decreased behavioral activity. Other investigators ascribed SWS (Herman et al., 1964), or both SWS and REM sleep to the tortoise (Vasilescu, 1970). Pyrethon and Dusan-Pyrethon (1968) studied single representatives from 3 reptilian orders (python, caiman and turtle), and imputed the presence of SWS in each of them, and also claimed to have observed REM sleep in the python. Finally, Karmanova and Churnosov (1972) reported diminished rather than increased slow wave activity during sleep in the swamp turtle.

In none of the foregoing studies were arousal thresholds measured, decreased responsiveness being a cardinal characteristic of sleep as defined earlier. However, Meglasson and Huggins (1979) very recently claimed that SWS was present in caimans, associated with

258

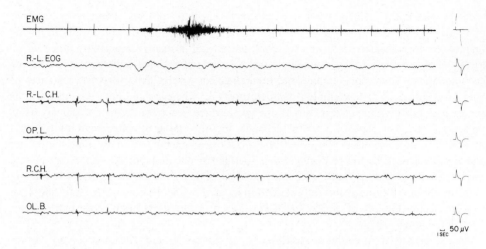

Fig. 1. Brief EMG arousal in the tortoise associated with cessation of spiking activity. Note that spiking returns as the EMG diminishes following the arousal. R, right; L, left; C.H., cerebral hemisphere; OP.L., optic lobe; OL.B., olfactory bulb. (From Walker and Berger, 1973, reproduced with permission.)

elevated arousal thresholds. The "high voltage slow EEG" which these authors considered to be SWS, consisted of 1 min sample periods during which as little as 15% of the record was occupied by delta waves greater than 50 μV. This is hardly comparable to avian or mammalian SWS, in which the record is typically dominated by 200–300 μV delta waves

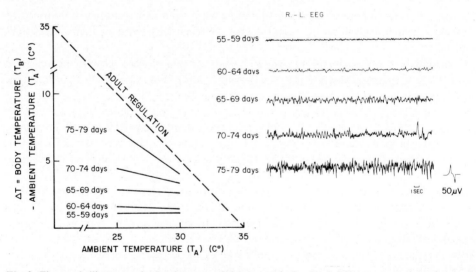

Fig. 2. The graph illustrates the development of thermoregulation for 5 different age groups of opossums. Body temperature (T_b) was measured at an ambient temperature of 25 and 30°C for each day of age. At a particular age, body insulation remains constant at both ambient temperatures and therefore, differences in body temperature above that of the ambient temperature ($\Delta T = T_b - T_a$) are directly related to thermoregulatory processes (Morrison and Petajan, 1962). For an animal to minimally thermoregulate it would be expected that ΔT would increase as ambient temperature is lowered. Note the correspondence between the development of thermoregulatory capabilities and the appearance of slow wave EEG activity. (From Walker 1978, reproduced with permission.)

(Walker and Berger, 1972). Moreover, their measurements of arousal thresholds were flawed by the adoption of respiratory activity and EEG desynchronization in response to electrical shock as the criteria for arousal, rather than in increased EMG activity or overt behavior. Finally, according to their Table I, activated EEG patterns (PTD, Level I) were more likely to be accompanied by a "sleep-like" posture than by postures of behavioral alertness. Therefore, we believe their claim that SWS originally evolved in reptiles is not justified by their data.

We observed two distinct electrophysiological states in the tortoise, *Testudo denticulata* (Walker and Berger, 1973): (1) a high tonic and/or phasic EMG associated with low voltage fast (LVF) frequency EEG activity (predominantly 6–10 cps, <40 μV) and a heart rate of 20–30 beats/min; and (2) a reduced tonic EMG, an EEG consisting of high voltage (60–150 μV) spiking superimposed upon LVF (predominantly 6–10 cps, <40 μV) activity and a decreased heart rate of 10–20 beats/min (Fig. 1). Spikes were evident over the olfactory bulb, cerebral hemispheres, and optic lobes and were manifested either singly or in irregular multiphasic bursts. Spikes were present during inactive periods but disappeared with increased muscle activity and/or movement (Fig. 1). Studies of arousal thresholds revealed no differences between the spiking and non-spiking electrophysiological states. Therefore, spiking activity in itself did not constitute a reliable index of sleep.

Similar spiking and non-spiking EEG activity has also been reported in the chameleon, iguana, turtle, crocodile and alligator (Flanigan, 1973; Flanigan et al., 1973, 1974, Meglasson and Huggins, 1979; Tauber et al., 1966; Van Twyver, 1973). On the basis of electrophysiological evidence, neither SWS nor REM sleep are, as such, recognizable in reptiles.

However, Flanigan and co-workers have argued for the presence of *behavioral* sleep in reptiles. Stereotyped resting postures constituted 85–95% of a 24 h period in their studies and appear to meet one of the behavioral criteria for sleep formulated by Pieron (1913), but in ectotherms such postures might simply reflect behavioral thermoregulation such as basking (Walker and Berger, 1973). Flanigan (1974) considered spiking activity associated with "behavioral sleep" as an analog of mammalian SWS, and presented evidence of responses in spiking activity similar to that of SWS during pharmacological intervention and "sleep deprivation" in mammals. However, such an interpretation would appear to be inconsistent with his records which exhibited spiking accompanying behavioral postures classified as wakefulness. Meglasson and Huggins (1979) did not observe any correlations between spiking patterns and behavioral postures in caimans. Thus, spiking activity in the reptilian EEG can be present during both wakefulness and behavioral sleep, merely differing in frequency between the various behavioral postures, whereas high amplitude slow wave EEG activity is normally confined to sleep in mammals. Studies other than our own also failed to find evidence of either electrophysiological or behavioral sleep in the sea turtle and alligator (Susic, 1972; Van Twyver, 1973).

Thus, although the status of sleep in reptiles remains controversial, we do not find the evidence sufficient to support the claim that an analog of mammalian SWS is present in reptiles.

Not all newborn mammals and birds are capable of thermoregulation through endothermy but rely upon maternal heat. Significant for the present hypothesis is the fact that those endotherms which lack complete thermoregulation at birth also lack SWS and independent studies of the ontogenesis of thermoregulation and of SWS indicated their simultaneous development. Therefore, we investigated the development of SWS and thermoregulation in an American marsupial, the opossum, *Didelphis virginiana* (Walker and Berger, 1980). The first signs of thermoregulation developed simultaneously with 1–3 cps high

260

voltage EEG slow waves at approximately 65 days of age (Fig. 2). As slow wave EEG activity increased gains were also made in thermoregulatory ability. Near-normal thermoregulatory capabilities were evident at 79 days together with the electrophysiological characteristics of SWS typical of adult opossums.

The increasing energetic cost of homeothermy in the developing opossum is illustrated by the fact that oxygen consumption increases approximately 1300% at low T_as between the ages of 75 and 85 days (Reynolds, 1952). However, during this same period body weight increases only 80%. Thus SWS develops at that point when it would appear most profitable to conserve energy.

The foregoing data on the phylogenesis and ontogenesis of SWS and thermoregulation are consistent with the hypothesis that SWS is uniquely associated with endothermy.

Sleep and metabolic rate

If SWS evolved to offset increased metabolic costs of endothermy, mammals with high metabolic rates might be expected to sleep more than those with low metabolic rates. Zepelin and Rechtschaffen (1974), in an extensive survey of the literature on sleep and metabolism in 53 mammals, found strong positive correlations between basal metabolic rate (BMR) and daily sleep amount. High correlations were also present between BMR and each of the component parts of sleep, SWS (Fig. 3) and REM sleep. Zepelin and Rechtschaffen attributed the correlation between BMR and REM sleep to the dependence of REM sleep on the prior occurrence of SWS and inferred that metabolic rate is a determinant of sleep time and "that sleep may fulfill an important function in the regulation of energy expenditures". In a further analysis, Allison and Cicchetti (1976) also included two ecological factors and

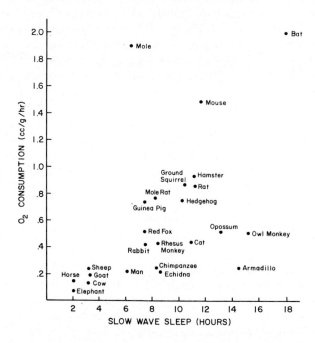

Fig. 3. Oxygen consumption values (either derived or estimated) and the amount of slow wave sleep in a 24 h period across 24 animals. (Based on data compiled by Zepelin and Rechtschaffen, 1974.)

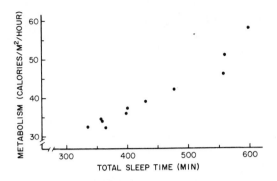

Fig. 4. Measurements of metabolism and total sleep time in males ranging from 3–79 years of age. The age groups consisted of 3–5, 6–9, 10–12, 13–15, 16–19, 20–29, 30–39, 40–49, 50–59, 60–69 and 70–79 years. To derive correlation coefficients between sleep measures, metabolic rate and age (see text) the mean values for each age group were used. Sleep times for each age group were obtained from Williams et al. (1974) and metabolic values for each age group were derived from Robertson and Reid (1952).

found high correlations between SWS and body weight; the latter is known to be strongly correlated with metabolic rate (Brody, 1945).

Close correlations between metabolic rates and amounts of sleep are also apparent within single species as exemplified in humans. Fig. 4 illustrates the remarkably high correlations between metabolic rate and total sleep time (TST) in groups of males ranging from 3 to 79 years of age ($r = +0.98$). There were also high correlations between the mean age of each group and metabolic rate (-0.83) as well as total sleep time (-0.83). Since age is correlated with both metabolic rate and sleep time, a partial correlation was performed to hold the effects of age constant. Even with age partialled out, a high correlation between sleep time and metabolic rate remained ($r = +0.92$). Metabolic rate also correlated strongly with the amount of NREM ($r = +0.95$) and REM sleep ($+0.96$). Again, these high correlations remained once the effects of age were partialled out (NREM, $r = +0.85$; REM, $r = +0.89$).

The strength of the relation between metabolic rate and sleep states is remarkable and could be taken to indicate that individuals with high metabolic rates sleep more than those with low rates, to partially offset the caloric cost.

Changes in the thermoregulatory system during sleep associated with lowered metabolism

During sleep, muscular activity and heart rate are reduced (Kleitman, 1963) and in humans metabolic rate decreased from 8–30% below resting waking levels (Brebbia and Altschuler, 1965; Jana, 1965; Magnussen, 1944; Milan and Evonuk, 1967; Robin et al., 1958). Haskell (1978) showed that in humans sleeping at a T_a of 21°C, oxygen consumption decreased as much as 40% below periods of intermittent wakefulness. Elsewhere (Heller et al., 1978), we have estimated that by sleeping and lowering its T_b by 2°C, a 100 g animal exposed to a T_a of 0°C without food can survive 5 days, a day longer than it would if it were in a state of relaxed wakefulness. By entering shallow torpor and lowering its T_b 10°C it can gain an additional 2 days and by hibernating and regulating its T_b at 7°C it can survive a 65-day fast. Although these calculations are gross approximations, they do point out the adaptive value of lowering metabolism and T_b during periods of food shortage, especially for small mammals which can only survive short fasts.

It has been argued that decreased metabolism during sleep results from muscular relaxation associated with sleep but is not a fundamental process of sleep itself (Kleitman, 1963; Moruzzi, 1966). However, this view is no longer tenable since recent evidence points to sleep-dependent adjustments in the thermoregulatory system that reduce metabolic rate (Heller and Glotzbach, 1977).

A fall in body and/or brain temperature in both humans and animals usually accompanies the onset of sleep (Abrams and Hammel, 1964; Adams, 1963; Day, 1941; Euler and Söderberg, 1958; Hammel et al., 1963; Kirk, 1931; Kreider and Iampietro, 1959; Kreider et al., 1958), regardless of the point in the circadian rhythm at which it occurs (Mills et al., 1978). Vasodilation with the onset of sleep resulting in increased heat loss, has been invoked as the cause of the fall in brain temperature (Baker and Hayward, 1967; Hayward and Baker, 1969). Vasomotor changes influence the rate of heat loss from the body and consequently T_b. More direct evidence of CNS thermoregulatory adjustments associated with sleep onset is the increase in sweating and frequency of panting in a neutral or warm environment (Euler and Söderberg, 1958; Geschickter et al., 1966; Ogawa et al., 1967; Parmeggiani and Sabattini, 1972; Satoh et al., 1965). When exposed to cold, decreased shivering with sleep onset was described in a primitive mammalian hibernator, the echidna (Allison et al., 1972), whereas increased shivering was observed during transition from wakefulness to sleep in the domestic cat (Parmeggiani and Sabattini, 1972). Neither skin nor body temperatures were recorded in the cat, a non-hibernator. On being exposed to extreme cold of $0-10°C$ an abrupt fall in skin temperature caused by vasodilation associated with sleep onset might stimulate thermal receptors that enhance shivering processes.

Studies of the relationship between hypothalamic temperature and thermoregulatory metabolic responses strongly support the conclusion that body temperature is regulated at a lower level during SWS than during wakefulness in both kangaroo rats and marmots (Glotzbach and Heller, 1976; Florant et al., 1978). Similar relations were observed during entrance into hibernation.

The foregoing findings of sleep-dependent regulated decreases in T_b and metabolism provide direct support for the hypothesis that SWS serves an energy-conserving function.

ELECTROPHYSIOLOGICAL AND THERMOREGULATORY SIMILARITIES BETWEEN SLEEP, SHALLOW TORPOR AND HIBERNATION

Sleep and hibernation are temporally and physiologically continuous in alpine ground squirrels

Several investigators have suggested that hibernation is entered from a state of sleep or may be an extension of sleep (e.g. Satinoff, 1970; South et al., 1969; Suomalainen, 1961; Twente and Twente, 1965). Electroencephalographic (EEG) sleep spindles prevalent in primates, felines, and, to a lesser extent, rodents, occurred during entrance into hibernation in the European hedgehog (Shtark, 1961), and in ground squirrels (Satinoff, 1970; Strumwasser, 1959) and sleep patterns typical of those in euthermia were described during hibernation entrance in marmots (South et al., 1969). Satinoff (1970), however, cited preliminary evidence that ground squirrels entered hibernation from a wakeful or drowsy state resembling the onset of SWS, but nevertheless suggested that hibernation might be the "deepest stage" of sleep. It should be remembered that entrance into hibernation is defined by a fall in T_b and the question of when hibernation begins may hinge on methods of definition. Since T_b can fall by as much as $2°C$ during euthermic sleep, if it then falls to still lower levels, the onset of hibernation could be construed as beginning at the onset of sleep itself (i.e. from wakefulness) at the initial point of T_b decline. Alternatively it could be considered as beginning at the point at which T_b declines below levels that normally occur during euthermic sleep.

We have recently completed extensive studies of the relationship between sleep and hibernation in alpine ground squirrels (*Citellus lateralis* and *beldingi*). Continuous records of brain temperature (T_{br}) and electrographic variables were obtained during euthermic periods both in the summer and winter and throughout entire episodes of hibernation in the winter (Walker et al., 1977). During the summer the animals were maintained on a 12 : 12 h light—dark photoperiod at a T_a of 23°C; in the winter they were exposed to continuous darkness at 6°C. Hibernation was entered through sleep states but the distribution of sleep states differed from that of both summer and winter euthermic sleep. Just prior to the bout of hibernation the animals slept an average of 53% during the total recording time of 5 h of which 22% was REM sleep (Fig. 5). During the initial decrease in brain temperature (T_{br}) from 35 to 25°C, total sleep time increased to 88% but REM sleep decreased to 10% of sleep time. REM sleep progressively decreased as T_{br} declined and only 2 instances of REM sleep were observed below a T_{br} of 27°C. The initial decrement in T_{br} occurred during sleep and never during wakefulness. Although subsequent brief periods of wakefulness (<2 min) did occur without disrupting the decline in T_{br}, any sustained periods of wakefulness were associated either with a decreased rate of decline or with an increase in T_{br}.

The EEG amplitude declined with decreased T_{br} so that classical sleep stages could not be identified below a T_{br} of approximately 25°C (Fig. 6), but even at T_{br}s as low as 10°C, the majority of the record was composed of 0–4 cps activity more characteristic of SWS than either REM sleep or wakefulness. Below T_{br}s of 10°C the EEG was isoelectric except for intermittent bursts of spindles. The exit from hibernation was characterized by massive EMG activity and an EEG resembling that of euthermic wakefulness. When T_{br} returned to approximately 33°C, EMG activity was reduced and the EEG was largely that of SWS with intermittent wakefulness.

The results of this study and that of South et al. (1969), show that the entrance into

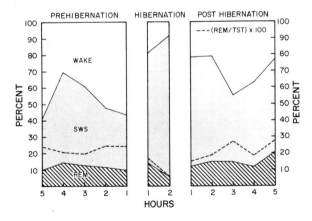

Fig. 5. Mean hourly percentages of wakefulness, SWS and REM sleep for 5 alpine squirrels (*C. lateralis* and *beldingi*) for recording periods prior to, during, and immediately following hibernation. Per cent sleep time occupied by REM sleep is represented by a dashed line (------). (From Walker et al., 1977, reproduced with permission.)

264

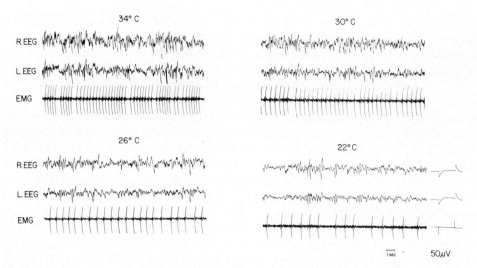

Fig. 6. Examples of slow wave EEG activity and heart rate from one alpine squirrel during one entry into hibernation at brain temperatures of 34, 30, 26 and 22°C. (From Walker et al., 1977, reproduced with permission.)

hibernation is characterized by sleep. There are also indicants that the deeper portions of hibernation are also sleep related because of the persistence of low voltage slow wave EEG activity at T_{br}s as low as 10°C and sleep-like spindle activity at even lower T_{br}s.

Pengelley and Fisher (1963) described an endogenous circannual cycle of hibernation in ground squirrels (*Citellus lateralis*) maintained under constant temperature of 22°C. Thus, low T_as are not necessary to induce hibernation. Because the EEGs of hibernating animals with T_{br}s of 6°C cannot be directly compared with those of euthermic animals, electrophysiological recordings of naturally occurring shallow hibernation at T_as of 22°C were obtained from ground squirrels (*Citellus lateralis*) during the winter so that they could be scored by conventional criteria for entire episodes of torpor (Walker, 1978).

The same measurements as in the previous study were recorded for 10–20 days from 4 golden-mantled ground squirrels (*Citellus lateralis*). Fourteen instances of 9–61 h ($\bar{X}$ = 24 h) periods of hibernation were observed where T_{br} dropped below euthermic levels at a rate of approximately 1°C/h but remained near or above the T_a of 22°C. In shallow hibernation T_{br}s ranged from 23 to 29°C, and the length of hibernation bouts was inversely related to T_{br}, averaging 46 h at a T_{br} of 23°C but only 11 h at a T_{br} of 29°C. This relationship held across the 4 animals, and also within 1 animal in which 6 separate bouts of hibernation were recorded, confirming similar findings of Twente and Twente (1965). These authors had shown that the length of dormancy, regardless of whether it was deep hibernation, shallow hibernation or sleep, was inversely proportional to the T_b of the animal. This similarity again suggests a functional relationship between sleep and torpor.

Entrances occurred most often in the late afternoon or early evening but could also occur at other times of the 24 h period. Although EEG amplitude, heart rate, and tonic EMG decreased together with T_{br} during entrance into shallow hibernation, classification of SWS, REM sleep and wakefulness was possible throughout entire bouts of hibernation according to conventional electrographic criteria (Fig. 7).

Sleep/wakefulness patterns were consistent across animals during shallow hibernation regardless of the time at which hibernation occurred and were similar to those previously

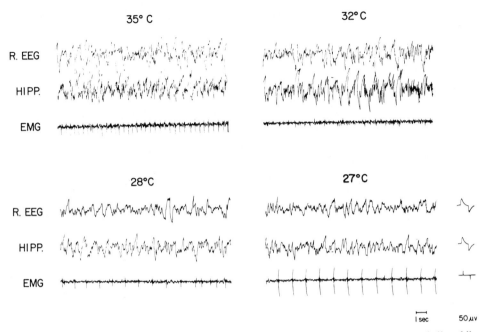

Fig. 7. Examples of SWS from a golden-mantled ground squirrel during the entrance into shallow hibernation. The electrophysiological characteristics of SWS at a T_{br} of 27°C are representative of that occurring during the majority of the bout of shallow hibernation. (From Walker, 1978, reproduced with permission.)

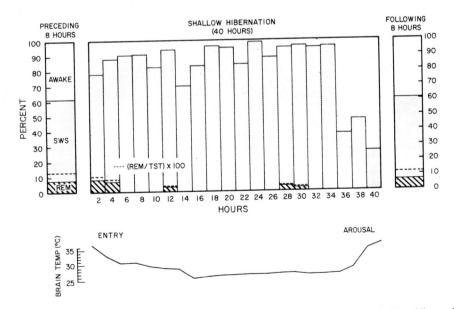

Fig. 8. Sleep and wakefulness percentages for 8 h prior to and following shallow hibernation plus bi-hourly sleep and wakefulness percentages and T_{br} measurements for a golden-mantled ground squirrel undergoing an entire bout of shallow hibernation. Note the similarity in the sleep and wakefulness percentages prior to and following shallow hibernation. (From Walker, 1978, reproduced with permission.)

described during entrance into deep hibernation. Per cent sleep time increased from 63% prior to entrance to 88% during entrance (Fig. 8). Episodes of wakefulness during the entrance were associated either with slowing of the descent in T_{br} or with a leveling off or increase in T_{br} if sustained for more than 2 min (Fig. 9). Both total sleep time (TST) and SWS increased whereas REM sleep decreased as T_{br} declined, so that REM sleep comprised only 8% of TST for the entire entrance and was absent at T_{br}s below 24°C (Fig. 10). This reduction in REM sleep was due to a reduced REM sleep frequency since the mean duration of REM sleep episodes remained constant.

During the deepest portions of shallow hibernation, electrophysiological activity alternated between brief episodes of wakefulness (mean duration 2.0 min) that comprised 11% of the record and longer periods of SWS (mean duration 15.0 min) that constituted the remainder of the record. Per cent sleep was high in both the light and dark portions of the 24 h period, and in both cases exceeded that observed during the major sleep period at night when animals were euthermic.

The spontaneous return to euthermia at the end of the hibernation period was characterized by increased wakefulness but with SWS still dominant (69%) and REM sleep absent, contrasted with the increased wakefulness and EMG activity characterizing non-provoked arousal from deep hibernation. When arousal was induced by sensory stimulation, electro-

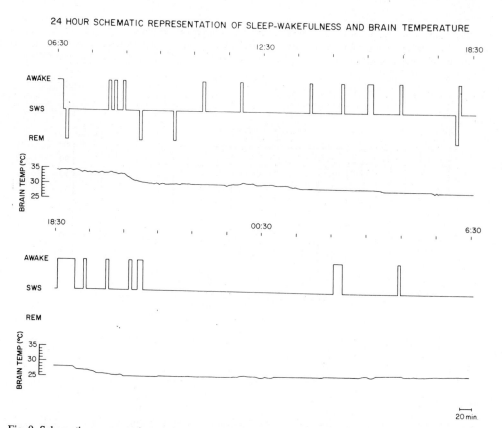

Fig. 9. Schematic representation of sleep and wakefulness plotted with changes in T_{br} as a golden-mantled ground squirrel enters shallow hibernation at a T_a of 22°C. Note that the last episode of REM sleep occurs at a T_{br} of approximately 28°C. (From Walker, 1978, reproduced with permission.)

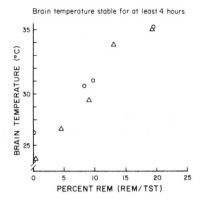

Fig. 10. Brain temperature related decreases in REM sleep as a percentage of sleep time for two golden-mantled ground squirrels ($\circ$ and $\triangle$) during the entrance into shallow hibernation. Percentage REM sleep was calculated only for periods where T_{br} remained stable for at least 4 h. (From Walker, 1978, reproduced with permission.)

physiological activity during return to euthermia was characterized by wakefulness; and T_{br} rose at a more rapid rate than when SWS was present during spontaneous arousals.

These observations of the behavioral and electrophysiological characteristics of SWS during hibernation of the alpine ground squirrel support the contention that sleep and hibernation are homologous. Moreover, there exists no clear-cut demarcation in the characterization of SWS during euthermia and that during shallow hibernation at T_{br}s above 22°C. Therefore, it is reasonable to assume that hibernation represents merely a "deeper" phase of SWS and not a qualitatively distinct functional state.

Sleep and shallow torpor (estivation) are homologous in desert ground squirrels

In order to investigate if there would also exist a physiological continuity between sleep and shallow torpor, the round-tailed ground squirrel (*Citellus tereticaudus*) was chosen as experimental animal. This species resides in a totally different ecological niche from that of its alpine relative (*Citellus lateralis*) and displays a temporally different form of dormancy. It lives in hot, dry desert regions and enters short periods of shallow torpor when food is scarce in the summer. This form of summer torpor has been called estivation.

Shallow torpor was induced by food deprivation in 4 round-tailed ground squirrels (*Citellus tereticaudus*) during the months of July and August (Walker et al., 1979). The animals were maintained at a T_a of 25 ± 0.5°C and on a 12 : 12 h light—dark photoperiod. Continuous electrophysiological and T_{br} recordings were obtained over a period of 10—26 days during which time 20 bouts of torpor occurred (at least 4 on each animal).

Animals first entered torpor after 2, 3, 5 and 19 days of food deprivation, respectively. Subsequent bouts followed at approximately 24- or 48-h intervals (Fig. 11). A distinct nocturnal pattern of torpor occurring at the usual sleep time was present in 3 animals. T_{br} decreased during the first half of the night (1°C/40—50 min); stabilized at 26—28°C for 1—4 h and then increased to euthermic levels over a period of approximately 1 h. Bouts lasted an average of 10 h, from initial decrease in T_{br} to return to euthermia. Return to euthermia was spontaneous and occurred during the last 2 h of the dark period (06.00—08.00 h). One adult animal that went 19 days without food before entering torpor exhibited

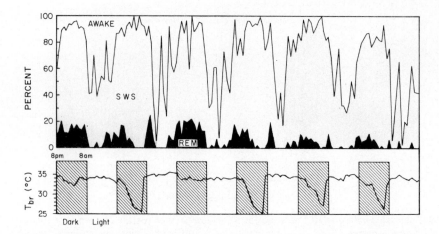

Fig. 11. Hourly sleep and wakefulness percentages and measures of T_{br} for a desert round-tailed ground squirrel over a 6-day period. Decreases in T_{br} indicate bouts of shallow torpor (or estivation). (From Walker et al., copyright 1979 by the American Association for the Advancement of Science.)

bouts of torpor during the night, but the timing and duration of other bouts were variable. Thus, the shortest bout began in the afternoon and lasted 8 h whereas the longest began in the early morning and lasted 18 h. As with alpine squirrels during shallow torpor, sleep and wakefulness could be identified according to conventional electrographic criteria at all T_{br}s (Fig. 12).

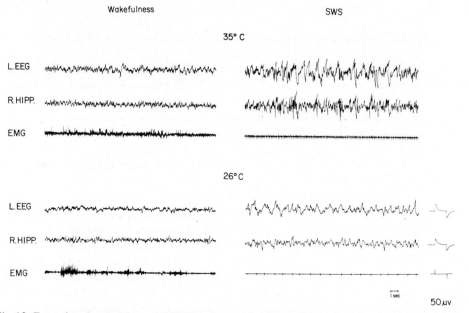

Fig. 12. Examples of wakefulness and SWS in the round-tailed ground squirrel at euthermic levels (T_{br} = 35°C) and during shallow torpor (T_{br} = 26°C). Note the correspondence between electrophysiological activity in shallow torpor and those for shallow hibernation. (From Walker et al., copyright 1979 by the American Association for the Advancement of Science.)

The changes in the distribution of sleep and waking states during entrance into shallow torpor in *Citellus tereticaudus* were similar to those previously described for *Citellus lateralis* and *Citellus beldingi* during their initial entrances into hibernation. As T_{br} declined, total sleep time increased from 66% prior to entrance to 92% during the entrance. Conversely, per cent of time spent in REM progressively decreased owing to a lengthening of the REM sleep cycle, so that REM sleep comprised only 6% of TST for the entire entrance, compared to the 17% that normally occurs during the 12 h dark period at euthermic T_{br}s. REM sleep occurred only occasionally at T_{br}s below 27°C.

During the deepest portion of the bout, when T_{br} remained stable between 26 and 28°C, electrophysiological activity alternated between brief episodes of wakefulness comprising only 7% of the record and long periods of uninterrupted sleep constituting the remaining 93% of the record. In contrast, the per cent sleep time normally observed at euthermic T_{br}s during a 12 h dark period was only 82%. On those occasions when torpor did occur during the day, sleep—wakefulness patterns were essentially the same as during nocturnal torpor, and comprised more total sleep and less REM sleep than during temporally-equivalent euthermic periods.

Bouts of torpor were usually terminated by an episode of increased wakefulness signalling an increase in T_{br} and a return to euthermia. During the return to euthermia, wakefulness increased to 39% but REM sleep remained absent. Shivering occasionally occurred during both wakefulness and SWS as T_{br} increased.

Therefore, the above results point to the physiological correspondence of shallow torpor and hibernation, i.e. changes in EKG, EMG and EEG activity during bouts of shallow torpor were the same as in shallow hibernation. Moreover, sleep patterns during entire bouts of shallow torpor in desert ground squirrels were qualitatively and quantitatively identical to those of shallow hibernation in alpine ground squirrels.

Sleep and daily torpor in pocket mice

Bartholomew and Cade (1957) reported that the pocket mouse (*Perognathus longemembris*) may engage in intense and coordinated behavior alternating with periods of behavioral quiescence as its T_b falls continuously from 34–27°C during entrance into torpor. The length of these periods of wakefulness was not recorded so it is unclear whether the mode of entrance into torpor in the pocket mouse differs from that observed in the ground squirrel. We studied sleep and torpor in the same species of pocket mice to determine if a process other than sleep for regulating T_b at lower levels exists in this species (Harris et al., 1979).

Torpor was induced by food deprivation in animals at T_as of 23–25°C exposed to a 12 : 12 h light : dark photoperiod. Contrary to Bartholomew and Cade (1957), we did not see or record any evidence of "periods of great activity" accompanying declines in T_{br}; moreover, electrophysiological activity and sleep patterns during these entrances into torpor were similar to those previously reported for ground squirrels. Entrance into torpor was predominantly through SWS. Any brief periods of wakefulness either halted the decline in T_{br} or raised it (Fig. 13). TST increased while REM sleep decreased dramatically or was absent during the entrance. Once T_{br} stabilized at about 25°C, torpor was composed of almost continuous SWS.

Daily shallow torpor occurring in some small mammals, such as pocket mice or round-tailed ground squirrels, has sometimes been interpreted as an extension or magnification of the euthermic circadian rhythms of T_b. However, in this study some bouts of torpor occurred independently, at times remote from the minor circadian decreases of T_b. There-

270

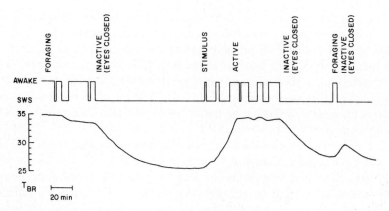

Fig. 13. Schematic representation of sleep and wakefulness plotted with visual observations and T_{br} as a pocket mouse (*Perognathus longemembris*) enters, arouses and then re-enters shallow torpor. Note that wakefulness is associated with an increase in T_{br}.

fore, the decreased T_b of torpor is associated more closely with sleep than with a pre-established circadian variation of T_b independent of sleep. Furthermore, the foregoing results show that the homology between sleep, shallow torpor and hibernation in 3 species of ground squirrel also extends to an unrelated species.

Continuity of thermoregulatory processes between SWS and hibernation

It is now known that hibernators still possess continuous thermoregulatory capabilities during deep torpor, and do not simply revert to a poikilothermic condition (Heller and Glotzbach, 1977). It is likely that a unitary regulatory mechanism is responsible for the entire range of T_bs exhibited by the hibernator. The concept of continuity of the thermoregulatory system over such a broad range of T_bs is supported by the demonstration of temperature-sensitive preoptic neurons in hibernators exhibiting continuous firing-rate curves over a temperature range of $30°C$ (Wünnenberg et al., 1976). Furthermore, the hypothalamic threshold to cold for a metabolic thermoregulatory response progressively decreases but continues to exist throughout the entrance (Heller et al., 1977) and during entire bouts of deep hibernation (Heller and Colliver, 1974; Florant and Heller, 1977) in a manner similar to, but of greater extent than that which occurs at the onset of SWS (Glotzbach and Heller, 1976). Recently, Florant et al. (1978) were able to measure the hypothalamic temperature threshold for metabolic heat production in the marmot during euthermic wakefulness and SWS; and at various T_bs $(25-10°C)$ during the entrance into hibernation. They found that when the values during the entrance into hibernation were extrapolated, they were continuous with those of euthermic SWS but not euthermic wakefulness.

These findings and the fact that hibernation is entered through SWS have led us to postulate that both shallow torpor and hibernation are a continuation of thermoregulatory adjustments initiated during SWS. Because of the thermoregulatory, electrophysiological and behavioral continuity among the above 3 states of dormancy, it is reasonable to assume that there is also a continuity of biological significance among these states, viz. energy conservation.

Hibernation and circannual rhythms of sleep

If hibernation is an extension of sleep one might expect there to be circannual rhythms of sleep proclivity in euthermic animals corresponding to endogenous circannual rhythms of hibernation previously demonstrated in marmots, chipmunks, and ground squirrels (Davis and Finnie, 1975; Heller and Poulson, 1970; Pengelley and Fisher, 1963). Moreover, the golden-mantled ground squirrel exhibits seasonal changes in body weight and food consumption even when high T_as prevent hibernation (Pengelley and Fisher, 1963). We recently found that there is a circannual rhythm of sleep in euthermic golden-mantled ground squirrels with its maxima coinciding with the hibernation season (Walker et al., 1980).

Several 24 h electrophysiological recordings were obtained on 4 animals at 2–3 month intervals over a 16 month period under the same environmental conditions present in the animal colony ($T_a = 22 \pm 0.5°C$, 12 : 12 h light : dark photoperiod). Since *Citellus lateralis* exhibits periods of shallow hibernation at room temperature during November–February, T_{br} was monitored to insure that electrophysiological recordings were obtained at comparable euthermic levels of 34–37°C throughout the 16 month period of study. Coded electrophysiological recordings were scored "blind" for sleep/wakefulness according to conventional criteria (Walker et al., 1977).

Fig. 14 shows the seasonal changes in per cent time spent asleep in a 24 h period for each animal. Although there was some variation, a consistent trend was present in all animals. Sleep increased in the fall, remained high during the winter, decreased in the spring and reached its lowest levels during the summer. May–June and August–September measurements of per cent sleep time for a 24 h period were both significantly less than during November–December (T = 6.58, $P < 0.01$; T = 3.85, $P < 0.05$, respectively) or during February–March (T = 9.46, $P < 0.01$; T = 2.65, $P < 0.05$, respectively). A trend analysis, using orthogonal polynomials, revealed a significant quadratic component ($P < 0.01$), again indicating the presence of a seasonal rhythm.

Despite the seasonal changes in sleep propensity under constant environmental conditions, the proportions of sleep spent in SWS and REM sleep remained remarkably stable throughout the year, as did the diurnal distribution of sleep and wakefulness.

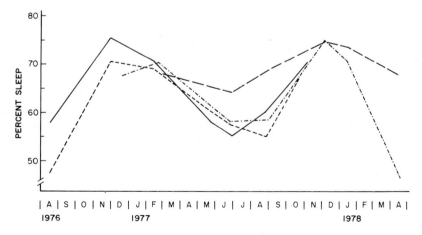

Fig. 14. Annual changes in percentage of a 24 h period spent asleep for 4 golden-mantled ground squirrels maintained at a temperature of 22°C and 12 : 12 h light : dark photoperiod. Animals were euthermic for the duration of all recording periods. (From Walker et al., 1980, reproduced with permission.)

The bear (Hock, 1960; Morrison, 1960; Nelson et al., 1973), some species of chipmunk (Cade, 1963; Heller and Poulson, 1970) and probably the badger, skunk and raccoon (Hudson and Bartholomew, 1964) exhibit a form of dormancy sometimes termed "seasonal sleep" in which T_b is maintained near euthermic levels at 33–34°C. The bear can survive in this condition up to 100 days without eating, undergoing only a 25% reduction in body weight (Nelson et al., 1973). The near euthermic T_bs and easy arousability to wakefulness point to this state as being an extended period of sleep. Possibly heterothermic mammals of today evolved from ancestors displaying similar patterns of extended sleep. Increased length of sleep, where T_b remains near euthermic levels, may be sufficient in itself to meet, or at least partially reduce, energy needs in ecological situations where food availability is seasonal, especially in larger mammals whose rate of heat loss is proportionally less than in small true hibernators. Increased selective pressure favoring a progressive lowering of T_b during SWS and/or an extension of time spent in this state in the course of evolution could account for the phenomena of daily torpor, seasonal hibernation, and seasonal sleep.

EVOLUTION OF ENDOTHERMY, SWS AND HIBERNATION

Endothermy

Paleontological and physiological considerations indicate that endotherms originally descended from large homeothermic reptiles such as therapsids, through reduction in body size coupled with the development of tachymetabolism and insulative fur (MacNab, 1978). States of torpidity in mammals have been viewed as either phyletically more recent than endothermy (Hudson, 1973) or alternatively, as a more primitive vestige of reptilian tolerance of low T_bs (Cade, 1963). The existence of continuous and precise thermoregulation of T_b during the entrance and throughout bouts of hibernation suggests that hibernation evolved either simultaneously with endothermy or as a subsequent adaptation of it. SWS involves a downward regulated adjustment of T_b qualitatively similar to that observed during hibernation, and thus could have represented an optimal pre-adaptation for the subsequent development of hibernation and daily torpor.

SWS

The presence of SWS, shallow torpor and hibernation in the echidna (Allison and Van Twyver, 1972; Allison et al., 1972) — one of three living endothermic nontherian * mammals — and the physiological homologies between these states indicate that they share a common evolutionary history. The absence of SWS in reptiles and its presence in therian ** and nontherian mammals points to the evolution of SWS early in mammalian history. Then, as now, it would have been selectively advantageous for small homeotherms to decrease energy expenditure during periods of inactivity. Although terrestrial habitats were relatively warm in the Jurassic and Cretaceous period, significant metabolic reductions could have been achieved by a slight lowering of T_b during inactive periods, especially during periods of food shortage, as was discussed earlier.

---

* Egg-laying mammals — monotremes.
** Placental and marsupial animals.

Torpor and hibernation

The appearance of more extreme forms of mammalian dormancy than euthermic sleep probably occurred long after the major adaptive radiation of mammals and birds. Substantial cooling of the earth's surface did not occur until the mid-to-late Tertiary period (Flohn, 1969) and resulted in increased seasonality with extended periods of both cold and food scarcity toward the polar regions. Animals in the harshest habitats would experience selective pressures favoring further modifications in existing processes of energy conservation.

Since SWS probably existed in its present form as an energy conserving state by this time, it represented an optimal condition for the emergence of additional patterns of dormancy. The further evolution of increased lengths of sleep time independently of, or in conjunction with, a greater SWS-related decline in T_b would have allowed homeotherms of differing sizes and highly divergent ecological niches to cope with their energy demands.

THE FUNCTION OF REM SLEEP

In this review we have focused on the function of SWS and have not paid much regard to the role of REM sleep in mammalian evolution. This is because a sufficient and consistent body of evidence has yet to be accumulated that delineates the primal biological function of REM sleep in the same manner as we believe now exists for SWS. Nevertheless, we note that the presence of REM sleep is not inconsistent with the foregoing conclusions concerning the function of SWS and that REM sleep itself probably conserved as much if not more energy than SWS in some animals. Studies of human metabolism indicate that metabolism during REM sleep is either equal to that of NREM sleep (Webb and Hiestand, 1975) or slightly higher (Brebbia and Altschuler, 1965; Haskell et al., 1978), but in any case tends to be lower than that of wakefulness. Only 3 preliminary studies on metabolism of REM sleep in the opossum, rat and ground squirrel, respectively, exist to date, but all of them indicate that it is lower than during SWS (Berger, 1975; Roussel and Bittel, 1979; Kilduff, personal communication). These differences in metabolism between humans and animals are mirrored by differences in thresholds of arousal. Thresholds during REM sleep in animals are higher than during SWS sleep (Van Twyver and Garrett, 1972) whereas in humans they are equal to those of stage 2 sleep (Rechtschaffen et al., 1966). A reduction in metabolism associated with loss of muscle tone during REM sleep in animals is consistent with extensive findings indicating a reversion to a poikilothermic condition during REM sleep (see Heller and Glotzbach, 1977 for a review). Animals exposed to high or low T_as maintain T_b regulation during sleep by markedly curtailing the frequency and length of REM episodes. Perhaps then REM sleep is a vestige of a reptilian poikilothermic state of waking inactivity, and can be regarded as "archisleep" in accord with Jouvet's (1961) original view of it. EMG activity is isoelectric in inactive reptiles (Fig. 1; Walker and Berger, 1973) as it is during REM sleep. Contrary to the assumption of Allison and Van Twyver (1970) that REM sleep first appeared in therian mammals, its absence in echidna might in fact indicate that in nontherians SWS completely eclipsed waking reptilian inactivity, as it almost did in birds, which have only sparse amounts of REM sleep. The high voltage spikes prominent during inactivity in reptiles (Fig. 3) might be analogs (or homologs) of ponto-geniculo-occipital (PGO) spikes of REM sleep. Consistent with this interpretation is evidence that EEG spiking activity in the tortoise is possibly generated in the optic lobe (Walker and Berger, 1973). Although

Flanigan et al. (1973) originally suggested that reptilian EEG spikes were similar to PGO spikes, Flanigan (1974) subsequently argued that they were analogs of mammalian and avian slow waves. Clearly, further studies are required to explore REM sleep's possible relation to reptilian inactivity.

SUMMARY

We have proposed that sleep, shallow torpor and hibernation in mammals and birds are homologous physiological processes. Phylogenetic and ontogenetic correlations between sleep and endothermy and sleep-dependent thermoregulatory adjustments associated with decreased metabolism are consistent with an energy-conserving role for sleep. Electrophysiological studies demonstrating physiological continuities between sleep, shallow torpor and hibernation, as well as seasonal changes in amounts of sleep, lead us to speculate that deeper states of dormancy evolved through a gradual extension of thermoregulatory adjustments initiated in all mammals during sleep.

ACKNOWLEDGEMENTS

We appreciate the collaboration of our colleagues Steve ↘. Glotzbach, H. Craig Heller, Ann Garber, D. Vance Harris and Ed Haskell in many phases of this research.
This research was supported by NIH Grant GM-23694.

REFERENCES

Abrams, R. and Hammel, H.T. (1964) Hypothalamic temperature in unanesthetized albino rats during feeding and sleep. *Amer. J. Physiol.*, 206: 641–646.

Adams, T. (1963) Hypothalamic temperature in the cat during feeding and sleep. *Science*, 139: 609–610.

Allison, T. and Cicchetti, D.V. (1976) Sleep in mammals: ecological and constitutional correlates. *Science*, 194: 732–734.

Allison, T. and Van Twyver, H. (1970) The evolution of sleep. *Nat. Hist.*, 79: 56–65.

Allison, T. and Van Twyver, H. (1972) Electrophysiological studies of the echidna *Tachyglossus aculeatus*. II. Dormancy and hibernation. *Arch. ital. Biol.*, 110: 184–194.

Allison, T., Van Twyver, H. and Goff, W.R. (1972) Electrophysiological studies of the echidna *Tachyglossus aculeatus*. I. Waking and sleeping. *Arch. ital. Biol.*, 110: 145–184.

Aserinsky, E. and Kleitman, N. (1953) Regularly occurring periods of eye motility and concomitant phenomena during sleep. *Science*, 118: 273–274.

Baker, M.A. and Hayward, J.N. (1967) Autonomic basis for the rise in brain temperature during paradoxical sleep. *Science*, 157: 1586–1588.

Bartholomew, G.A. and Cade, T.J. (1957) Temperature regulation, hibernation, and aestivation in the little pocket mouse, *Perognathus longimembris*. *J. Mammal.*, 38: 60–72.

Berger, H. (1969) Über das Elektroenkephalogramm des Menschen. *Arch. Psychiat. Nervenkr.*, 87: 527–570.

Berger, R.J. (1969) The physiological characteristics of sleep. In *Sleep Physiology and Pathology*, A. Kales (Ed.), Lippincott, Philadelphia, pp. 66–79.

Berger, R.J. (1975) Bioenergetic functions of sleep and activity rhythms and their possible relevance to aging. *Fed. Proc.*, 34: 97–102.

Berger, R.J., Taub, J.M. and Walker, J.M. (1973) Sleep as a biological adaptive process. In *The Nature of Sleep*, U.J. Jovanovic (Ed.), Gustav Fischer Verlag, Stuttgart, pp. 252–255.

Berger, R.J. and Walker, J.M. (1972) Sleep in the burrowing owl (*Speotyto cunicularia hypugaea*). *Behav. Biol.*, 7: 183–194.

Brebbia, D.R. and Altschuler, K.Z. (1965) Oxygen consumption rate and electroencephalographic stages of sleep. *Science*, 150: 1621–1623.

Brody, S. (1945) *Bioenergetics and Growth*, Hafner, New York, pp. 352–403.

Cade, T.J. (1963) Observations on torpidity in captive chipmunks of the genus Eutamias. *Ecology*, 44: 255–261.

Davis, H., Davis, P.A., Loomis, A.L., Harvey, E.N. and Hobart, G. (1937) Changes in human brain potentials during the onset of sleep. *Science*, 86: 448–450.

Davis, H., Davis, P.A., Loomis, A.L., Harvey, E.N. and Hobart, G. (1938) Human brain potentials during the onset of sleep. *Neurophysiol.*, 1: 24–38.

Davis, D.E. and Finnie, E.P. (1975) Entrainment of circannual rhythm in weight of woodchucks. *J. Mammal.*, 56: 199–203.

Day, R. (1941) Regulation of body temperature during sleep. *Amer. J. Dis. Child.*, 61: 734–746.

Dement, W.C. and Kleitman, N. (1957) Cyclic variations in EEG during sleep and their relation to eye movements, body motility, and dreaming. *Electroenceph. clin. Neurophysiol.*, 9: 673–690.

Euler, C.V. and Söderberg, U. (1958) Co-ordinated change in temperature thresholds reflexes for thermoregulatory reflexes. *Acta physiol. scand.*, 42: 112.

Flanigan, W.F., Jr. (1973) Sleep and wakefulness in Iguanid lizards *Ctenosaura pectinata* and *Iguana iguana*. *Brain, Behav. Evol.*, 8: 401–436.

Flanigan, W.F., Jr. (1974) Sleep and wakefulness in chelonian reptiles. II. The red-footed tortoise, *Geochelone carbonaria*. *Arch. ital. Biol.*, 112: 253–277.

Flanigan, W.F., Jr., Wilcox, R.H. and Rechtschaffen, A. (1973) The EEG and behavioral continuum of the crocodilian, *Caiman sclerops*. *Electroenceph. clin. Neurophysiol.*, 34: 521–538.

Flanigan, W.F., Jr., Knight, C.P., Hartse, K.M. and Rechtschaffen, A. (1974) Sleep and wakefulness in chelonian reptiles. I. The box turtle, *Terrapene carolina*. *Arch. ital. Biol.*, 112: 227–252.

Flohn, H. (1969) Ein geophysikalisches Eiszeit-Model. *Eiszeitalter Gyw.*, 20: 204.

Florant, G.L. and Heller, H.C. (1977) CNS regulation of body temperature in euthermic and hibernating marmots (*Marmota flaviventris*). *Amer. J. Physiol.*, 232: R203–R208.

Florant, G.L., Turner, B.M. and Heller, H.C. (1978) Temperature regulation during wakefulness, sleep, and hibernation in marmots. *Amer. J. Physiol.*, 235: R82–R88.

Geschickter, E.H., Andrews, P.A. and Bullard, R.W. (1966) Nocturnal body temperature regulation in man: a rationale for sweating in sleep. *J. appl. Physiol.*, 21: 623–630.

Glotzbach, S.F. and Heller, H.C. (1976) Central nervous regulation of body temperature during sleep. *Science*, 194: 537–539.

Hammel, H.T., Jackson, D.C., Stolwijk, J.A.J., Hardy, J.D. and Strømme, S.B. (1963) Temperature regulation by hypothalamic proportional control with an adjustable set point. *J. appl. Physiol.*, 18: 1146–1154.

Harris, D.V., Walker, J.M. and Berger, R.J. (1979) Torpor in the pocket mouse (*Perognathus longimembris*). In *3rd Int. Congr. Sleep Res.*, Tokyo, Japan.

Haskell, E.H. (1978) *Effects of Sleep at Altered Ambient Temperatures on Electrophysiological Sleep and Thermoregulatory Mechanisms in Human Subjects, and in Ground Squirrels (Citellus lateralis)*. Ph.D. Thesis, University of California, Santa Cruz.

Haskell, E.H., Palca, J.W., Walker, J.M., Berger, R.J. and Heller, H.C. (1978) The influence of ambient temperature on electrophysiological sleep in humans. *Sleep Res.*, 7: 169.

Hayward, J.N. and Baker, M.A. (1969) A comparative study of the role of the cerebral arterial blood in the regulation of brain temperature in five mammals. *Brain Res.*, 16: 417–440.

Heller, H.C. and Colliver, G.W. (1974) CNS regulation of body temperature during hibernation. *Amer. J. Physiol.*, 227: 583–589.

Heller, H.C., Colliver, G.W. and Beard, J. (1977) Thermoregulation during entrance into hibernation. *Pflügers Arch. ges. Physiol.*, 369: 55–59.

Heller, H.C. and Glotzbach, S.F. (1977) Thermoregulation during sleep and hibernation. *Environmental Physiology II. Int. Rev. Physiol.*, 15: 147–188.

Heller, H.C. and Poulson, T.L. (1970) Circadian rhythms. II. Endogenous and exogenous factors controlling reproduction and hibernation in chipmunks (Eutamias) and ground squirrels (Spermophilus). *Comp. biochem. Physiol.*, 33: 357–383.

Heller, H.C., Walker, J.M., Florant, G.L., Glotzbach, S.F. and Berger, R.J. (1978) Sleep and hibernation:

electrophysiological and thermoregulatory homologies. In *Strategies in Cold: Natural Thermogenesis and Torpidity,* L. Wang and J.W. Hudson (Eds.), Academic Press, New York, pp. 225–265.

Herman, H., Jouvet, M. and Klein, M. (1964) Etude polygraphique du sommeil chez la tortue. *C.R. Soc. Biol. (Paris),* 258: 2175–2178.

Hobson, J.A. (1967) Electrographic correlates of behavior in the frog with special reference to sleep. *Electroenceph. clin. Neurophysiol.,* 22: 113–121.

Hock, R.J. (1960) Seasonal variations in physiologic functions of arctic ground squirrels and black bears. *Bull. Mus. comp. Zool.,* 101: 289–299.

Hudson, J.W. (1973) Torpidity in mammals. In *Comparative Physiology of Thermoregulation, Vol. 3,* G.C. Whittow (Ed.), Academic Press, New York, pp. 97–165.

Hudson, J.W. and Bartholomew, G.A. (1964) Terrestrial animals in dry heat: estivators. In *Handbook of Physiology: Adaptation to the Environment, Vol. 4,* D.B. Dill, E.F. Adolph and C.G. Wilbur (Eds.), Springer-Verlag, pp. 541–550.

Jana, H. (1965) Energy metabolism in hypnotic trance and sleep. *J. appl. Physiol.,* 20: 308–310.

Jouvet, M. (1961) Telencephalic and rhombencephalic sleep in the cat. In *The Nature of Sleep,* G.E.W. Wolstenholm and M. O'Connor (Eds.), Little Brown, Boston, pp. 188–206.

Karmanova, I.G. and Churnosov, E.V. (1972) Electrophysiological investigations of natural sleep and wakefulness of turtles and chickens. *Zh. Evoliutsionnoi biokhimii i fiziologu,* 8: 59–65.

Kirk, E. (1931) Untersuchungen über den Einfluss des normalen Schlafes auf die Temperatur der Füsse. *Scand. Arch. Physiol.,* 61: 71–78.

Kleitman, N. (1963) *Sleep and Wakefulness.* University of Chicago Press, Chicago.

Kreider, M.B., Buskirk, E.R. and Bass, D.E. (1958) Oxygen consumption and body temperatures during the night. *J. appl. Physiol.,* 12: 361–366.

Kreider, M.B. and Iampietro, P.F. (1959) Oxygen consumption and body temperature during sleep in cold environments. *J. appl. Physiol.,* 14: 765–767.

Loomis, A.L., Harvey, E.N. and Hobart, G.A. (1937) Cerebral states during sleep as studied by human brain potentials. *J. exp. Psychol.,* 21: 127–144.

Lucas, E., Sterman, M.B. and McGinty, D.J. (1969) The salamander EEG: a model of primitive sleep and wakefulness. *Psychophysiology,* 6: 230.

Magnussen, G. (1944) *Studies on the Respiration during Sleep. A Contribution to the Physiology of the Sleep Function,* H.K. Lewis, London.

MacNab, B.K. (1978) The evolution of endotherms in the phylogeny of mammals. *Amer. Naturalist,* 112: 1–21.

Meglasson, M.D. and Huggins, S.E. (1979) Sleep in a crocodilian, *Caiman sclerops. Comp. biochem. Physiol.,* 63: 561–567.

Milan, F.A. and Evonuk, E. (1967) Oxygen consumption and body temperatures of Eskimos during sleep. *J. appl. Physiol.,* 22: 565–567.

Mills, J.N., Minors, D.S. and Waterhouse, J.M. (1978) The effect of sleep on human circadian rhythm. *Chronobiol.,* 5: 14–27.

Morrison, P. (1960) Some interrelations between weight and hibernating functions. *Bull. Mus. comp. Zool.,* 124: 75–90.

Morrison, P. and Petajan, J.H. (1962) The development of temperature regulation in the opossum, *Didelphis marsupialis virginiana. Physiol. Zool.,* 35: 52–65.

Moruzzi, G. (1966) The functional significance of sleep with particular regard to the brain mechanisms underlying consciousness, In *Brain and Conscious Experience,* J.C. Eccles (Ed.), Springer Verlag, Berlin, pp. 345–388.

Nelson, R.A., Wahner, H.W., Jones, J.D., Ellefson, R.D. and Zollman, P.E. (1973) Metabolism of bears before, during, and after winter sleep. *Amer. J. Physiol.,* 224: 491–496.

Ogawa, T., Satoh, T. and Takagi, K. (1967) Sweating during night sleep. *Jap. J. Physiol.,* 17: 135–148.

Ookawa, T. (1972) Avian wakefulness and sleep on the basis of recent electroencephalographic observations. *Poultry Sci.,* 51: 1565–1574.

Ookawa, T. and Gotoh, J. (1965) Electroencephalogram of the chicken recorded from the skull under various conditions. *J. comp. Neurol.,* 124: 1–14.

Parmeggiani, P.L. and Sabattini, L. (1972) Electromyographic aspects of postural, respiratory, and thermoregulatory mechanisms in sleeping cats. *Electroenceph. clin. Neurophysiol.,* 33: 1–13.

Pengelley, E.T. and Fisher, K.C. (1963) The effects of temperature and photoperiod on the yearly hibernating behavior of captive golden-mantled ground squirrels (*Citellus lateralis tescorum*), *J. canad. Zool.,* 41: 1103–1121.

Pieron, H. (1913) *La problème physiologique du sommeil,* Masson, Paris.

Pyrethon, J. and Dusan-Pyrethon, D. (1968) Etude polygraphique du cycle veille-sommeil chez trois geures de reptiles. *C.R. Soc. Biol. (Paris),* 162: 181–186.

Rechtschaffen, A., Hauri, P. and Zeitlin, M. (1966) Auditory awakening thresholds in REM and NREM sleep stages. *Percept. mot. Skills,* 22: 927–942.

Reynolds, H.C. (1952) Studies on reproduction in the opossum (*Didelphis virginiana virginiana*), *Univ. Calif. Publ. Zool.,* 52: 232–284.

Robertson, J.D. and Reid, D.D. (1952) Standards for the basal metabolism of normal people in Britain. *Lancet,* 1: 940–943.

Robin, E.D., Whaley, R.D., Crump, C.H. and Travis, D.M. (1958) Alveolar gas tensions, pulmonary ventilation and blood pH, during physiological sleep in normal subjects. *J. clin. Invest.,* 37: 981–989.

Rojas-Ramirez, J.A. and Tauber, E.S. (1970) Paradoxical sleep in two species of avian predator (Falconiformes). *Science,* 167: 1754–1755.

Roussel, B. and Bittel, J. (1979) Thermogenesis and thermolysis during sleep and waking in the rat. *Pflügers Arch. ges. Physiol.,* 382: 225–231.

Satinoff, E. (1970) Hibernation and the central nervous system. In *Progress in Physiological Psychology, Vol. 3,* E. Stellar and J.M. Sprague (Eds.), Academic Press, New York, pp. 201–236.

Satoh, T., Ogawa, T. and Takagi, K. (1965) Sweating during daytime sleep. *Jap. J. Physiol.,* 15: 523–531.

Segura, E.T. (1966) Estudios electroencefalograficos en anfibos. *Acta physiol. lat.-amer.,* 16: 277–282.

Shtark, M.B. (1961) An electrophysiological study of hibernation. *Fiziol. Zh. (Leningr.),* 47: 1–226.

Snyder, F. (1966) Toward an evolutionary theory of dreaming. *Amer. J. Psychiat.,* 123: 121–142.

Snyder, F. (1969) Sleep and REM as biological enigmas. In *Sleep Physiology and Pathology,* A. Kales (Ed.), Lippincott, Philadelphia, pp. 266–280.

South, F.E., Breazile, J.E., Dellmann, H.D. and Epperly, A.D. (1969) Sleep, hibernation and hypothermia in the yellow-bellied marmot (*M. flaviventris*). In *Depressed Metabolism,* X.J. Mosacchia and J.F. Saunders (Eds.), Elsevier, New York, pp. 277–312.

Strumwasser, F. (1959) Thermoregulatory, brain and behavioral mechanisms during entrance into hibernation in the squirrel, *Citellus beecheyi. Amer. J. Physiol.,* 196: 15–22.

Suomalainen, P. (1961) Hibernation and sleep. In *The Nature of Sleep,* G.E.W. Wolstenholme and M.O. O'Connor (Eds.), Little, Brown, Boston, pp. 307–316.

Susic, V. (1972) Electrographic and behavioral correlations of the rest–activity cycle in the sea turtle, *Caretta caretta* L. (Chelonia). *J. exp. biol. Ecol.,* 10: 81–87.

Tauber, E.S., Roffwarg, H.P. and Weitzman, E.C. (1966) Eye movements and electroencephalogram activity during sleep in diurnal lizards. *Nature (Lond.),* 212: 1612–1613.

Tauber, E.S., Rojas-Ramirez, J. and Hernandez-Peon, R. (1968) Electrophysiological and behavioral correlates of wakefulness and sleep in the lizard (*Ctensosaura pectinata*). *Electroenceph. clin. Neurophysiol.,* 24: 424–443.

Tradardi, V. (1966) Sleep in the pigeon. *Arch. ital. Biol.,* 104: 516–521.

Twente, J.W. and Twente, J.A. (1965) Regulation of hibernating periods by temperature. *Proc. nat. Acad. Sci. (Wash.),* 54: 1058–1061.

Van Twyver, H. (1973) Polygraphic studies of the American alligator. *Sleep Rev.,* 2: 89.

Van Twyver, H. and Allison, T. (1972) A polygraphic and behavioral study of sleep in the pigeon (*Columba livia*). *Exp. Neurol.,* 35: 138–153.

Van Twyver, H. and Garrett, W. (1972) Arousal threshold in the rat determined by meaningful stimuli. *Behav. Biol.,* 7: 205–215.

Vasilescu, E. (1970) Sleep and wakefulness in the tortoise (*Emys orbicularis*). *Rev. Romaine de Biol., Series de Zoologie,* 15: 177–179.

Walker, J.M. (1978) *Sleep, Daily Torpor, and Hibernation: Continuous Processes of Energy Conservation,* Ph.D. Thesis, University of California, Santa Cruz.

Walker, J.M. and Berger, R.J. (1972) Sleep in the domestic pigeon (*Columba livia*). *Behav. Biol.,* 7: 195–203.

Walker, J.M. and Berger, R.J. (1973) A polygraphic study of the tortoise (*Testudo denticulata*): absence of electrophysiological signs of sleep. *Brain Behav. Evol.,* 8: 453–467.

Walker, J.M. and Berger, R.J. (1980) The ontogenesis of sleep states, thermogenesis and thermoregulation in the Virginia opossum. *Develop. Psychobiol.,* in press.

278

Walker, J.M., Garber, A., Berger, R.J. and Heller, H.C. (1979) Sleep and estivation (shallow torpor): continuous processes of energy conservation. *Science,* 204: 1098–1100.

Walker, J.M., Glotzbach, S.F., Berger, R.J. and Heller, H.C. (1977) Sleep and hibernation in ground squirrels (*Citellus* spp.): Electrophysiological observations. *Amer. J. Physiol.,* 233: R213–R221.

Walker, J.M., Haskell, E.H., Berger, R.J. and Heller, H.C. (1980) Hibernation and circannual rhythms of sleep. *Physiol. Zool.,* 53: 8–11.

Webb, P. and Hiestand, M. (1975) Sleep metabolism and age. *J. appl. Physiol.,* 38: 257–262.

Williams, R.L., Karacan, I. and Hursch, C.J. (1974) *EEG of Human Sleep: Clinical Applications,* Wiley, New York.

Wünnenberg, W., Merker, G. and Spedula, E. (1976) Thermosensitivity of preoptic neurons in a hibernator (golden hamster) and non-hibernator (guinea pig). *Pflüg. Arch. ges. Physiol.,* 363: 119–123.

Zepelin, H. and Rechtschaffen, A. (1974) Mammalian sleep, longevity and energy metabolism. *Brain Behav. Evol.,* 10: 425–470.

Sleep as a Restorative Process:
Human Clues

Department of Psychiatry, University of Edinburgh, Scotland (U.K.)

INTRODUCTION

This chapter and that of Dr. K. Adam, which follows, examine the proposition that sleep is for growth and tissue restoration, and that sleep provides optimal conditions for protein synthesis. Protein synthesis and degradation proceed all the time, but they are not always equal. The metabolic conditions of wakefulness allow degradation to have priority, as indeed would be essential to cope with emergencies. In sleep it would seem that the balance between degradation and synthesis can shift in favour of synthesis.

The proposition that sleep is associated with tissue restoration does not deny that sleep as a behaviour may be advantageous in its own right. It would be expected that in evolution species would so evolve that their sleep habits would be optimal for survival. Species that are constantly liable to being killed by other animals will survive better if they stay awake more. The belief that sleep is associated with tissue restoration does not rest upon assumptions about the length of time needed to be spent in sleep either by the individual or the species. It would merely be expected that there would be a broad relationship of longer or more intensely restorative sleep to counter-balance greater waking degradation.

Shakespeare's Macbeth called sleep "chief nourisher in life's feast". In modern times, the Nobel laureate, W.R. Hess (1965) wrote of how, "At the height of maximal activity . . . a negative balance ensues" and how the resultant fatigue and consequent sleep brought about "restorative processes . . . during the functional relaxation with the compensation of defects in the structural organization, either of the cell membranes or conditions within the cell". Human defects after sleep loss have been easiest to demonstrate for brain function and so some modern writers have tended to assume that it was for the brain alone that sleep provided restoration. Thus, Feinberg et al. (1967) wrote: "Sleep is a function of the rate of waking brain metabolism . . . need for rest or restitution of neurones . . .", in contrast to Kety (1960) who had suggested the "possibility that . . . in sleep, the brain is the servant of the body . . . the need for sleep . . . perhaps in the muscular system, the heart, kidneys . . .".

More mitoses with sleep

In fact, there has been evidence for over 40 years that bodily growth and renewal is faster during the time of sleep. Blumenfeld (1938) studied mitoses in the rat kidney and, using statistical methods uncommon in his day, reported a significantly higher rate of mitoses by day than by night. Rats, it will be remembered, normally sleep by day when it is light. In contrast, humans sleep in the nighttime and Cooper (1939) reported that in the skin of human infants the mitotic rate was significantly greater by night than by day. A much faster rate of skin renewal through mitosis during the sleep period of mice was reported by Halberg et al. (1965), while Fisher (1968) described the same phenomenon for human adults. More recently, Valk and Van den Bosch (1978), making precise measurement of ulnar length, concluded that most of the bone's growth in boys took place in the night.

I was led to propose some years ago that: "living organisms show rhythms of motor activity and motor inactivity ... wakefulness and sleep ... sleep, when energy expenditure is internally directed, for synthesis of molecules required for growth and repair" (Oswald, 1973). The time relation between the motor activity and inactivity periods and the decreases and increases of tissue renewal seemed apparent, but my own ideas about the internal direction of energy for synthesis were muddled, and Kirstine Adam saw the mechanisms more clearly (Adam and Oswald, 1977).

Species metabolic rate correlates with sleep

Among the papers that encouraged a renewed interest in the restorative function of sleep was that of Zepelin and Rechtschaffen (1974), who drew data about sleep from studies of 53 mammalian species. They looked to see whether longer sleep in a species correlated with longer life-span, but found no relationship. They also looked at the relationship between sleep and metabolic rate. In some cases there were metabolic data available but they also relied upon the high linear correlation between body weight and total metabolism of the animal per day, from which could be calculated the metabolic rate per unit body weight. They found a positive correlation of 0.64 ($P < 0.001$) between the habitual daily duration of sleep and the metabolic rate of the species. Animals with a higher rate of oxidative metabolism were thus found to sleep longer on average, as if in compensation. Zepelin and Rechtschaffen found a correlation between the duration of slow-wave sleep and metabolic rate, and this was later confirmed by Allison and Cicchetti (1976). It is clear that, on an interspecies basis, the more bodily work done in daily activity, the greater the duration of sleep, and especially of slow-wave sleep.

Slow-wave sleep is worth more

In the course of a night's sleep there are cyclical changes, with a period of about 100 min in the adult human. At one time these were thought of as recrudescences of light sleep but it was realized that there were two kinds of sleep that alternated (Oswald, 1962). One is known as orthodox or non-rapid-eye-movement (NREM) sleep, and the other as paradoxical or rapid-eye-movement (REM) sleep. Human orthodox sleep is divided into 4 stages, according to the electroencephalogram, and stages 3 and 4 are called slow-wave sleep, or SWS. If sleep is disturbed selectively so that subjects are deprived especially of paradoxical sleep, then, as Dement (1960) showed, and many others since, when unbroken sleep is allowed there appears to be compensation in time for some of the paradoxical sleep lost. Likewise, as Agnew et al. (1964) first showed, selective deprivation of slow-wave sleep, carried out by disturbing the sleeper so that he remains in stage 2, leads later to more slow-wave sleep, as if in compensation. We need sleep, and it looks as if we need both kinds of sleep.

The fact that there are two different kinds of sleep has led to ideas that they might have different roles in the restorative process. I earlier suggested that the chief function for slow-wave sleep might be for general bodily restitution and that paradoxical sleep might be in some way "chiefly for brain repair" (Oswald, 1969; Oswald, 1970). Hartmann (1973) wrote a book on the functions of sleep and suggested that slow-wave sleep was "responsible for anabolism and production of macromolecules" and that paradoxical sleep "may make use of some of these macromolecules in processes of restoration and reconnections". However, it has been easier to see a link between SWS and the need for restoration.

Simple lack of sleep causes sleep onset to occur more quickly (Agnew and Webb, 1971) and causes subsequent relative enhancement of the proportion of SWS, either after deliberate deprivation of sleep for several days and nights (Berger and Oswald, 1962; Williams et al., 1964), or even within a single day, when, as Agnew and Webb (1968) wrote, "the degree and the amount of stage 4 is a function of the time since prior sleep" (see also Karacan et al., 1970; Webb and Agnew, 1971). As Dement and Greenberg (1966) put it, SWS is "worth more".

Hormones: anabolic during sleep, catabolic during wakefulness

• The greatest encouragement for a return of interest to sleep's restorative role came with the Japanese discovery of a link between SWS and the large nocturnal secretion of human growth hormone (GH). The secretion actually depends (in undrugged states) upon the presence of SWS (Sassin et al., 1969; Schnure et al., 1971). The effect of this sleep-released growth hormone would be, as Parker et al. (1969) put it, "to enhance amino acid incorporation and diminish their diversion to gluconeogenesis . . . effect on growth and repair in sleep so sleep has an anabolic function".

Growth hormone (GH) stimulates amino acid uptake into tissues, promotes protein and RNA synthesis (Korner, 1965) and has other actions, such as the stimulation of human red blood cell formation indirectly through potentiation of erythropietin (Golde et al., 1977). It raises blood-free fatty acids, the subsequent degradation of which provides energy for cellular work, thereby saving amino acids from catabolism and increasing their availability for protein synthesis during sleep. In contrast to the high levels of GH during sleep, corticosteroids are low in the night and only rise as the morning approaches. Corticosteroids stimulate protein catabolism. As a consequence of this harmonious inverse relationship there is even greater net protein synthesis during human sleep, as demonstrated by Rudman et al. (1973) who injected GH and found significantly greater nitrogen retention after a dose just before bedtime than after a dose at 08.00 h when corticosteroids are high.

Whereas the growth hormone release is sleep-dependent, the rise of corticosteroids at the end of the night's sleep is part of a circadian rhythm and if the time for sleep and wakefulness are abruptly altered, then the rise of corticosteroid secretion still occurs at the original clock time, and will only be changed by the passage of days and weeks under a new time schedule of sleep and wakefulness (Weitzman et al., 1975). Consequently, in the man who starts night-shift working, the normal relation between the secretions of growth hormone and corticosteroids is lost, and this fact alone would make the night-shift worker's sleep less restorative. During the first week after starting night-shift, the circadian rhythm of high daylight adrenaline output persists (Åkerstedt, 1977), and this too would reduce the restorative value of the daytime sleep, while persisting low values of adrenaline at night would make the worker less efficient at his job.

It is not only GH that is sleep-dependent, but also the large rise in human prolactin secretion at night (Sassin et al., 1973), as well as luteinizing hormone and testosterone during early puberty (Boyar et al., 1974; Rubin et al., 1976) and all 4 hormones are anabolic in their actions. Adult men have their highest testosterone at night, and human plasma vasopressin too is highest at night (George et al., 1975); vasopressin stimulates brain protein synthesis in the rat (Benetato et al., 1972).

In sharp contrast is the waking pattern of hormones, with high levels of secretion of the catecholamines and corticosteroids, both of which are strongly catabolic. Catecholamine secretion, as manifested by excretion, is lowest in sleep, while during wakefulness it rises and is highest if there is greater physical activity (Townshend and Smith, 1973). Corticosteroids too are lowest in sleep and are greater during a day of activity than a day of waking rest (Weitzman et al., 1975).

INCREASED METABOLIC DEMAND IS ASSOCIATED WITH MORE RESTORATIVE SLEEP

If sleep is for restoration, then we could expect that extra degradation by day, through increased metabolic demands, would lead to compensation through more restorative sleep at night. The first clear indicator of this phenomenon came from the work of Hobson (1968) with cats. After moderate exercise on a treadmill, the cats fell asleep more quickly and they had more synchronized (slow-wave) sleep. In man it would seem that increased metabolic demand by day is indeed associated with more restorative sleep at night, or at least by sleep of longer duration, by more slow-wave sleep, and by more growth hormone.

Physical exercise causes subsequent sleepiness and impairs performance on tests of alertness (Lubin et al., 1976). In association with greater waking exercise, Moses et al. (1977) and Walker et al. (1978) reported a longer duration of sleep in man. Investigations of athletes have found that extra exercise is associated with more slow-wave sleep (Baekeland and Lasky, 1966; Zloty et al., 1973; Maloletnev and Telia, 1975; Shapiro et al., 1975; Griffin and Trinder, 1978), while my colleagues and I found that greater physical exercise among non-athletes caused more nocturnal growth hormone secretion and that the catabolic corticosteroids during sleep were reduced to even lower levels than normal (Adamson et al., 1974).

The total human daily energy expenditure is proportional to body weight, since a heavy body requires more energy in order that it may be carried around all day. This increased metabolic demand by day among people who are overweight is associated with longer total sleep (Crisp and McGuiness, 1976; Adam, 1977). Human body temperature rises during the day as a function of the raised metabolic rate (Timbal et al., 1972) and it falls again during nocturnal sleep. When body temperature and catecholamines are highest, psychomotor efficiency is greatest (Fröberg et al., 1972; Frankenhaeuser, 1975). Some people have a higher metabolic rate and higher temperatures during the day than others. Taub and Berger (1976) studied a group of 10 healthy young men who habitually slept around 10 h per night and compared them with a group of healthy young men who habitually slept between 7 and 8 h per night. The longer sleepers had higher daytime body temperatures, faster reaction times and fewer errors, suggesting that they had by day a higher metabolic rate and that their longer sleep by night was for compensation.

Thyroid hormone raises the metabolic rate and whereas patients who are hypothyroid have no slow-wave sleep (Kales et al., 1967), patients with hyperthyroidism have an unusually high proportion of SWS among their total sleep and more nocturnal growth hormone (Dunleavy et al., 1974). After days during which normal men had had higher thyroxine secretion they had more SWS at night (Johns et al., 1975).

Acute starvation too increases metabolic demands, for instead of using food we burn up our body tissues, including muscle and fat. This increased metabolic demand of acute starvation increases slow-wave sleep and the secretion of nocturnal growth hormone (Parker et al., 1972; MacFadyen et al., 1973; Karacan et al., 1973). If instead there is chronic intake of a drug used for slimming purposes, such as fenfluramine, there has been found to be increase of slow-wave sleep and possibly of nocturnal growth hormone (Lewis et al., 1971; Dunleavy et al., 1973).

Loss of sleep for prolonged periods is itself stressful and there is a higher excretion of catecholamines (Fröberg et al., 1972). The increased metabolic demand causes increased breakdown of body protein, as manifested by greater nitrogen excretion (Scrimshaw et al., 1966); sleep deprivation causes, as already mentioned, a subsequent increased proportion of slow-wave sleep, and, in monkeys, an increase of sleep-related growth hormone secretion when sleep eventually is allowed (Jacoby et al., 1975). Even during a short nap within a single day, human GH secretion is greater with greater elapsed time since sleep (Karacan et al., 1974).

. We thus see recurring themes that imply a special role for slow-wave sleep, and we may recall the earlier conclusions about the pattern of catabolic hormones by day and anabolic hormones by night, the growth hormone being especially associated with slow-wave sleep. However, there are reasons more fundamental than the hormone pattern why sleep, and slow-wave sleep in particular, should favour anabolism, namely the relationship to cellular work (see too the next chapter).

UNRESPONSIVENESS AND LOW CELLULAR WORK

If one asks what are the fundamental features of sleep, it can be said that they are *inertia* and *unresponsiveness*. Through sleep the central nervous system enforces rest, with a generalized low rate of cellular work. The inertia can provide rest for the greater part of the body, but it is only the unresponsiveness of sleep that allows the central nervous system to rest. Bodily immobility alone will not restore the brain, nor the impairment of skilled performance caused by sleep loss: "bedrest is not a substitute for sleep" (Lubin et al., 1976). Wakefulness is a state of high responsiveness, a high rate of cellular work and a consequent high rate of oxidative metabolism. Sleep is a state of unresponsiveness, with a low rate of cellular work and hence of low oxidative metabolism.

Responsiveness and work lowest in slow-wave sleep

If we consider human responsiveness to meaningful sounds, Williams et al. (1966) demonstrated that, compared with wakefulness, responsiveness is lower during stage 1, lower still during stage 2, lowest of all during stages 3 and 4 (SWS), and at a rather higher level, comparable to stage 2, during paradoxical sleep. The pattern of responsiveness of the scratch reflex in patients with itchy skins is exactly the same, with sleep being a time of low responsiveness and SWS being again the time of most profound unresponsiveness (Savin et al., 1975). The same relationships are again true of the incidence of another form of rhythmic activity during sleep, tooth-grinding (Satoh and Harada, 1973). Precisely the same relationships within the different sleep stages, as compared with wakefulness, are found for the reflexes that maintain human blood pressure (Coccagna et al., 1971). Eye blink reflexes too follow the same relationships, with lowest responsiveness during stages 3 and 4 sleep, although in the report by Erkulvrawatr et al. (1978) the frequency of blink reflexes rose as high during paradoxical sleep as during wakefulness, but their latency was longer.

The relationship of these variations in responsiveness in the different sleep stages to cellular work is clear if one considers oxygen consumption. Benedict (1915) had shown that whole body heat production is reduced during sleep compared with resting wakefulness. Since then there have been a number of studies that have have shown that oxygen consumption is lower during sleep than wakefulness, but most of these have not made minute to minute observations of sleep or taken note of the variations with movements during sleep. A satisfactory report in this regard is that of Brebbia and Altshuler (1968). They found a major fall in oxygen consumption between resting wakefulness and stages 1 and 2 sleep, and that the further small fall between stage 2 and SWS was statistically highly significant, with, once again, the rate of whole body oxygen consumption being slightly higher during REM sleep, and similar then to that during stage 2.

In sleep there is a low rate of cerebral activation from the brain stem reticular formation and the consequent unresponsiveness provides the hallmark of sleep (Steriade, 1970). Responsiveness depends on high levels of activation, with a greater rate of movement of potassium and other ions out of and back into brain cells, and more work by the ion pumps that undertake most of the cellular work of the brain. Direct measurements of oxygen consumption in the dog brain have shown that it is significantly lower during sleep than during wakefulness (Ingvar, 1974) and cerebral blood flow, usually an indicator of oxidative metabolism, in man is at its lowest during slow-wave sleep, being then some 35% below resting awake levels (Derman et al., 1979).

The unresponsiveness of sleep thus ensures a low rate of cellular work throughout the body and the brain, and as a consequence there is low oxygen consumption during sleep. Responsiveness is lowest during SWS, and so is oxygen consumption. This time of lowest rate of cellular work, in slow-wave sleep, is the same time that Dement and Greenberg (1966) concluded was "worth more" for restorative purposes.

A high rate of cellular work and higher body temperatures characterize wakefulness, in which there is a capacity for extremely high rates of degradation, at whatever cost, in order to cope with emergencies. In order to restore the balance there would have to be other times when synthesis outweighed degradation and the time of lowest cellular work, i.e. during sleep, might be expected to allow the balance between degradation and synthesis to shift in favour of maximal protein synthesis. Why this is inevitably so is described in the next chapter.

PARADOXICAL SLEEP

As earlier mentioned, in 1969 I myself, and in 1973 Hartmann, proposed that paradoxical sleep had some special role for synthetic functions in the brain. It had been possible to point to high proportions of paradoxical sleep associated in time with presumed brain repair after episodes of poisoning (Haider and Oswald, 1970; Oswald et al., 1973). There was also known to be a large proportion of active sleep (which appears to be the equivalent of paradoxical sleep in the new-born, including the premature infant) at a time when brain growth is very rapid. Conversely, when the brain synthetic mechanisms are failing to renew the substance of the brain, so that it is actually shrinking in senility, there is a disproportionate fall in the time spent in paradoxical sleep (Feinberg et al., 1967). The proportion of sleep spent in paradoxical sleep is low in association with low rates of cognitive processing among adult mental defectives (Feinberg, 1968). Human memory traces or engrams are strengthened during sleep and, although there is still some controversy, the weight of evidence favours paradoxical sleep as being particularly important for the protein synthesis that is presumably needed to strengthen the memory trace (Idzikowski, 1978; Barondes, 1970). All these general relationships seemed to point to paradoxical sleep as a time especially for brain synthetic processes.

When making my earlier suggestion, however, I failed to realize the problem posed by the high cerebral blood flow during paradoxical sleep, higher indeed than during resting wakefulness (Townsend et al., 1973). In general, the blood flow through a tissue is proportional to the rate of oxidative metabolism, and if oxidative metabolism is higher during paradoxical sleep than during resting wakefulness then, unless there is compartmentalization, it is not compatible with a relatively high rate of net protein synthesis in brain cells. Also to be considered is the report by Adam (1977) that the proportion of sleep spent in paradoxical sleep among adults in later middle-age, when they are of stable weight and regular life habits, and when they have been allowed to become thoroughly accustomed to the laboratory, is proportional to gross body weight and therefore to total daily bodily work. In paradoxical sleep the muscles are flaccid and therefore paradoxical sleep is the time of maximal rest for the muscles which carry the body weight around all day. Since the body weight of mental defectives is highly correlated with their intelligence (when the body fails to grow so too does the brain: Mosier et al., 1965), the relationship between less paradoxical sleep and lower IQ in mental defectives could be explicable in terms of their body weight, and not their cognitive processing. At the present time, therefore, paradoxical sleep remains paradoxical!

CONCLUSIONS

The traditional belief that sleep is associated with tissue restoration is once more in favour among many scientists, and there is supporting evidence from studies of tissue renewal, for example, by mitosis. Across species there is a positive correlation between greater duration of sleep and the need for more restoration, owing to a higher daily metabolic rate. In the human, increased metabolic demand leads to longer total sleep, more slow-wave sleep and more growth hormone, again suggesting compensatory restoration.

Whereas the hormone pattern of wakefulness promotes catabolism, the hormone pattern of sleep favours anabolism. More fundamentally, sleep is a time of inertia and unresponsiveness, the latter ensuring rest, not only for the body, but also for the brain. The unresponsiveness is associated with a low rate of oxygen consumption because of a low rate of cellular work. The low rate of cellular work during sleep in turn requires less degradation, and would thus allow more net protein synthesis. Human slow-wave sleep is the time of most extreme unresponsiveness, of lowest work and it is "worth more". The role of paradoxical sleep remains unclear.

REFERENCES

Adam, K. (1977) Brain rhythm that correlates with obesity. *Brit. med. J.,* 2: 234–4.
Adam, K. and Oswald, I. (1977) Sleep is for tissue restoration. *J. roy. Coll. Physicians.,* 11: 376–388.
Adamson, L., Hunter, W.M., Ogunremi, O.O., Oswald, I. and Percy-Robb, I.W. (1974) Growth hormone increase during sleep after daytime exercise. *J. Endocr.,* 62: 473–478.

Agnew, H.W. and Webb, W.B. (1968) The displacement of stage 4 and REM sleep within a full night of sleep. *Psychophysiology,* 5: 142–148.

Agnew, H.W. and Webb, W.B. (1971) Sleep latencies in human subjects: age, prior wakefulness, and reliability. *Psychonom. Sci.,* 24: 253–254.

Agnew, H.W., Webb, W.B. and Williams, R.L. (1964) The effects of stage four sleep deprivation. *Electroenceph. clin. Neurophysiol.,* 17: 68–70.

Åkerstedt, T. (1977) Inversion of the sleep–wakefulness pattern: effects on circadian variations in psychophysiological activation. *Ergonomics,* 20: 459–474.

Allison, T. and Cicchetti, D.V. (1976) Sleep in mammals: ecological and constitutional correlates. *Science,* 194: 732–734.

Baekeland, F. and Lasky, R. (1966) Exercise and sleep patterns in college athletes. *Percept. mot. Skills,* 23: 1203–1207.

Barondes, S.H. (1970) Cerebral protein synthesis inhibitors block long-term memory. *Int. Rev. Neurobiol.,* 12: 177–206.

Benedict, F.G. (1915) Investigations at a nutrition laboratory of the Carnegie Institution of Washington. *Science,* 42: 75–84.

Benetato, G.R., Bordeianu, A. and Butculescu, I. (1972) Effect of vasopressin on protein metabolism in the hypothalamus. *Rev. roum. Physiol.,* 9: 177–182.

Berger, R.J. and Oswald, I. (1962) Effects of sleep deprivation on behaviour, subsequent sleep and dreaming. *J. ment. Sci.,* 108: 457–465.

Blumenfeld, C.M. (1938) Periodic and rhythmic mitotic activity in the kidney of the albino rat. *Anat. Rec.,* 72: 435–443.

Boyar, R.M., Rosenfeld, R.S., Kapen, S., Finkelstein, J.W., Roffwarg, H.P., Weitzman, E.D. and Hellman, L. (1974) Human puberty: simultaneous augmented secretion of luteinizing hormone and testosterone during sleep. *J. clin. Invest.,* 54: 609–618.

Brebbia, D.R. and Altshuler, K.Z. (1968) Stage related patterns and nightly trends of energy exchange during sleep. In *Computers and Electronic Devices in Psychiatry,* N.S. Kline and E. Laska (Eds.), Grune and Stratton, New York, pp. 319–335.

Coccagna, G., Mantovani, M., Brignani, F., Manzini, A. and Lugaresi, E. (1971) Arterial pressure changes during spontaneous sleep in man. *Electroenceph. clin. Neurophysiol.,* 31: 277–281.

Cooper, Z.K. (1939) Mitotic rhythm in human epidermis. *J. invest. Derm.,* 2: 289–300.

Crisp, A.H. and McGuiness, B. (1976) Jolly fat: relation between obesity and psychoneurosis in general population. *Brit. med. J.,* 1: 7–9.

Dement, W. (1960) The effects of dream deprivation. *Science,* 131: 1705–1707.

Dement, W. and Greenberg, S. (1966) Changes in total amount of stage four sleep as a function of partial sleep deprivation. *Electroenceph. clin. Neurophysiol.,* 20: 523–526.

Derman, S., Karacan, I., Meyer, J.S. and Sakain, F. (1980) Regional cerebral blood flow of normal volunteers during sleep. *Sleep Res.,* 8: in press.

Dunleavy, D.L.F., Oswald, I., Brown, P. and Strong, J.A. (1974) Hyperthyroidism, sleep and growth hormone. *Electroenceph. clin. Neurophysiol.,* 36: 259–263.

Dunleavy, D.L.F., Oswald, I. and Strong, J.A. (1973) Fenfluramine and growth hormone release. *Brit. med. J.,* 3: 48.

Erkulvrawatr, S., Feldman, R.G., Sax, D.S. and Ohr, J.T. (1978) Cyclic alterations of blink reflexes: an EEG and EMG study during wakefulness and sleep. *Clin. Electroenceph.,* 9: 173–180.

Feinberg, I. (1968) Eye movement activity during sleep and intellectual function in mental retardation. *Science,* 159: 1256.

Feinberg, I. (1974) Changes in sleep cycle patterns with age. *J. psychiat. Res.,* 10: 283–306.

Feinberg, I., Koresko, R.L. and Heller, N. (1967) EEG sleep patterns as a function of normal and pathological aging in man. *J. psychiat. Res.,* 5: 107–144.

Fisher, L.B. (1968) The diurnal mitotic rhythm in the human epidermis. *Brit. J. Derm.,* 80: 75–80.

Frankenhaeuser, M. (1975) Sympathetic-adrenomedullary activity, behaviour and the psychosocial environment. In *Research in Psychophysiology,* P.H. Venables and M.J. Christie (Eds.), John Wiley, London, pp. 71–94.

Fröberg, J., Karlsson, C.G., Levi, L. and Lidberg, L. (1972) Circadian variations in performance, psychological ratings, catecholamine excretion, and diuresis during prolonged sleep deprivation. *Int. J. Psychobiol.,* 2: 23–36.

George, C.P.L., Messerli, F.H., Genest, J., Nowaczynski, W., Boucher, R., Kuchel, O. and Rojo-Ortega, M. (1975) Diurnal variation of plasma vasopressin in man. *J. clin. Endocr.,* 41: 332–338.

Golde, D.W., Bersch, N. and Li, C.H. (1977) Growth hormone: species-specific stimulation of erythropoiesis in vitro. *Science*, 196: 1112–1113.

Griffin, S.J. and Trinder, J. (1978) Physical fitness, exercise and human sleep. *Psychophysiology*, 15: 447–450.

Haider, I. and Oswald, I. (1970) Late brain recovery processes after drug overdose. *Brit. med. J.*, 2: 318–322.

Halberg, F., Galichi, J.H., Ungar, F. and French, L.A. (1965) Circadian rhythmic pituitary adrenocorticotropic activity, rectal temperature and pinnal mitoses of starving, dehydrated C mice. *Proc. Soc. exp. Biol. N.Y.*, 118: 414–419.

Hartmann, E.L. (1973) *The Functions of Sleep*, Yale University Press, New Haven.

Hess, W.R. (1965) Sleep as a phenomenon of the integral organism. In *Sleep Mechanisms*, K. Akert, C. Bally and J.P. Schadé (Eds.), Elsevier, Amsterdam, pp. 3–8.

Hobson, J.A. (1968) Sleep after exercise. *Science*, 162: 1503–1505.

Idzikowski, C.J. (1978) Sleep and memory in humans. In *Practical Aspects of Memory*, M.M. Gruneberg, P.G. Morris and R.N. Sykes (Eds.), Academic Press, London, pp. 311–318.

Ingvar, D.H. (1974) Sleep and intracranial pathology: introduction. In *Sleep*, P. Levin and W.P. Koella (Eds.), Karger, Basel, pp. 164–169.

Jacoby, J.H., Smith, E., Sassin, J.F., Greenstein, M. and Weitzman, E.D. (1975) Altered growth hormone secretory pattern following prolonged sleep deprivation in the rhesus monkey. *Neuroendocrinology*, 18: 9–15.

Johns, M.W., Masterton, J.P., Paddle-Ledinek, J.E., Patel, Y.C., Winikoff, D. and Malinek, M. (1975) Variations in thyroid function and sleep in healthy young men. *Clin. Sci. molec. Med.*, 49: 629–632.

Kales, A., Heuser, G., Jacobson, A., Kales, J.D., Hanley, J., Zweizig, J.R. and Paulson, M.J. (1967) All night sleep studies in hypothyroid patients before and after treatment. *J. clin. Endocr.*, 27: 1593–1599.

Karacan, I., Rosenbloom, A.L., Londono, J.H., Salis, P.J., Thornby, J.I. and Williams, R.L. (1973) The effect of acute fasting on sleep and the sleep-growth hormone response. *Psychosomatics*, 14: 33–37.

Karacan, I., Rosenbloom, A.L., Londono, J.H., Williams, R.L. and Salis, P.J. (1974) Growth hormone levels during morning and afternoon naps. *Behav. Neuropsychiat.*, 6: 67–70.

Karacan, I., Williams, R.L., Finley, W.W. and Hursch, C.J. (1970) The effects of naps on nocturnal sleep: influence on the need for stage-1 REM and stage 4 sleep. *Biol. Psychiat.*, 2: 391–399.

Kety, S. (1960) General discussion. In *The Nature of Sleep*, G.E.W. Wolstenholme and M. O'Connor (Eds.), Churchill, London, p. 394.

Korner, A. (1965) Growth hormone control of biosynthesis of protein and ribonucleic acid. *Recent Progr. Hormone Res.*, 21: 205–236.

Lewis, S.A., Oswald, I. and Dunleavy, D.L.F. (1971) Chronic fenfluramine administration: some cerebral effects. *Brit. med. J.*, 3: 67–70.

Lubin, A., Hord, D.J., Tracy, M.L. and Johnson, L.C. (1976) Effects of exercise, bedrest and napping on performance decrement during 40 hours. *Psychophysiology*, 13: 334–339.

MacFadyen, U.M., Oswald, I. and Lewis, S.A. (1973) Starvation and human slow-wave sleep. *J. appl. Physiol.*, 35: 391–394.

Maloletnev, V.I. and Telia, Z.A. (1975) The influence of exercise on the night sleep in man. *Bull. Acad. Sci. Georgian SSR*, 77: 449–452.

Moses, J., Lubin, A., Naitoh, P. and Johnson, L.C. (1977) Exercise and sleep loss: effects on recovery sleep. *Psychophysiology*, 14: 414–416.

Mosier, H.D., Grossman, H.J. and Dingman, H.F. (1965) Physical growth in mental defectives. A study in an institutionalized population. *Pediatrics*, 36: 317–462.

Oswald, I. (1962) Sleep mechanisms: recent advances. *Proc. roy. Soc. Med.*, 55: 910–912.

Oswald, I. (1969) Human brain protein, drugs and dreams. *Nature (Lond.)*, 223: 893–897.

Oswald, I. (1970) Sleep, the great restorer. *New Scientist*, 46: 170–172.

Oswald, I. (1973) Is sleep related to synthetic purpose? In *Sleep: Physiology, Biochemistry, Psychology, Pharmacology, Clinical Implications*, W.P. Koella and P. Levin (Eds.), Karger, Basel, pp. 225–228.

Oswald, I., Lewis, S.A., Tagney, J., Firth, H. and Haider, I. (1973) Benzodiazepines and human sleep. In *The Benzodiazepines*, S. Garattini, E. Mussini and L.O. Randall (Eds.), Raven Press, New York, pp. 613–625.

288

Parker, D.C., Sassin, J.F., Mace, J.W., Gotlin, R.W. and Rossman, L.G. (1969) Human growth hormone release during sleep: electroencephalographic correlation. *J. clin. Endocr.*, 29: 871–874.

Parker, D.C., Rossman, L.G. and Vanderlaan, E.F. (1972) Persistence of rhythmic human growth hormone release during sleep in fasted and nonisocalorically fed normal subjects. *Metabolism*, 21: 241–252.

Rubin, R.T., Poland, R.E. and Tower, B.B. (1976) Prolactin-related testosterone secretion in normal adult men. *J. clin. Endocr.*, 42: 112–116.

Rudman, D., Freides, D., Patterson, J.H. and Gibbas, D.L. (1973) Diurnal variation in the responsiveness of human subjects to human growth hormone. *J. clin. Invest.*, 52: 912–918.

Sassin, J.F., Frantz, A.G., Kapen, S. and Weitzman, E.D. (1973) The nocturnal rise of human prolactin is dependent on sleep. *J. clin. Endocr.*, 37: 436–440.

Sassin, J.F., Parker, D.C., Johnson, L.C., Rossman, L.G., Mace, J.W. and Gotlin, R.W. (1969) Effects of slow wave sleep deprivation on human growth hormone release in sleep: preliminary study. *Life Sci.*, Part I, 8: 1299–1307.

Sassin, J.F., Parker, D.C., Mace, J.W., Gotlin, R.W., Johnson, L.C. and Rossman, L.G. (1969) Human growth hormone release: relation to slow-wave sleep and sleep–waking cycles. *Science*, 165: 513–515.

Satoh, T. and Harada, Y. (1973) Electrophysiological study on tooth-grinding during sleep. *Electroenceph. clin. Neurophysiol.*, 35: 267–275.

Savin, J.A., Paterson, W.D., Oswald, I. and Adam, K. (1975) Further studies of scratching during sleep. *Brit. J. Derm.*, 93: 297–302.

Schnure, J.J., Raskin, P. and Lipman, R.L. (1971) Growth hormone secretion during sleep: impairment in glucose tolerance and nonsuppressibility by hyperglycemia. *J. clin. Endocr.*, 33: 234–241.

Scrimshaw, N.S., Habicht, J.P., Pellet, P., Piché, M.L. and Cholakos, B. (1966) Effects of sleep deprivation and reversal of diurnal activity on protein metabolism of young men. *Amer. J. clin. Nutr.*, 19: 313–319.

Shapiro, C.M., Griesel, R.D., Bartel, P.R. and Jooste, P.L. (1975) Sleep patterns after graded exercise. *J. appl. Physiol.*, 39: 187–190.

Steriade, M. (1970) Ascending control of thalamic and cortical responsiveness. *Int. Rev. Neurobiol.*, 12: 87–144.

Taub, J.M. and Berger, R.J. (1976) Effects of acute sleep pattern alteration depend upon sleep duration. *Physiol. Psychol.*, 4: 412–420.

Timbal, J., Colin, J., Boutelier, C. and Guieu, J.D. (1972) Bilan thermique de l'homme en ambiance controlée pendant 24 heures. *Pflügers Arch. ges. Physiol.*, 335: 97–108.

Townsend, R.E., Prinz, P.N. and Obrist, W.D. (1973) Human cerebral blood flow during sleep and waking. *J. appl. Physiol.*, 35: 620–625.

Townshend, M.M. and Smith, A.J. (1973) Factors influencing the urinary excretion of free catecholamines in man. *Clin. Sci.*, 44: 253–265.

Valk, I.M. and Van den Bosch, J.S.G. (1978) Intradaily variation of the human ulnar length and short term growth – a longitudinal study in eleven boys. *Growth*, 42: 107–111.

Walker, J.M., Floyd, T.C., Fein, G., Cavness, C., Lualhati, R. and Feinberg, I. (1978) Effects of exercise on sleep. *J. appl. Physiol.*, 44: 945–951.

Webb, W.B. and Agnew, H.W. (1971) Stage 4 sleep: influence of time course variables. *Science*, 174: 1354–1356.

Weitzman, E.D., Boyar, R.M., Kapen, S. and Hellman, L. (1975) The relationship of sleep and sleep stages to neuroendocrine secretion and biological rhythms in man. *Recent Progr. Hormone Res.*, 31: 399–446.

Williams, H.L., Hammack, J.T., Daly, R.L., Dement, W.C. and Lubin, A. (1964) Responses to auditory stimulation, sleep loss and the EEG stages of sleep. *Electroenceph. clin. Neurophysiol.*, 16: 269–279.

Williams, H.L., Morlock, H.C. and Morlock, J.V. (1966) Discriminative responses to auditory signals during sleep. *Psychophysiology*, 2: 208–215.

Zepelin, H. and Rechtschaffen, A. (1974) Mammalian sleep, longevity, and energy metabolism. *Brain Behav. Evol.*, 10: 425–470.

Zloty, R.B., Burdick, J.A. and Adamson, J.D. (1973) Sleep of distance runners. *Activ. nerv. sup. (Praha)*, 15: 217–221.

Sleep as a Restorative Process and a Theory to Explain Why

KIRSTINE ADAM

Department of Psychiatry, University of Edinburgh, Edinburgh, Scotland (U.K.)

· INTRODUCTION

A few years ago Oswald (1969) saw evidence for sleep as a time for restoration and repair of the body and the brain. Restoration or repair must, like growth, depend on protein synthesis. I shall present evidence to support this proposition from nearly 60 reports showing that rates of protein synthesis or of mitotic division are higher at the time of rest and sleep. In addition I shall present a theory, based on fundamental principles, to explain why this should be so.

Oscillations about a mean are inherent in any system subject to feedback control, and this is true of all living systems. In the simplest organisms there are oscillations between food-engulfing activity on the one hand and inactivity with assimilation on the other. There will also be oscillations between a state in which degradative chemical processes are accelerated and one in which synthetic processes are enhanced. I propose that it is the differing energy demands of the activity/inactivity rhythm that chiefly determine the degradative/synthetic rhythm, such that the synthetic period inevitably coincides with the inactive or rest period, and that this is equally true in higher organisms in which a central nervous system ensures rest's integrity through positive unresponsiveness during sleep, and that such relationships, present throughout the animal kingdom, rely upon a fundamental metabolic co-ordinator, the "cellular energy charge". The energy charge is a measure of the available free energy in the form of adenosine triphosphate (ATP).

Fig. 1 summarizes in simple terms the proposition that, as cellular work is reduced energy

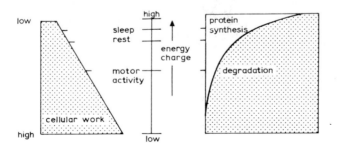

Fig. 1. Differences in cellular work (and so energy charge) during motor activity, rest and sleep and the resulting differences in the rates of degradative processes and protein synthesis.

charge reaches higher levels and so protein synthesis will be favoured and degradative processes will diminish. Cellular work includes the processes involved in the production of heat, motor activity, the maintenance of ion gradients, and active transport systems — all of which use up ATP and so tend to lower the energy charge. The demands of cellular work are thus in competition for ATP with the needs of synthesis.

Feeding must play a vital role in this interplay, since food supplies the substrates for energy production as well as the building materials for the synthesis of structural and storage macromolecules. The intracellular fate of the digestion products from food depends upon the metabolic balance within cells. In higher forms of life, the assimilation of ingested food also depends upon the hormonal environment, for the endocrine systems of the body exert powerful effects on metabolic processes in general, and influence the requirements for the various nutrients. In man at least, the normal hormonal pattern complements the more fundamental rhythms associated with the sleeping/waking cycle.

ACTIVITY/INACTIVITY RHYTHMS AND THE ENERGY CHARGE

Rates of synthesis and degradation controlled by energy charge

To sustain life an organism has to maintain a chemical composition that differs from its surroundings and to do so it must expend energy. It must repair its structural molecules and it must reproduce, both of which involve biosynthetic, energy-using processes, reproduction requiring cell-division as well. The necessary energy is furnished by the catabolism of food and fuel stores to yield ATP and is released by cleavage of the terminal phosphate(s), leaving ADP or AMP (the adenosine di- and monophosphates). These energy-releasing reactions are enzymatically coupled to synthetic reactions, to supply the energy that drives them. The adenine nucleotides, AMP, ADP and ATP, accept, store and transfer chemical potential energy and constitute a link among all the cell's activities. ATP is also used up to do cellular work. This includes the maintenance of chemical gradients (e.g. Na^+/K^+ pumps), active transport, and energy for heat production and for motor activity. Hence, the adenine pool is a link between activity/inactivity rhythms and the catabolic/anabolic balance of the cell.

To achieve co-ordination, some universal, internal signal must operate to enhance or inhibit the cell's chemical activities, all of which can be broadly divided into energy-yielding (ATP-producing) reactions and energy-using (ATP-depleting) processes. It is the energy state of the cell that provides that signal. Its influence on metabolic pathways has been defined by Atkinson (1968), who proposes that the energy charge, EC = (ATP + ADP/2)/ATP + ADP + AMP, of a cell varies within a range up to unity. Lower values of EC favour ATP-producing pathways, while high values of EC promote ATP-utilizing sequences.

The loci of control are regulatory enzymes that are sensitive to the levels of the adenine nucleotides and that catalyze the irreversible steps in biochemical sequences. Every pathway has at least one such step, without which no net flux could occur. Irreversible steps mean that the end-product of a synthetic sequence is not degraded by the reverse of the synthetic pathway, and hence the rates of synthesis and degradation can be controlled by a single signal, which modifies the activities of the regulatory enzymes in both synthetic and degradative pathways simultaneously. The EC level provides such a signal and affects these pathways in opposite ways. Degradative pathways yield ATP and so raise the EC of a cell. A higher level of EC then acts as a signal to reduce the rate of degradation. Synthetic pathways depend on ATP to drive them and are promoted by higher levels of EC. If EC falls, it is a

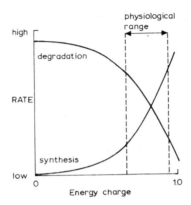

Fig. 2. Typical curves of the rates of reaction of control enzymes in synthetic and degradative pathways in response to different levels of cellular energy charge.

signal to increase degradation and curtail synthesis as the system tries to restore a higher EC, which is thermodynamically more stable (Goldbeter, 1974). Oscillations in the rates of synthesis and degradation are inevitable because of these feedback control mechanisms.

Fig. 2 shows the typical response to changes in EC of the rates of reaction of regulatory enzymes in synthetic and degradative pathways. The control enzymes have response curves with steeper slopes in the region of higher EC and physiological values lie in the highly responsive "cross-over" portion of the graphs (Chapman et al., 1971; Atkinson, 1970) where small changes in EC can disproportionately alter the relative rates of synthesis and degradation. In addition, both types of EC response curves can be modified by the concentration of the biosynthetic end-product in such a way that if, for example, a synthetic end-product were in short supply, then the responsiveness to EC of the control enzymes in the synthetic pathway would be increased and synthesis enhanced (Fig. 3).

A prediction from this theory is that, even under constant conditions, energy production (degradation) and synthetic processes will, in broad terms, exhibit predictable rhythmic variations which are oppositely phased so that when one rhythm has a peak the other shows a trough.

In living organisms these spontaneous rhythms will be perturbed through the variable demands of cellular work over the sleeping/waking rhythm. Cellular work must be done to

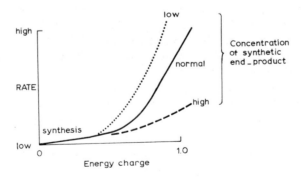

Fig. 3. Typical rate of reaction of a synthetic pathway in response to different levels of cellular energy charge and the modification of this response by high and low concentrations of synthetic end-product.

sustain life, but in doing so it uses up ATP and lowers EC, and will thus stimulate degradative processes and impair those of synthesis. Inactivity (and therefore sleep) reduces the rate at which ATP is used up to do cellular work and I shall also present evidence that the rate of heat production and the activity of the brain Na^+/K^+ ATPase ion pump are both reduced during sleep. Therefore, EC can rise and so synthesis is stimulated and degradation reduced.

Protein synthesis, growth and activity

The concept of energy charge was originally applied to intermediary metabolism, but other processes too are sensitive to EC. The sensitivity of steps in protein synthesis to changes in adenine nucleotides, (Freudenberg and Mager, 1971; Walton and Gill, 1975; Rupniak and Quincey, 1975; Ayuso-Parrilla and Parrilla, 1975; Mendelsohn et al., 1977) are of particular interest, as are the changes in EC that are synchronized with growing and non-growing phases of *E. coli* (Chapman et al., 1971). Such synchronized changes illustrate how EC correlates with anabolic processes.

It is proposed that the simple organism's oscillations between rest and activity, and thus in the amount of cellular work done, must induce concomitant oscillations in EC and so, in turn, in other cellular processes. Motor activity demands ATP and hence, motility and food-gathering will lower EC, promote degradative processes, temporarily suppress biosynthesis and result in a relatively low concentration of protein. After taking in sufficient nourishment it would be economical to rest. The EC would then rise and conditions would be optimal for the biosynthetic processes previously curtailed, and these would be even greater because of the added signal of low protein concentration.

Evidence that motility does inhibit synthetic processes can be seen in an experiment where the unicellular *Stentor coeruleus* was cut in half, such that each half received an equal share of the macronucleus, but only one half had the ciliary apparatus. Subsequent onset of mitotic activity occurred much earlier in the cilia-free end (Guttes and Guttes, 1959). Presumably, the EC must have risen during the enforced rest of the non-ciliated end and acted as a trigger for synthetic processes.

Synthesis during rest in higher organisms

In complex organisms, although motility and responsiveness to the environment are not characteristics of each cell, the same principles apply. Responsiveness, through the information-carrying system, is energy-consuming, and so tends to lower the EC. The house cricket, *Acheta domesticus,* has a 24 h rhythm of RNA and protein synthesis in its brain and sub-oesophageal ganglion, with synthesis being highest when the insects are inactive. Their activity increases sharply with the onset of darkness, whereupon synthesis of RNA and protein in the brain falls to its lowest value (Cymborowski and Dutkowski, 1969, 1970).

Higher organisms store fuel foods to allow prolonged activity without feeding. As in simple organisms, the optimal time for synthetic processes would be during a rest/sleep period following feeding. Many higher animals are observed to rest/sleep after feeding and, indeed, feeding and sleeping have been shown in many investigations to be inter-related (e.g. Crisp and Stonehill, 1976; Danguir and Nicolaidis, 1979).

During activity, the energy-requiring, biosynthetic pathways would be suppressed by a downward shift in the EC, which would stimulate catabolic processes in tissues directly involved (e.g. muscles). Even more tissues would be influenced if their substrates for ATP production and synthesis of macromolecules were diverted as fuel for motor activity. Contracting muscle in vitro has a lower ATP concentration than resting muscle, despite a tripling in the rate of oxidative metabolism (Crabtree and Newsholme, 1972; Newsholme and Start, 1973). Likewise, brief exercise considerably reduces the EC of rat skeletal muscle in vivo (Wojciechowska et al., 1975). The concentration of ATP in biopsies taken from human muscle after 2 min of exercise is 25% less than from resting controls (Karlson and Saltin, 1970). Conversely, the in vivo rates of protein synthesis in rat diaphragm muscle (Rebolledo and Gagliardino, 1971) and myocardium (Rau and Meyer, 1975) are highest during the resting/sleeping period. It has been shown in man that exercise enhances the output of alanine from muscle and its subsequent re-uptake by the liver where it is a gluconeogenic precursor (Ahlborg et al., 1974). As examples of tissues linked indirectly: the rate of protein synthesis falls in the hypothalamus if rats exercise (Bordeianu and Butculescu, 1971), protein synthesis in rat skin is at its highest (Chekulaeva, 1969) and the highest rate of cartilage matrix synthesis in mice (Simmons, 1968) both occur in the daylight, when these rodents rest and sleep.

The effect of 30 min of exercise on the incorporation rate of radioactive methionine into liver, kidney, heart and muscle protein was studied in groups of rats (Mateev et al., 1967). Control rats were compared with experimental rats sacrificed during exertion, and with rats sacrificed at 30 min intervals up to 5 h following the period of exercise. The rate of amino acid incorporation into protein was greatly decreased, both during the exercise period, and for several hours after the exertion had ceased.

In man, exercise inhibits skin mitosis for many hours afterwards (Fisher, 1968), and under certain circumstances has been shown to induce protein catabolism by Molé and Johnson (1971), who found a paradoxical effect of surfeit feeding on protein metabolism: it was anabolic at rest but catabolic following exercise.

Peaks in mitotic rate in frog crystalline lens epithelium coincide with episodes of motor inactivity, whereas troughs are associated with active periods (Kuznetsov et al., 1972). It is important to distinguish such phenomena from the hypertrophy of tissues that results from increased use. The latter involves the activation of genetic material in the nucleus, with increased formation of RNA, and subsequently of proteins many hours later (Meerson, 1975).

Mitosis and ATP

Mitosis depends upon synthesis, whether for tissue maintenance or for the propagation of the species. There is a strong relationship between mitotic activity and higher concentrations of ATP (Guttes and Guttes, 1959). A fall in ATP below a critical level inhibits mitosis (Epel, 1963). A positive correlation between the rhythm of ATP level and cell division has been shown for *Tetrahymena pyriformis* (Plesner, 1964). Moreover, most tissues have a 24 h variation of mitotic rate, with the maximum occurring during the resting/sleeping period, when ATP and EC levels are presumably at their highest. Examples are listed in Table I.

It could be that through evolution the rhythms of energy-dependent mitotic proliferation became entrained to the variations in energy state associated with the rest/activity cycle. The hormones of higher organisms are sophisticated additions to more primitive controls but where investigated they are found to be complementary (Bullough, 1948; Sigelman et al., 1954; Fisher, 1968; Vonnahme, 1974).

TABLE I

MITOSES MAXIMAL DURING THE TIME OF REST AND SLEEP

Species	Tissue	Reference
Ectodermal tissues:		
Man	Epidermis	Cooper and Schiff (1938); Scheving (1959); Fisher (1968)
Mouse	Epidermis	Halberg et al. (1965)
Rat	Epidermis	Chekulaeva (1969)
Rat	Healing epidermis	Gololobova (1960)
Rat	Corneal epithelium	Sigelman et al. (1954)
Mouse	Corneal epithelium	Vasama and Vasama (1958)
Frog	Crystalline lens epithelium	Kuznetsov et al. (1972)
Rat	Pineal parenchyma	Renzoni and Quay (1964)
Rat	Anterior pituitary	Nöuet and Kujas (1975)
Hamster	Cheek pouch epithelium	Brown and Berry (1968); Izquierdo and Gibbs (1972)
Rat	Sebaceous gland cells	Bertalanffy (1957)
Rat	Lacrimal, parotid and submandibular glands	Vonnahme (1974)
Pregnant mice	Mammary alveolar epithelium	Echave Llanos and Piezzi (1963)
Rat	Lip epithelium	Bertalanffy (1960)
Rat	Buccal mucosa	Bertalanffy (1960)
Rat	Anal epithelium	Bertalanffy (1960)
Guinea pig	Tympanic membrane	Reeve (1977)
Mesodermal tissues:		
Man	Bone marrow	Mauer (1965)
Rat	Epiphyseal cartilage	Simmons (1964)
Rat	Bone marrow	Clark and Korst (1969); Hunt and Perris (1974); Uryadnitskaya (1974)
Mouse	Bone marrow	Clark and Korst (1969)
Rat	Kidney tubules	Shavipov (1967); Saetran (1972)
Rat	Thymus	Hunt and Perris (1974); Kirk (1972)
Rat	Inner enamel epithelium incisor teeth	Gasser et al. (1972a)
Endodermal tissues:		
Rat	Liver parenchyma	Vonnahme (1974); Jaffe (1954)
Mouse	Liver	Barnum et al. (1958)
Rat	Tongue	Gasser et al. (1972b)
Mouse	Squamous epithelium of tongue and oesophagus	Burns et al. (1976)
Rat	Rectal mucosa after injury	Reeve (1975)
Rat	Gastric epithelium	Clark and Baker (1962)
Rat	Lung interalveolar septa	Romanova (1966)
Rat	Duodenum	Scheving et al. (1972)
Mouse	Duodenum	Scheving et al. (1972)
Mouse	Colon	Chang (1971)

FEEDING AND SYNTHESIS

Feeding also induces oscillations in metabolism, and in higher organisms it is the liver that has to deal with the influxes of nutrients so that the variations in the blood levels of the various nutrients are not too great.

When a protein meal is fed to dogs, more than half of the incoming amino acids are degraded to urea, a small proportion are retained as liver protein, some are secreted as plasma proteins and only about a quarter of the incoming load passes into the general circulation as free amino acids (Elwyn, 1970).

The 24 h rhythm of net protein synthesis in rat liver (Richardson and Rose, 1971) is the only instance that I could find in the literature of a peak in synthetic rate occurring during the activity period. It may readily be understood why this organ should be the only exception for, in response to an increased amino acid supply, protein synthesis in the liver is accelerated, while protein breakdown is reduced (Munro et al., 1975) which results in the accumulation of enzymes with short half-lives involved in the metabolism of the incoming nutrients. In consequence there are diurnal rhythms in the synthesis of liver enzyme proteins, and in the accumulation and breakdown of liver RNA, which are both related to the intermittent intake of meals containing protein (Munro et al., 1975). However, the rate of cell division in liver is maximal at the usual time for rest and sleep (see Table I for refs.) and so presumably structural repair processes in liver are accelerated at this time.

The plasma levels of amino acids are also affected by dietary carbohydrate through an insulin-dependent mechanism. Within about an hour of consuming carbohydrates, the levels of most plasma amino acids decrease, owing to deposition in muscle through insulin-mediated transport (Munro et al., 1959). Muscle represents the major depot for retention of free amino acids in the body (Munro, 1970), but deposition of amino acids in muscle does not necessarily lead to an increase in protein synthesis rate, as protein synthesis depends on many things, and especially on the intracellular ATP levels.

SLEEP PROMOTES SYNTHETIC PROCESSES

Sleep is more than rest

Rest reduces cellular work and thus reduces ATP depletion, but sleep is more than merely rest. It is a state of unresponsiveness brought about by active nervous mechanisms, a highly evolved form of rest that ensures that the whole body, including the nervous system, has an opportunity to recuperate.

Less energy is expended when asleep than when awake. In man, for instance, the rate of heat production is greater during quiet rest than when asleep (Benedict, 1915), and in those animals that have been studied, heat output is greater during the waking period than at the time of sleep (Besch and Woods, 1977). Energy expenditure, measured as oxygen consumption, is lower during sleep than when awake (Brebbia and Altshuler, 1968). This means that less cellular work is done when asleep, and EC should therefore rise. It has now been shown that in a variety of tissues EC is higher during sleep, and that the rise in EC is *sleep dependent* (Durie et al., 1978).

Sleep is not a uniform state, there are two types of sleep that alternate: NREM, or "orthodox" sleep, and REM or "paradoxical" sleep. Human NREM sleep is divided into stages 1–4, according to electroencephalographic criteria. Stages 3 and 4 are called slow wave sleep (SWS). The stages differ in their degrees of responsiveness, with stage 2 being a less responsive state than stage 1, SWS being a state of least responsiveness, while REM sleep is about equal to stage 2 (Fig. 4). These relationships are true for responses to auditory stimuli (Williams et al., 1964), blood pressure reflexes (Coccagna et al., 1971), and scratching by patients with itchy skins (Savin et al., 1975). In harmony with the differing

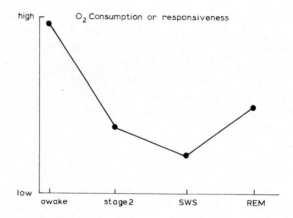

Fig. 4. In stages 3 and 4 (slow wave) sleep, responsiveness is lowest to auditory signals, scratching is least, blood pressure is lowest, and whole-body oxidative metabolism is lowest; the demands of cellular work, that compete with the needs of synthesis, are at their lowest.

degrees of responsiveness, the same relationships hold true for the rates of oxygen consumption that accompany these sleep stages. Human metabolic rate is some 10% lower in stage 2 than in wakeful rest, with a further 2% fall during SWS (Brebbia and Altshuler, 1968); and from this one can understand why SWS is thought to be "worth more" for restoration. The reduction in cellular work in SWS may mean that EC is even higher in SWS than in the other stages of sleep, so that synthetic processes would be further enhanced. In addition, this rise in EC would be in the portion of the response curve (Fig. 2) where small changes in EC lead to disproportionately large changes in the rate of synthesis.

Sleep for growth and repair

In an analysis of data from 53 species, Zepelin and Rechtschaffen (1974) found a positive correlation between daily sleep durations and metabolic rates. Their interpretation was in terms of energy conservation, but, it can be seen from another viewpoint: the higher the rate of metabolism (and hence degradation) during the active period, the longer would be the sleeping period needed for compensatory synthesis. In individual men the customary duration of sleep correlates positively with waking body temperatures, and hence presumably with waking metabolic rate (Taub and Berger, 1976). Growth too depends upon synthetic functions and in one investigation it was found that a group of children of short stature had grown only one-third as fast during times of poor sleep as during times of good sleep (Wolff and Money, 1973).

Growth and repair necessarily depend on net protein synthesis and therefore, on a positive nitrogen balance. Rudman et al. (1973) found that more nitrogen was retained in humans deficient in growth hormone (GH) following an injection of GH at 23.00 h, than after a similar dose at 08.00 h suggesting that subsequent sleep facilitated nitrogen retention and presumably growth in GH deficient children. On the other hand, sleep deprivation for 2 nights in 19 young men led to a significant increase in nitrogen excretion on the second day of deprivation, which continued at high levels during the first post-deprivation day, and on the second post-deprivation day fell to below baseline levels (Scrimshaw et al., 1966). Nitrogen intake was constant throughout this study. Sleep deprivation must be stressful

(Kuhn et al., 1969) and therefore elevated corticosteroids probably contributed to the increased nitrogen excretion. Nevertheless, the results suggest that sleep deprivation enhanced protein and/or amino acid catabolism. The apparent time delay before nitrogen excretion increased following the commencement of sleep deprivation was probably a reflection of the inertia in urea excretion. Growth and repair, of course, also depend on the ingestion of a diet adequate in both energy and protein, but the fate of ingested food depends on the metabolic conditions prevailing during the assimilative period. These metabolic conditions depend on the short- and long-term nutritional status, the extent of motor activity, the time of the day or night and the hormonal environment, factors which are inevitably interdependent.

In man, more amino acids are excreted in the urine during the hours 08.00–11.00 h than between 02.00 and 05.00 h, even during total starvation, (Tewksbury and Lohrenz, 1970) and the same pattern is found for the degradation of tryptophan (Rapoport and Beisel, 1968). Normal subjects have been shown to have a 24 h rhythm in their plasma amino acid levels, with peaks during the day and with lowest levels around 02.00 h. The rhythm persisted in subjects fed a protein-deficient diet (Wurtman et al., 1968a). The latter condition distinguishes the tyrosine amino acid rhythm from the rhythm of activity of the hepatic enzyme, tyrosine transaminase, which is extinguished by a protein deficient diet (Wurtman et al., 1968b). The biological significance of the rhythm of amino acid levels is unclear, but it may represent a stimulation of the uptake of amino acids into tissues at certain times of the 24 h. It is thus interesting that alteration of the sleeping period from 22.00–06.00 h to 10.00–18.00 h caused a rapid shift (within 48 h) in the peak plasma amino acid concentration to 04.00 h, i.e. into the new activity period (Feigin et al., 1968).

The hormones of sleep

The large nocturnal secretion of human GH (Takahashi et al., 1968; Honda et al., 1969), is dependent upon the presence of sleep and especially of SWS (Sassin et al., 1969; Schnure et al., 1971). This itself reveals sleep to be a time that facilitates anabolic processes in man, since GH stimulates amino acid uptake into tissues, promotes protein and RNA synthesis (Korner, 1965) and has wide inter-reactions, such as stimulating red blood cell formation indirectly through erythropoietin (Peschle et al., 1972). It raises blood free fatty acids, the subsequent degradation of which is a source of cellular energy (ATP), thereby saving amino acids from catabolism and increasing their availability for protein synthesis during sleep.

Corticosteroids reduce net protein synthesis (Ardeleanu and Sterescu, 1973; Friedman and Strang, 1966) and nocturnal GH comes at that time in the 24 h when corticosteroids are lowest (Weitzman et al., 1971). Consequently, even greater protein synthesis occurs during human sleep, as demonstrated by Rudman et al. (1973) who injected GH and found significantly greater nitrogen retention after a dose at 23.00 h than after a dose at 08.00 h.

Three other sleep-dependent hormones are known: prolactin (Sassin et al., 1973), luteinizing hormone and testosterone (Boyar et al., 1972, 1974; Rubin et al., 1973, 1976); all 4 hormones released by sleep are thus hormones that promote anabolism.

Slow wave sleep for compensatory restoration

It has been suggested that sleep, and slow wave sleep in particular, may have compensatory features for the degree of waking activity. This is reviewed by Oswald in this book. I would like to add that, based on the argument I put forward earlier, SWS will also be most strongly associated with anabolic repair because cellular work is predicted to be at its lowest during SWS and EC therefore likely to be highest with the result that synthetic processes are further accelerated.

SLEEP AND THE BRAIN

Sleep – a state of unresponsiveness

It is the brain that controls sleep, and it is brain functions such as the power to sustain attention that are most obviously impaired by sleep deprivation. Although the mature brain no longer grows, it still needs synthetic activity. It rivals the liver in its high rate of turnover of proteins and nucleic acids, consistent with its role in information processing, storage and retrieval, which rely on synthetic activity over and above the protein synthesis required for enzymes and renewal of structural components. The benefit of sleep is most obvious for the brain, since during mere rest the nervous system remains highly responsive to the environment, whereas in sleep it becomes relatively unresponsive (Steriade, 1970). The responsiveness of the wakeful cortex depends upon sustained ascending activation from the mesencephalic reticular formation, and the high levels of extracellular K^+ thus caused (Katzman and Grossman, 1975). These higher levels of K^+ are closely coupled to higher energy consumption by the ATPase ion pump (Bachelard, 1975a; Jöbsis et al., 1975; Lowry, 1975). Higher extracellular K^+ implies that intracellular K^+ levels have been lowered. Cerebral protein synthesis is sensitive to *intracellular K^+* concentration. For instance, a rise in intracellular K^+ concentration from 25 to 80 mM resulted in a 6-fold increase in the rate of protein synthesis (Roberts and Zomzely, 1966).

Sleep deprivation impairs mental functions, and as the deprivation continues there is an increasing "pressure" to sleep, which suggests some mounting deficit in cerebral recharging or repair. Fig. 3 enables one to understand why, after prolonged sleep-deprivation (when the concentration of proteins and therefore of end-products would be lower) restoration can be accomplished in fewer hours than were actually lost.

Synthesis and energy charge

Brain protein synthesis is at its highest rate at a time of the 24 h when rats are normally asleep (Richardson and Rose, 1971; Rose et al., 1969; Gordon and Scheving, 1968; Dainat and Rebière, 1978). The cat has several sleep periods, and with each of these there is a rise in the protein content of perfusates from the brain (Drucker-Colín et al., 1975a). Jones (1971) found that brain ATP levels of golden hamsters were higher during sleep.

The parallelism that exists between the rate of RNA synthesis and the ATP concentration in brain slices, and the fact that ATP concentration for optimal amino acid incorporation by microsomal and ribosomal preparations is more critical in the cerebral cortex than in similar preparations from liver (Zomzely et al., 1964), both suggest that the cell content of available ATP is the regulating factor in brain protein synthesis (Itoh and Quastel, 1969).

The protein and RNA content of supra-optic nuclei was higher in sleeping than in waking rats, while the latter in turn had a higher content than sleep-deprived animals (Doemin and Rubinskaya, 1974). Van den Noort and Brine (1970) measured the ATP, ADP and AMP concentrations in rat brain after 13 h of sleep-deprivation and after 1 h of subsequent sleep. Calculations of EC using their results give a value of only 0.77 after 13 h of sleep deprivation but 0.83 after the 1 h of sleep. Sleep deprivation may be stressful and so a more recent study measured the levels of ATP, ADP and AMP in the forebrain and cerebellum of mice that were asleep, and in those that were *spontaneously* awake at the *same time of day* (Durie et al., 1978). Again, EC was higher in the sleeping mice (forebrain EC = 0.92; cerebellum EC = 0.90) than in those that were awake (ECs = 0.79 and 0.78 respectively). The rise in EC associated with sleep is in the highly responsive portion of the curve; Fig. 3 illustrates how protein synthesis in the brain would differ under these two conditions and how there could be additional enhancement of protein synthesis during sleep at a time when end-product concentration would presumably be low.

NREM–REM sleep cycles and protein synthesis

The different physiology of NREM and REM sleep suggests that they differ in function, but a causal relationship has been proposed because NREM always precedes REM sleep (Hartmann, 1973). The leading ATP user of the brain is the Na^+/K^+ ATPase ion pump (Bachelard, 1975a), the rate of activity of which is determined by the rate of neuronal firing (Lowry, 1975). During SWS the majority of neurones have a much reduced firing-rate compared with waking (McGinty et al., 1974). As a result of this low rate, ATP depletion would be reduced and EC level would rise, whereas during subsequent REM sleep the higher firing rates (McGinty et al., 1974) would lower intracellular ATP and stimulate brain glycolysis and respiration. The firing rate of many neurones during REM sleep approximates to waking but this is not in response to the outside world and may represent transfer of information among neurones.

The amount of REM sleep seems to be correlated with the intensity of brain synthetic activity (Oswald, 1969, 1970, 1976; Stern and Morgane, 1974). If higher rates of protein synthesis occur during REM sleep itself in conjunction with the higher rate of cell firing, this would imply compartments of ATP pools between, for example, neurones and glia, or intracellular compartments within neurones, as there is for glucose transport (Bachelard, 1975b).

In higher organisms, protein is synthesized at the rate of two amino acids per sec, which means that it takes 1–2 min to synthesize a medium-sized protein molecule (Dintzis, 1961), in addition to the time required to initiate the process. Oscillations have been found in the rate of protein synthesis in a remarkable diversity of tissues (Brodsky, 1975). There is a theoretical minimum oscillation period of the order of minutes, because of the inertia in the protein synthetic machinery (Goodwin, 1963). The REM periods of most species last only a few minutes, and this is so short a time that the onset of a REM period could hardly be the primary initiator of any increased brain protein synthesis associated with that period. Possibly, peak rates of brain protein synthesis might coincide with the onset of REM periods, conditions for stimulating the peaks having been generated during the preceding SWS, when cell firing would have been at a minimum and when, therefore, EC would have risen.

It has been assumed by many (e.g. Drucker-Colín et al., 1975a) that REM sleep stimulates protein synthesis, but could it not be the other way round, with peaks in protein level or rate of synthesis stimulating the occurrence of REM sleep? There is some evidence to suggest that this may be the case. For instance, prolonged fasting in adult rats greatly reduced the conversion of glucose to protein (Barkai et al., 1974) and feeding deoxyglucose (which cannot be metabolized) caused a decrease in amount of REM sleep in rats (Panksepp et al., 1973). Injection of bovine GH into rats resulted in a temporally related increase in REM sleep and increased levels of whole brain soluble proteins (Drucker-Colín et al., 1975b). In contrast, a similar molecular weight protein, thyrotropin, had no effect on the amount of REM sleep. Anisomycin reduced the amount of sleep, and REM sleep in particular. There was also a time-dependent decrease in brain protein levels. Administration of GH at the same time as the antibiotic returned sleep to control levels.

In humans the effect on sleep patterns of administering glucocorticoid has been investigated by Gillin et al. (1972). They found a dose-related reduction in the amount of REM sleep. Corticosteroids are known readily to penetrate into the brain tissue (Peterson and Chaikoff, 1963) and as these hormones promote protein catabolism (Ardeleanu and Sterescu, 1973; Friedman and Strang, 1966) it could be that a reduction in net protein synthesis led to the decrease in REM sleep. So there does appear to be some evidence to support the proposition that peaks in brain protein concentration may stimulate REM sleep. And it is tempting to speculate with Brodsky (1975) that oscillations in the rate of protein synthesis are in fact the main cause of NREM–REM cycles.

SUMMARY

I propose that the rest/activity cycle of simple organisms and the sleeping/waking rhythm of higher animals induce concomitant fluctuations in cellular energy charge. In turn, the metabolic balance alters such that degradative processes are stimulated during wakefulness and activity, whereas restorative, synthetic processes are inevitably favoured during inactivity and sleep. This hypothesis is presented in broad terms, to apply at all levels of biological integration.

Feeding also induces oscillations in metabolism. In simple organisms, food gathering and motor activity go hand in hand, and the assimilative, synthetic phase is associated with the resting period. Higher organisms do not always rest or sleep after feeding and have evolved complex systems for storage and retrieval of nutrients, which allow them to remain active for relatively long periods of time. Nevertheless, I believe the same general principles apply.

REFERENCES

Ahlborg, G., Felig, P., Hagenfeldt, L., Hendler, R. and Wahren, J. (1974) Substrate turnover during prolonged exercise in man. Splanchnic and leg metabolism of glucose, free fatty acids, and amino acids. *J. clin. Invest.,* 53: 1080–1090.

Ardeleanu, A. and Sterescu, N. (1973) Some aspects of cerebral protein metabolism in relation to age and species. Hormonal influences. *Rev. roum. Physiol.,* 10: 369–377.

Atkinson, D.E. (1968) The energy charge of the adenylate pool as a regulatory parameter. Interaction with feedback modifiers. *Biochemistry,* 7: 4030–4034.

Atkinson, D.E. (1970) Enzymes as control elements in metabolic regulation. In *The Enzymes,* P.D. Boyar (Ed.), *Vol. 1,* Academic Press, New York and London, pp. 461–489.

Ayuso-Parrilla, M.S. and Parrilla, R. (1975) Control of hepatic protein synthesis. Differential effects of ATP levels on the initiation and elongation steps. *Europ. J. Biochem.,* 55: 593–599.

Bachelard, H.S. (1975a) Energy utilized by neurotransmitters. In *Brain Work,* D.H. Ingvar and N.A. Lassen (Eds.), Munksgaard, Copenhagen, pp. 79–81.

Bachelard, H.S. (1975b) How does glucose enter brain cells? In *Brain Work,* D.H. Ingvar and N.A. Lassen (Eds.), Munksgaard, Copenhagen, pp. 126–141.

Barkai, A., Mahadik, S. and Rapport, M.M. (1974) Flow in vivo of glucose carbon to brain protein in rats: effect of starvation. *J. Neurochem.,* 22: 511–516.

Barnum, C.P., Jardetzky, C.D. and Halberg, F. (1958) Time relations among metabolic and morphologic 24 h changes in mouse liver. *Amer. J. Physiol.,* 195: 301–310.

Benedict, F.G. (1915) Investigations at a nutrition laboratory of the Carnegie Institution of Washington. *Science,* 42: 75–84.

Bertalanffy, F.D. (1957) Mitotic activity and renewal rate of sebaceous gland cells in the rat. *Anat. Rec.,* 129: 231–241.

Bertalanffy, F.D. (1960) Mitotic rates and renewal times of the digestive tract epithelia in the rat. *Acta anat. (Basel),* 40: 130–148.

Besch, E.L. and Woods, J.E. (1977) Heat dissipation biorhythms of laboratory animals. *Lab. Animal Sci.,* 27: 54–59.

Bordeianu, A. and Butculescu, I. (1971) Autoradiohistographic study of protein synthesis of brain during exertion. *Rev. roum. Physiol.,* 8: 541–545.

Boyar, R., Finkelstein, J., Roffwarg, H., Kapen, S., Weitzman, E. and Hellman, L. (1972) Synchronization of augmented luteinizing hormone secretion with sleep during puberty. *New Engl. J. Med.,* 287: 582–586.

Boyar, R.M., Rosenfeld, R.S., Kapen, S., Finkelstein, J.W., Roffwarg, H.P., Weitzman, E.D. and Hellman, L. (1974) Simultaneous augmented secretion of luteinizing hormone and testosterone during sleep. *J. clin. Invest.,* 54: 609–618.

Brebbia, D.R. and Altshuler, K.Z. (1968) Stage related patterns and nightly trends of energy exchange during sleep. In *Computers and Electronic Devices in Psychiatry,* N.S. Kline and E. Laska (Eds.), Grune and Stratton, New York, pp. 319–335.

Brodsky, W. (1975) Protein synthesis rhythm. *J. theor. Biol.,* 55: 167–200.

Brown, J.M. and Berry, R.J. (1968) The relationship between diurnal variation of the number of cells in mitosis and of the number of cells synthesizing DNA in the epithelium of the hamster cheek pouch. *Cell Tiss. Kinet.,* 1: 23–33.

Bullough, W.S. (1948) Mitotic activity in the adult male mouse *mus musculus* L. The diurnal cycles and their relations to waking and sleeping. *Proc. roy. Soc. B.,* 135: 212–233.

Burns, E.R., Scheving, L.E., Fawcett, D.F., Gibbs, W.M. and Galatzan, R.E. (1976) Circadian influence on the frequency of labeled mitoses method in the stratified squamous epithelium of the mouse esophagus and tongue. *Anat. Rec.,* 184: 265–274.

Chang, W.W.L. (1971) Renewal of the epithelium in the descending colon of the mouse. 3. Diurnal variation in the proliferative activity of epithelial cells. *Amer. J. Anat.,* 131: 111–119.

Chapman, A.G., Fall, L. and Atkinson, D.E. (1971) Adenylate energy charge in *E. coli* during growth and starvation. *J. Bact.,* 108: 1072–1086.

Chekulaeva, L.I. (1969) The diurnal rhythm of protein metabolism in skin epidermis. *Tsitologiia,* 11: 632–635.

Clark, R.H. and Baker, B.L. (1962) Effect of adrenalectomy on mitotic proliferation of gastric epithelium. *Proc. Soc. exp. Biol. (N.Y.),* 111: 311–315.

Clark, R.H. and Korst, D.R. (1969) Circadian periodicity of bone marrow mitotic activity and reticulocyte counts in rats and mice. *Science,* 166: 236–237.

Coccagna, G., Mantovani, M., Brignani, F., Mancina, A. and Lugaresi, E. (1971) Arterial pressure change during spontaneous sleep in man. *Electroenceph. clin. Neurophysiol.,* 31: 277–281.

Cooper, Z.K. and Schiff, A. (1938) Mitotic rhythm in human epidermis. *Proc. Soc. exp. Biol. (N.Y.),* 39: 323–324.

Crabtree, B. and Newsholme, E.A. (1972) The activities of phosphorylase, hexokinase, phosphofructokinase, lactate dehydrogenase and glycerol 3-phosphate dehydrogenase in muscles from vertebrates and invertebrates. *Biochem. J.,* 126: 49–58.

Crisp, A.H. and Stonehill, E. (1976) *Sleep, Nutrition and Mood,* John Wiley, Chichester, England.

Cymborowski, B. and Dutkowski, A. (1969) Circadian changes in RNA synthesis in the neurosecretory cells of the brain and subesophageal ganglion of the house cricket. *J. insect Physiol.,* 15: 1187–1197.

Cymborowski, B. and Dutkowski, A. (1970) Circadian changes in protein synthesis in the neurosecretory cells of the central nervous system of *Acheta domesticus. J. insect Physiol.,* 16: 341–348.

Dainat, J. and Rebière, A. (1978) Daily variations of the in vivo (^{3}H) leucine incorporation into the cerebellar and cerebral proteins of the normal and hypothyroid young rat. *Experientia (Basel),* 34: 264–265.

Danguir, J. and Nicolaidis, S. (1979) Dependence of sleep on nutrients' availability. *Physiol. Behav.*, 22: 735–740.

Dintzis, H.M. (1961) Assembly of the peptide chains of hemoglobin. *Proc. nat. Acad. Sci. (Wash.)*, 47: 247–261.

Doemin, N.N. and Rubinskaya, N.L. (1974) The protein and RNA content in neurones and their glial cell satellites of the rat brain supra-optic nucleus after REM sleep deprivation lasting 24 h. *Dokl. Akad. Nauk SSSR, Otd. Biokh.*, 214: 940–942.

Drucker-Colín, R.R., Spanis, C.W., Cotman, C.W. and McGaugh, J.L. (1975a) Changes in protein levels in perfusates of freely moving cats: relation to behavioural state. *Science*, 187: 963–965.

Drucker-Colín, R.R., Spanis, C.W., Hunyadi, J., Sassin, J.F. and McGaugh, J.L. (1975b) Growth hormone effects on sleep and wakefulness in the rat. *Neuroendocrinol.*, 18: 1–8.

Durie, D.J.B., Adam, K., Oswald, I. and Flynn, I.W. (1978) Sleep: cellular energy charge and protein synthetic capability. *IRCS Med. Sci.*, 6: 351.

Echave Llanos, J.M. and Piezzi, R.S. (1963) 24 h rhythm in the mitotic activity of normal mammary epithelium on normal and inverted lighting regimens. *J. Physiol. (Lond.)*, 165: 437–442.

Elwyn, D. (1970) The role of the liver in regulation of amino acid and protein metabolism. In *Mammalian Protein Metabolism, Vol. 4*, H.N. Munro (Ed.), Academic Press, New York and London, pp. 523–584.

Epel, D. (1963) The effects of carbon monoxide inhibition on ATP level and the rate of mitosis in the sea urchin egg. *J. Cell Biol.*, 17: 315–319.

Feigin, R.D., Klainer, A.S. and Beisel, W.R. (1968) Factors affecting circadian periodicity of blood amino acids in man. *Metab. clin. Exp.*, 17: 764–775.

Fisher, L.B. (1968) The diurnal mitotic rhythm in the human epidermis. *Brit. J. Derm.*, 80: 75–80.

Friedman, M. and Strang, L.B. (1966) Effect of long term corticosteroids and corticotrophin on the growth of children. *Lancet*, 2: 568–572.

Freudenberg, H. and Mager, J. (1971) Studies on the mechanism of the inhibition of protein synthesis induced by intracellular ATP depletion. *Biochim. biophys. Acta (Amst.)*, 232: 537–555.

Gasser, R.F., Scheving, L.E. and Pauly, J.E. (1972a) Circadian rhythms in the cell division rate of the inner enamel epithelium and in the uptake of ^{3}H-thymidine by the root tip of rat incisors. *J. dent. Res.*, 51: 740–746.

Gasser, R.F., Scheving, L.E. and Pauly, J.E. (1972b) Circadian rhythms in the mitotic index of the basal epithelium and in the uptake rate of ^{3}H-thymidine by the tongue of the rat. *J. Cell Physiol.*, 80: 437–441.

Gillin, J.C., Jacobs, L.S., Fram, D.H. and Synder, F. (1972) Acute effect of glucocorticoid on normal human sleep. *Nature (Lond.)*, 237: 398–399.

Goldbeter, A. (1974) Modulation of the adenylate energy charge by sustained metabolic oscillations. *FEBS Lett.*, 43: 327–330.

Gololobova, M.T. (1960) 24 hour rhythm of cell multiplication in rat epidermis during healing of skin wounds. *Byull. éksp. Biol. Med.*, 50: 118–122.

Goodwin, B. (1963) *Temporal Organization in Cells. Theory of Cellular Control Processes*, Academic Press, London and New York.

Gordon, P. and Scheving, L.E. (1968) Covariant 24 h rhythm for acquisition and retention of avoidance learning and brain protein synthesis in rats. *Fed. Proc.*, 27: 223.

Guttes, E. and Guttes, S. (1959) Regulation of mitosis in *Stentor coeruleus*. *Science*, 129: 1483.

Halberg, F., Galicich, J.H., Ungar, F. and French, L.A. (1965) Circadian rhythmic pituitary adrenocorticotropic activity, rectal temperature and pinnal mitosis of starving, dehydrated C mice. *Proc. Soc. exp. Biol. (N.Y.)*, 118: 414–419.

Hartmann, E. (1973) *The Functions of Sleep*, Yale University Press, New Haven, Conn.

Honda, Y., Takahashi, K., Takahashi, S., Azumi, K., Irie, M., Sakuma, M., Tsushima, T. and Shizume, K. (1969) Growth hormone secretion during nocturnal sleep in normal subjects. *J. clin. Endocr.*, 29: 20–29.

Hunt, N.H. and Perris, A.D. (1974) Ca^{2+} and the control of circadian mitotic activity in rat bone marrow and thymus. *J. Endocr.*, 62: 451–462.

Itoh, T. and Quastel, J.H. (1969) Ribonucleic acid biosynthesis in adult and infant rat brain in vitro. *Science*, 164: 79–80.

Izquierdo, J.N. and Gibbs, S.J. (1972) Circadian rhythms of DNA synthesis and mitotic activity in hamster cheek pouch epithelium. *Exp. Cell Res.*, 71: 402–408.

Jaffe, J.J. (1954) Diurnal mitotic periodicity in regenerating rat liver. *Anat. Rec.,* 120: 935–954.

Jöbsis, F., Rosenthal, M., Lamanna, J., Lothnan, E., Cordingly, G. and Somjen, G. (1975) Metabolic activity in epileptic seizures. In *Brain Work,* D.H. Ingvar and N.A. Lassen (Eds.), Munksgaard, Copenhagen, pp. 185–196.

Jones, P.C.T. (1971) On the nature of biological clocks. *Experientia (Basel),* 27: 1014–1015.

Karlson, J. and Saltin, B. (1970) Lactate, ATP and CP in working muscles during exhaustive exercise in man. *J. appl. Physiol.,* 29: 598–602.

Katzman, R. and Grossman, R. (1975) Neuronal activity and potassium movement. In *Brain Work,* D.H. Ingvar and N.A. Lassen (Eds.), Munksgaard, Copenhagen, pp. 149–166.

Kirk, H. (1972) Mitotic activity and cell degeneration in the mouse thymus over a period of 24 hrs. *Z. Zellforsch.,* 129: 188–195.

Korner, A. (1965) Growth hormone control of biosynthesis of protein and ribonucleic acid. *Recent Progr. Hormone Res.,* 21: 205–236.

Kuhn, E., Brodan, M., Brodonová, M. and Ryšánek, K. (1969) Metabolic reflection of sleep deprivation. *Activitas nervosa sup. (Praha),* 11: 165–174.

Kuznetsov, E.V., Chugunov, YuD. and Brodskii, V. Ya. (1972) Diurnal rhythms in the locomotor and mitotic activity of frogs under natural conditions. *Soviet J. Ecology,* 3: 10–15.

Lowry, O.H. (1975) Energy metabolism in brain and its control. In *Brain Work,* D.H. Ingvar and N.A. Lassen (Eds.), Munksgaard, Copenhagen, pp. 48–63.

Mateev, D., Sheytanov, M., Anghelova, P. and Hristov, T. (1967) Effect of physical work on intensity of protein synthesis in young and old white rats. *C.R. Acad. Bulgare Sci.,* 20: 1221–1224.

Mauer, A.M. (1965) Diurnal variation of proliferative activity in human bone marrow. *Blood,* 26: 1–7.

McGinty, D.J., Harper, R.M. and Fairbanks, M.K. (1974) Neuronal unit activity and the control of sleep states. In *Advances in Sleep Research, Vol. 1,* E.D. Weitzman (Ed.), Spectrum, New York, pp. 173–216.

Meerson, F.Z. (1975) Role of synthesis of nucleic acids and protein in adaptation to the external environment. *Physiol. Rev.,* 55: 79–123.

Mendelsohn, S.L., Nordeen, S.K. and Young, D.A. (1977) Rapid changes in initiation-limited rates of protein synthesis in rat thymic lymphocytes correlate with energy charge. *Biochem. Biophys. Res. Comm.,* 79: 53–60.

Molé, P.A. and Johnson, R.E. (1971) Disclosure by dietary modification of an exercise-induced protein catabolism in man. *J. appl. Physiol.,* 31: 185–190.

Munro, H.N. (1970) Free amino acid pools and their role in regulation. In *Mammalian Protein Metabolism, Vol. 4,* H.N. Munro (Ed.), Academic Press, New York and London, pp. 299–386.

Munro, H.N., Black, J.G. and Thomson, W.S.T. (1959) The mode of action of dietary carbohydrate on protein metabolism. *Brit. J. Nutr.,* 13: 475–485.

Munro, H.N., Hubert, C. and Baliga, B.S. (1975) In *Alcohol, Nutrition and Protein Synthesis, Vol. 1,* M. Rothschild, M. Oratz and S.S. Schreiber (Eds.), Pergamon, New York, p. 33.

Newsholme, E.A. and Start, C. (1973) *Regulation in Metabolism.* John Wiley, London, New York, Sydney and Toronto, p. 109.

Nouët, J.C. and Kujas, M. (1975) Variations of mitotic activity in the adenohypophysis of male rats during a 24 h cycle. *Cell Tiss. Res.,* 164: 193–200.

Oswald, I. (1969) Human brain protein, drugs and dreams. *Nature, (Lond.),* 223: 893–897.

Oswald, I. (1970) Sleep, the great restorer. *New Scientist,* 46: 170–172.

Oswald, I. (1976) The function of sleep. *Postgrad. med. J.,* 52: 15–18.

Panksepp, J., Jalowiec, J.E., Zolovick, A.J., Stern, W.C. and Morgane, P.J. (1973) Inhibition of glycolytic metabolism and sleep–waking states in cats. *Pharmacol. Biochem. Behav.,* 1: 117–119.

Peschle, C., Rappaport, I.A., Sasso, G.F., Gordon, A.S. and Condorelli, M. (1972) Mechanism of growth hormone (GH) action on erythropoises. *Endocrinology,* 91: 511–517.

Peterson, N.A. and Chaikoff, L.L. (1963) Uptake of intravenously injected (4-^{14}C) cortisol by adult rat brain. *J. Neurochem.,* 10: 17–23.

Plesner, P. (1964) ATP rhythm correlates with rhythm of cell division in *Tetrahymena pyriformis. C.R. Trav. Lab. Carlsberg,* 34: 1–76.

Rapoport, M.I. and Beisel, W.R. (1968) Circadian periodicity of tryptophan metabolism. *J. clin. Invest.,* 47: 934–939.

Rau, E. and Meyer, D.K. (1975) A diurnal rhythm of incorporation of L-(^{3}H)leucine in myocardium of the rat. *Recent Adv. Stud. Cardiac Struct. Metab.,* 7: 105–110.

304

Rebolledo, O.R. and Gagliardino, J.J. (1971) Circadian variations of the protein metabolism in muscle. *J. interdisciplin. Cycle Res.*, 2: 101–108.

Reeve, D.R.E. (1975) A study of mitotic activity and the diurnal variation of the epithelial cells in wounded rectal mucous membrane. *J. Anat. (Lond.)*, 119: 333–345.

Reeve, D.R.E. (1977) Some observations on the diurnal variation of mitosis in the stratified squamous epithelium of wounded tympanic membrane. *Cell Tiss. Res.*, 182: 253–263.

Renzoni, A. and Quay, W.B. (1964) Daily karyometric and mitotic rhythms of pineal parenchymal cells in the rat. *Amer. Zool.*, 4: 416–417.

Richardson, K. and Rose, S.P.R. (1971) A diurnal rhythmicity in incorporation of lysine into rat brain regions. *Nature (New Biol.)*, 233: 182–184.

Roberts, S. and Zomzely, C.E. (1966) Regulation of protein synthesis in the brain. In *Protides of the Biological Fluids*, H. Peeters (Ed.), Elsevier, Amsterdam, London and New York, pp. 91–102.

Romanova, L.K. (1966) Diurnal periodicity of mitotic cell division in the interalveolar septa of rat lungs. *Bull. exp. Biol. Med.*, 61: 689–691.

Rose, C.M., Chou, C., Zigmond, M.J. and Wurtman, R.J. (1969) Diurnal rhythms in metabolism of tyrosine and synthesis of protein and norepinephrine. *Fed. Proc.*, 28: 690.

Rubin, R.T., Gouin, P.R., Kales, A. and Odell, W.D. (1973) Luteinizing hormone, follicle stimulating hormone and growth hormone secretion in normal adult men during sleep and dreaming. *Psychosom. Med.*, 35: 309–321.

Rubin, R.T., Poland, R.E. and Tower, B.B. (1976) Prolactin-related testosterone secretion in normal adult men. *J. clin. Endocr.*, 42: 112–116.

Rudman, D., Freides, D., Patterson, J.H. and Gibbas, D.L. (1973) Diurnal variation in the responsiveness of human subjects to HGH. *J. clin. Invest.*, 52: 912–918.

Rupniak, H.T.R. and Quincey, R.V. (1975) Small changes in energy charge affect protein synthesis in reticulocyte lysates. *FEBS Lett.*, 58: 99–101.

Saetren, H. (1972) The diurnal variation of the first mitotic wave released among rat kidney tubule cells by partial nephrectomy. *Acta Path. microbiol. scand.*, 80: 736–742A.

Sassin, J.F., Parker, D.C., Mace, J.W., Gotlin, R.W., Johnson, L.C. and Rossman, L.G. (1969) H.G.H. release: relation to slow-wave sleep and sleep–waking cycles. *Science*, 165: 513–515.

Sassin, J.F., Frantz, A.G., Kapen, S. and Weitzman, E.D. (1973) The nocturnal rise of human prolactin is dependent on sleep. *J. clin. Endocr.*, 37: 436–440.

Savin, J.A., Paterson, W.D., Oswald, I. and Adam, K. (1975) Further studies of scratching during sleep. *Brit. J. Derm.*, 93: 297–302.

Scheving, L.E. (1959) Mitotic activity in the human epidermis. *Anat. Rec.*, 135: 7–14.

Scheving, L.E., Burns, E.R. and Pauly, J.E. (1972) Circadian rhythms in mitotic activity and ^{3}H-thymidine uptake into the duodenum: effect of isoproterenol on the mitotic rhythm. *Amer. J. Anat.*, 135: 311–318.

Schnure, J.J., Raskin, P. and Lipman, R.L. (1971) Growth hormone secretion during sleep: impairment in glucose tolerance and nonsuppressibility by hyperglycemia. *J. clin. Endocr.*, 33: 234–241.

Scrimshaw, N.S., Habicht, J.P., Pellet, P., Piche, M.L. and Cholakos, B. (1966) Effects of sleep deprivation and reversal of diurnal activity on protein metabolism of young men. *Amer. J. clin. Nutr.*, 19: 313–319.

Sharipov, F.Kh. (1967) Changes in diurnal rhythm of mitotic activity of the convoluted tubules of compensatory and regeneration hypertrophy of the kidney in rats. *Bull. exp. Biol. Med.*, 64: 1117–1119.

Sigelman, S., Dohlman, C.H. and Friedenwald, J.S. (1954) Mitotic and wound-healing activities in the rat corneal epithelium. Influence of various hormones and endocrine glands. *Arch. Ophthal. (Chic.)*, 52: 751–757.

Simmons, D.J. (1964) Circadian mitotic rhythm in epiphyseal cartilage. *Nature (Lond.)*, 202: 906–907.

Simmons, D.J. (1968) Daily rhythm of S^{35} incorporation into epiphyseal cartilage in mice. *Experientia (Basel)*, 24: 363–364.

Steriade, M. (1970) Ascending control of thalamic and cortical responsiveness. *Int. Rev. Neurobiol.*, 12: 87–144.

Stern, W.C. and Morgane, P.J. (1974) Theoretical view of REM sleep function. Maintenance of catecholamine systems in the central nervous system. *Behav. Biol.*, 11: 1–32.

Takahashi, Y., Kipnis, D.M. and Daughaday, W.H. (1968) Growth hormone secretion during sleep. *J. clin. Invest.*, 47: 2079–2090.

Taub, J.M. and Berger, R.J. (1976) Effects of acute sleep pattern alteration depend upon sleep duration. *Physiol. Psychol.,* 4: 412–420.

Tewksbury, D.A. and Lohrenz, F.N. (1970) Circadian rhythm of human urinary amino acid excretion in fed and fasted states. *Metabolism,* 19: 363–371.

Uryadnitskaya, T.I. (1974) 24 h variations in the proliferative activity of the rat bone marrow cells. *Byull. éksp. Biol. Med.,* 78: 105–108.

Van den Noort, S. and Brine, K. (1970) Effect of sleep on brain labile phosphates and metabolic rate. *Amer. J. Physiol.,* 218: 1434–1439.

Vasama, R. and Vasama, R. (1958) On the diurnal cycle of mitotic activity in the corneal epithelium of mice. *Acta anat. (Basel),* 33: 230–237.

Vonnahme, F.J. (1974) Circadian variation in cell size and mitotic index in tissues having a relatively low proliferation rate in both normal and hypophysectomized rats. *Int. J. Chronobiol.,* 2: 297–309.

Walton, G.M. and Gill, G.N. (1975) Nucleotide regulation of a eukaryotic protein synthesis initiation complex. *Biochim. biophys. Acta (Amst.),* 390: 231–245.

Weitzman, E.D., Fukushima, D., Nogeire, C., Roffwarg, H., Gallagher, T.F. and Hellman, L. (1971) Twenty-four hour pattern of the episodic secretion of cortisol in normal subjects. *J. clin. Endocr.,* 33: 14–22.

Williams, H.L., Hammack, J.T., Daly, R.L., Dement, W.C. and Lubin, A. (1964) Responses to auditory stimulation sleep loss and the EEG stages of sleep. *Electroenceph. clin. Neurophysiol.,* 16: 269–279.

Wojciechowska, F., Karon, H. and Blawacka, M. (1975) The effect of short-lasting intensive physical exercise on ATP content in the rat muscle and liver. *Acta physiol. pol.,* 26: 313–316.

Wolff, G. and Money, J. (1973) Relationship between sleep and growth in patients with reversible somatotropin deficiency. *Psychol. Med.,* 3: 18–27.

Wurtman, R.J., Rose, C.M., Chou, C. and Larin, F.F. (1968a) Daily rhythms in the concentration of various amino acids in human plasma. *New Engl. J. Med.,* 279: 171–175.

Wurtman, R.J., Shoemaker, W.J. and Larin, F. (1968b) Mechanism of the daily rhythm in hepatic tyrosine transaminase activity: Role of dietary tryptophan. *Proc. nat. Acad. Sci. (Wash.),* 59: 800–807.

Zepelin, H. and Rechtschaffen, A. (1974) Mammalian sleep, longevity and energy metabolism. *Brain Behav. Evol.,* 10: 425–470.

Zomzely, C.E., Roberts, S. and Rapaport, D. (1964) Regulation of cerebral metabolism of amino acids III. Characteristics of amino acid incorporation into protein of microsomal and ribosomal preparations of rat cerebral cortex. *J. Neurochem.,* 11: 567–582.

The Cognitive Activity of Sleep

DAVID B. COHEN

University of Texas at Austin, Austin, Texas (U.S.A.)

INTRODUCTION

Inferences about cognitive capacity are typically based on measures of physiological, mental and motoric events, but measurement of these is restricted or made ambiguous by sleep. For example, a reliable motor response to a discriminative stimulus suggests the occurrence of perception and recognition. However, sleeping organisms are biologically unprepared for motor responsiveness, which is incompatible with energy conservation (Meddis, 1977; Walker and Berger, 1980) and optimal tissue repair (Adam, 1980; Oswald, 1980; Adam and Oswald, 1977). Biological or experimental conditions which minimize the motivation, capacity or opportunity for motor activity may therefore lead to false inferences about underlying events. Likewise, the ambiguity of physiological responsiveness, and the unreliability of memory complicate investigations of the nature and significance of cognitive activity during sleep.

Momentary responsiveness to the environment is only one facet of the problem. Another is the extent to which the organism is permanently modified by cognitive processes during sleep. Does sleep *permit* new learning? Does sleep *protect* recent learning by reducing interference from new learning? Does sleep *reinforce* recent learning by repetition or coding? More speculatively, is it possible that sleep *generates* new learning, perhaps by re-working recent and old learning in the crucible of dream consciousness? Even if it were possible to determine the cognitive capacity during sleep, its biological significance would remain questionable. Do responsiveness, inventiveness and change during sleep enhance the adaptability of the individual and, thus, the survival of the species, or are they inconsequential epiphenomena of brain activity?

I have organized my discussion of research on the cognitive activity of sleep into 3 sections. In the first I discuss evidence that sleeping organisms are capable of detecting and recognizing relatively familiar information. In the second, I consider the capacity to retain some permanent trace of the mental experiences during sleep, whether induced by external stimulation or generated spontaneously. In the third section, I discuss research bearing on the assumption that the rapid-eye-movement (REM) period plays a special role in the reinforcement and adaptive integration of waking experience.

RESPONSIVENESS DURING SLEEP

Physiological and motoric responsiveness

The capacity to detect and discriminate external stimulation while asleep can be demonstrated at the physiological level. For example, the complexity of cortical (e.g., K-complex) and cardiac response is influenced by the meaningfulness of the stimulus, e.g. personal name, or shock-conditioned stimulus (Beh and Barratt, 1965; Minard et al., 1968; Oswald et al., 1960). Such findings clearly indicate the cognitive nature of responsiveness, i.e. the capacity of the sleeping brain to utilize long-term memory to interpret impinging information.

While the capacity for recognizing external events might seem self-evident, given the high neuronal activity during sleep, the importance of such a capacity is *not* so evident. It is in any case a factor of less importance to survival than are safe sleeping conditions, appropriate awakening thresholds, or occasional awakenings to assess the environment (Allison and

TABLE I

DETERMINANTS OF AWAKENING THRESHOLD *

A. Operational definition of responsiveness:
  (1) EEG measures (e.g. alpha, K-complex, evoked potential);
  (2) manual operation (e.g. operating on a thumb switch);
  (3) speech;
  (4) dream incorporation.

B. Method of stimulus presentation:
  (1) method of constant stimuli (i.e. measure percentage of positive responses);
  (2) method of limits, i.e gradual increase in intensity (measure threshold intensity).

C. Nature of stimulus:
  (1) meaningful
     (a) verbal—nonverbal
     (b) awakening "required" vs not "required";
  (2) meaningless;
  (3) modality (e.g. visual, auditory, tactile);
  (4) complex − simple.

D. Temporal factors:
  (1) time of night (e.g. real time, early vs late REM periods, etc.);
  (2) duration of accumulated sleep time prior to stimulus presentation;
  (3) time since last body movement.

E. Biological state factors:
  (1) stage of sleep;
  (2) body temperature;
  (3) phasic events (e.g. K-complex, spindle, eye movement, etc.);
  (4) need state (e.g. pre-sleep manipulation of hunger; prior sleep or REM deprivation).

F. Individual differences (normal and abnormal):
  (1) situational;
  (2) dispositional
     (a) intelligence
     (b) temperament
     (c) attitudes, values, interests
     (d) sex.

* From Cohen (1979b) p. 82.

Cicchetti, 1976; Snyder, 1966; Webb, 1974). At least in humans, however, extended wakefulness in the course of a night's sleep is a last resort, and frequent sleep stage changes or periodic wakefulness probably imply a defect in brain mechanisms. Powerful, instinctively regulated inhibition of brain stem activating systems is the rule, to which cognitive elaboration of significant information may contribute by "absorbing" information that could otherwise elicit arousal. The special significance of REM sleep in this regard is apparent in the extraordinary variability of its auditory awakening thresholds, i.e. the thresholds are higher for awakenings which yield dream reports referring to the waking stimuli (Bradley and Meddis, 1974). Such incorporations are more likely in REM than in NREM sleep (Rechtschaffen et al., 1966).

The complexity of the interrelationship between physiological responsiveness during sleep and transition to wakefulness, the information processing of sleep, and the nature of stimuli and other events are suggested by the material in Table I. The combination of data on physiological responsiveness during sleep and auditory awakening thresholds thus indicates that a surprising amount of external information can be processed during sleep. However, given the protected and insulated conditions associated with human sleep in modern society, relatively few demands appear to be made on such a capacity.

How useful are the indices of physiological responsiveness (e.g. heart and respiratory rate, phasic EEG, galvanic skin response (GSR), body temperature) for making inferences about information processing during sleep? They are certainly better indicators of sensory detection threshold than are motor events or experimental reports, the usefulness of which is somewhat compromised by, respectively, instinct-imposed limitations and unreliability of reporting. Nevertheless, physiological indices too appear to be of limited usefulness, for the following reasons. First, the full complexity of responses to any but the simplest stimulus is generally lost or degraded in its physiological expression, at least as conventionally recorded. Second, physiological measures do not correlate very well with experiential reports (Cohen, 1979b; Rechtschaffen, 1973). Third, physiological measures also do not correlate well with auditory arousal thresholds (Rechtschaffen et al., 1966). Thus, despite their objectivity, measures of physiological responsiveness constitute a limited resource.

The capacity of the sleeping organism to detect and recognize external information can also be observed in motor behavior, although this form of expressiveness is typically limited to relatively simple reactions. Nevertheless, by forcing the sleep instinct to compete with an experimentally induced motive, cognitive capacity can be revealed even by motoric activity, as in the work of Williams et al. (1966) in which simple stimuli (tones) and simple motor responses (pressing a microswitch attached to the hand) were used. Pre-sleep instructions to make a response to a stimulus administered while asleep yielded decreasing performance as a function of stages 1 through 4 and REM. In slow wave sleep (stages 3 and 4) and in REM very few responses at all were obtained. However, when punishment (abrupt and unpleasant awakening to loud noise, bright light plus threat of shock) for not responding was imposed, overall responding increased dramatically for REM sleep, but only slightly for stages 3 and 4. Apparently, the enhancement of performance can be made specific to REM sleep when the motive to respond during REM is selectively increased. This can be done by combining REM deprivation during the first half of the night with punishment (abrupt awakening) for not responding during the otherwise uninterrupted sleep of the second half of the night (Salamy, 1971). Common to these studies by Williams and Salamy (op. cit.) is the use of simple stimuli and responses about which the subject has been instructed prior to sleep. Under such conditions, it is clear that recent learning — in this case of stimulus—response contingencies — is capable of motoric expression during sleep, *given the right conditions.*

By exploiting motor capacity it may even become possible to study sleep cognition (dreaming?) in higher animals. For example, young, socially isolated monkeys could be trained to make a response to a stimulus the consequence of which is access to a playmate. The effect of extinction (i.e. response to the stimulus no longer affords the opportunity for social contact) on response production during REM could be assessed. Elevation of the response frequency over baseline and training periods would be consistent with hypotheses about the importance of incentive-related cognitive processes during REM. Other interesting questions could be pursued, such as: what would be the effect on the electro-cortical and electro-ocular properties of REM? Would the amount of REM or the frequency of REM periods change? What would be the effect of REM deprivation on accommodation to the extinction situation? If theories about the special significance of REM for emotional adaptation are correct, then surely the physiological, motoric and mental properties of REM should be maximally altered by challenges to the personal and social self.

Mental responsiveness

Much of the research on cognitive responsiveness during sleep has focused on the transformation of external stimuli during dreaming. Such a stimulus introduced during sleep may be of two types: (1) the significance of which is experimentally conditioned prior to sleep; and (2) the meaning of which is long-established through personal experience. The potential usefulness of the former has been discussed by Antrobus (1977) and Cohen (1979b). Auditory stimuli of little inherent interest or personal significance could, prior to sleep, be conditioned to elicit discrete cognitive responses about attributes or concepts. During subsequent sleep, differential responsiveness to such cues might permit strong inferences about differential weighing of cognitions, and how these may be modified by individual differences in gender, age and personality.

The potential usefulness of stimuli whose meaning is long-established through personal experience, is illustrated in the work of Berger (1963) and Castaldo and Holzman (1967, 1969). Berger (1963), also reported that personal names elicited 4 kinds of incorporation that could be matched better than chance to the original stimulus. There was *assonance* (e.g., "Robert" transformed into rabbit), *association* (e.g. dreaming about what the stimulus-person might do), *direct reference* to the name, and *direct representation* of the person named. Measurement of responsiveness to the stimulus is thus complicated by the peculiarities of the cognitive system, e.g. condensation of A and B (e.g. arm/chair to form AB (e.g. charm), selection of B only (e.g. chair), or transformation of A and B into C (e.g. armistice). The apparently extraordinary impact of one's name or voice on REM mentation (Berger, 1963; Castaldo and Holzman, 1967, 1969) has yet to be exploited from a theoretical or clinical perspective. For example, how would the cognitive elaboration of the subject's own name introduced during REM be different in individuals differing in self-esteem? Would there be a difference in affective intensity, symbolic elaboration or ability to recall the dream? Further, would individuals with low self-esteem learn during sleep to press microswitches if the consequence were elimination of such a stimulus? On the other hand, would high self-esteem subjects try to eliminate stimuli associated with pre-sleep failures?

Experimental research might also contribute to the clinical investigation of symbol formation. For example, the meaning and personal significance of stimuli chosen on the basis of theoretical or clinical considerations could be explored by repeated stimulation across REM periods and across nights. Rather than starting from the manifest content of a dream to infer significance, one would control *latent* content. Thus, theoretical assumptions about REM in general, plus clinical knowledge of a particular individual would, eventually, become paramount considerations in the selection of stimuli. The idea of making some sort of experimental inroad into the latent content of dreaming is not entirely far-fetched for at least two reasons. First, individuals are capable of comprehending verbal information introduced during REM (Evans et al., 1970). Second, latent content is defined as a motivating thought which, in analysis, is rendered into words. Thus, the use of powerful verbal stimuli as an analogue of naturally occurring processes would not be entirely artifactual.

There is often a tenuous relationship between experimental interventions, especially of the pre-sleep sort, and predictable forms of dream content. For example, exciting or stressful films observed prior to sleep have little specifiable influence on dream content (Foulkes and Rechtschaffen, 1964; Foulkes et al., 1969). However, more attention to theoretical assumptions about what is an effective (e.g. ego threatening) situation and what REM sleep is about might yield more reliable and interesting experience—dream relationships (Witkin, 1969).

LEARNING DURING SLEEP

As with recognition of old information, the learning of new information can be inferred from physiological and motor behavior during sleep. For example, investigations have achieved classical conditioning of K-complexes to tones (Beh and Barrett, 1965) and operant conditioning of hand movement (Granda and Hammack, 1961), both in response to a shock unconditioned stimulus (UCS). The work of Williams et al. (1966) and of Salamy (1971) discussed above is also consistent with the idea that some types of learning are possible during sleep, especially when the clues are familiar.

In the light of the reported success at producing sleep conditioning, the inability to achieve reliable habituation to simple stimuli (e.g. tones) in the EEG and autonomic indices of sleep, especially REM sleep (Johnson et al., 1975) is curious. Perhaps it illustrates a peculiar economy of attention to meaningful things. If so, we should expect that habituation, especially during REM sleep, might occur to stimuli previously conditioned to an organismically (e.g. shock) or personally (e.g. failure) significant event.

Memory of sleep experiences

Individuals can reliably estimate the duration of prior sleep intervals, the accuracy being greatest for REM sleep. It is improved by a clearly recallable stimulus marker presented during a period of awakening prior to the onset of the sleep interval (Carlson et al., 1978), or by a well-recalled dream from which time course can be inferred (Dement and Kleitman, 1957). Thus, time is loosely preserved in the pace of salient cognitive events during sleep.

Short-term memory for simple stimuli (e.g. numbers) administered during sleep is a function of the cortical activity of the stage from which the subject is awakened. Thus, the probability of accurate recall or recognition is greatest for information presented during stages 1, 2 and REM, and is least during stages 3 and 4 (Lasaga and Lasaga, 1973). However, in order for more complicated information (e.g. short sentences) to be transferred from short-term to long-term *state-independent* memory, cortical arousal in the form of alpha or beta rhythms must occur (Lehmann and Koukkou, 1973). Thus, the more complex the information, and the more difficult the retrieval task (e.g. recall as opposed to recognition), the longer must be the arousal subsequent to stimulation.

The following conclusions can be drawn about sleep learning. First, short-term memory for simple stimuli is possible even in stages 3 and 4, though it is more reliable in stages, 1, 2 and REM. However, novel and complex stimuli are apt to induce higher frequencies in the EEG, a shift to a "lighter" sleep stage, or even a brief awakening. Second, relatively complex input, like verbal information, may achieve long-term storage in the form of *state-dependent* responsiveness if the learning occurs in the context of a fairly active EEG, such as in REM sleep. It is not likely that this information will be retrievable after sleep, however, unless it is followed immediately by awakening, which permits the recapture of information through cues still in short-term memory. Third, the recall of complex verbal information requires EEG activation during initial processing. Thus, reliable and useful learning of complex information is unlikely if presented during *uninterrupted* (i.e. alpha-free) sleep and not followed by an arousal. Lehman and Koukkou (1973) hypothesize that the EEG "tells us about the state of the gate between short-term memory and long-term memory. The specific function of writing memory material into state-independent long-term memory is possible only during wakefulness EEG, i.e., with dominant scalp EEG frequencies of 8 Hz or higher. Many functions of the central nervous system become less efficient with the slowing of the EEG, but the writing down of long-term memory appears to be particularly sensitive. In turn, reading of old memory material persists during EEG slowing" (p. 47).

Dreaming may be thought of as a "reading of old memory material". The fact that a dream can be retrieved suggests that it is at least a form of short-term memory. The fact that such a dream experience is lost if it occurs earlier in a period of sleep or prior to an awakening characterized by tension and distraction (Cohen, 1979a), suggests either that transfer to long-term store is impeded during sleep (e.g. similar to the loss of material that is "shadowed" in attention experiments), or that it is stored in long-term memory whose retrieval is state-dependent. Either possibility would be the result of a characteristic lack of reflection on what is happening during sleep, what Rechtschaffen (1978) calls the "single-mindedness of dreams".

Dream experiences are largely the product of a reorganization of information already known, rather than the product of an ad hoc accommodation to external stimuli. Thus, it may be easier for these novel products to attain long-term storage and to have an indirect influence despite failure of overt recall. For example, amnesic patients may show progressive improvement over a number of trials on a task for which they have no recognition memory (Wickelgren, 1979). Sleep learning may be akin to incidental learning (Bransford, 1979). For example, a stimulus word presented to the unattended ear while the subject concentrates on a semantically ambiguous sentence presented to the other ear can influence the meaning of the subsequently recalled sentence despite non-recall of the stimulus word. Similarly, a stimulus word presented during REM sleep may influence the direction of the dream despite non-recall of the stimulus. In both cases, the stimulus is encoded outside of normal waking consciousness and therefore under minimal voluntary control; it cannot be recalled, and thus cannot be used. Finally, in both cases, evidence for encoding comes from indirect effects on thought, affect and behavior. The possibility that a kind of incidental learning during sleep has an indirect and unconscious influence on waking behavior is strongly implied, if not required, by theories emphasizing the adaptive significance of REM sleep (e.g. Breger, 1967; Dewan, 1969; Greenberg and Pearlman, 1974).

Influence of sleep experiences

Anecdotal evidence abounds on the value of dreaming for problem solving (e.g. see Krippner and Hughes, 1970). However, empirical evidence that dreaming has a detectable consequence on subsequent behavior, even in the absence of dream recall, is surprisingly scarce considering its theoretical import.

Bokert (1965) found evidence that thirst manipulations, induced prior to sleep, were associated with enhanced thirst-related words in REM dreams. More interesting, subjects showing evidence of such preoccupation reported less thirst, and they drank less in the morning than subjects not showing such evidence. An analogous finding, obtained in a very different type of experiment, was reported by Cohen and Cox (1975). Male subjects were exposed to pre-sleep manipulations, one of which was designed to maximize ego threat (minimal information, social isolation, perfunctory treatment, and induced failure on an "IQ test"). Subjects in this condition who showed evidence of dreaming about the "problem" (incorporators) reported significantly more positive mood in the morning compared to their pre-sleep reports. Non-incorporators, having about the same bad pre-sleep mood as the incorporators, showed no such change. Moreover, although incorporators and non-incorporators did not differ immediately prior to post-sleep debriefing in willingness to return to the laboratory for additional studies, incorporators showed a dramatic increase in willingness when questioned a month later. These results on the apparent influence of dreaming on post-sleep effect and attitude are shown in Fig. 1.

Evidence that what one dreams about may influence post-sleep mood (Kramer and Roth, 1973) is consistent with the view that dreaming may, under certain (e.g. non-traumatic) conditions, influence post-sleep events in a beneficial way. Under certain stressful conditions, however, dreaming may have the opposite effect as de Koninck and Koulack (1975) reported in an experimental investigation of the effect of film-induced stress on dreaming. The combination of pre-sleep film plus soundtrack played during sleep produced dream incorporations of the film material, but this appeared to have a negative effect on mood assessed post-sleep. At best then, the few available studies are consistent with the view that dreaming may have *some* effect, although not necessarily a felicitous one. A major challenge to dream research would be to determine under what conditions, and for which subjects, dreaming about some problem has a positive or negative effect on post-sleep behavior.

Hypotheses about the nature of information processing have emphasized accommodation

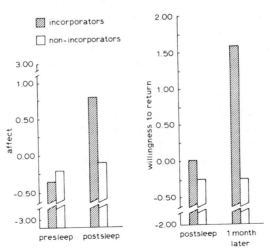

Fig. 1. Changes in effect and attitude for incorporator and non-incorporator subjects in the ego-threat condition of the Cohen and Cox (1975) study (from Cohen (1976) p. 353).

to the environment. Flow charts invariably begin with a sensory information detector/ buffer. Selection and reinforcement of information (in short-term memory) precedes the long-term phase. The guiding influence of past experience is considered, but the accent is on new information. While it may be useful to assess the cognitive capacities of the sleeping individual within the context of such models (see Williams, 1973), the evidence suggests that recognition of personally relevant information, and cognitive reinforcement and extension of information already "in the system", predominates during sleep over learning novel and extrinsic information (Bertini, 1973). Yet, it is just this sort of thing which defies flow chart modelling and controlled observation. Further, it raises a curious philosophical question. (I say philosophical because I do not see how it can be either operationally defined or empirically tested.) Let us assume that the incidental learning paradigm for sleep learning can be used to tell us something about the naturally occurring condition of sleep. If so, does a dream constructed entirely from long-term memory, like that constructed in part out of impinging external information (e.g. systematically controlled by the experimenter), constitute a form of new learning? If so, then the individual has something new that he didn't have prior to the construction of the dream even though he produced the dream out of prior knowledge and through mechanisms constrained by prior knowledge. The dreamer is then like, for instance, the playwright who knows more about the play once he produces it than he did when it was merely a set of ideas. If the product of an autochthonous dream constitutes a form of new learning, then the accretion of knowledge produced during sleep may periodically supplement the accretion of knowledge arising out of wakefulness. Do ontogenetically older (infantile?) patterns of thinking, periodically active during the 24 h cycle, reinforce instinctive behavior and temperamental dispositions which would fade out otherwise, or which we would prefer to disallow (Jouvet, 1980)? Or is the dream process merely a periodic reaffirmation of material which needs no reinforcement through new learning?

THE SPECIAL SIGNIFICANCE OF REM SLEEP

The dramatic physiological and oneiric properties of REM sleep have inspired much research and theory concerning its special significance. From reviews by Fishbein and Gutwein (1977) and by McGrath and Cohen (1978), a set of major experimental strategies for studying the special significance of REM sleep has been distilled. In the first, an attempt is made to demonstrate a link between REM processes and adaptive behavior, by showing that the two are correlated and that both are correlated to similar CNS events. Thus, new learning or stimulating environments may induce changes in REM characteristics which may permit inferences about the active contribution of REM to memory consolidation or the like. Conversely, REM deprivation (RD) may be used to produce opposite effects on brain and behavior, and thus allow inferences about the importance of normally occurring REM sleep. Thus, in the first strategy, one looks at the effect of learning on REM characteristics, while in the second, one focuses on the effect of RD on learning and memory.

A third strategy is to show that a neurophysiological abnormality may affect both the characteristics of REM and the capacity for learning or memory. For example, there is evidence that experimental lesions of the locus coeruleus may have two effects. First, there may be as much as a 50% reduction of phasic (e.g. eye movement or PGO spike) activity in REM. Second, there appears to be a prolongation of the period during which new memory traces are susceptible to disruption by subsequent electro-convulsive shock (ECS) (Fishbein and Gutwein, 1977). Evidence for a correlation between change or disruption of normal

REM processes on the one hand, and the loss or lability of memory on the other, would constitute strong evidence for the hypothesis that REM sleep contributes to the new learning.

A final strategy includes some agent or activity which can simulate the effects of REM or modify the effects of RD. For example, Hartmann and Stern (1972) reported that the active avoidance learning deficit produced by 4 days of prior RD could be reduced by introducing L-DOPA before behavioral testing. This finding is consistent with the hypothesis that REM sleep restores or prepares the catecholamine systems underlying learning (Hartmann, 1973).

The effect of learning on undisturbed REM sleep, the effect of RD on learning, and the modification of such effects through the experimental manipulation of physiology provide converging evidence for hypotheses about the nature and importance of REM sleep. Of the various strategies described above, RD has been the one used most frequently. The remainder of this chapter is therefore devoted to an analysis of information processing during sleep from the RD perspective.

Hypotheses about REM function

An outline and schematic representation of hypotheses on REM function is provided by Table II and Fig. 2.

Biological hypotheses about REM functions have emphasized facilitation of CNS maturation during gestation and early infancy (Allison et al., 1972; Ephron and Carrington, 1966; Roffwarg et al., 1966). In these theories, it is the stimulation of neural growth which is important, rather than the processing of information. Thus, for example, post-learning increments of REM sleep could be a consequence rather than a cause of memory fixation during pre-sleep learning, a "restoration of neurons involved in learning" (Bloch et al., 1977, p. 268).

Psychobiological hypotheses about REM, on the other hand, have emphasized consolidation and integration of recent learning, especially that which is complex, affectively significant, and for which the organism is instinctively unprepared (Breger, 1967; Dewan, 1969; Greenberg and Pearlman, 1974; Hartmann, 1973). Thus, recent information becomes integrated with old programs especially during sleep. The result would be an elaborated cognitive map, a reinforced sense of self, enhanced affective adjustment, greater interpersonal skill and inventiveness (Breger, 1967; Dewan, 1969; Foulkes, 1967; Fiss, 1969; Greiser et al., 1972; Krippner and Hughes, 1970). Collectively, these ideas boil down to two

TABLE II
FUNCTIONS HYPOTHESIZED FOR REM SLEEP

A. Facilitation of the endogenous substrate (preparatory function):
(1) stimulation of maturation of CNS during early ontogeny;
(2) periodic reafferentation of CNS after slow wave sleep;
(3) activation of genome-determined circuits underlying fixed action patterns crucial to species survival but rarely activated during wakefulness (reinforcement of phylogenetic "memory").

B. Facilitation of information processing (consolidation/adaptation):
(1) consolidation/adaptation with respect to recent (labile) memory (reprogramming);
(2) vigilance: detection and cognitive elaboration of perceptual/mnemonic information in order to preserve sleep or to promote wakefulness and effective action;
(3) learning: achievement of long-term storage (relatively state-dependent) for induced or spontaneous cognitive products (dreams) which can then influence post-sleep behavior and adjustment.

316

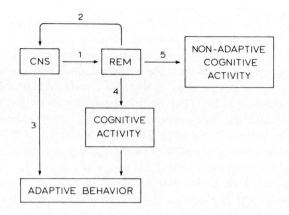

Fig. 2. Schematic representation of the major hypotheses regarding the function of REM sleep, which is an instinctive expression of brain function (arrow 1), as indicated by its ubiquity and resistance to change. The hypothesis that REM sleep facilitates CNS function and, thus, indirectly adaptive behavior, is indicated by arrows 2 and 3. The hypothesis that REM sleep contributes to adaptive behavior by providing a unique set of conditions that promote the reinforcement or elaboration of recent learning is indicated by arrow 4. Arrow 5 indicates the possibility that the cognitive activity of REM is merely an inconsequential response to subcortical events or a non-specific expression of an aroused CNS.

general hypothetical functions of REM sleep as illustrated in Fig. 2: (a) a preparatory function arising from autochthonous neural activation/reorganization (arrow 2) which facilitates subsequent adjustments, e.g. new learning, skilled performance (arrow 3); and (b) a sensory information processing function, which also promotes learning and other adaptive adjustments (arrow 4) (McGrath and Cohen, 1978). Fig. 2 represents the additional assumption that the cognitive activity of REM sleep may contribute little or nothing to the reinforcement or reorganization of memory, and thus be inconsequential for day-to-day adaptations (arrow 5).

REM deprivation methodology

Like REM sleep, REM deprivation may influence behavior either by adding something unique (a positive effect) or by eliminating something (a negative effect). Table III is an out-

TABLE III

EFFECTS OF REM SLEEP AND REM SLEEP DEPRIVATION (RD)

Conditions	Effects	
	Positive	Negative
REM	Neural activation, reorganization ↓ CNS facilitation, memory consolidation, emotional adaptation.	Reduced input/output responsiveness ↓ Energy conservation, reduced interference of STM-to-LTM.
RD	Enhanced REM drive, CNS excitation, physiological stress.	Lost/reduced CNS function, lost opportunity for cognitive activity of REM (CNS essentially normal).

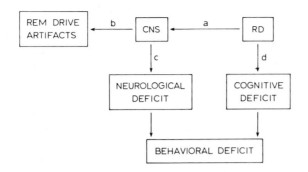

Fig. 3. Effect of REM deprivation (RD). Note that there are basically 3 effects possible. First, there is a direct effect upon CNS function (a) producing excessive drive and, consequently, "artifacts" such as fatigue and sleep disruption, stress, etc. (b). Second, there is a possible loss of an essential CNS function (c) leading to behavioral deficits. Third, RD may simply eliminate cognitive activity of REM (in an otherwise normal CNS) that normally facilitates memory and/or emotional adaptation (d). In the use of RD techniques to investigate the hypothetized preparatory function or the hypothetized cognitive/information processing function, an essential requirement is obviously the elimination or control of REM "drive artifacts".

line of assumptions or facts about the effects of, respectively, the presence or absence of REM. Fig. 3 describes the hypothetical effects resulting from RD, just as Fig. 2 describes the hypothetical functions of REM. Again, broadly speaking, there are 3 possibilities, one clearly inconsequential or epiphenomenal from the perspective of REM theory, the others (i.e. respectively, "biological" and "cognitive/informational") highly relevant to REM theory.

First, RD produces enhanced REM drive (i.e. persistent reduction of latencies to onset of given REM period) and, consequently stress due to multiple awakenings, loss of sleep, biorhythmic disruption, etc. Second, assuming that REM sleep has a CNS preparatory function, RD may produce a decrement in one or another CNS function. Third, RD might eliminate a unique, or at least highly specialized, cognitive activity, e.g. for consolidating labile memory traces or for facilitating adaptation to emotional experiences. The first effect, namely enhanced REM drive is clearly an epiphenomenon from the perspective of REM theory. It merely indicates that REM is very hard to suppress without producing physiological disturbances. Controlling for (and in some rare instances, successfully eliminating) REM drive is a major problem, the typical strategy being the introduction of the same amount of "artifact" into a REM-non-deprived group. Problems of ecological validity and generalizability remain, however, not to mention the basic question of whether it is really possible to control or eliminate REM drive without introducing still other side-effects.

Assuming we could somehow circumvent the problem of REM-drive effects, behavioral deficits produced by RD would be attributable to CNS defect (interference with a preparatory function) or to loss of specialized cognitive activity *. Comparing behavioral defects caused by RD occurring either *prior* to or *subsequent* to new learning can be used to assess these two hypotheses (see McGrath and Cohen, 1978). For example, if RD prior to new learning had no effect on long-term memory, while RD subsequent to the same learning did have an adverse effect, the hypothesis that cognitive activity of REM facilitates consolidation/adaptation would be favored. Nevertheless, despite elaborative controls and

---

* In effect, this assumption means that we can control for all artifacts of RD, such that the only functional difference between RD and RND control groups is the absence of REM in the former.

sophisticated experimental designs, effects produced by RD do not *necessarily* represent the obverse of normally occurring REM sleep, since RD does more than merely eliminate REM sleep. For example, it disrupts circadian and ultradian rhythms as well as enhancing REM drive. Inferences drawn from RD data about the normal process of REM sleep will therefore not always be straight-forward and convincing. This point will be reiterated below.

The ideal RD experiment should include: (1) effective suppression of REM sleep; (2) control of non-specific physiological effects; and (3) separation of learning vs performance effects. I will briefly discuss each of these requisites. For more detailed analyses of these and other problems *, several comprehensive reviews of the RD literature are available (Ellman et al., 1978; Fishbein and Gutwein, 1977; McGrath and Cohen, 1978; Vogel, 1975).

REM deprivation of mice and rats (the usual subjects of animal research on cognitive effects of RD) has typically been accomplished by taking advantage of the postural muscular atonia characteristic of REM sleep. Small pedestals, surrounded by water, permit non-REM (NREM) sleep but inhibit REM, producing frequent awakenings whenever the animal's head falls into the water. REM suppressant drugs (e.g. amphetamines) have also been used, sometimes in conjunction with pedestal or hand awakenings. Corresponding control groups are, respectively, placed on large pedestals, given non-suppressant drugs, and awakened only during NREM. With human subjects, the usual method is to awaken subjects either at the onset of each REM period (RD) or during stage 2-NREM (RND).

Differential RD is easily documented in the human RD studies by electrophysiological monitoring. On the other hand, most animal research has not employed EEG monitoring of sleep, raising some questions about differential attainment of REM in the RD vs RND groups, especially when RD is carried out for 24 h or less (Vogel, 1975). In addition, it has been pointed out (Hicks et al., 1976; McGrath and Cohen, 1978) that loss of REM sleep is a function of the ratio of weight to pedestal size, which in turn is related to the degree of confinement and stress, two major artifacts which have concerned reviewers.

Differential RD is not sufficient to test hypotheses about the functions of REM sleep, since it is necessary to control for numerous other factors. Much of the concern about control stems from the possibility that RD may produce a unique condition, the effects of which are not necessarily the obverse of REM. For example, animal research indicates that two kinds of generalized physiological effects are produced by confinement, sleep disruption and other discomforts inherent in RD treatments: (1) physiological stress (as expressed in weight loss, adrenal hypertrophy, etc.); and (2) hyperexcitability of the CNS (e.g. lowered thresholds for convulsions, electrocortical self-stimulation, shock-induced fighting, drug-induced aggressive and sexual behavior). This physiological "noise" may create considerable obstacles to interpreting the effects of RD on learning because of its complex facilitating (excitability) and interfering (distractability) effects **

There are other potential complications. RD may interfere with learning and thus with

---

* For example, it is desirable to control for number and distribution of awakenings, total sleep time, weight loss and confinement.

** A novel approach to control for RD artifact has been utilized in a series of studies by Pearlman (reviewed in McGrath and Cohen, 1978). Comparison is made of the effects of RD immediately after or delayed for 3 h after learning trials. Other notable features of the research are: use of drugs to induce selectively the RD, use of RND as well as delayed RD as comparison groups for assessing immediate RD effect on easy vs difficult tasks, the learning trials of each distributed over more than one day (mixed RD design; see Table IV). It is thus possible to assess, in this case for rats, the effect of immediate RD on "unprepared" learning relative to delayed RD, RND, and "prepared" learning conditions.

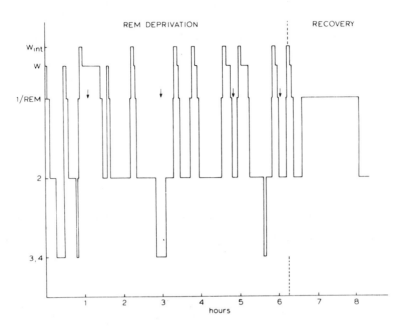

Fig. 4. REM deprivation (6 h) and recovery sleep. RD produced 8 REM periods, i.e. twice the number expected. W_{int} indicates that part of wakefulness constituting the experimenter–subject interchange. W refers to wakefulness in the absence of interview. Arrows indicate the onset of each of 4 REM periods for the same subject during an equivalent period of time of a separate night of uninterrupted sleep.

performance on any subsequent behavioral tests conducted in either RD or RND conditions. However, RD could facilitate or permit learning that is RD state-dependent. If so, then performance deficits would be expected to occur when behavioral assessment of learning is carried out during subsequent RND conditions (Joy and Prinz, 1969). It is also conceivable that RD interferes with the behavioral manifestation of learning, but not with the learning itself. If so, then the manifestation of that (latent) learning would require RND conditions of testing. In addition, we should expect RD performance deficits on tasks initially learned during RND conditions. In sum, RD may interfere with new learning, permit or even facilitate state-dependent learning, or interfere with performance on tests of learning. Studies reporting the presence or absence of RD effects do not always permit a choice between these alternative explanations.

Generalizability is a major problem for RD research. When RD is produced by awakenings at the onset of each REM period, REM latencies diminish dramatically for most subjects, sometimes rather early during the first night of RD. Fig. 4 shows the sleep "architecture" of a male subject given 6 h of RD. Normally about 4 REM periods would be expected to occur during this period. We have found that during the sixth and seventh hours of the first night of RD, the number of awakenings required to produce RD (i.e. to keep the amount of REM sleep per episode down to 1.0–1.5 min, which is a reliable lower limit), may reach 15 or more awakenings (Cohen et al., 1978). Even assuming that one could control for such a massive assault on the integrity of sleep by control (NREM) awakenings, what could be concluded about the normal function of REM from differences in post-sleep behavior in RD and RND groups? A balance obviously needs to be struck so that differential effects can be produced with a *minimum* of RD and its presumed side-effects.

TABLE IV

SUMMARY OF RESULTS GENERATED BY RESEARCH BASED ON RD PARADIGMS APPROPRI-
ATE TO TESTING THE HYPOTHESIS THAT REM SLEEP MEDIATES COMPLEX ADAPTIVE
BEHAVIOR

Name	General paradigm	Purpose	Subjects	Outcome *		
				+	0	−
Prior RD	RD–Train	Role of REM in preparing learning	Rats	5	4	1
			Mice	2	2	0
			Humans	2	1	0
			Total	9	7	1
Subsequent RD	Train–RD–Test	Role of REM in retention/emotional adaptation	Rats	3	5	0
			Mice	4	0	0
			Humans	6	4	0
			Total	13	9	0
Mixed RD	Train–RD–Train and/or Test–RD–Train and/or Test . . .	Related to either preparation or retentation/ adaptation	Rats	12	2	0
			Mice	0	1	0
			Total	12	3	0

* Results either favor, fail to support, or contradict the hypothesis.

Effects of REM deprivation

Detailed reviews of the results of REM deprivation studies (Ellman et al., 1978; Fishbein and Gutwein, 1977; McGrath and Cohen, 1978) will not be replicated here. It will suffice to summarize the overall findings and implications. The overriding hypothesis is that RD interferes with the capacity, or opportunity, for information processing necessary for learning, memory and adaptation. RD has been carried out in 3 ways: prior to new learning, subsequent to new learning, or during the acquisition phase of new learning. Table IV is a rough box score of results from these "prior", "subsequent" and "mixed" designs, based on the data discussed in the McGrath and Cohen (1978) review. The numbers in the Table IV are merely suggestive because the results of any study are subject to interpretation, and because the quality or reliability of each study varies.

At first glance, it would appear from the table that there is a significant effect of RD subsequent to new learning, especially when distributed across many sleep periods with REM (mixed design). This would in turn suggest that consolidation of (rather than preparation for) new learning is affected by REM sleep.

Unfortunately, such conclusions are premature because the data base is insufficient *. I have already discussed some of the methodological points raised by reviewers regarding adequacy of differential RD and sufficiency of control. There is an additional set of considerations that further underscores the highly preliminary state of the data. These con-

---

* In fact, the range of conclusions stemming from recent reviews of the RD literature varies from the optimistic (Fishbein and Gutwein, 1977; Greenberg and Pearlman, 1974) to the cautiously optimistic (McGrath and Cohen, 1978) to the critical (Ellman et al., 1978) to the sceptical (Vogel, 1975).

siderations boil down to two major categories: situation and individual. For both theoretical and empirical reasons, it is reasonable to suppose that the importance of REM sleep is a function of the task to be learned. Dewan (1969) and Greenberg and Pearlman (1974) have argued that REM sleep facilitates the learning of two kinds of information: (1) complex and difficult; and (2) affectively significant. Thus, RD should not adversely affect the learning or recall of word lists in humans and light-signalled bar press responses in rats. However, RD should adversely affect recall of failure-related information in humans and latent learning in rats. Thus, selection and control of the difficulty/affectivity of the task is an important consideration. Perhaps the apparent reliability of results from mixed RD paradigms is a function of the inherently greater difficulty, or vulnerability to interference, of learning that can be distributed over a number of days rather than massed in one or more trials. On the other hand, failure to consider, or to adequately select and control for, task difficulty/affectivity (Greenberg and Pearlman, 1974) may account for the relatively less impressive findings in the RD studies of human subjects.

The personality of the subject, like the nature of the task, may be a factor in the strength of RD results, and thus in the apparent importance of REM sleep. For example, if REM sleep facilitates emotional adaptation, then the effects of RD on REM drive and post-sleep behavior may be particularly marked in individuals who tend to suppress disturbing effects, i.e. "repressors". While there are some findings consistent with this assumption (Cohen, 1977), more recent, unpublished findings from our laboratory have failed to confirm it unambiguously. Specifically, whereas REM deprivation induced enhanced REM pressure in repressors under test-failure conditions (as compared to repressors in either success or neutral conditions), it did not adversely affect post-sleep performance. If REM sleep is specialized — and potentially motivated — for a particular type of psychological "work", then those psychological conditions associated with intensification of REM (e.g. longer or more phasically active REM periods, greater RD-induced REM pressure, etc.) should be associated with relatively greater behavioral deficits subsequent to REM deprivation. The literature has yet to demonstrate a consistent relationship between changes in waking behavior induced by RD.

Overall then, RD subsequent to new learning may interfere with performance on complex and affective tasks. This would be consistent with the hypothesis that information processing during REM sleep is especially suited to the transfer of labile recent memory into a more permanently retrievable form. Serious questions remain however, about the reliability and strength of the results, and thus about the importance of this hypothetical function. These in turn raise questions about methodology (e.g. differential RD, relevance of task, species and individual differences, learning vs performance deficits, etc.) and ecological validity (e.g. disruption of normal sleep patterns, effects due to a "RD syndrome" vs effects due to absence of REM).

Perhaps the biggest problem with the deprivation approach to the question of special significance is the focus on *necessity* of REM. The fact is that decrement or loss of function due to REM deprivation, especially in the human studies, has been modest when the experiments were adequately controlled, and in most cases could be attributed to the side-effects of deprivation rather than to the loss of REM. A more productive approach might be to focus on the enhancement or alteration of behavior immediately following REM, which could be done in a non-deprivation situation. For example, there is evidence that sleep following wakefulness during which learning has taken place is characterized by heightened REM time and/or more REM periods (Arkin et al., 1978; Fishbein and Gutwein, 1977; McGrath and Cohen, 1978). In addition, there is some evidence that the number of REM

322

periods induced by REM deprivation can be increased by imposing REM antithetical cognitive activity (e.g. verbal, numerical) during awakenings timed to occur at the onset of each REM period (Cohen et al., 1978). Collectively, these findings are consistent with the view that challenging learning conditions will intensify the information processing of subsequent REM sleep (Greenberg and Pearlman, 1974). However, for some reason, the effect of stimulation-induced changes in REM on post-sleep behavior has not been given the same research emphasis as the effect of psychological stimulation in REM per se (Cohen, 1979b). If REM sleep contributes to waking behavior, then the consequences of changes in REM should be of equal interest as the antecedents. Our current research efforts are devoted to this question of the effects of experimentally influenced REM cognition on subsequent behavior.

ACKNOWLEDGEMENT

This chapter was supported, in part, by Grant MH26613 from the National Institute of Mental Health, U.S.A.

REFERENCES

Adam, K. (1980) Sleep as a restorative process and a theory to explain why. In *Adaptive Capabilities of the Nervous System, Progress in Brain Research, Vol. 53*, M.A. Corner et al. (Eds.), Elsevier, Amsterdam, pp. 289–305.

Adam, K. and Oswald, I. (1977) Sleep is for tissue restoration. *J. roy. Coll. Physicians*, 11: 376–388.

Allison, T. and Cicchetti, D.V. (1976) Sleep in mammals: ecological and constitutional correlates. *Science*, 194: 732–734.

Allison, T., von Twyver, H. and Goff, W.R. (1972) Electrophysiological studies on the echidna, *Tachyglossus aculeatus*. I. Waking and sleep. *Arch. ital. Biol.*, 110: 145–184.

Antrobus, J.S. (1977) The dream as a metaphor: an information-processing and learning model. *J. ment. Imagery*, 2: 327–338.

Arkin, A.M., Antrobus, J.S. and Ellman, S.J. (1978) *The Mind in Sleep: Psychology and Psychophysiology*. Lawrence Erlbaum, Hillsdale, New Jersey.

Beh, H.C. and Barratt, P.E.H. (1965) Discrimination and conditioning during sleep as indicated by the electroencephalogram. *Science*, 147: 1470–1471.

Berger, R.J. (1963) Experimental modification of dream content by meaningful verbal stimuli. *Brit. J. Psychiat.*, 109: 722–740.

Bertini, M. (1973) REM sleep as a psychophysiological "agency" of memory organization. In *Sleep: Physiology, Biochemistry, Psychology, Pharmacology, Clinical Implications*, W.P. Koella and P. Levin (Eds.), Karger, Basel, Switzerland, pp. 61–62.

Bloch, V., Hennevin, E. and Leconte, P. (1977) Interaction between post-trial reticular stimulation and subsequent paradoxical sleep in memory consolidation processes. In *Neurobiology of Sleep and Memory*, R.R. Drucker-Colín and J. McGaugh (Eds.), Academic Press, New York, pp. 255–272.

Bokert, E. (1965) The effects of thirst and related auditory stimulation on dream reports. Paper presented to the Association for the Psychophysiological Study of Sleep, Washington, D.C.

Bradley, C. and Meddis, R. (1974) Arousal threshold in dreaming sleep. *Physiol. Psychol.*, 2: 109–110.

Bransford, J.D. (1979) *Human Cognition: Learning, Understanding and Remembering*, Wadsworth, Belmont, California.

Breger, L. (1967) Function of dreams. *J. abnorm. soc. Psychol.*, 72: 1–28.

Carlson, V.R., Feinberg, I. and Goodenough, D.R. (1978) Perception of the duration of sleep intervals as a function of sleep stage. *Physiol. Psychol.*, 6: 497–500.

Castaldo, V. and Holzman, P.S. (1967) The effect of hearing one's voice on sleep mentation. *J. nerv. ment. Dis.*, 144: 2–13.

Castaldo, V. and Holzman, P.S. (1969) The effect of hearing one's own voice on dream content: a replication. *J. nerv. ment. Dis.*, 148: 74–82.

Cohen, D.B. (1976) Dreaming: experimental investigation of representational and adaptive properties. In *Consciousness and Self-Regulation: Advances in Research, Vol. 1*, G.E. Schwartz and D. Shapiro (Eds.), Plenum, New York.

Cohen, D.B. (1977) Neuroticism and dreaming sleep: a case for interactionism in personality research. *Brit. J. soc. Clin. Psychol.*, 16: 153–163.

Cohen, D.B. (1979a) Remembering and forgetting dreaming. In *Functional Disorders of Memory*, J.F. Kihlstrom and F.J. Evans (Eds.), Lawrence Erlbaum, Hillsdale, New Jersey.

Cohen, D.B. (1979b) *Sleep and Dreaming: Origins, Nature and Functions*, Pergamon Press, Oxford, England.

Cohen, D.B. and Cox, C. (1975) Neuroticism in the sleep laboratory: implications for representational and adaptive properties of dreaming. *J. abnorm. soc. Psychol.*, 84: 91–108.

Cohen, D.B., McGrath, M.J., Bell, L.W., Hanlon, M.J. and Simon, N. (1978) REM motivation induced by brief REM deprivation: the influence of cognition, gender, and personality. *J. Personality soc. Psychol.*, 36: 741–751.

Dement, W. and Kleitman, N. (1957) The relation of eye movements during sleep to dream activity: an objective method for the study of dreaming. *J. exp. Psychol.*, 53: 339–346.

Dewan, E.M. (1969) The programming (P) hypothesis for REMs. In *Phys. Sci. Res. Papers*, N. 388, Air Force Cambridge Research Laboratories, Project 5628.

Ellman, S.J., Spielman, A.J., Luck, D., Steiner, S.S. and Halperin, R. (1978) REM deprivation: a review. In *The Mind in Sleep: Psychology and Psychophysiology*, A.M. Arkin, J.S. Antrobus and S.J. Ellman (Eds.), Lawrence Erlbaum, Hillsdale, New Jersey, pp. 419–457.

Ephron, H.A. and Carrington, P. (1966) Rapid eye movement sleep and cortical homeostasis. *Psychol. Rev.*, 75: 500–526.

Evans, F.J., Gustafson, L.A., O'Connell, D.N., Orne, M.T. and Shor, R.E. (1970) Verbally induced behavioral responses during sleep. *J. nerv. ment. Dis.*, 150: 171–187.

Fishbein, W. and Gutwein, B.M. (1977) Paradoxical sleep and memory storage processes. *Behav. Biol.*, 19: 425–464.

Fiss, H. (1969) The need to complete one's dreams. In *The Meaning of Dreams: Recent Insights from the Laboratory*, J. Fisher and L. Breger (Eds.), California Mental Health Research Symposium, No. 3, Bureau of Research, California Department of Mental Hygiene, Sacramento, California.

Foulkes, D. (1967) Dreams of the male child: Four case studies. *J. Child Psychol.*, 8: 81–87.

Foulkes, D. and Rechtschaffen, A. (1964) Presleep determinants of dream content: effects of two films. *Percept. mot. Skills*, 19: 983–1005.

Foulkes, D., Larson, J.D., Swanson, E.A. and Rardin, M. (1969) Two studies of childhood dreaming. *Amer. J. Orthopsychiat.*, 39: 627–643.

Granda, A.M. and Hammack, J.T. (1961) Operant behavior during sleep. *Science*, 133: 1485–1486.

Greenberg, R. and Pearlman, C.A. (1974) Cutting the REM nerve: an approach to the adaptive role of REM sleep. *Perspect. biol. Med.*, 17: 513–521.

Greiser, C., Greenberg, R. and Harrison, R.H. (1972) The adaptive function of sleep: the differential effects of sleep and dreaming on recall. *J. abnorm. soc. Psychol.*, 80: 280–286.

Hartman, E. (1973) *The Functions of Sleep*. Yale University Press, New Haven.

Hartmann, E. and Stern, W.C. (1972) Desynchronized sleep deprivation: learning deficit and its reversal by increased catecholamines. *Physiol. Behav.*, 8: 585–587.

Hicks, R.A., Thomsen, D., Pettey, B. and Okeida, A. (1976) REM sleep deprivation and exploration in rats. *Psychol. Rep.*, 38: 567–570.

Johnson, L.C., Townsend, R.E. and Wilson, M.R. (1975) Habituation during sleep and waking. *Psychophysiology*, 12: 574–584.

Jouvet, M. (1980) Paradoxical sleep and the nature–nurture controversy. In *Adaptive Capabilities of the Nervous System, Progress in Brain Research, Vol. 53*, Elsevier, Amsterdam, pp. 331–346.

Joy, R.M. and Prinz, P.N. (1969) The effect of sleep altering environments upon acquisition and retention of conditional avoidance response in the rat. *Physiol. Behav.*, 4: 809–814.

Koninck, J.M. de, and Koulack, D. (1975) Dream content and adaptation to a stressful situation. *J. abnorm. soc. Psychol.*, 84: 250–260.

Kramer, M. and Roth, T. (1973) The mood regulating function of sleep. In *Sleep: Physiology, Biochemistry, Psychology, Pharmacology, Clinical Implications*, W.P. Koella and P. Levin (Eds.), S. Karger, Basel, Switzerland, pp. 563–571.

Krippner, S. and Hughes, W. (1970) Dream and human potential. *J. humanist. Psychol.,* 10: 1–20.

Lasaga, J.I. and Lasaga, A.M. (1973) Sleep learning and progressive blurring of perception during sleep. *Percept. mot. Skills,* 37: 51–62.

Lehmann, D. and Koukkou, M. (1973) Learning and EEG during sleep in humans. In *Sleep, Physiology, Biochemistry, Psychology, Pharmacology, Clinical Implications,* W.P. Koella and P. Levin (Eds.), S. Karger, Basel, Switzerland, pp. 43–47.

McGrath, M.J. and Cohen, D.B. (1978) REM sleep facilitation of adaptive waking behavior: a review of the literature. *Psychol. Bull.,* 85: 24–57.

Meddis, R. (1977) *The Sleep Instinct.* Routledge and Kegan Paul, London.

Minard, J., Loiselle, R., Ingledue, E. and Dautilich, C. (1968) Discriminative electroculogram deflections (EOGDs) and heart-rate (HR) pauses elicited during maintained sleep by stimulus significance. *Psychophysiology,* 5: 232.

Oswald, I. (1980) Sleep as a restorative process: human clues. In *Adaptive Capabilities of the Nervous System, Progress in Brain Research, Vol. 53,* M.A. Corner et al. (Eds.), Elsevier, Amsterdam, pp. 279–288.

Oswald, I., Taylor, A.M. and Treisman, M. (1960) Discriminative responses to stimulation during human sleep. *Brain,* 83: 440–453.

Rechtschaffen, A. (1973) The psychophysiology of mental activity during sleep. In *The Psychophysiology of Thinking,* J. McGuigan and R.A. Schoonover (Eds.), Academic Press, New York, pp. 153–205.

Rechtschaffen, A. (1978) The single-mindedness and isolation of dreams. *Sleep,* 1: 97–109.

Rechtschaffen, A., Hauri, P. and Zeitlin, M. (1966) Auditory awakening thresholds in REM and NREM stages. *Percept. mot. Skills,* 22: 927–942.

Roffwarg, H.P., Muzio, J. and Dement, W.C. (1966) The ontogenetic development of the human sleep–dream cycle. *Science,* 152: 604–618.

Salamy, J. (1971) Effects of REM deprivation and awakening on instrumental performance during stage 2 and REM sleep. *Biol. Psychiat.,* 3: 321–330.

Snyder, F. (1966) Toward an evolutionary theory of dreaming. *Amer. J. Psychiat.,* 123: 121–136.

Vogel, G.W. (1975) A review of REM sleep deprivation. *Arch. Gen. Psychiat.,* 32: 749–761.

Walker, J.M. and Berger, R.J. (1980) Sleep as an adaptation for energy conservation functionally related to hibernation and shallow torpor. In *Adaptive Capabilities of the Nervous System, Progress in Brain Research, Vol. 53,* Elsevier, Amsterdam, pp. 255–278.

Webb, W.B. (1974) Sleep as an adaptive response. *Percept. mot. Skills.,* 38: 1023–1027.

Wickelgren, W.A. (1979) Chunking and consolidation: a theoretical synthesis of semantic networks, configuring in conditioning, S-R versus cognitive learning, normal forgetting, the amnesic syndrome and the hippocampal arousal syndrome. *Psychol. Rev.,* 86: 44–60.

Williams, H.L. (1973) Information processing during sleep. In *Sleep: Physiology, Biochemistry, Psychology, Pharmacology, Clinical Implications,* W.P. Koella and P. Levin (Eds.), S. Karger, Basel, Switzerland, pp. 36–43.

Williams, H.L., Morlock, H.C. and Morlock, J.V. (1966) Instrumental behavior during sleep. *Psychophysiology,* 2: 208–216.

Witkin, H.A. (1969) Presleep experience and dreams. In *The Meaning of Dreams: Recent Insights from the Laboratory,* J. Fisher and L. Breger (Eds.), California Mental Health Research Symposium No. 3. Bureau of Research, California department of Mental Hygiene, Sacramento, California.

Paradoxical Sleep Deprivation in Animal Studies: Some Methodological Considerations

A.M.L. COENEN and Z.J.M. VAN HULZEN

*Department of Comparative and Physiological Psychology, University of Nijmegen, 6525 GG Nijmegen
(The Netherlands)*

INTRODUCTION

Deprivation of paradoxical sleep (PS) is used extensively in animals as a method for investigating the possible role of PS in behavioural processes. Two hypotheses, based mainly on this approach, have received much attention in the current literature. The information processing hypothesis of PS (Jouvet, 1965; Gaarder, 1966; Moruzzi, 1966) relates PS to learning and memory processes, whereas the neural excitability hypothesis (Cohen and Dement, 1965) assigns PS a more general role of reducing brain excitability.

THE INFORMATION PROCESSING HYPOTHESIS

Several lines of evidence are in agreement with the idea that PS is a state conducive to information processing (Drucker-Colín and McGaugh, 1977). Unfortunately, research devoted to delineating more precisely the role of PS in learning and memory processes has provided inconsistent results. The reasons responsible for the discrepancies between studies may be at least partly methodological.

A variety of PS deprivation paradigms has been employed in studying the information processing hypothesis of PS. In the first paradigm, PS deprivation is applied for a short period of time (e.g. 3 h) immediately following learning, and the retention is measured after a period of rest. According to the consolidation hypothesis of PS (Greenberg and Pearlman, 1974; Hennevin and Leconte, 1977) a deficit in retention is produced by the absence of PS during the critical consolidation period. In the second paradigm, animals are deprived of PS for a long period of time (e.g. 72 h) following learning, and at one of several intervals after the deprivation period an electroconvulsive shock (ECS) is administered to the animals. They are allowed to recover from the acute effects of PS deprivation and ECS before retention testing takes place. An impairment of retention is interpreted in terms of the memory facilitation hypothesis of PS (Fishbein and Gutwein, 1977), according to which an already established memory trace is rendered unstable by long-term PS deprivation and susceptible to disruption. Finally, in studies using the third paradigm, long-term PS deprivation is applied prior to learning and an ECS is administered at various intervals after training. Again, a recovery period is allowed prior to the retention test. The memory facilitation hypothesis of PS accounts for a retention deficit by assuming that long-term PS deprivation delays the conversion of labile into stable memory, thereby prolonging the susceptibility

326

period of memory. Subsequent consolidation may take place when PS is permitted to occur during the interval between training and ECS.

For the purpose of depriving animals of PS two instrumental techniques are currently available. The "arousal" technique consists of waking animals each time the onset of PS is identified from electrophysiological indices. Although this technique requires much labour, it can easily be performed for a short period of time. However, after a few hours the number of awakenings needed to prevent an animal from entering PS increases rapidly (Morden et al., 1967). For long-term PS deprivation it is common to use the "watertank" technique. Animals are placed on small platforms surrounded by water. Under these circumstances when they enter PS, muscular atonia accompanying PS results in their touching the water and awakening. Inevitably, any technique of PS deprivation is more or less confounded with unintended effects, for which appropriate controls have to be designed. An obvious control for the arousal technique is the "yoked" control in which arousal takes place concurrently, irrespective of the sleep–waking activity of the control animal. The control most frequently adopted for the watertank technique is the large platform control, the adequacy of which has been thoroughly discussed in recent reviews (Vogel, 1975; Ellman et al., 1978).

Studies concerning the effects of short-term PS deprivation following learning on the retention have used the watertank technique for depriving animals of PS rather than the arousal technique. Most of these studies have reported an impairment of retention (e.g. Pearlman and Greenberg, 1973; Leconte et al., 1974). In order to control for non-specific effects accompanying the technique a delayed platform was chosen. This is understandable in view of the fact that differences in the degree of PS deprivation only gradually develop between the large and small platform conditions. However, the adequacy of the delayed platform control within this paradigm has been questioned (e.g. Vogel, 1975). What has

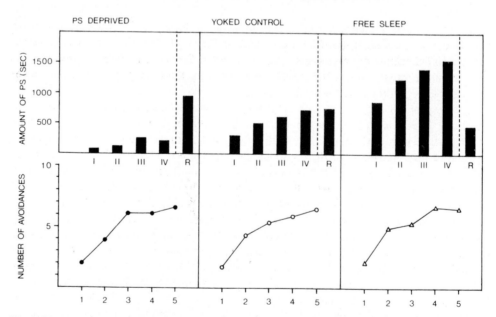

Fig. 1. Mean number of avoidances in the 5 training sessions of shuttle-box avoidance (Arabic numerals) and mean amount of PS during the 4 intersession intervals (Roman numerals) and the recovery sleep (R). The intersession intervals lasted 2 h and 45 min and the recovery sleep was monitored for 1 h. (From Van Hulzen and Coenen, 1979, reprinted by permission.)

been neglected is the fact that this control is not suitable for non-specific effects of the technique which potentially modulate memory storage processes, but only for proactive effects influencing subsequent retention.

In a recent study (Van Hulzen and Coenen, 1979), the arousal technique was used to deprive rats of PS during shuttle-box avoidance distributed over the light period of the diurnal cycle. Yoked control animals were taken as control for possible confoundings of the technique, whereas free sleep rats were left undisturbed during the intervals between sessions. It appeared that distributed shuttle-box avoidance proceeded normally irrespective of the almost total absence of PS during the intersession intervals (Fig. 1). Apparently, memory storage processes are not dependent on the presence of PS immediately following a period of learning, which violates the consolidation hypothesis of PS.

The watertank technique of PS deprivation has also been adopted for studies on the effects on retention of long-term PS deprivation prior or subsequent to learning. Commonly, the large platform is chosen as control for non-specific concomitants of the technique (e.g. stress, sleep loss, confinement, wetness). For studies in mice this control has been abandoned, because these animals tend to sit at the edge of the large platform and are almost as deprived of PS as the experimental animals (Fishbein and Gutwein, 1977). In order to circumvent this problem of control, Fishbein and his associates have designed experiments which are based on the combined effects of PS deprivation and ECS. The important variable to change is the interval between termination of PS deprivation and administration of ECS. Both in the pre-learning (e.g. Linden et al., 1975) and post-learning deprivation studies (e.g. Fishbein et al., 1971) an impairment of retention was found depending on the time between PS deprivation and ECS. One-trial passive avoidance was mostly used as the learning task in this type of study. One post-learning deprivation experiment in rats that used one way shuttle-box avoidance yielded similar results (Wolfowitz and Holdstock, 1971). The interpretion of these findings was that the state produced by long-term deprivation is detrimental to memory conversion and memory maintenance processes in the sense that they are rendered susceptible to disruption. In a recent study in mice (Shiromani et al., 1979) short-term PS deprivation, by means of the watertank technique, was applied subsequent to learning and an ECS was administered immediately thereafter. This treatment appeared ineffective in impairing retention, suggesting that short-term PS deprivation is not enough to produce a labile memory trace. The finding that memory processes are susceptible to disruption immediately after long-term PS deprivation may be alternatively interpreted by proposing that long-term PS deprivation increases central neural excitability, in which state amnesic agents are rendered more effective (Fishbein et al., 1971). This alternative interpretation is reminiscent of the neural excitability hypothesis of PS. Alterations in neural excitability induced by long-term PS deprivation may influence a variety of behavioural processes, in particular those with drive-motivational components (Vogel, 1975). It is in this context that one might consider possible effects of long-term PS deprivation on learning. There is some evidence that acquisition of avoidance learning is influenced by long-term PS deprivation (Albert et al., 1970; Plumer et al., 1974), although it is difficult to establish whether learning or performance variables are affected.

THE NEURAL EXCITABILITY HYPOTHESIS

In studying the behavioural consequences of long-term PS deprivation in the light of the neural excitability hypothesis of PS, the watertank technique has been employed for PS

328

deprivation and the large platform taken as control. Several studies in rats have reported an increase in locomotor activity after long-term PS deprivation (Albert et al., 1970; Ogilvie and Broughton, 1976; Hicks and Moore, 1979), in contrast to studies in mice (Fishbein and Gutwein, 1977) in which no differences in activity level were found. The increased locomotor activity observed in the rat after long-term PS deprivation may be due to the restriction of movement imposed on the animal on the small platform rather than to PS deprivation per se. It has been observed that mice are quite active on small platforms placed in cages with wire-mesh lids, whereas rats do not exhibit much activity under these circumstances (Fishbein and Gutwein, 1977). In other words, in this type of experiment restriction of movement is at least one variable for which the large platform may not be adequate as control.

It seems imperative to use an alternative technique of PS deprivation in conjunction with the watertank technique in order to be sure whether the behavioural effects of the deprivation treatment are due to PS deprivation per se. Therefore, a PS deprivation technique was developed (Van Hulzen and Coenen, in preparation) starting from the principle that the occurrence of PS is invariably preceded by slow-wave sleep (SWS). Animals staying in their home cages are allowed to sleep for only brief periods of time (too short to permit PS to occur) by producing postural imbalance in the animals at regular intervals. This is accomplished by an apparatus which moves the animals' cages backwards and forwards like a pendulum, forcing the animals to regularly walk downwards to the other side of their cages. Control rats are placed in a pendulum adjusted in a way that no imbalance is produced in the animals. They can therefore obtain sleep and PS while swinging. Using this technique it is possible to effectively deprive rats of PS for 72 h; only a few episodes of PS were detected in the animals during this period. The recovery sleep at the beginning of the dark phase of the illumination cycle was monitored for 3 h. Rats spent about 31% of total time in PS and 9% in SWS (Fig. 2), whereas baseline values were 6% and 11% respectively.

A preliminary study of the effects of 72 h of PS deprivation on locomotor activity was carried out in Wistar rats weighing between 275 and 375 g. The number of crossings in a shuttle-box was used as index of locomotor activity. The crossings were noted during a 15 min period at the beginning of the dark period immediately following the deprivation treat-

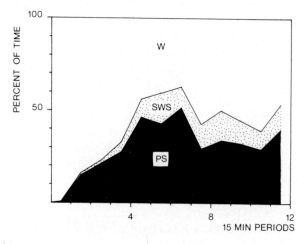

Fig. 2. Recovery sleep after 72 h of PS deprivation at the beginning of the dark phase of the illumination cycle. Mean percentages of PS, SWS and wakefulness (W), expressed in total time, are plotted in 15 min periods.

TABLE I

MEANS AND S.D. OF THE CROSSINGS IN THE SHUTTLE-BOX FOR THE 5 TREATMENT GROUPS

The data were analyzed statistically using MANOVA planned comparison tests (n per group = 12). The comparisons were: (1) group A plus B plus C plus D vs group E; (2) group A plus B vs group C plus D; (3) group A vs group B; and (4) group C vs group D. The second and fourth comparisons were found to be significant: $F(1, 55) = 4.74, P < 0.05$ and $F(1,55) = 6.64, P < 0.05$, respectively.

	Pendulum experimental (A)	Pendulum control (B)	Platform experimental (C)	Platform control (D)	Free sleep control (E)
15 min period	31.2 ± 8.5	33.7 ± 9.1	43.7 ± 15.0	33.4 ± 5.9	36.0 ± 7.8

ment. Two PS deprivation groups were studied: a "pendulum" experimental group and a "platform" experimental group. Animals of the latter group were placed on 6.2 cm diameter platforms. In addition, 3 control groups were run: a "pendulum" control, a "platform" control (diameter 12.8 cm) and a "free sleep" control. Table I summarizes the results.

The platform experimental group showed significantly more crossings in the shuttle-box than the platform control group, whereas no significant differences were found between the pendulum experimental and the pendulum control group. These results suggest that a non-specific effect of the small platform, probably its restriction of movement, was responsible for the increased locomotor activity in the platform experimental group. Consequently, other behavioural effects of this PS deprivation technique may be contaminated by changes in locomotor activity.

REFERENCES

Albert, I., Cicala, G.A. and Siegel, J. (1970) The behavioural effects of REM sleep deprivation in rats. *Psychophysiology*, 6: 552–560.

Cohen, H. and Dement, W. (1965) Sleep: changes in threshold of electroconvulsive shock in rats after deprivation of "paradoxical" phase. *Science*, 150: 1318–1319.

Drucker-Colín, R.R. and McGaugh, J.L. (1977) *Neurobiology of Sleep and Memory*, Academic Press, New York.

Ellman, S.J., Spielman, A.J., Luck, D., Steiner, S.S. and Halperin, R. (1978) REM-deprivation: a review. In *The Mind in Sleep: Psychology and Psychophysiology*, A.M. Arkin, J.S. Antrobus and S.J. Ellman (Eds.), John Wiley, New York, pp. 419–457.

Fishbein, W. and Gutwein, B.M. (1977) Paradoxical sleep and memory storage processes. *Behav. Biol.*, 19: 425–464.

Fishbein, W., McGaugh, J.L. and Swarz, J.R. (1971) Retrograde amnesia: electroconvulsive shock effects after termination of rapid eye movement sleep deprivation. *Science*, 172: 80–82.

Gaarder, K.A. (1966) A conceptual model of sleep. *Arch. gen. Psychiat.*, 14: 253–260.

Greenberg, R. and Pearlman, C. (1974) Cutting the REM-nerve: an approach to the adaptive role of REM-sleep. *Perspect. biol. Med.*, 17: 513–521.

Hennevin, E. et Leconte, P. (1977) Etude des relations entre le sommeil paradoxal et les processus d'acquisition. *Physiol. Behav.*, 18: 307–319.

Hicks, R.A. and Moore, J.D. (1979) REM-sleep deprivation diminishes fear in rats. *Physiol. Behav.*, 22: 689–692.

Jouvet, M. (1965) Paradoxical sleep. A study of its nature and mechanisms. In *Sleep Mechanisms, Progress in Brain Research, Vol. 18*, K. Akert, C. Bally and J.P. Schadé (Eds.), Elsevier, Amsterdam, pp. 20–62.

Leconte, P., Hennevin, E. and Bloch, V. (1974) Duration of paradoxical sleep necessary for the acquisition of conditioned avoidance in the rat. *Physiol. Behav.,* 13: 675–681.

Linden, E.R., Bern, D. and Fishbein, W. (1975) Retrograde amnesia: prolonging the fixation phase of memory consolidation by paradoxical sleep deprivation. *Physiol. Behav.,* 14: 409–412.

Morden, B., Mitchell, G. and Dement, W. (1967) Selective REM sleep deprivation and compensation phenomena in the rat. *Brain Res.,* 5: 339–349.

Moruzzi, G. (1966) The functional significance of sleep with particular regard to the brain mechanisms underlying consciousness. In *Brain and Conscious Experience,* J.C. Eccles (Ed.), Springer-Verlag, Berlin, pp. 345–388.

Ogilvie, R.D. and Broughton, R.J. (1976) Sleep deprivation and measures of emotionality in rats. *Psychophysiology,* 13: 249–260.

Pearlman, C.A. and Greenberg, R. (1973) Posttrial REM sleep: a critical period for consolidation of shuttle-box avoidance. *Anim. Learn. Behav.,* 1: 49–51.

Plumer, S.I., Matthews, L., Tucker, M. and Cook, T.M. (1974) The water-tank technique: avoidance conditioning as a function of water level and pedestal size. *Physiol. Behav.,* 12: 285–287.

Shiromani, P., Gutwein, B.M. and Fishbein, W. (1979) Development of learning and memory in mice after brief paradoxical sleep deprivation. *Physiol. Behav.,* 22: 971–978.

Van Hulzen, Z.J.M. and Coenen, A.M.L. (1979) Selective deprivation of paradoxical sleep and consolidation of shuttle-box avoidance. *Physiol. Behav.,* 23: 821–826.

Vogel, G.W. (1975) A review of REM sleep deprivation. *Arch. gen. Psychiat.,* 32: 749–761.

Wolfowitz, B.E. and Holdstock, T.L. (1971) Paradoxical sleep deprivation and memory in rats. *Commun. Behav. Biol.,* 6: 281–284.

Paradoxical Sleep
and the Nature–Nurture Controversy

MICHEL JOUVET

Department of Experimental Medicine, Claude Bernard University, Lyon (France)

INTRODUCTION

Individual differences in behaviour between animals of the same species are common knowledge. Since Locke and his "Tabula Rasa" postulate, individual differences in behaviour have been explained by different environmental conditions. This explanation was also given by Watson (1924) and became an axiom of experimental psychology. However, it also became evident that the concept of "average individual responses" to a stimulus was a fiction. Tryon (1934) opened a new way of understanding individual differences in behaviour when he began the analysis of the genetic variance for maze learning behaviour. This analysis was most welcomed by evolutionary biologists. As stated by Mayr (1958): "Striking individual differences have been described for predatory–prey relations, for the reactions of birds to mimicking or to warning colourations, for child care among primates and for maternal behaviour in rats. It is generally agreed by observers that much of this individual difference is not affected by experience but remains essentially constant through the entire life-time of the individual . . .". In fact, such striking individual differences had been also described 30 years previously by Pavlov (1927): "The type and degree of pathological disturbance that develops from some definite cause was found in all cases to be determined primarily by the character of the individual nervous system of the animals . . .".

These short citations from the long lasting "nature vs nurture" controversy (see Hirsch, 1962; Diamond, 1974) are a good introduction to ask the following naïve questions:

(1) Since there are both genetic and epigenetic (environmental) factors responsible for individual differences in behaviour, how and when do they interact?

(2) It can be easily admitted that the genetic factors are predominant during ontogenesis. But is this process terminated at the end of the maturation of the central nervous system? Do the numerous synaptic connections between the billions of neurones responsible for idiosyncratic behaviour remain unaltered during the entire life-span?

Yet, after the end of maturation of the central nervous system (CNS), epigenetic stimuli alter the pattern of organization of the CNS both in its structural and biochemical aspects (see refs. in Gottlieb, 1976). How, then, can we explain that animals which have been raised in the same environment may show different behaviours in response to the same stimuli? Epigenetic stimuli usually need numerous repetitions in order to alter the synaptic organization established at the end of maturation. Why should genetic programming mechanisms not also need to be reinforced through reprogrammation in order to maintain, re-establish or "stabilize" those synaptic pathways which are responsible for individual differences in behaviour? The answer to these questions depends upon solving the following problems:

(1) How could a genetic reprogramming operate in an adult animal; does the mature brain periodically "regress" to immaturity? Are there modifiable synapses which can be activated or stabilized by some endogenous stimulating mechanism, and when could such a mechanism occur?

(2) If such a mechanism exists, how can we demonstrate its existence? The inter-individual or phenotypic (P) variance in behaviour can be partitioned into components:

$$\sigma P^2 = \sigma G^2 + \sigma E^2 + \sigma I^2$$

where G represents heredity, E the environment and I their interaction (Hirsch, 1962). In the case of genetic reprogramming (G′) we have one more component:

$$\sigma P^2 = \sigma G^2 + \sigma G'^2 + \sigma E^2 + \sigma I^2 .$$

On the one hand, if we could suppress G′ in an individual from a heterogeneous genetic population, the comparison of the possible alteration of its behaviour with the average behaviour of the other members of the population will be difficult, since the very concept of "average behaviour" is a myth. On the other hand, it would be easier to measure the effect of G′ in different pure strains of animals, since its suppression might be expected to decrease the phenotypic variance of behaviour which exists between the two populations.

In this speculative essay, we shall review the experimental evidence in favour of the hypothesis that an endogenous genetic programming occurs during paradoxical sleep (PS) in mammals. Firstly, the steps are outlined which would be necessary (at least theoretically) for a periodical "read out" of the innate endogenous mechanism that would programme the brain for specific individual behaviour or "typology". Such a mechanism would obey some internal laws (that shall be called here "synchronistic organization"). It would also necessitate some relationship with the epigenetic history of the organism ("diachronistic organization"). Secondly, some of the mechanisms of PS which could fit this model will be summarized.

A THEORETICAL MODEL OF PERIODIC GENETIC PROGRAMMING OF THE CENTRAL NERVOUS SYSTEM *

Synchronistic organization of the model

How could a genetic reprogramming operate in a mature nervous system? There are several theoretical possibilities:

(a) some humoral factor(s) either in the blood or in the CSF may stimulate or de-repress the DNA of some neurones, which then enter into mitosis, divide and start making new programmed connections. This mechanism would contradict the dogma that mature neurones do not divide, as neuroblasts do, but well established dogma sometimes have to be modified. It has indeed recently been shown by Lundberg and Mollgard (1979) that transplants of foetal brain or liver may induce mitosis in neurones of the *mature* rat brain. α-Foeto-protein would be a putative factor for such an effect. It remains of course to be

---

* This model differs from the model which has been proposed earlier (Jouvet, 1978) in as much as it emphasizes *selective* mechanisms, whereas the first model was based upon *instructive* mechanisms.

proven that this protein (or a similar one) could cross the blood-brain or the blood—CSF barrier in the adult brain;

(b) reprogramming of the specific genetic synaptic circuitry responsible for individual specificity of behaviour does not necessitate the building of new circuitry. Special classes of neurones established late in ontogeny, like Jacobson type II neurones (Jacobson, 1970), might synthesize proteins which would be incorporated in the membrane as receptors. The stimulation of these receptors by some endogenous stimulating mechanism could reprogramme the genetic organization of behaviour via the same "stabilizing mechanisms" which occur during learning involving epigenetic stimulation. In this case, we have to postulate the existence of some endogenous pacemaker or generator which would impinge upon those neurones (see Fig. 1).

Since "genetic programming" is related to behaviour, an *organization of stereotyped innate activity* in the pyramidal and extrapyramidal motor system should result, so that "rehearsal" (maintenance, facilitation or induction) of genetically programmed behaviour might occur. Thus, the descending volleys would necessarily impinge upon the moto-.neurones.

Since motoneurones are submitted to the influences of a genetic programming, two consequences should ensue:

(a) in some experiments on animals of pure genetic strain it should be possible to distinguish *certain genetic components* in the firing of motoneurons which fall directly under the control of the generator during the programming period;

(b) there would also have to be some mechanism which *suppresses overall muscular* activity during the programming of the perceptual and motor systems. Otherwise, the organism would be subject to some uncontrolled stereotyped behaviour which is possibly very inadaptive during either wakefulness or sleep.

In order to achieve this genetic "readout" without too much "external noise", a mecha-

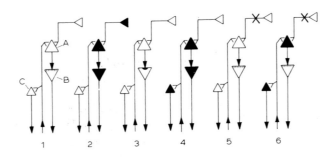

Fig. 1. Theoretical model of a genetic reprogramming during PS. 1: a neurone (B) responsible for the genetic reprogramming (Golgi type II) has synthesized a protein from the genome located in the nucleus of the perikaryon. This protein is incorporated into the membrane as a labile receptor (hatched area). 2: during PS, the PGO system (upper right in black) impinges directly or indirectly upon the interneurone A. This will stimulate and stabilize the receptor of neurone B. 3: this stabilization persists during the waking period following PS. 4: as long as the receptor is functional, epigenetic stimuli (ascending fibre) will be able to activate both non-specific arousal (C) and the idiosyncratic behavioural responses. 5: if PS is suppressed (crosses) and if PGO programming does not occur, the receptor protein is not stabilized and neurone B cannot be activated. 6: in such a case the epigenetic stimulus will not trigger the hereditary specific behavioural response, but only non-specific arousal or orientating responses. Chloramphenicol could act upon the synthesis of the post-synaptic receptor of neurone B. This would explain the uncoupling between PGO activity and multi-unit activity, depending upon the output of neurone B (see text).

nism is required that would *inhibit the arrival of external inputs*. Thus, most of the synapses submitted to the "programming" would be ready for any "integrative process" as may occur during epigenetic attention.

Finally, since at the time of hereditary programming the brain cannot receive and respond to external (and possibly internal) incoming stimuli due to the inhibition of afferent impulses, and since muscular activity is also inhibited, a *protective mechanism* must exist that enables this process to occur when and only when the organism is not threatened by potentially dangerous stimuli, i.e. at a time when the waking mechanisms are no longer stimulated, thus *during sleep*.

Diachronistic organization of the model

Genetic programming should, of course, be predominant during ontogenesis, i.e. during the period of that genetic readout which structurally programs the CNS. Programming should then decrease with maturation, since it can only occur during sleep.

In order to be effective, periodic programming must be related to the previous epigenetic stimuli that impinge upon the CNS during waking, since learning may have somewhat altered the previous genetic reprogramming. For example, there should be some mechanism that adapts the duration of the genetic readout to the number of significant external or internal (hormonal) stimuli which have induced some epigenetic alterations of the synapses.

However, the genetic readout, being mostly related "forward to experience", is not necessarily adaptive to the latest historical situation of the individual. In such a case, the periodic reprogrammation may or may not be in accordance with the processing of new information. In some cases, it may facilitate the acquisition of long-term memory, but in others, it may have no effect, or may even inhibit or destroy certain epigenetic memory traces. Thus, suppression of genetic programming may either impair, facilitate or have no effect upon learning, but it should always decrease the phenotypic variance in behaviour among individuals belonging to different genetic strains of the same species.

ARE THE MECHANISMS OF PARADOXICAL SLEEP SUITABLE FOR A PERIODIC GENETIC PROGRAMMING OF THE CNS?

In this section, the neurophysiological mechanisms of paradoxical sleep, which might be explained by a theoretical model of genetic programming, will be summarized.

Synchronistic mechanisms

Protein synthesis and paradoxical sleep. The possible, but very unlikely possibility that mitosis of adult central neurones might be triggered by PS has not yet been examined. However, the hypothesis that protein synthesis occurs during PS (and could play a role in genetic reprogramming), is indirectly supported by the following evidence.

(a) A protein or peptide factor may be necessary for PS (Fig. 2). PS can be selectively suppressed by several inhibitors of protein synthesis which do not alter either waking or slow wave sleep, e.g. cycloheximide (Pegram et al., 1973) and chloramphenicol (Petitjean et al., 1975; Rojas-Ramirez et al., 1977). Moreover, chloramphenicol administered to a *p*-chlorophenylalanine (PCPA)-pretreated cat suppresses the occurrence of PS which otherwise follows a subsequent injection of 5-hydroxytryptophan (5-HTP) or γ-hydroxybutyrate (Petit-

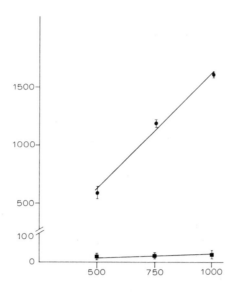

Fig. 2. Suppression of paradoxical sleep by chloramphenicol. Ordinate: duration (min) of the suppression of PS after the oral administration of chloramphenicol (black circles). Absence of effect of thioamphenicol (black squares). Mean ± S.D. (5 cats). Abscissa: dose (g) for a 3 kg cat.

jean, personal communication). The possible inhibitory action of chloramphenicol upon mitochondrial protein synthesis is unlikely to be the explanation, since thioamphenicol (which also has a similar action upon mitochondria) does not alter PS (Petitjean et al., 1975). However, the fact that a peptide, mediated through the blood or CSF, is necessary for PS does not necessarily indicate that the protein synthesis required for genetic reprogramming of synaptic circuitry occurs *during* PS;

(b) PS dependent protein synthesis can occur in the brain. A high molecular weight protein has been found in the brain of PCPA-pretreated cats (Bobillier et al., 1973) after restoration of SWS and PS by means of 5-HTP. The results obtained by Drucker-Colín et al. (1975) also suggest that protein is released in the brain stem of the cat during PS. Moreover, the administration of *low* doses of chloramphenicol (insufficient to suppress PS) results in the uncoupling of ponto—geniculo—occipital (PGO) activity and multiple unit activity recorded in several regions of the brain stem (Drucker-Colín et al., 1979). If this finding were to be verified by recordings from single neurones it would have important theoretical significance, since it would imply that the programming of the CNS by the PGO generator does not activate the putative, genetically programmed post-synaptic receptors of Golgi type II neurones. In such a case, chloramphenicol would inhibit the synthesis of certain post-synaptic receptors according to the hypothesis of Ramirez (1973) (Fig. 1).

The PGO system as an endogenous programming mechanism. According to the experimental data, obtained mainly in the cat during the last 20 years, the concept of a ponto-geniculo-occipital (PGO) system, where high voltage slow PGO waves can be recorded during PS, has emerged and can be briefly summarized as follows.

(a) The "generator" of PGO activity is located in a cluster of neurones located in the dorsolateral part of the pontine reticular formation. There are two bilaterally symmetrical "generators", each of which may be subdivided into two components: the one for programming the rostral part of the brain is situated in the region of the nucleus parabrachialis

336

lateralis and dorso-lateralis tegmenti; the second lies in the region of the Kolliker–Fuse nucleus, and is related to eye movements during PS (Sakai, 1979). These generators of PGO activity are not unlike any other pacemaker system, since PGO activity can still be recorded both *periodically* and *spontaneously* in the "isolated pons preparation", where the region of the generator is isolated by prepontine and midbulbar transsections (Matsuzaki, 1969). The chief neurotransmitter of PGO activity is still unknown, but there is indirect evidence supporting the role of cholinoceptive synapses in the generation of PGO activity (see Jouvet, 1972).

(b) The pathways which convey PGO information from the pons to the lateral geniculate nucleus have been delimitated by the lesion technique. An ipsilateral pathway ascends from each generator, impinges upon the lateral geniculate nucleus and the visual cortex, and crosses the midline in the suprachiasmatic commissure to reach the contralateral geniculate body (Laurent et al., 1974). Pontine generators send excitatory influences also to the contralateral oculomotor nuclei through pauci-synaptic connections (Cespuglio et al., 1975a).

What are the targets of the PGO programming? Chronic microelectrode recording from single cells or of integrated multi-unit activity (MUA) from the cat's brain during PS, in combination with macroelectrode recording of PGO, have provided us with an abundance of data concerning most of the cortical and subcortical structures. Thus, it has been shown that MUA in the pontine and mesencephalic reticular formation, the red nucleus, the pyramidal tract, etc. is correlated with PGO activity. At the cortical level, 40% of the visual cortex neurones are influenced – inhibited or excited – by PGO activity (see Steriade and Hobson, 1976). Moreover, the work of Steriade (1978) has provided us with new information concerning the possible nature of the cortical cells which enter into play during PS. In a series of careful studies, Steriade and his associates found that large output cells (Golgi type I) were active during waking, while Golgi type II interneurones in the parietal association areas were silent. In contrast, these interneurones discharged at high frequency during PS in "spectacularly close temporal relation with the rapid-eye-movements". Although PGO activity was not recorded in these experiments, it is most likely that the discharges of these Golgi type II cells were under the influence of the ascending PGO activity, since ocular motricity during

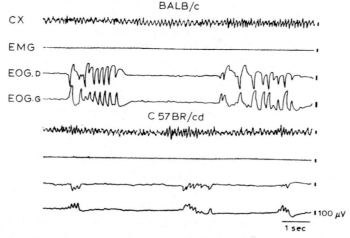

Fig. 3. The patterns of rapid-eye-movement recorded during PS from the right and left electro-oculogram (EOG-D-G) are strikingly different in BALB/c and C57BR/cd mice. CX, frontal cortex. EMG of the neck muscle. Calibration: 1 sec, 100 μV. (From Cespuglio et al., 1975a.)

waking had no such effect. Thus, Golgi type II interneurones (which develop later than Golgi type I cells in ontogenesis) could be a good candidate for the reinforcement of typology by genetic programming (see Fig. 1). Their activation by the PGO system during PS would permit the control of a very large proportion of the cortical and subcortical neurones.

Evidence for a genetic coding of the pattern of PGO activity (Fig. 3). Genetic studies of PS are not easy since they can be performed only in mice, the only "dreaming" mammals in which inbred strains are available. Unfortunately, it is very difficult to record central PGO activity in mice, but the analysis of the rapid-eye-movements (REM) during PS may provide an indirect, but accurate index of the PGO pattern. Thus, the patterns of REM in two inbred strains, C57BR and BALB/C, during PS are strikingly different in animals kept for a long time in the same environment (Cespuglio et al., 1975b). The analysis of the pattern of REM in the F1 hybrids and in the back cross, which necessitates the use of a large computer, is not yet finished, so we do not have enough data to specify and analyze the nature of the genetic mechanisms which are probably involved in the control of PGO patterning. Different patterns of organization of PGO pattern have also been registered in two subspecies of baboons (*Papio papio* and *Papio hamadryas*) by Bert (1975).

To sum up, the PGO system may be compared, on the one hand, to an endogenous stimulating system which influences a large proportion of brain cells during PS (an influence which may be mediated in part through the excitation of Golgi type II interneurones). On the other hand, the pattern of PGO activity appears to be controlled by genetic factors in inbred strains of mice. The analogy between the PGO system and the hypothetical endogenous genetic programming system, as proposed above, is therefore not unlikely.

What is the "on line" result of the PGO programming upon behaviour?

According to the synchronistic organization of the model, a genetic reprogramming would validate or "stabilize" the synapses involved in that repertoire of performances which is responsible for the idiosyncrasy of behaviour (i.e. *individual* differences) within a non-inbred population, or for *typological* differences among inbred populations. We should therefore be able, in principle, to observe the "on line" result of this programming during PS, but this is of course impossible during physiological PS, since the total inhibition of muscular tone which prevents gross body movements is in fact one of the major criteria of PS. However, thanks to microelectrode recordings, various anatomical methods, and local lesion with thermocoagulation or kainic acid, it has been possible to delimit quite precisely the neural systems which are responsible for postural atonia (Sakai, 1979; Sakai et al., 1979; Sastre et al., 1979). This has made possible very discrete lesions which selectively suppress postural atonia, which has permitted us to unveil the dramatic "oneiric" behaviours which correspond to the on-line behavioural result of the PGO programming.

The postural atonia system

The powerful inhibitory mechanism responsible for postural atonia during PS is commanded by a bilateral cluster of neurones located medially to the locus coeruleus α (peri-locus coeruleus α). These neurones, which are most probably cholinoceptive, are connected with the magnocellular nucleus of the medulla through a descending ipsilateral pathway. From this latter nucleus, which belongs to the inhibitory bulbar formation of Magoun and Rhines (1946), reticulo-spinal influences exert a powerful pre- and post-synaptic inhibition upon the motoneurones. The alternative hypothesis that the giganto-cellular nucleus of the fronto-tegmental field of the pontine tegmentum is responsible for postural atonia, PGO

338

activity and fast cortical activity during PS (Hobson et al., 1974a, b; McCarley and Hobson, 1971) has been recently invalidated, since its total destruction with in situ injection of kainic acid does not alter these tonic or phasic components of PS (Sastre et al., 1979).

The oneiric behaviour

The system controlling the inhibition of muscle tone during PS does not belong to the "generator" responsible for PGO coding, nor to the system responsible for fast cortical activity during PS. It is therefore possible to destroy it in the cat without interfering with the central programming that occurs during PS. Thus, the *bilateral* destruction of a small portion of the locus coeruleus complex, or of its descending pontine pathway, is followed by the appearance of complex motor behaviour during PS (Sastre, 1978; Sastre and Jouvet, 1979).

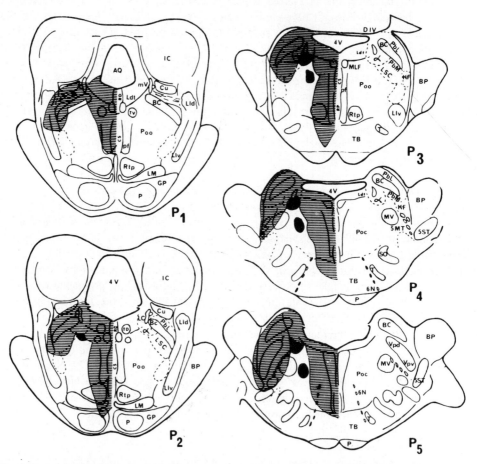

Fig. 4. Frontal section of the pons of the cat in the Horsley–Clarke coordinates P1–5. The solid areas indicate the (unilateral) localization of those (bilateral) lesions which selectively suppress postural atonia during PS. The dorsal lesion coincides with the medial part of locus coeruleus α and peri-locus coeruleus α. The ventral lesion corresponds to the interruption of a descending lateral tegmento–reticular pathway which terminates in the magno-cellular nucleus of the medulla. The horizontal hatching corresponds to electrolytic lesions which do not suppress postural atonia. PGL, n. parabrachialis lateralis; Ldt, n. lateralis tegmenti dorsalis; PGM, n. parabrachialis medialis; KF, n. Kolliker–Fuse; PoC, n. pontis caudalis; BP, brachium pontis; 5MT, motor nucleus of trigeminal nerve; BC, brachium conjunctivum; 4V, fourth ventricle. (Modified from Sastre, 1978.)

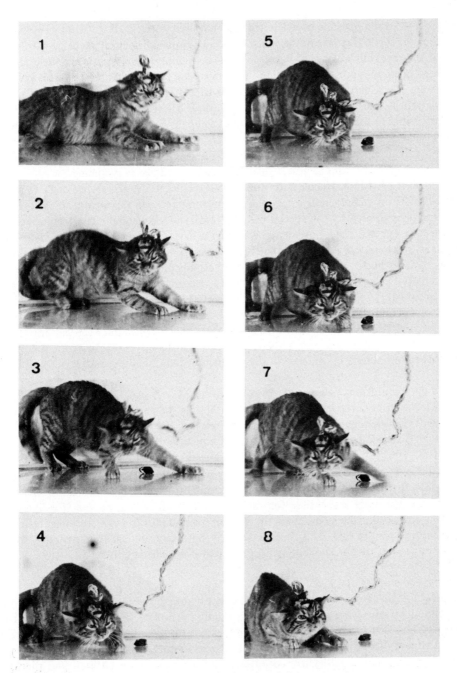

Fig. 5. Oneiric fright behaviour during PS 3 weeks after bilateral destruction of the region of locus coeruleus α. (From Sastre, 1978.)

While there is no alteration of behaviour during waking or slow wave sleep, the onset of PS – which is characterized by fast cortical activity, PGO activity and extreme myosis – leads to an *increase* of muscle tone. The cat will then raise its head and display "orienting behaviour" towards some laterally or vertically situated absent stimulus. Afterwards, it may "follow" some invisible object in its cage and even "attack" it, or it may display rage behaviour, or fright (Fig. 5). We have also observed grooming or drinking behaviour (on the floor of the cage) but we have so far not observed any sexual behaviour in the male cats that have been operated upon. The duration of these stereotyped oneiric behaviours is very variable. If the attack behaviour is too violent, this will often awaken the animal briefly, after which it usually goes back to sleep. Pursuit behaviour has been observed to last up to 3 min. It is impossible to predict what kind of stereotyped behaviour will occur at the beginning of each episode of PS, *but there is a distinct overall statistical organization for each cat.* Some cats may display up to 60% of aggressive behaviour whereas others display only 20% of such behaviour and present, for example, a relatively high percentage of grooming.

The oneiric behaviour which occurs during PS is related to the occurrence of PGO activity (Sastre, 1978). In fact, there is a very close correlation between the activity of each pontine generator (as indicated by the special PGO pattern in the ipsilateral lateral geniculate) and the orienting eye and head movements. Watching behaviour, which is so characteristic in the still cat without any eye or head movements, is not accompanied by any PGO activity. Complex behaviours such as pursuit or attack are accompanied by a very complex pattern of PGO activity. Since PGO activity *precedes* the occurrence of eye movements and other muscular activity, we must conclude that the central PGO activity is either responsible for central programming or that it occurs simultaneously with it. The neurophysiological mechanisms responsible for oneiric behaviour are not yet known, but either the pattern of PGO activity is "instructive" and can actually *organize* the stereotyped activity or, more probably, this pattern *selects* certain genetically programmed motor subsystems.

Control of afferent stimuli during PS

This mechanism occurring during PS (but not during the period of slow wave sleep which precedes it) is well-documented (see refs. in Pompeiano, 1970) and is not unlike the afferent control mechanism that has been postulated during attention and distraction (Hernandez-Peon et al., 1961). It has been verified in the somesthetic, auditory and the visual systems. In this latter system, moreover, it has been shown that the PGO activity itself is directly responsible for the control of visual afferent sensitivity. We still do not know the exact mechanisms which are responsible for such controls in other systems, but it is likely that they too come from the pons, since the control over auditory inputs still operates during PS in chronic pontile cats. This mechanism may be responsible, at least partially, for the striking increase in the threshold of auditory arousal which characterizes PS.

Sleep and the priming of PS

Under normal circumstances, PS does not appear during waking. It has to be "primed" by a period of slow wave sleep (SWS). This priming period of sleep can occur only if the waking system of the brain stem is no longer excited by potentially dangerous external or internal stimuli (acoustic or olfactory signals from predators, pain, etc.). Thus, the amount of PS in mammals is significantly correlated with a safety factor (Allison and Cicchetti, 1976). Among the mechanisms which enter into play during waking, the noradrenergic neurones which ascend within the dorsal norepinephrine bundle are in part responsible for the tonic EEG activation of the cortex (see Jouvet, 1972). The overall decrease of unitary activity in the rostral part of the locus coeruleus which occurs at the beginning of PS (Chu and Bloom, 1974) and which belongs to the gating mechanisms of PGO waves, may therefore be the electrical index signalling the dampening of an important subsystem belonging to the waking mechanisms. How the slow wave sleep mechanisms contribute to the priming of PS, is still not known. Apparently, the rostral raphe system is active during waking but silent during PS, since unit activity in the nucleus raphe dorsalis stops completely at the beginning of PS (McGinty and Harper, 1976). Thus, this nucleus could also be involved in controlling the gate for releasing PGO activity. Since the activity of, presumably serotonin (5-HT)-containing, neurones of the nucleus raphe magnus *increases* during PS (Cespuglio et al., 1978), the caudal raphe system might inhibit the rostral raphe so as to open the gate. The presence of peptides together with 5-HT in the raphe neurones (Chan-Palay et al., 1978; Hökfelt et al., 1978) would be in accordance with the hypothesis that peptide factor(s) are also involved in PS mechanisms (see above).

Summing up, the onset of PS (which is the most dangerous part of the sleep—waking cycle, since the organism is blind, deaf and paralyzed) is protected by at least two mechanisms. The first one is passive: the decrease of activity of the waking system in the absence of potentially external or internal dangerous stimuli; the second is active: the intervention of serotoninergic mechanisms, which are first involved in SWS and then open the "gating mechanisms" that control PGO activity.

Diachronistic organization of PS

PS and the ontogenesis of the central nervous system (Fig. 6)

The high amount of PS or of a "PS-like state" during early maturation of the CNS is a most striking phenomenon which has been verified in ovo in the chick (see Corner, 1977), in utero in the guinea pig, and post-natally in the rat, kitten and newborn baby (see Jouvet-Mounier et al., 1970; Roffwarg et al., 1966). Apparently, when the CNS is still undergoing maturational processes, during which a strict genetic programming takes place in order to organize the "hardwired" multiple synaptic connections among different systems, PS, or a PS-like state occupies 50—60% or more of the total time. It is also quite possible that such a process is diffuse in this very early period, when most of the neurones have not yet made their synaptic connections. It is only when the maturational processes become terminated

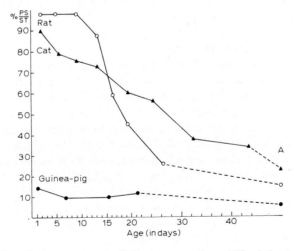

Fig. 6. Paradoxical sleep during ontogenesis. Ordinate: proportion of PS relative to total sleep duration (TS). Abscissa: age (in days). A, adult. Immature newborn mammals, such as the rat or the cat, have a much greater proportion of PS than mature newborns, such as the guinea-pig. However, a similar increase of PS can be recorded in utero in foetal guinea-pigs when their CNS is still undergoing maturation. (From Jouvet-Mounier et al., 1970.)

(e.g. when there is no more division of neuroblasts) that the formation of synaptic connections by the pontine PGO generator enables this endogenous pacemaker system to start periodically programming the Golgi type II interneurones which have only just appeared (Jacobson, 1970).

PS, phylogenesis and adaptivity

In order to be adaptive, the genetic programming occurring during PS should be in some relationship with previous events (immediate past history) and should also serve to prime or to organize subsequent behaviour. Indeed, a periodic programming mechanism will be acting upon an altered nervous system every time the latter has been submitted to epigenetic stimuli. Thus, there will be many more possibilities of interaction between "nature and nurture", so that *the range of modifiability of innate behaviour could be increased.*

Such a possibility would not exist in animals that do not undergo PS, as most probably is the case in poikilothermic animals (amphibians, fishes, reptiles). In these lower vertebrates, PS or a PS-like state might exist in ovo (see Corner, 1977), but the genetic programming would be over at the end of maturation. The innate patterns of behaviour are then fixed for the entire life-span within the genetic structures of the CNS, with little or no further possibility of modification in these lower vertebrates. However, selective synaptogenesis still exists in the adult animals, as a consequence of which the optic nerve fibres in adult amphibians, for example, are able to regenerate after being sectioned. This phenomenon, which does not exist in birds or mammals, has been used as a model for the restoration of visual function after transplantation of the eye in numerous experiments (see Gottlieb, 1976). In such a case, the genome of the nerve cells contains all the information needed to maintain synaptogenesis of innate circuitry even after the end of the maturative period. This process does not permit much flexibility, however, and it is well known that innate behaviour is much more rigid in lower vertebrates than in higher forms.

The appearance of homeothermia in higher vertebrates which gives more liberty to the organism, was accompanied by an increase in complexity of the brain. PS, may have been evolved in order to permit more variance, and thus more degrees of freedom, in the expression of genetically controlled behaviour.

Relation of PS to previous epigenetic events

Epigenetic events may act upon PS by controlling its duration. This control is proven by the well-known related phenomena which create the "need" for PS, its "rebound" after a previous deprivation, and the "reimbursement of the debt" which occurs. These phenomena demonstrate that there are some regulatory mechanisms tending to determine the quantities of PS and of PGO waves as biological constants (respectively, 180 min and 16,000 per diem in the cat). Two processes may increase the quantity of PS: the first one shortens the duration of the intervals between PS while the second increases the duration of PS episodes. Both processes enter into play during the rebound of PS (which never exceeds 60% of sleeping time, whatever the duration of deprivation (Vimont-Vicary et al., 1966). It is possible that the periodicity of PS depends upon the metabolism of the 5-HT neurones which prime PS. Indeed, the durations of intervals between PS become increased when 5-HT metabolism is decreased (as after injections of PCPA, monoamine oxidase inhibitors, or destruction of the raphe system), while they become shortened when its metabolism increases (as after PS deprivation or lesion of the isthmus, see Jouvet, 1972). The mechanism responsible for the increase in duration of PS episodes is unknown, but it could be related either to the increased protein synthesis possibly occurring during PS deprivation or to the putative

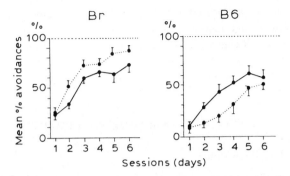

Fig. 7. Effect of pharmacological PS deprivation by α-methyl-DOPA on the performance of an active avoidance task in a Y maze in two C57 strains: C57BR(BR) and C57BL/6(B6). Administration of α-methyl-DOPA (100 mg/kg) provokes complete suppression of PS for 9—11 h. Daily injection immediately after each training session over the first 5 days caused a delay in acquisition of an active avoidance task in BR mice. Treated B6 mice exhibited a significant facilitation of acquisition. Similar results were obtained by instrumental PS deprivation for 10 h. Dotted lines, controls; solid lines, treated mice. (Modified from Kitahama et al., 1976.)

executive cholinergic and/or cholinoceptive mechanisms.

Interestingly enough, only the first of the two processes enters into play when PS increases during learning (see Hennevin and Leconte, 1971). In such a case, the regulatory mechanism is only responsible for the decrease of the intervals between PS episodes, *but it does not act upon PS itself.*

Relationship of PS with subsequent behaviour

This final section concerns the very controversial subject of PS deprivation (see Vogel, 1975). For the time being, it is impossible to suppress PS selectively without serious non-specific side effects (stress, total sleep disturbances, etc.). A review of the literature concerning the effects of PS deprivation upon learning shows an almost equal number of positive and negative findings. This discrepancy may result partly from genetic factors. The interaction between PS deprivation and learning in different genetic strains has been extensively studied (Kitahama, 1979; Kitahama and Valatx, 1979; Kitahama et al., 1980) and the results obtained with C57 mice can be summarized as follows. C57BR and C57BL/6 have the same genetic origin. They also have a similar amount of SWS and PS, the same circadian variation of the sleep—waking cycle, and they present an identical recovery of PS after deprivation ("reimbursement" of 60% of the PS "debt"). However, these two strains differ both in their activity in the open field and in their learning ability in active avoidance tasks in Y mazes: C57BR show a "reminiscence effect" which does not exist in C57BL/6. Neither of these two strains show such an effect for positive reinforcement (Destrade et al., 1976). Instrumental PS deprivation (lasting either 10 or 24 h) or pharmacological PS suppression with chlorimipramine or α-methyl DOPA supresses the reminiscence effect in C57BR, facilitates learning in C57BL/6 in some conditions, or else has no effect (Fig. 7). Moreover, PS deprivation has no significant effect on the high open field activity of C57BR, whereas it significantly increases the low activity of C57BL/6 (Kitahama, 1979). Thus, the *phenotypic variance between C57BR and C57BL/6 for both maze avoidance learning and open field activity is significantly reduced by PS deprivation.*

These results do not prove, of course, that PS is responsible for a genetic reprogramming process which would increase the phenotypic variance among different genetic strains. It could be objected that factors other than PS deprivation are responsible for these effects (an objection which cannot be rejected at the present time). Moreover, one might explain these results by postulating that PS deprivation alters learning only in "fast" learners (as the C57BR), while "slow" learners (C57BL/6) cannot be so impaired. However, inhibition of protein synthesis which cycloheximide (which acts upon intrinsic learning mechanisms and also suppresses PS) does considerably impair learning in both of the C57 strains.

WHAT IS PROGRAMMED DURING PS?

If we come back to the formula

$$\sigma P^2 = \sigma G^2 + \sigma G'^2 + \sigma E^2 + \sigma I^2$$

in which G' represents PS, i.e. the periodic endogenous stimulation of hereditarily programmed synapses (possibly Golgi type II interneurones), while G represents the genetic blue-print established during maturation (mostly with Golgi type I neurones), we can see that the best experimental possibilities for studying the effect of PS supression would be to keep both G and environment as well controlled as possible (e.g. by using inbred genetic strains and isolation experiments). Will PS suppression decrease the phenotypic variance among strains of mice with respect to nest building or maternal behaviours, or between a gun and a sporting dog as concerns hunting tactics? If certain innate behaviours necessitate a genetic reprogramming during PS in order to stabilize the templates for recognition of innate releasing stimuli and for rehearsal of fixed motor patterns (as has been discussed earlier, see Jouvet, 1978), it follows that severe alterations in the development of these behaviours may well occur. If the genetic programming of "typology" is valid in man, then the 100 min of dreaming which occur every night may be as important as the action of the cultural environment which surrounds us during waking. Would PS deprivation in man, in diminishing our hereditary programmation, increase the relative weight of the social and cultural influences, and what are the limits? This question might have some important ethical consequences.

ACKNOWLEDGEMENTS

This work has been performed with the help of INSERM Grant U 52, CNRS Grant LA 162 and DRET Grant 77 093.

REFERENCES

Allison, T. and Cicchetti, D.V. (1976) Sleep in mammals: ecological and constitutional correlates. *Science*, 194: 732–734.

Bert, J. (1975) Caractères génériques et caractères spécifiques de l'activité de pointes "ponto-géniculo-occipitales" (PGO) chez deux babouins, *Papio hamadryas* et *Papio papio*. *Brain Res.*, 88: 362–366.

Bobillier, P., Froment, J.L., Seguin, S. et Jouvet, M. (1973) Effects de la p. chlorophenylalanine et du 5-hydroxytryptophane sur le sommeil et le métabolisme central des monoamines et des protéines chez le chat. *Biochem. Pharmacol.*, 22: 3077–3090.

Cespuglio, R., Laurent, J.P. et Jouvet, M. (1975a) Etude des relations entre l'activité ponto–géniculo–occipitale (PGO) et la motricité oculaire chez le chat sous réserpine. *Brain Res.*, 83: 319–335.

Cespuglio, R., Musolino, R., Debilly, G., Jouvet, M. et Valatx, J.L. (1975b) Organisation différente des mouvements oculaires rapides du sommeil paradoxal chez deux souches consanguines de souris. *C.R. Acad. Sci. (Paris)*, 280: 2681–2684.

Cespuglio, R., Gomez, M.E., Walker, E. and Jouvet, M. (1978) Single unit recordings of the nuclei raphe dorsalis and magnus during sleep–waking cycle. In *Sleep Research, Vol. 7,* M. Chase, M.M. Mitler and P. Walter (Eds.), Brain Research Institute, Univ. of California. Los Angeles, 26.

Chan-Palay, V., Jonsson, G. and Palay, S.L. (1978) Serotonin and substance P coexist in neurons of the rat's central nervous system. *Proc. nat. Acad. Sci. (Wash.),* 75: 1582–1586.

Chu, N.S. and Bloom, F.E. (1974) Activity patterns of catecholamine-containing pontine neurons in the dorsal-lateral tegmentum of unrestrained cats. *J. Neurobiol.,* 5: 544–577.

Corner, M.A. (1977) Sleep and the beginnings of behavior in the animal kingdom-studies of ultradian motility cycles in early life. *Progr. Neurobiol.,* 8: 279–296.

Destrade, C., Jaffard, R., Deminiere, J.M. et Cardo, B. (1976) Effets de la stimulation de l'Hippocampe sur la réminiscence chez deux lignées de souris. *Physiol. Behav.,* 16: 237–243.

Diamond, S. (1974) Four hundred years of instinct controversy. *Behav. Gen.,* 4: 237–252.

Drucker-Colín, R.R., Spanis, C.W., Cotman, C.W. and McGaugh, J.L. (1975) Changes in protein levels in perfusates of freely moving cats: relation to behavioral state. *Science,* 187: 963–964.

Drucker-Colín, R.R., Zamora, J., Bernal-Pedraza, J. and Sosa, B. (1979) Modification of REM sleep and associated phasic activities by protein synthesis inhibitors. *Exp. Neurol.,* 63: 458–467.

Gottlieb, G. (Ed.) (1976) *Neural and Behavioral Specificity: Studies on the Development of Behavior and the Nervous System, Vol. 3,* Academic Press, New York, 352 pp.

Hennevin, E. et Leconte, P. (1971) La fonction du sommeil paradoxal. Faits et hypothèses. *Ann. Psychol.,* 2: 489–519.

Hernandez-Peon, R., Brust-Carmona, H., Penaloza-Rojas, J. and Bach-Y-Rita, G. (1961) The efferent control of afferent signals entering the central nervous system. *Ann. N.Y. Acad. Sci.,* 89: 866–882.

Hirsch, J. (1962) Individual differences in behavior and their genetic basis. In *Roots of Behavior,* E.L. Bliss (Ed.), Harper.

Hobson, J.A., McCarley, R.W., Freedman, R. and Pivik, R.T. (1974a) Time course of discharge rate changes by cat pontine brain stem neurons during sleep cycle. *J. Neurophysiol.,* 37: 1297–1309.

Hobson, J.A., Pivik, R.T., McCarley, R.W. and Freedman, R. (1974b) Selective firing by cat pontine brain stem neurons in desynchronized sleep. *J. Neurophysiol.,* 37: 497–511.

Hökfelt, T., Ljungdahl, A., Steinbusch, H., Verhofstad, A., Nilsson, G., Brodin, E., Pernow, B. and Goldstein, M. (1978) Immunochemical evidence of substance P-like immunoreactivity in some 5-hydroxytryptamine containing neurons in the rat central nervous system. *Neurosci.,* 3: 517–538.

Jacobson, M. (1970) Development, specification and diversification of neuronal connections. In *The Neurosciences, 2nd Study Program,* F.O. Schmitt (Ed.), The Rockefeller University Press, New York, pp. 116–129.

Jouvet, M. (1972) The role of monoamines and acetylcholine-containing neurons in the regulation of the sleep-waking cycle. *Ergebn. Physiol.,* 64: 165–305.

Jouvet, M. (1978) Does a genetic programming of the brain occur during paradoxical sleep? In *Cerebral Correlates of Conscious Experience, INSERM Symposium 6,* P. Buser and A. Buser-Rougeul (Eds.), Elsevier/North-Holland Biomedical Press, Amsterdam, pp. 245–261.

Jouvet-Mounier, D., Astic, L. and Lacote, D. (1970) Ontogenesis of the states of sleep in rat, cat and guinea pig during the first post-natal month, *Develop. Psychobiol.,* 2: 216–239.

Kitahama, K. (1979) *Etude Neuro-Psycho-Pharmaco-Génétique sur la Relation Sommeil-Apprentissage,* Ph.D. Thesis, Claude Bernard University, 203 pp.

Kitahama, K. and Valatx, J.L. (1979) Genetic study of instrumental and pharmacological paradoxical sleep deprivation in mice; strain differences. *Neuropharmacology,* in press.

Kitahama, K., Valatx, J.L. and Jouvet, M. (1980) A possible role for paradoxical sleep in the phenomenon of "reminiscences" in C57BR mice. *Physiol. Behav.,* in preparation.

Laurent, J.P., Cespuglio, R. et Jouvet, M. (1974) Délimitation des voies ascendantes de l'activité ponto–géniculo–occipitale chez le chat. *Brain Res.,* 65: 29–52.

Lundberg, J.J. and Mollgard, K. (1979) Mitotic activity in adult rat brain induced by implantation of pieces of fetal rat brain and liver. *Neurosci. Lett.,* 13: 265–270.

Magoun, H.W. and Rhines, R. (1946) An inhibitory mechanism in the bulbar reticular formation. *J. Neurophysiol.,* 9: 165–171.

Matsuzaki, M. (1969) Differential effects of sodium butyrate and physostigmine upon the activities of para-sleep in acute brain stem preparations. *Brain Res.,* 13: 247–265.

Mayr, E. (1958) Behavior and Systematics. In *Behavior and Evolution,* A. Roe and G.G. Simpson (Eds.), Yale University Press, New Haven.

McCarley, R.W. and Hobson, J.A. (1971) Single neuron activity in cat giganto-cellular tegmental field: selectivity of discharge in desynchronized sleep. *Science,* 174: 1250–1251.

McGinty, D.J. and Harper, R.M. (1976) Dorsal raphe neurons: depression of firing during sleep in cats. *Brain Res.,* 101: 569–575.

Pavlov, I.P. (1927) *Conditioned Reflexes: An Investigation of the Physiological Activity of the Cerebral Cortex,* University Press, London, Oxford.

Pegram, V., Hammond, D. and Bridgers, W. (1973) The effect of protein synthesis inhibition on sleep in mice. *Behav. Biol.,* 3: 377–382.

Petitjean, F., Sastre, J.P., Bertrand, N., Cointy, C. and Jouvet, M. (1975) Suppression du sommeil para-doxal par le chloramphenicol. Absence d'effet du thiamphenicol. *C.R. Soc. Biol. (Paris),* 280: 1236–1239.

Pompeiano, O. (1970) Mechanism of sensorimotor integration during sleep. *Progr. physiol. Psychol.,* 3: 1–179.

Ramirez, C. (1973) Synaptic plasma membrane protein synthesis: selective inhibition by chloramphenicol in vivo. *Biochem. biophys. Res. Commun.,* 50: 452–458.

Roffwarg, H.P., Muzio, J.N. and Dement, W.C. (1966) Ontogenetic development of the human sleep–dream cycle. *Science,* 52: 604–619.

Rojas-Ramirez, J.A., Aguilar-Jimenez, E., Posadas-Andrews, A., Bernal-Pedraza, J.G. and Drucker-Colín, R.R. (1977) The effects of various protein synthesis inhibitors on the sleep–wake cycle of rats. *Psychopharmacology,* 53: 147–150.

Sakai, K. (1980) Some anatomical and physiological properties of pontomesencephalic tegmental neurons with special reference to the PGO waves and postural atonia during Paradoxical Sleep in the cat. In *The Reticular Formation Revisited. IBRO Monogr. Series, Vol. 6,* M. Brazier (Ed.), Raven Press, New York.

Sakai, K., Kanamori, N. et Jouvet, M. (1979) Activités unitaires spécifiques du sommeil paradoxal dans la formation réticulée bulbaire chez le chat non restreint. *C.R. Acad. Sci. (Paris),* 289: 557–561.

Sastre, J.P. (1978) *Effets des Lésions du Tegmentum Pontique sur l'Organisation des États de Sommeil chez le chat. Analyse des Mécanismes des Comportements Oniriques.* Thèse Neurophysiol., Lyon, pp. 256.

Sastre, J.P. et Jouvet, M. (1979) Le comportement onirique du chat. *Physiol. Behav.,* 22: 979–989.

Sastre, J.P., Sakai, K. et Jouvet, M. (1979) Persistance du sommeil paradoxal chez le chat après destruc-tion de l'aire giganto-cellulaire du tegmentum pontique par l'acide kaïnique. *C.R. Acad. Sci. (Paris),* 289: 959–964.

Steriade, M. (1978) Cortical long-axoned cells and putative interneurons during the sleep–waking cycle. *Behav. Brain Sci.,* 3: 465–483.

Steriade, M. and Hobson, J.A. (1976) Neuronal activity during the sleep–waking cycle. In *Progress in Neurobiology, Vol. 6,* G. Kerkut and J.W. Phillis (Eds.), Pergamon Press, New York, pp. 1–376.

Tryon, R.C. (1934) Individual differences. In *Comparative Psychology,* F.A. Moss (Ed.), Prentice Hall, Englewood Cliffs, N.J.

Vimont-Vicary, P., Jouvet-Mounier, D. et Delorme, F. (1966) Effets EEG et comportementaux des priva-tions de sommeil paradoxal chez le chat. *Electroenceph. clin. Neurophysiol.,* 20: 439–449.

Vogel, G.W. (1975) A review of REM sleep deprivation. *Arch. gen. Psychiat.,* 32: 749–764.

Watson, J.B. (1924) *Behaviorism.* Norton, New York.

Does Rapid-Eye-Movement Sleep Play a Role in Brain Development?

M.A. CORNER, M. MIRMIRAN, H.L.M.G. BOUR, G.J. BOER, N.E. van de POLL, H.G. van OYEN and H.B.M. UYLINGS

Netherlands Institute for Brain Research, Amsterdam (The Netherlands)

INTRODUCTION

In the preceding article, Jouvet (1980) has presented a plausible case for supposing that "active" (i.e., rapid-eye-movement) sleep (AS) could be an important factor in the normal maturation and maintenance of neural organization. The fact that AS is present for a large percentage of the time at early stages of development, and that its phasic motor manifestations are much more intense and frequent than in adult animals, indeed makes a compelling argument for pursuing this line of reasoning. Furthermore, AS may be physiologically related in certain respects to prenatal spontaneous motility mechanisms (Corner, 1977, 1978), and it has been proposed that the latter too play a significant role in neurogenesis (Changeux and Mikoshiba, 1978).

GENERAL THEORETICAL CONSIDERATIONS

A variety of developmental processes such as outgrowth of neurites, formation of synapses, and polarization of excitable membranes could in principle be responsive to neuronal bio-electric activity. Exogenous (i.e. sensory) stimulation produces well-documented morphological and physiological effects upon brain development (see Mistretta and Bradley, 1978) but concerning the possibility of *endogenous* stimulation effects, we still know next to nothing. The following general hypotheses, however, seem worthwhile considering.

(1) Endogenously generated nerve impulses could facilitate genetic "readout" during the development of neuronal networks which mediate innate behaviors. Such a function has been postulated for early embryonic neuromotor activity (see Changeux and Mikoshiba, 1978) as well as for AS in fetal and neonatal animals (Jouvet, 1979, 1980).

(2) Bioelectric activity generated spontaneously within the central nervous system could interact, directly or indirectly, with afferent stimulation so as to modulate neuronal growth responses to sensory experience. There is some recent evidence that this may be the case with respect to monoaminergic control over neocortical plasticity, in animals exposed to visual stimulation during specific periods of development (Pettigrew, 1978).

(3) Spontaneous neuronal discharges can modify the synthesis and/or release of neurohormones (e.g. Lincoln, 1978), and there is a number of hormones known to exert a more or less powerful effect upon normal brain maturation (see Balázs, 1974; Boer et al., 1980; Flerkó, 1971).

AN EXPERIMENTAL APPROACH TO THE PROBLEM

The most straightforward way of beginning was to employ the "defect" strategy traditionally used by experimental embryologists for analyzing developmental mechanisms (see Weiss, 1969) – i.e. the suspected causal factor, AS in our case, is eliminated as completely and selectively as possible. We opted for a pharmacological method of AS deprivation, since the antidepressant drug, chlorimipramine (Anafranil), has proven to be highly effective in this regard, and to have only a minimal effect upon the overall amounts of sleep and wakefulness (Mirmiran et al., 1980a, b).

In infant rats during the second and third weeks of postnatal life, AS was experimentally reduced to the adult level, either by twice-daily injections of 15 mg/kg chlorimipramine in saline (series A) or by a single daily injection of 25 mg/kg suspended in an oil-dépôt vehicle (series B). In each series there was a control group consisting of an equal number of equivalent specimens injected with the vehicle only. The loss of AS (Fig. 1) was almost completely compensated for by increased quiet sleep (QS), with the remainder being accounted for by a relatively large number of short awakenings during QS. The experimental rats of series A showed a slight retardation in body weight (Mirmiran et al., 1980b) which was not observed in series B (Fig. 2; but cf. Table I). All of the studied groups displayed apparently normal behavior in the nest.

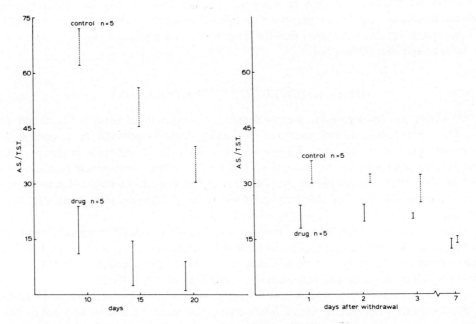

Fig. 1. Left: Active sleep (AS) as percentage of total sleep time (TST), measured in control rats and during chronic chlorimipramine treatment (series B, see text for details). One control and one experimental animal were recorded simultaneously from 09.00 h onwards. After 1 h in the 9–10-day-olds, 2 h in the 14–15-day-olds, and 3 h in the 19–20-day-olds, each pair was returned to the nest for feeding. This procedure was repeated until all 5 animals had been recorded (in the youngest group each pup was then recorded for a second time). Injections took place (see text for details) between 11.00 and 12.00 h. Right: AS percentage during the week following cessation of chronic chlorimipramine treatment. The vertical bars indicate the range of values observed in each series of measurement.

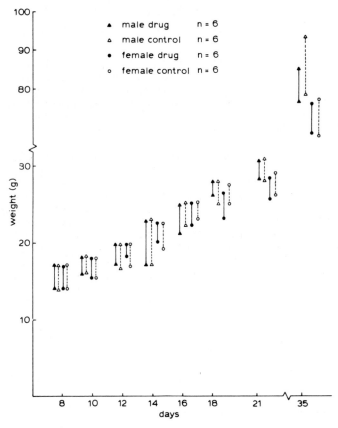

Fig. 2. Body weights (range of measured values) in control and drug-treated rats of series B during the injection period and 2 weeks later.

The absence of well-founded conceptual guidelines concerning the functional significance of AS during development brought us to examine a wide range of behaviors and brain regions after the animals reached maturity. Such a survey seemed to be required before we could, with any logical justification, either concentrate upon the most probable areas of AS involvement or, alternatively, conclude that AS is unlikely to have any ontogenetic significance.

Behavioral tests

Consequences of the drug-regimen for behavior were assessed in male rats from series A, starting at 70 days and lasting until 9—10 months of age. The test-battery included: open-field activity, sexual behavior, mouse killing, passive avoidance learning, and operant tasks for, respectively, spatial (left-right alternation) and temporal (20 sec differential reinforcement of low rate, DRL) discrimination learning. Significant differences between the control and the experimental groups were found on the following tests.

(1) Open-field behavior, during 2 min in a circular enclosure on 5 consecutive days, showed abnormally low levels of ambulation (Fig. 3) and rearing in the treated group. This effect occurred during the later part of the test period, when these activities are supposed to be exploratory in nature. Defecation occurred more frequently, but not significantly so. All

TABLE I

REGIONAL BRAIN WEIGHTS OF 15-MONTH-OLD RATS, TREATED NEONATALLY WITH CHLOR-IMIPRAMINE (SERIES B)

Dissection of brain regions was carried out within 15 min after sacrifice of each animal; each region was weighed immediately after isolation, and then frozen in liquid nitrogen for later biochemical procedures (see Table II). Mean recovery of the sum of brain regional weights was 96%, and the data are presented as mean ± S.E.M. Differences were tested statistically using Student's t-test.

	Male		Female	
	Control (n = 4)	Experimental (n = 5)	Control (n = 5)	Experimental (n = 6)
Body (g)	346 ± 35	332 ± 26	244 ± 11	219 ± 2 *
Brain (g)	1.95 ± 0.04	1.93 ± 0.02	1.74 ± 0.01	1.84 ± 0.02 *
Cerebral cortex (mg)	736 ± 20	725 ± 19	659 ± 14	696 ± 11 **
Cerebellum (mg)	276 ± 10	265 ± 4	247 ± 2	253 ± 4
Bulbus olfactorius (mg)	67 ± 7	78 ± 5	57 ± 4	63 ± 8
Colliculi (mg)	58 ± 4	64 ± 4	63 ± 4	60 ± 2
Hypothalamus (mg)	42 ± 1	52 ± 2 *	45 ± 1	43 ± 1
Hippocampus (mg)	118 ± 3	128 ± 4	107 ± 5	122 ± 2 *
Medulla oblongata (mg)	222 ± 6	226 ± 4	200 ± 2	206 ± 1
Residue (mg)	347 ± 13	324 ± 5	299 ± 10	319 ± 10

* Significant at the level of $P \leqslant 0.05$.
** Significant at the level of $P < 0.10$.

these effects may be interpreted as signs of heightened anxiety (Denenberg, 1969).

(2) Masculine sexual behavior appeared to be normal in its motivational aspects (latency and frequency of mounts) but was severely deficient in its consummatory aspects (intromissions and, even more so, ejaculations: Fig. 4). Series B males at 5 months showed similar disturbances. Neither the post-mortem histology (at 12 months of age, in series A) of receptors on the glans penis, nor the testosterone levels in the blood plasma, gave any indication that a disturbance of gonadal hormone production — either prepuberal or in adulthood — could be a factor in this behavioral syndrome (Beach et al., 1969).

(3) Left—right alternation learning was carried out faster in the experimental than in the control group, without there being any difference in response accuracy. A similar but not statistically significant tendency was observed in the DRL test.

Mouse-killing and passive avoidance learning were the behavioral tests which failed to indicate any difference between treated and control animals.

Sleep organization

Series A male animals were implanted at 11 months of age with EEG, EMG and EOG electrodes for making standard polygraphic recordings. Although their total sleep time (TST) was normal, the experimental rats turned out to have significantly more AS than did the controls: range 11–16%, vs 5–10% (n = 5 in each group). This difference resulted mainly from a higher frequency of AS epochs (3.6 vs 1.9/h of recording time) and, to a lesser extent, from a longer average duration of such epochs (68.4 sec vs 46.0 sec). In addition, 40% of the AS periods in the treated group were characterized by unusually frequent and intense muscular twitches (Fig. 5), such as are normally seen only in infant rats or during the

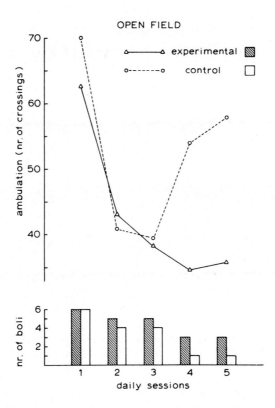

Fig. 3. Graphic representation of ambulation and defecation in an open-field test (series A male rats) during 2 min on 5 subsequent days. Ambulation was recorded by counting the number of crossings of concentric circles in a circular field which was subdivided into 19 sectors. The field was situated in a sound-isolated room, with the air-conditioning providing a constant background noise. Illumination consisted of a 20 W incandescent light bulb 80 cm above the test field.

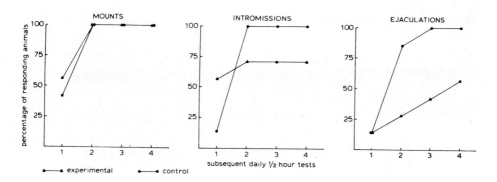

Fig. 4. The incidence of mounts, intromissions and ejaculations in experimental and control male rats (series A, see text) presented as a cumulative percentage of animals in the two groups which displayed each of these behavioral parameters. The animals were tested with females brought into behavioral estrus by injection of 50 μg estrogen plus 1 mg progesterone per rat.

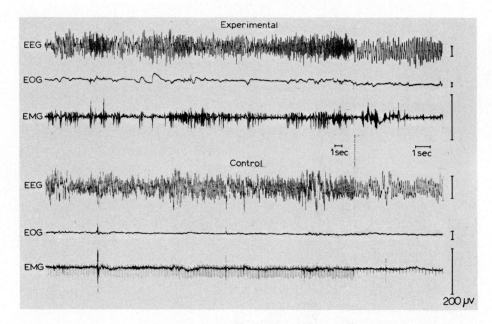

Fig. 5. Polygraphic registrations of AS in control and in experimental (male) rats at 11 months of age (series A, see text). EEGs were recorded from the dorsal hippocampus, EMGs from the dorsal neck muscles, and EOGs from the left orbit.

"rebound" period following acute AS deprivation (Fig. 6). These abnormal AS epochs could occur directly following wakefulness, and were on the whole much longer (90 sec median) than either "normal" epochs in the same animals (30 sec median) or AS epochs in controls

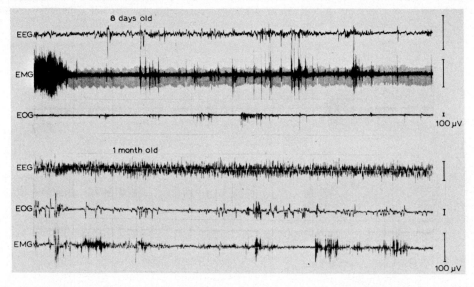

Fig. 6. Vigorous spontaneous motility during AS in, respectively, a normal infant animal (above) and in a juvenile rat during the "rebound" phase following acute AS-deprivation (below). Suppression of AS was achieved by an i.p. injection of 300 mg/kg α-methyl DOPA in the morning, followed 12 h later by a dose of 200 mg/kg. The polygraph recording was made 12 h after the second injection.

TABLE II

DNA AND PROTEIN DATA OF THE BRAIN AREAS AFFECTED IN WEIGHT BY NEONATAL TREATMENT WITH CHLORIMIPRAMINE

The frozen brain parts (see Table I) were homogenized in water, and then diluted for making duplicate DNA (ethidium bromide method: Boer, 1975) and protein assays (Folin method: Lowry et al., 1951). Data are presented as mean ± S.E.M. for absolute or relative amounts (per wet weight).

	Male		Female	
	Control	Experimental	Control	Experimental
Cerebral cortex				
DNA (μg)	1130 ± 65	950 ± 45**	890 ± 50	940 ± 50
(μg/mg)	1.55 ± 0.12	1.31 ± 0.05**	1.34 ± 0.07	1.36 ± 0.08
protein (mg)	109 ± 6	110 ± 3	85 ± 4	90 ± 3
(mg/mg)	0.150 ± 0.010	0.152 ± 0.002	0.129 ± 0.03	0.129 ± 0.03
protein/DNA (mg/mg)	96 ± 4	116 ± 5*	96 ± 3	94 ± 6
Hippocampus				
DNA (μg)	154 ± 8	159 ± 12	149 ± 12	179 ± 7**
(μg/mg)	1.31 ± 0.04	1.23 ± 0.05	1.39 ± 0.08	1.45 ± 0.06
protein (mg)	18.8 ± 0.6	20.0 ± 0.7	16.4 ± 0.8	19.0 ± 0.6*
(mg/mg)	0.160 ± 0.009	0.156 ± 0.003	0.153 ± 0.004	0.153 ± 0.004
protein/DNA (mg/mg)	122 ± 8	126 ± 7	109 ± 9	106 ± 4
Hypothalamus				
DNA (μg)	76 ± 5	89 ± 4*	74 ± 3	76 ± 3
(μg/mg)	1.83 ± 0.13	1.73 ± 0.03	1.64 ± 0.04	1.75 ± 0.04
protein (mg)	6.2 ± 0.3	7.3 ± 0.3*	6.2 ± 0.3	6 ± 0.2
(mg/mg)	0.148 ± 0.002	0.142 ± 0.003	0.137 ± 0.005	0.138 ± 0.003
protein/DNA (mg/mg)	81 ± 6	82 ± 2	83 ± 4	78 ± 3

* $P \leqslant 0.05$.
** $P < 0.10$.

(35 sec median). EEG "activation" (i.e. the ratio of θ to δ wave mean amplitudes in the hippocampus during AS) was also greater than normal: θ/δ values ranged from 1.6 to 2.4 in experimental, vs 1.0 to 1.2 in control animals.

At 15 months of age, the sleep of each animal in series B was observed behaviorally during five 1 h periods on different days. AS was indicated by the presence of rapid-eye-movements, twitching of the extremities and/or shallow and irregular breathing, together with closed eyes and a recumbent body position. Both the male and the female control animals displayed an average of 1.5 AS epochs/h observation time, with a mean duration of 50–60 sec. In the experimental females, the incidence of AS was about the same as in the controls (1.3 epochs/h, also lasting 50–60 sec on average). Experimental males, in contrast, showed the same type of sleep abnormality as was described above for the males of series A: a much higher incidence (2.6/h) of relatively long-lasting (75 sec) AS epochs, in 60% of which the frequency and intensity of phasic movements were distinctly greater than normal. It is interesting to note that 5 such epochs (1.5%) were also observed in the drug-treated *female* rats, as opposed to zero in the control animals of both sexes ($P < 0.02$, χ^2 test).

Brain structure

At 15 months of age, the brains of series B rats were examined for possible changes induced as a result of early AS deprivation (i.e. chronic chlorimipramine treatment). Using the procedure of Patel et al. (1978), several regions were dissected out and weighed (Table I). Despite their lower body weight, a significant increase above control values for total brain weight is to be found in the experimental female animals, attributable for the most part to enlargement of the hippocampus and cerebral cortex. In contrast, overall brain weight in males does not seem to have been affected. There is, however, a striking increase in the hypothalamus, alone, of all the areas studied.

Measurements of DNA and protein of the affected areas (Table II) show that, in the experimental group, the female hippocampus and the male hypothalamus contain more cells, but that cell density (DNA/wet weight) and cell size (protein/DNA) are not significantly different from the control values. Very remarkable, however, is the effect upon the male (but not the female) cerebral cortex: although no weight change can be observed (Table I), there is a drastic decrease in the number of cells (−16%) in the group which had been neonatally treated with chlorimipramine. Moreover, some of the cells present must be considerably larger than normal (+20% on the average), since the total protein content is about the same as in the cerebral cortex of control male rats.

RESEARCH PERSPECTIVES

The behavioral, physiological and anatomical abnormalities described above defy interpretation at the present time, but they do indicate that AS might indeed play a significant part in normal brain maturation. Even as regards the *negative* findings, a possible interpretation is that the AS deprivation was not early, prolonged or deep enough for its potential impact to be fully manifested, or else that any latent damage was neutralized by the compensatory increase in AS which developed at an unknown time after cessation of the drug injections. Before any such conclusions can be drawn, however, one or more suitable controls will need to be carried out. After all, chlorimipramine works by blocking monoamine (especially serotonin) re-uptake at nerve endings throughout the brain (e.g. Carlsson, 1969; Lidbrink et al., 1971) and therefore could directly affect many functions other than AS. Suitable experimental procedures will undoubtedly become available as more becomes known about the mechanisms underlying the various phenomena which occur during sleep (for review, see Steriade and Hobson, 1976).

SUMMARY

In summary, a first attempt has been made, using the strategy of the defect-experiment, to test the hypothesis that active sleep (AS) is important for the normal development of the central nervous system. AS was suppressed in rat pups throughout the second and third weeks of life, by means of daily injections of chlorimipramine. No AS rebound occurred during the week following discontinuation of the drug, but in adulthood the experimental male animals all showed a sizeable increase and intensification of AS. Specific effects on the open-field test suggest an abnormally high anxiety level in the drug-treated males (females have not yet been tested); their sexual performance was also severely deficient. Post-mortem brain examination revealed a selective enlargement of the hypothalamus in experimental male rats, together with reduced cell number in the cerebral cortex. In females, it was the hippocampus and cerebral cortex which were clearly enlarged, so much so as to cause a significantly higher total brain weight in the experimental group. It may be concluded that disturbances in monoamine metabolism can drastically reduce AS during infancy, and lead to specific brain and behavior abnormalities in later life. A *causal* role for AS suppression in this "chlorimipramine syndrome" is conceivable, but may be concluded only if suitable controls lead to a replication of the present results.

ACKNOWLEDGEMENTS

The authors wish to thank Ms. S.M. van der Zwan, Mr. H. Pronker and Ms. C.M.H. van Rheenen-Verberg for their technical assistance, as well as Ms. J. Sels for typing the manuscript.

REFERENCES

Balász, R. (1974) Hormonal influence on brain development. *Biochem. Soc. Spec. Publ.,* 1: 39–57.

Beach, F., Noble, R. and Orndoff, R. (1969) Effects of perinatal androgen treatment on responses of male rats to gonadal hormones in adulthood. *J. comp. physiol. Psychol.,* 68: 490–497.

Boer, G.J. (1975) A simplified microassay of DNA and RNA using ethidium bromide. *Analyt. Biochem.,* 65: 225–231.

Boer, G.J., Swaab, D.F., Uylings, H.B.M., Boer, K., Buijs, R.M. and Velis, D.N. (1980) Neuropeptides in rat brain development. In *Adaptive Capabilities of the Nervous System, Progress in Brain Research, Vol. 53,* M.A. Corner et al. (Eds.), Elsevier, Amsterdam, pp. 207–227.

Carlsson, A. (1969) Demonstration of extraneuronal 5-HT accumulation in brain following membrane-pump blockade by chlorimipramine. *Brain Res.,* 12: 456–460.

Changeux, J.P. and Mikoshiba, K. (1978) Genetic and "epigenetic" factors regulating synapse formation in vertebrate cerebellum and neuromuscular junction. In *Maturation of the Nervous System, Progress in Brain Research, Vol. 48,* M.A. Corner et al. (Eds.), Elsevier, Amsterdam, pp. 43–67.

Corner, M.A. (1977) Sleep and the beginnings of behavior in the animal kingdom — studies of ultradian motility cycles in early life. *Progr. Neurobiol.,* 8: 279–295.

Corner, M.A. (1978) Spontaneous motor rhythms in early life – phenomenological and neurophysiological aspects. In *Maturation of the Nervous System, Progress in Brain Research, Vol. 48*, M.A. Corner et al. (Eds.), Elsevier, Amsterdam, pp. 349–364.

Denenberg, V.H. (1969) Open field behavior in the rat: what does it mean? *Ann. N.Y. Acad. Sci.,* 159: 852–859.

Drucker-Colin, R. (1979) Protein molecules and the regulation of REM sleep: possible implications for function. In *The Function of Sleep*, R. Drucker-Colin, M., Shkurovich and M.B. Sterman (Eds.), Academic Press, New York, pp. 99–112.

Flerkó, B. (1971) Steroid hormones and the differentiation of the central nervous system. In *Current Topics in Experimental Endocrinology, Vol. 1*, L. Martin and V.H.T. James (Eds.), Academic Press, New York, pp. 41–80.

Jouvet, M. (1979) Does a genetic programming of the brain occur during paradoxical sleep? In *Cerebral Correlates of Conscious Experience, INSERM Symp. Vol. 6*, P. Buser and A. Rougeul-Buser (Eds.), North-Holland, Amsterdam, pp. 245–261.

Jouvet, M. (1980) Paradoxical sleep and the nature–nurture controversy. In *Adaptive Capabilities of the Nervous System, Progress in Brain Research, Vol. 53*, M.A. Corner et al., (Eds.), Elsevier, Amsterdam, pp. 331–346.

Lidbrink, P., Jonsson, G. and Fuxe, K. (1971) The effect of imipramine-like drugs and antihistamine drugs on uptake mechanisms in the central NA and 5-HT neurons. *Neuropharmacology,* 10: 521–536.

Lincoln, D.W. (1978) Investigation of hypothalamic function: anatomical and physiological studies. In *The Endocrine Hypothalamus*, S. Jeffcoate and J. Hutchinson (Eds.), Academic Press, New York, pp. 35–74.

Lowry, O.H., Rosebrough, N.J., Farr, A.L. and Randall, R.J. (1951) Protein measurement with the Folin phenol reagent. *J. biol. Chem.,* 193: 265–275.

Mistretta, C.M. and Bradley, R.M. (1978) Effects of early sensory experience on brain and behavioral development. In *Early Influences, Studies Develop. Behav. Nerv. Syst., Vol. 4*, G. Gottlieb (Ed.), Academic Press, New York, pp. 215–247.

Mirmiran, M., Bour, H.L. and Corner, M.A. (1980a) Pharmacological suppression of paradoxical sleep during postnatal development in the rat. In *Sleep-1978*, L. Popoviciu et al. (Eds.), Edit. Médicale, Bucharest, in press.

Mirmiran, M., Corner, M.A. and Bour, H.L. (1980b) Pharmacological suppression of active (REM) sleep in infant rats: effect on adult sleep patterns. In *Ontogenesis of the Brain, Vol. 3*, S. Trojan et al. (Eds.), Charles University Press, Prague, in press.

Patel, A.J., Del Vecchio, M. and Atkinson, D.J. (1978) Effect of undernutrition on the regional development of transmitter enzymes: glutamate decarboxylase and choline acetyltransferase. *Develop. Neurosci.,* 1: 41–53.

Pettigrew, J.D. (1978) The paradox of the critical period for striate cortex. In *Neuronal Plasticity*, C.W. Cotman (Ed.), Raven Press, New York, pp. 311–330.

Steriade, M. and Hobson, J.A. (1976) Neuronal activity during the sleep–waking cycle. *Progr. Neurobiol.,* 6: 155–376.

Weiss, P.A. (1969) *Principles of Development (Rev. Ed.)*, Hafner, New York.

SECTION IV

Aggressive Behavior as Social Adaptation

(edited by N.E. van de Poll)

Biological Substrates of Aggression

K.E. MOYER

Department of Psychology, Carnegie Mellon University, Pittsburgh, Pa. 15213 (U.S.A.)

INTRODUCTION

In this paper an attempt will be made to develop a physiological model of aggression, and then to examine some of the implications of that model for aggression control.

It should first be pointed out that aggression is not a unitary construct. There are a number of different kinds of aggressive behavior. Although this may not ultimately be the most useful classification, I have suggested that the following kinds of aggression exist: predatory, inter-male, fear-induced, maternal, instrumental, irritable, and sex-related (Moyer, 1968). Each of these above types of aggression, with the exception of instrumental, has different underlying neural and hormonal determinants. It is obvious that no single model can fit each of these in detail. It is possible, however, to identify mechanisms or types of mechanisms that are similar for all or most of the different types of aggression. The basic premise of this model is that in the brains of animals and humans there are neural systems that, when fired in the presence of a relevant target, result in aggressive or destructive behavior towards that target. In the case of humans, the actual aggressive behavior may be controlled, but the individual will still have the appropriate feelings of hostility. There is now abundant evidence to support that premise. (See Moyer, 1976 for details.)

DISCUSSION

Some of the most fundamental work in this area has been done by John Flynn at Yale, who has carried out extensive studies with cats using the implanted electrode technique. The cats used by Flynn were non-predatory and would not normally attack rats. Some, in fact, would live with a rat for months and not molest it. If an electrode implanted in the cat's lateral hypothalamus is electrically activated, however, the animal will ignore the experimenter standing there, but it will immediately attack and kill an available rat. The kill will be very precise, resulting from a bite in the cervical region of the spinal cord in the manner of typical predatory aggression of the feline. If, on the other hand, the electrode is located in the medial hypothalamus, and the cat is stimulated in the presence of the rat, it will ignore the rat, and turn and attack the experimenter. The attack on the experimenter will be highly directed, not at all similar to the random attacks of a decerebrate animal. This cat appears as though it intends to do the experimenter harm, and in fact may well do so. (Egger and Flynn, 1963.)

One particularly interesting experiment that illustrates a number of things was carried out by Robinson et al. (1969). They took a small rhesus monkey and implanted an electrode in the anterior hypothalamus. They then put the animal in a primate chair, activated the electrode, and showed that the monkey did not become aggressive, either towards inanimate objects or towards the experimenter. It was then put in a cage with another monkey, one that was larger and dominant to the experimental animal, together with the dominant monkey's female consort. When stimulated in this situation, the experimental subject attacked only the dominant male monkey, sparing the female. This appeared to be a valid primate attack, because the dominant monkey reacted by counterattacking just as viciously as it usually would if attacked by a submissive animal. The stimulation-induced attacks were so intense, however, that the formerly dominant animal ultimately became submissive to the experimental monkey. This experiment shows first that the particular brain stimulation used resulted in one specific kind of aggression, which I have called "inter-male", i.e. the specific tendency for one male to attack another. Secondly, the experiment demonstrates that aggressive behavior is stimulus bound: in the absence of the relevant stimulus, even though stimulated time and again, the subject showed no irritability or increased tendency to attack other targets.

It is important not to generalize too quickly from one species to another, and one must be particularly cautious in generalizing to man. However, there is now good evidence that man, for all of his encephalization, has not escaped from the neural determinants of his aggressive behavior. There are now several hundred people who have electrodes implanted in their brains, with wires attached to small sockets cemented to the skull. These patients can be brought into the laboratory, plugged in, and precise areas deep in the brain can be electrically stimulated.

A case reported by King (1961) is particularly instructive. The patient was a very mild-mannered woman who was a generally submissive, kindly and friendly person. An electrode was implanted in the amygdala, and, when stimulated with a current of 5 mA, she became hostile and aggressive. She said, in an angry manner, such things as, "Take my blood pressure. Take it now". She also said, "Quit holding me! I'm getting up! You'd better get somebody else if you want to hold me! I'm going to hit you!". She then raised her arm as if to strike the experimenter, who then wisely turned down the current. It was possible to turn this woman's anger on and off with the flick of the switch. She later confirmed having felt anger, and also reported being upset about the fact that she had been angry. She did not report pain or any other discomfort, but she simply was "turned on" angry. Similar findings have been reported by other investigators (Sem-Jacobsen, 1968; Heath, 1964).

There are a number of pathological processes in the human brain which result in the activation of the neural systems for feelings of hostility. For instance, tumors with an irritative focus frequently result in increased irritability and rage attacks if they are located in particular portions of the brain. It is important to note that not all brain tumors produce pathological aggression. Many, in fact, produce apathy and somnolence. However, if they develop in such a way as to impinge upon and activate the neural systems for aggressive behavior, the syndrome of pathological aggressivity may appear. Tumors in the septal region, the temporal lobe, and the frontal lobe have produced this reaction. In 1962, Sano reported on 1800 cases of brain tumor and most frequently found the irritability syndrome in those that involved the temporal lobe and the anterior hypothalamus. There are other brain dysfunctions which increase the probability of feelings of hostility and irritability, including diffuse brain lesions, senile dementia, chronic brain syndrome, encephalitis, rabies and some forms of epilepsy. There is also evidence from several sources that, like many other systems

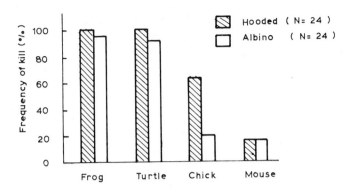

Fig. 1. The frequency with which the hooded and albino rats killed each of the 4 test animals shown in the figure.

in the brain, suppressor systems exist which are antagonistic to the aggression systems. That evidence will be covered in detail later.

It is fortunate that neither in humans nor in animals is aggression very frequent. Thus, in order to understand the physiology of aggression, we must understand what it is that turns these neural systems on and off. Perhaps one of the best ways of thinking about this is in terms of thresholds for activating the systems. In certain circumstances the threshold for eliciting aggression is very high, and in that case it takes a great deal of provocation to activate them. There are other circumstances in which the threshold is much lower, so that the individual has an increased tendency to behave aggressively. Some of the variables that influence the thresholds of neural systems involved in aggression appear to be hereditary. For example, we have shown in my laboratory that some strains of rats are more often aggressive towards small chickens than are other strains (Bandler and Moyer, 1970).

It is also possible, as Lagerspetz (1964) has shown, to take a large population of mice and select from them the aggressive and non-aggressive animals. Within a relatively few generations it is possible to breed a highly aggressive strain of mice which will attack each other immediately when put together. If the non-aggressive animals are bred, on the other hand, a strain can be developed that will not fight whatever is done to them. Obviously, we do not have any comparable data on human beings, but if there are specific neural systems for different kinds of aggressive behavior, it follows that the propensity to develop different thresholds for each type of aggression is inherited. Neurological differences must be inherited in much the same way as differences in the shapes of noses are.

Another significant variable that contributes to differences in the threshold level for aggression is blood chemistry. It has been known for centuries, of course, that one can take the raging bull and convert it into a gentle steer by the operation of castration, which reduces the level of testosterone in the blood stream. The formal work on this problem was done in 1947 by Elizabeth Beeman, and has been repeatedly confirmed in many laboratories. Beeman, working with a strain of mice that would fight when put together, castrated the animals of the experimental group prior to puberty. When those mice were put together after reaching sexual maturity they did not fight at all, whereas the control group showed the usual amount of aggression characteristic of that strain. She then carried the experiment a step further and implanted pellets of testosterone subcutaneously in the castrated mice. When the testosterone had become effective they fought at the same level as did the control animals. Surgical removal of the testosterone pellets caused the mice once again to become docile. It was thus possible to manipulate the aggressive behavior of these mice simply by changing the testosterone level.

There are a variety of other blood chemistry changes that influence the thresholds for aggression. For example, there is a period during the week before menstruation when a significant percentage of women feel irritable, hostile and are easily aroused to anger (Dalton, 1959, 1960, 1961, 1964). Those who have had inadequate training in impulse control sometimes behave and act upon those impulses. In fact, one study that was conducted on 249 female prison inmates showed that 62% of the crimes of violence were committed in the pre-menstrual week, as opposed to only 2% in the post-menstrual week (Morton et al., 1953).

There also appears to be good clinical evidence that some individuals show an irritable, aggressive reaction when their blood chemistry is altered by a sudden drop in blood sugar, i.e. hypoglycemia (Kepler and Moersch, 1937; Wilder, 1943). Furthermore, at least one controlled study supports the clinical findings. Bolton (1973) spent considerable time with a very hostile tribe of Peruvian Indians, called the Quolla. Bolton hypothesized that the exceptionally high level of social conflict and hostility in the society could be partly explained by the tendency to hypoglycemia among the community residents. Peer ratings of aggressiveness (which had an acceptable reliability) were studied in relationship to blood sugar levels, as determined by a 4 h glucose tolerance test. A χ^2 analysis of the data showed a statistically significant relationship between aggression ranking and the change in blood glucose levels during the test. In view of all of the other possible causes of aggressive behavior, which could easily have confounded the results of this study, this remarkable finding indicates that the relationship between hypoglycemia and aggression must be a powerful one.

Our discussion so far has been concerned with physiology. It should be obvious, however, that learning has an important influence on behavior that we label aggressive, just as it does on any other category of behavior. With the proper use of reward and punishment, an animal can be taught either to overeat or to starve to death. By the same method, animals and humans can be taught to respectively exhibit or inhibit their tendencies to hostile behavior. It is clear that aggressive acts which are rewarded will have a higher probability of recurring than those that are not, while those that are punished will become less likely to recur later. Since human beings learn better and faster than all other animals, it is reasonable to expect that the internal impulses to aggressive behavior would be more subject to modification by experience in humans than in any other animal. Also, because of man's additional ability to manipulate symbols, and to substitute one symbol for another, one would expect to find a considerable diversity in the stimuli which will elicit or inhibit activity in the aggression systems. One would also expect that the modes of expression of aggression would be more varied, diverse, and less stereotyped in humans than in other animals. It is also important to remember that learned behaviors interact with the internal impulses to aggressive behavior. Thus, an individual who has a relatively low threshold for the activation of his neural hostility systems will require more training than will other individuals in order to achieve a given degree of aggression control.

Much can be learned about the mechanisms underlying aggression by studying possible physiological approaches to aggression control. There is no doubt that some of the most important methods for the control of hostile and antisocial behavior involve training, re-education, and social change. That is, the external environment is manipulated in some way in order to alter the individual's behavior or his potential for aggression. However, it should also be possible (although not necessarily desirable) to bring about such changes by influencing the internal milieu, i.e. by changing the individual's physiological state.

If there are neural systems which are active during, and responsible for aggressive behavior, it should also be possible to reduce or eliminate aggressive tendencies by interrupting or interfering with them directly. There is now abundant evidence that such a procedure is possible, and as might be suspected when dealing with neural systems rather than neural centers, there are several different brain areas which may be lesioned in order to reduce aggressive tendencies. For instance, one can take the wild cat *Lynx rufus rufus* which will attack with the slightest provocation, and make it permanently tame by bilaterally burning out the amygdala. (Schreiner and Kling, 1953.) The same thing can be done with the wild Norway rat, one of the few animals which will attack without apparent provocation (Woods, 1956).

Just as there are wild cats, wild rats and wild monkeys, so there are wild people, individuals who presumably have so much "spontaneous" activity in the neural systems which underlie aggressive behavior that they are a constant threat to themselves and to those around them. These are individuals who are confined to the back wards of mental hospitals under either constant sedation or constant restraint. The homicidal propensities of even these people can be reduced, however, if appropriate brain lesions are made to interrupt the functioning of the irascibility systems. There are a number of surgeons now who have done essentially the same operation on humans as described above for the cat and the rat. That is, a complete or partial bilateral amygdalectomy. The Japanese investigator Narabayashi and his colleagues, for example, report that they obtained 85% success in the reduction of violent behavior following a bilateral amygdalectomy (Narabayashi et al., 1963). Heimburger in Indiana reports a 92% increase in docility in extremely violent patients through the same operation. Not only was it possible to put such individuals in the open wards, i.e. take them out of isolation, but two of his patients have been released into society and appear to be making a reasonable adjustment (Heimburger et al., 1966).

There can be no doubt that a number of different brain lesions can reduce the tendency of an individual to both feel and express hostility. This fact is of considerable theoretical significance, since it confirms many of the findings on animals and substantiates predictions from the model described above. As a practical therapy for the control of aggressive behavior, however, it leaves much to be desired, because, among other reasons, there are very few individuals for whom such a drastic approach would be indicated. Furthermore, a serious problem with the use of lesions for the control of aggression is that when the operation is unsuccessful, as sometimes is the case, the patient's brain is permanently damaged to no avail. Surgery should therefore be a last resort therapy only to be used after all other types of control, both psychological and physiological, have been tried. There is evidence that in some of the hospitals around the world in which aggression control operations are performed, relatively little care is taken to ensure that brain surgery is, indeed, the "last resort therapy" that it should be (Valenstein, 1973).

The control of aggressive behavior can also be achieved by the activation of those neural systems which send inhibitory fibers to the aggression systems. Delgado (1963) has convincingly shown that vicious rhesus monkeys can be tamed by the stimulation of aggression-suppressing areas of the brain. In order to eliminate the need for restraint and the necessity for connecting wires to the head, a technique was developed by which the brain of the subject could be stimulated by remote, radio control. The monkey wore a small stimulating device on its back which was connected by leads under the skin to the electrodes which were implanted in various locations in the brain. The leads were connected through a very small switching relay that could be closed by an impulse from a miniature radio receiver which was bolted to the animal's skull. The transmitter was some distance away, and it was thus possible to study the monkeys while permitting them to roam freely in the caged area.

In one experiment the subject was the aggressive boss monkey that dominated the rest of the colony with his threatening behavior and overt attacks. A radio-controlled electrode was implanted in this monkey's caudate nucleus. When the radio transmitter was activated the boss monkey received stimulation in the caudate nucleus with the result that his spontaneous aggressive tendencies were blocked. His territoriality then diminished and the other monkeys in the colony reacted to him differently, making fewer submissive gestures and showing less fear. During caudate nucleus stimulation, it was even possible for the experimenter to enter the cage and catch the monkey with his bare hands. During one phase of the experiment, the button for the transmitter was placed inside the cage near the feeding tray and thus becoming available to all of the monkeys in the colony. One small monkey learned to stand next to the button and watch the boss monkey. Every time the latter would start to threaten and become aggressive the little monkey would push the button and calm him down (Delgado, 1963). I'll leave it to the reader to decide what the political implications of this experiment are, but I must say that it's the first experimental evidence I know of, in support of St. Matthew's prediction that "the meek shall inherit the earth".

Man also has neural systems in the brain which, when activated, function to block ongoing aggressive behavior. Heath (1954) has reported on an extremely hostile patient who had an electrode implanted in the septal region. This patient could be brought into the room raging, threatening, swearing and struggling, but as soon as the septal region was electrically stimulated (without his knowledge, of course) he relaxed, became docile and assumed a positive attitude. Furthermore, he was quite unable to account for the sudden change in his behavior. When the stimulating electrode was in the septal area, the patient might tell a dirty joke or reveal plans to seduce the waitress down at the corner bar, but there are other suppressor areas that do not elicit sexually-toned responses. Heath (1977) has recently reported a significant reduction in pathological violence and aggression in a number of patients after repeated stimulation in the vermal region of the cerebellum. Aggression-suppressing effects of brain stimulation may be rather prolonged. Sem-Jacobsen and Torkildsen (1960) report that stimulation in either the ventromedial frontal lobes or in the central area of the temporal lobe had a calming effect on a violent manic patients. When both points were stimulated in rapid succession the calming, anti-hostility effect was greater and of some duration.

The suppression of aggression by electrical stimulation is, undoubtedly, of considerable theoretical importance, but, as with brain lesions, is not yet a rational or useful therapeutic technique. Although the surgical risk of mortality through electrode implants is even lower than that of stereotaxic brain lesions, and in fact can be considered negligible, there are some serious side effects which demand a great deal more research before electrical stimulation of the brains of humans can be considered to be risk free. No data are available on humans, but it has been shown in mice, rats, cats and monkeys that repeated, brief, subthreshold stimulation of amygdala results in a progressive lowering of seizure threshold and ultimately in behavioral convulsions. This decrease in seizure threshold resulting from brain stimulation has been referred to as the "kindling" effect. Goddard (1972), who has studied this phenomenon in some detail, concludes that "kindling" is a permanent transynaptic change resulting from the stimulation, and is not due to tissue damage or scar formation.

Until it becomes possible to circumvent the "kindling" effect, any procedure which involves repeated electrical stimulation of the human brain places the patient at risk.

Our physiological model of aggressive behavior indicates that the neurological systems for aggressive behavior can be sensitized by certain chemical factors in the blood stream, primarily hormones. An understanding of endocrinological and other blood chemical influences upon aggression should lead to rational therapies for certain kinds of hostility in humans. The woman, for example, who suffers from periodic hyper-irritability every month, has a physician who either isn't aware of her problem or doesn't keep up on the literature. There are a variety of therapeutic measures now which can be taken to alleviate that particular problem. There are also violent individuals for whom the object of aggression is the same as the object for sexual behavior, including some men who commit brutal sex murders. Aggressive behavior which is directly associated with sexual behavior, either heterosexual or homosexual, can most generally be controlled by reducing or blocking the androgens in the blood stream, e.g. by castration. While there is considerable evidence that this operation is effective in reducing the level of sexual arousal regardless of its direction, it is a drastic and irreversible therapy. To make matters worse, there are also a variety of physical and psychological side effects. It has nevertheless been offered to sex criminals as an alternative to prison in some countries (Bremer, 1959).

More recently some investigators have attempted to block the effects of the male hormone by giving either estrogenic or progestogenic hormones or anti-androgenic drugs. Although a great deal more work needs to be done, and the problem of side effects must be considered, these techniques do show promise (Chatz, 1972; Blumer and Migeon, 1973). Although there is currently no drug which is a completely specific anti-hostility agent, a sizeable number of preparations, including the tranquilizers, are available, which greatly reduce aggressive tendencies as one component of their action. Most of the major tranquilizers, such as chlorpromazine, appear to have an anti-hostility effect over and above their sedative action. This also appears to be true of many of the minor tranquilizers, including librium and valium. However, the problem of predicting which drug will be effective in inhibiting hostility in a given individual is a very difficult problem. Aggressive behavior has many causes and can result from a variety of neural endocrine dysfunctions. So it is perhaps not surprising that no diagnostic tests are yet available which permit a truly rational pharmacotherapeutic approach to hostility control. It is nevertheless already possible to reduce, or even eliminate much of the irrational nonadaptive hostility found in many psychotic, neurotic or ostensibly normal individuals (Moyer, 1976).

The control techniques discussed above are powerful, but their limitations should be clearly understood. These methods would be ineffective in controlling the aggressive actions of a "trigger man" for Murder Incorporated or those of a bomber pilot over North Vietnam. Both are engaged in instrumental aggression, and neither may have any feeling of hostility towards his victims. When his radar indicates that it is time to press his bomb release button, the pilot may do so without the slightest feeling of antagonism, although his bombs may destroy the homes and lives of hundreds of people. He has behaved as he has been trained to behave, and emotional responses may not be involved at all. The "trigger man" for Murder Incorporated kills because he is financially rewarded for killing. He may not know his victim and may feel no animosity towards him whatsoever. These individuals have engaged in learned behavior, and there is no physiological manipulation known that can selectively effect learned responses. Further, with the current state of the art, no such method is likely to be found in the near future. It is not even clear where to start looking for that type of method. That kind of control must await major, and as yet quite unpredictable breakthroughs.

The distinction between instrumental aggression and aggressive behavior containing an affective component has important implications for the abuse potential of the physiological control of aggression. The use of physiological controls could, in fact, even be counterproductive for leadership which wishes to control the rebellious tendencies of a subject population. One reaction to oppression, political or otherwise, is to become angry and, as a result of that anger, to evolve a plan (which may well involve aggressive behavior) to alleviate the oppression. Another reaction to oppression is to recognize it as such intellectually and to come to the conclusion that the oppression must be eliminated. A plan, which too may involve aggressive behavior, is then worked out. Anti-hostility drugs in the water supply or other physiological measures will affect only the anger, but will have no influence on the intellectual processes involved in the aggressive plans. In fact, if the anger is controlled, the plans may become more effective because they will not involve the impulsive quality that often results from the urgency of anger. Furthermore, because the emotional component will not function as a distractor, the intellectual processes may function all the more efficiently.

REFERENCES

Bandler, R.J. and Moyer, K.E. (1970) Animals spontaneously attacked by rats. *Commun. Behav. Biol.,* 5: 177–182.

Beeman, E.A. (1947) The effect of male hormone on aggressive behavior in mice. *Physiol. Zool.,* 20: 373–405.

Blumer, D. and Migeon, C. (1973) Treatment of impulsive behavior disorders in males with medroxy-progesterone acetate. *Annual Meeting of the American Psychiatric Association.*

Bolton, R. (1973) Aggression and hypoglycemia among the Qolla: a study in psychobiological anthropology. *Ethnology,* 12: 227–257.

Bremer, J. (1959) *Asexualization.* Macmillan, New York.

Chatz, T.L. (1972) Management of male adolescent sex offenders. *Int. J. Offender Ther.,* 2: 109–115.

Dalton, K. (1959) Menstruation and acute psychiatric illness. *Brit. Med. J.,* 1: 148–149.

Dalton, K. (1960) Schoolgirls' misbehavior and menstruation. *Brit. Med. J.,* 2: 1647–1649.

Dalton, K. (1961) Menstruation and crime. *Brit. Med. J.,* 3: 1752–1753.

Dalton, K. (1964) *The Premenstrual Syndrome* Thomas, Springfield, Ill.

Delgado, J.M.R. (1963) Cerebral heterostimulation in a monkey colony. *Science,* 141: 161–163.

Egger, M.D. and Flynn, J.P. (1963) Effect of electrical stimulation of the amygdala on hypothalamically elicited attack behavior in cats. *J. Neurophysiol.,* 26: 705–720.

Goddard, G.V. (1972) Long term alteration following amygdaloid stimulation. In B. Eleftheriou (Ed.), The Neurobiology of the Amygdala, Plenum, New York, 1972, pp. 581–596.

Heath, R.G. et al. (1954) *Studies in Schizophrenia,* Harvard University Press, Cambridge, Mass., pp. 83–84.

Heath, R.G. (1964) Developments toward new physiologic treatments in psychiatry. *J. Neuropsychiat.,* 5: 318–331.

Heath, R.G. (1977) Modulation of emotion with a brain pace maker. *J. nerv. ment. Dis.,* 165: 300–317.

Heimburger, R.F., Whitlock, C.C. and Kalsbeck, J.E. (1966) Stereotaxic amygdalotomy for epilepsy with aggressive behavior. *J. Amer. Med. Assoc.,* 198: 165–169.

Kepler, E.J. and Moersch, F.P. (1937) The psychiatric manifestations of hypoglycemia. *Amer. J. Psychiat.,* 14: 89–110.

King, H.E. (1961) Psychological effects of excitation in the limbic system. In *Electrical Stimulation of the Brain,* D.E. Sheer (Ed.), University of Texas Press, Austin, pp. 477–486.

Lagerspetz, K. (1964) Studies on the aggressive behavior of mice. *Ann. Acad. Sci. fenn. B,* 131: 1–131.

Morton, J.H., Addition, H., Addison, R.G., Hunt, L. and Sullivan, J.J. (1953) A clinical study of premenstrual tension. *Amer. J. Obstet. Gynec.,* 65: 1182–1191.

Moyer, K.E. (1968) Kinds of aggression and their physiological basis. *Commun. Behav. Biol.,* 2: 65–87.

Moyer, K.E. (1976) *The Psychobiology of Aggression.* Harper and Row, New York, p. 117.

Narabayashi, H., Nagao, T., Saito, Y., Yoshido, M. and Nagahata, M. (1963) Stereotaxic amygdalotomy for behavior disorders. *Arch. Neurol. (Chic.), 9*: 1–16.

Robinson, B.W., Alexander, M. and Bowne, G. (1969) Dominance reversal resulting from aggressive responses evoked by brain telestimulation. *Physiol. Behav.,* 4: 749–752.

Schreiner, L. and Kling, A. (1953) Behavioral changes following rhinencephalic injury in cat. *J. Neurophysiol.,* 16: 643–658.

Sem-Jacobsen, C.W. (1968) *Depth-Electrographic Stimulation of the Human Brain and Behavior,* Thomas, Springfield, Ill.

Sem-Jacobsen, C.W. and Torkildsen, A. (1960) Depth recording and electrical stimulation in the human brain. In E.R. Ramey and D.S. O'Doherty (Eds.), *Electrical Studies on the Unanesthetized Brain,* Harper and Row, New York, pp. 275–290.

Valenstein, E.S. (1973) *Brain control,* Wiley, New York.

Wilder, J. (1943) Psychobiological problems in hypoglycemia. *Amer. J. dig. Dis.,* 10: 428–435.

Woods, J.W. (1956) "Taming" of the wild Norway rat by rhinencephalic lesions. *Nature (Lond.),* 178: 869.

Adaptive Aspects of Neuronal Elements in Agonistic Behavior

P.R. WIEPKEMA *, J.M. KOOLHAAS and R. OLIVIER-AARDEMA

University of Groningen, Department of Zoology, Haren, (The Netherlands)

INTRODUCTION

Normally each organism is well equipped with numerous characteristics serving to achieve an optimal survival and reproduction in a specific environment. Such an environment is by no means a uniform and static set of conditions, but rather a composite of many divergent compartments needed for, for example, food intake, parental care, resting, etc. Furthermore these compartments may change over time as a result of factors such as day—night cycles, climatic events, etc. It is to such a dynamic and complex environment that living organisms have become adapted.

Animals interact continuously with their environment, the perception of which is deter-mined and restricted by the capability of their receptors to sense a specific internal and external milieu. This interaction implies both behavioral reactions to relevant changes perceived in this environment and behavioral actions that change it. For instance, in spring a male stickleback reacts with migratory behavior to changes in its external environment (e.g. increasing day length), while later on it actively changes its new environment when building a nest needed for reproduction.

All these amazing interactions between individual organisms and their environment indicate the exceptional capability of the central nervous system (CNS) and this introduces our main question, namely, what sort of functions must the brain perform in order that an animal behaves adequately in its dynamic environment. Our interest is in the neural regulation of the occurrence of larger behavioral entities or systems (like food intake behavior, aggressive behavior, sexual behavior and so on) under more or less natural conditions. One of the functions the brain has to fulfil then is to release or to inhibit a given system, when specific qualities of the internal and external environment support or oppose its performance. We shall focus upon one system, aggressive behavior, and the role which two neural substrates, hypothalamus and amygdala, may play when integrating its occurrence with internal and external factors.

BEHAVIORAL SYSTEMS

We first have to define the concept "behavior system" and more specifically, the aggressive behavior system. The definition has been rooted in ethology and is strongly influ-

---

* Present address: Zodiac, Marijkeweg 40, Agricultural University, Wageningen, The Netherlands.

370

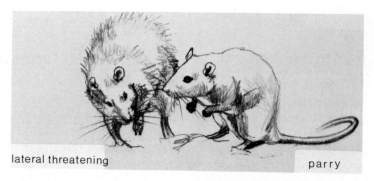

lateral threatening   parry

Fig. 1. Lateral threatening of a male rat towards a parrying conspecific. (From Timmermans, 1978.)

enced by the research of people like Lorenz (1937), Tinbergen (1950) and their colleagues or pupils (e.g. Baerends, 1976).

It was especially Lorenz who called attention to the idea that normal behavior consists for a large part of stereotyped movements and postures that are repeated over and again. These actions (Erbkoordinationen according to Lorenz) are called behavior elements. The gluing movement of a nest-building stickleback or the lateral threatening posture of a male rat (Fig. 1) exemplify such elements, which can be readily quantified in terms of frequencies and/or durations while also the sequential patterning can be analyzed quantitatively (cf. Colgan, 1978; Hazlett, 1977). This latter type of analysis clearly shows that in general, certain behavior elements are associated in time more than one would expect by chance only. Such non-random associations of behavior elements are defined as behavior systems. Since such systems often appear to serve a specific function they are named accordingly, e.g. food intake or nest building or territorial behavior and so on.

A critical and warning comment with respect to these behavior systems is appropriate here. Mostly, if not always, the systems have been defined on the basis of the behavior of many conspecifics in one or more conditions and therefore they represent an average picture. Actually, however, individuals may depart considerably from this global picture in their particular behavior structure (e.g. Baerends and Kruijt, 1973; Vodegel, 1978). Moreover the external conditions may be such that only parts of these behavior systems occur. For instance, the feeding system will present itself in a much more complete form when food has to be looked for, as compared to the situation in which food is offered at a well known time and place. We shall return to this point later on when discussing the functional role of the hypothalamus.

All these average systems consist of a number of elements that in themselves need not be specific for the system. What is specific is the association of just these elements and their often typical sequential patterning. This latter phenomenon, indicating a directionality in the performance of these behavior systems, has led to a distinction already made by Tinbergen (1951), namely in appetitive behavior, being the variable introductory part of the system, followed by an often very stereotyped consummatory part of the system.

A good example of such a system is feeding behavior of many species. This system includes a number of variable searching elements followed by stereotyped final ones like grasping the food and ingesting it (De Ruiter, 1967). It can be represented as a hierarchically organized regulatory system as has been done for other behavior systems, (for instance incubation behavior of herring gulls, Baerends, 1976). The regulatory aspect of feeding

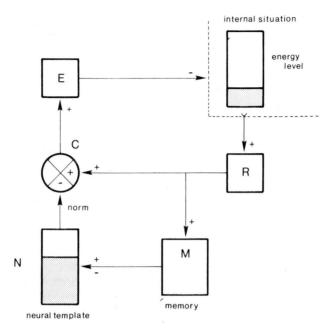

Fig. 2. Feeding behavior as a regulatory system. Receptors (R) perceive an existing internal energy level, that is compared in C with the appropriate norm (N). A difference in C activates feeding behavior (E), that increases the energy level and diminishes the difference in C. Experience in memory (M) may modulate N (cf. Fig. 4).

behavior is demonstrated by the fact that its performance results in a relative constancy of a complex set of internal parameters over longer periods of time. If we assume that feeding behavior is started when the actual values of these parameters deviate or threaten to deviate from a corresponding standard, one can state that feeding is directed at the homeostasis of specific properties of the internal environment (cf. Fig. 2).

At first sight, things seem to be more complex with respect to aggressive behavior, since its patterning seems to be much more diverse than feeding behavior. Moreover, it occurs in a wide variety of external situations. However, the difference might only be an apparent one, caused mainly by the fact that feeding has been investigated under relatively uniform conditions.

Aggressive behavior does occur in many different circumstances and it has been categorized accordingly (Moyer, 1968, 1980; Archer, 1976). Since this classification is based upon the hypothesis that aggressive patterns may differ widely with respect to behavioral organization and/or underlying physiological mechanisms, it is important to avoid mixing up heterogeneous phenomena and to restrict oneself to one type of aggressive behavior. For our purpose we have selected aggressive behavior that shows the formal characteristics of the earlier defined behavior systems: the presence of a variable introductory part followed by a stereotyped consummatory one (cf. Mogenson and Huang, 1973; Hogan and Roper, 1978). Such an aggressive system is the collection of behavior elements performed by a territory owner or a dominant male towards conspecific intruders or rivals, in the rat, *R. norvegicus*, under relatively free conditions (Calhoun, 1962; Telle, 1966; Timmermans, 1978; Lore and Flanelly, 1977). Quite another type of aggressive behavior is the shock-induced one, being an immediate reaction to some aversive stimulus and missing a variable introductory part.

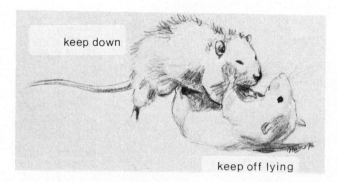

Fig. 3. Keep down of a dominant male rat. (From Timmermans, 1978.)

Wild rats live in colonies set up in the neighborhood of some (common) feeding area. Each colony may be divided into a number of territories inhabited by one dominant male and a number of adult females with their young. The territory itself is an area in and around a more or less complex system of burrows. An important point is that a male territory owner not only fights when he happens to meet an intruder, but that he also seems to look for possible strangers in his area. He may do so by patrolling his territory or by standing guard at a critical place.

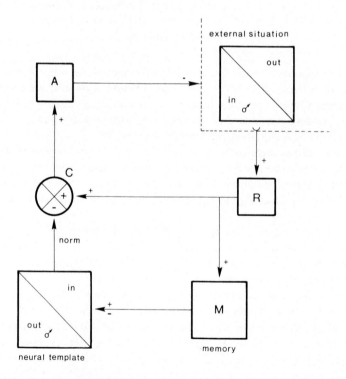

Fig. 4. Agonistic behavior as a regulatory system. Receptors (R) perceive an actual territorial situation, that is compared in C with the appropriate norm (N). A difference in C activates agonistic behavior (A), that changes the external situation in such a way that the difference in C becomes minimal. Experience in memory (M) may modulate N. (cf. Fig. 2).

Aggressive behavior performed may consist of variable searching behavior (patrolling), followed by approach, investigating, threatening postures, fighting, keeping down (Fig. 3) or chasing when an intruder is detected. The exact patterning of this behavior largely depends on which conspecific the intruder may be and where he is met. Since this behavior system may contain elements of approach and retreat, or attack and flight, it is often called agonistic behavior.

As in the case of feeding, this territorial agonistic behavior can be described as a hierarchically organized regulatory system, in this case however, directed at the homeostasis of certain aspects of the external environment, e.g. at the standard "no strange male(s) in a well-defined area" (Fig. 4). This behavior system (and thereby the homeostatic process) depends not only on a number of internal conditions (hormonal processes, availability of glucose and so on), but also on the experience of the male with former intruders inside its territory, its neighbors, etc. Much of this territorial agonistic behavior of the adult male rat is observed very clearly when a strange conspecific male is put into its home cage. These home males are often kept for weeks in isolation or together with one or more adult females in a large cage that is also used for testing. However, male rats may also perform agonistic behavior when they are put together in the same large observation cage. It is under all these conditions that most of the ethologically relevant brain research on territorial behavior of rats has been done (Adams, 1971, 1976; Blanchard et al., 1975; Koolhaas, 1975, 1978; Kruk et al., 1979; Lehman and Adams, 1977; Olivier, 1977a, b, Veening, 1975).

HYPOTHALAMUS AND MOTIVATED AGONISTIC BEHAVIOR

The hypothalamus is well known for two main functions: (1) it regulates many properties of the internal environment through its influence on the hypophysis and because of its involvement in the autonomic nervous system; and (2) it regulates in some way or another the occurrence of behavior systems such as feeding, agonistic, sexual behavior, etc.

Some years ago, Mogenson and Huang (1973) reviewed neurological aspects of motivated behavior and attributed to the hypothalamus an important role for intergrating overt behavior and visceral—endocrine aspects of the organism. In the present chapter we will try to make more explicit what such an integration might mean with respect to motivated agonistic behavior.

Although the first descriptions of the involvement of the hypothalamus in agonistic behavior (cats, Hess and Bruegger, 1943) are now rather dated, and even though many investigators have followed and enlarged this line of research, surprisingly few experiments have been performed in which this agonistic behavior was tested in the presence of one or more conspecifics imitating a more or less natural social context.

Lateral hypothalamus
One of the first reports dealing with such a situation has been published by Robinson et al. (1969); they found that electrical stimulation of the lateral or anterior hypothalamus of subordinate male rhesus monkeys could elicit agonistic behavior. If this behavior was performed repeatedly towards a dominant conspecific a dominance reversal resulted. The stimulation-bound behavior was largely similar to what occurs during spontaneous intraspecific fighting. The stimulated male who took the initiative in a fight never attacked the female that was also present during the agonistic encounter. This latter finding obtained a broader meaning when Alexander and Perachio (1973) showed that the occurrence of this

374

electrically-induced agonistic behavior strongly depended on which conspecific was present. Males were more often attacked than females, and subordinate males more often than dominant ones. Recently Lipp and Hunsperger (1978) found that familiarity with the environment is an important cue with respect to the elicitation of hypothalamically-induced agonistic behavior among marmosets. Panksepp (1971) and Woodworth (1971) reported that intraspecific agonistic behavior could be induced in rats also during electrical stimulation of the hypothalamus. Woodworth made the interesting observation that such stimulation-bound male attackers would stop their attack when the opponent was in a submissive posture, just like during spontaneous fights.

Similar data were obtained by one of us (Koolhaas, 1975, 1978), who tested stimulation-bound attack behavior of a male rat in its large home cage. Normally such a male will try to drive away any other adult male when put into this cage. Such territorial behavior is characterized by approach, investigating, piloerection, lateral threatening, frontal threatening, fighting and chasing when the intruder is a smaller male. The roles may become reversed if the intruder is a larger male; under such conditions the home male may avoid the intruder (Olivier, 1977a). When the incoming conspecific is an estrous female, approach followed by sexual behavior will occur, but practically no agonistic behavior. Brain stimulation of the same hypothalamic location in a given home male could lead to territorial agonistic behavior towards a subordinate intruder, as well as eventually to avoidance of a dominant intruder. Towards an estrous female some agonistic behavior may occur during stimulation, but sexual behavior was strongly diminished.

This stimulation-bound territorial behavior could be elicited from a specific hypothalamic area. Outside this area stimulation may facilitate reactive or defensive fighting, for instance when being investigated by an intruder. This latter type of agonistic behavior is typical of the subordinate male. It is characterized by the absence of introductory behavior (like approach, investigating and lateral threatening) and by the immediate (reflexive) occurrence

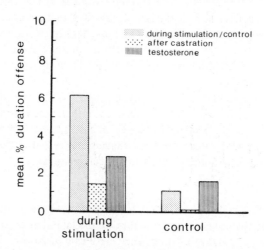

Fig. 5. Effect of castration and testosterone replacement on agonistic behavior elicited during lateral hypothalamic stimulation. Data of 5 male rats, each observed 5 times either during stimulation of the lateral hypothalamus (left) or without that stimulation (control, right). Duration of each observation 10 min, stimulation 10 sec on, 10 sec off, and so on. Ordinate: per cent of total observation time spent in offense (sum of lateral threatening, clinch and keep down). Abscissa: before or after castration and after castration + testosterone treatment.

of frontal threatening and biting when touched or investigated. It has been distinguished from territorial agonistic behavior – focused upon in this chapter – by several authors (Blanchard et al., 1977; Lehman and Adams, 1977; Olivier, 1977a). Intraspecific agonistic behavior sites in the hypothalamus never facilitated feeding and vice versa.

The important point is again that activation of specific places in the (lateral) hypothalamus facilitated agonistic behavior, the form and intensity of which strongly depended on the type of conspecific presented. In fact such data run entirely parallel with existing reports in the cat or opossum in the way aggressive behavior is determined by the presence of lifeless objects, non-conspecifics or conspecifics (Flynn et al., 1970; Roberts et al., 1967).

Recently we found (Fig. 5) that this hypothalamically-induced agonistic behavior of male rats was significantly reduced one week after castration. Treatment of these castrates with testosterone (500 μg testosterone proprionate/rat/day) restored the electrically-induced agonistic behavior, albeit not to the original level. Therefore stimulation-bound agonistic behavior seems to depend on a normal testosterone level in a similar way to that reported by Schuurman (1980) for spontaneous territorial behavior in male rats.

Obviously, in the (lateral) hypothalamus of male rats, and perhaps of other species too, territorial agonistic behavior can be facilitated completely if internal and external environmental aspects lend themselves to that behavior. In fact a similar conclusion can be drawn with respect to the relationship between other hypothalamic sites and feeding behavior (Hoebel, 1976).

Ventromedial hypothalamus

In contrast to these behavioral effects of the lateral hypothalamus, other parts of the hypothalamus, when stimulated, may stop the performance of behavior systems. For this reason Pribram (1971) distinguished a lateral "go" and a medial "stop" mechanism located in the hypothalamus. Such a "stop" function has been demonstrated by Veening (1975) who found that weak electrical stimulation of the ventromedial nucleus of the hypothalamus terminated ongoing agonistic (or feeding) behavior of male rats in their home cage. With respect to feeding behavior such a "stop" function is corroborated by the common finding that lesioning the medial hypothalamus leads to hyperphagia (cf. Hoebel, 1976).

Until now such a disinhibition of territorial agonistic behavior following medial hypothalamic lesions has not been reported generally. In most experiments such lesions led to an increase of reactive or defensive agonistic behavior (cf. Colpaert, 1975), but not of the territorial form we are interested in. This negative finding may be caused by the fact that in most studies the median hypothalamic lesions were too large to justify general conclusions as is suggested by the work of Olivier (1977a, b). This author found a dramatic difference between the agonistic behavior of male rats tested in their home cage following either anterior or posterior median hypothalamic lesions. The former males showed an enhanced reactive agonistic behavior when being investigated by a conspecific, whereas the latter approached male intruders, and attacked them much more than before. These latter animals were not difficult to handle in contrast to the animals which received anterior lesions. A similar differentiation of the median hypothalamus along an anterior–posterior axis has been suggested recently by Albert and Wong (1978).

The specificity of these posterior lesions is supported by the finding that such animals did not become hyperphagic, while their sexual behavior was similar to that of intact male rats. The disinhibited agonistic behavior of the posterior lesioned males was directed at males only and never at estrous females. Therefore there are good arguments for assuming that, at least in rats (and perhaps in other species too) lesions in the (median) hypothalamic structures may inhibit territorial agonistic behavior in a similar way as has been assumed with respect to feeding behavior. Current experiments performed by M. van der Berg in our laboratory have revealed that this disinhibited agonistic behavior is also testosterone-dependent. One week after castration the enhanced territorial behavior of posterior lesioned males is strongly diminished, whereas it is restored after one week of testosterone treatment.

Taking all these data together it is tempting to conclude that at the level of the hypothalamus behavior systems may be inhibited or facilitated. Obviously this hypothalamic influence depends on all those internal and external factors that normally control the occurrence of these behaviors (cf. Prop-van den Berg et al., 1977).

The intriguing point is then what sort of criteria may be applied at the hypothalamic level that terminate or release complete behavior systems. A plausible answer presents itself if we think of the intimate relationship between the hypothalamus and the regulation of the internal environment. Parameters of the interal milieu "perceived" at the hypothalamic level may be used as signals either to terminate or to release behavior systems, for instance blood glucose availability, blood androgen level, osmotic value of ECF and others. This assumption does not imply that, for instance, electrical stimulation of the lateral hypothalamus leading to agonistic behavior simply imitates a high androgen effect on the hypothalamus. If this was so, this stimulation effect would be independent of the existing androgen level. Obviously this is not the case. Since androgen-sensitive elements seem to be localized elsewhere in the hypothalamus (preoptic area, Bermond, 1978), an important question is then how specifically the lateral hypothalamic activity involved depends on the actions of these preoptic elements.

Of course we must be aware of a very complex constellation of internal environmental factors that determine which behavior systems are needed or permitted to perform. However, it might be that at the hypothalamic level the nervous system may say "yes" or "no" with respect to the occurrence of specific behavior systems on the basis of actual species-specific and critical values of the internal milieu.

Once a decision has been made, for instance "go", the behavior system is facilitated both in its sensory and its motoric aspects, as has been shown to be probable by Flynn et al. (1970).

A comment is needed on the concept of behavior systems. The foregoing discussion might have suggested that systems facilitated by hypothalamic stimulation always consist of introductory behavior followed by stereotyped consummatory patterns. This is not the case, however, since hypothalamic stimulation often facilitates only fragments of larger systems (see Roberts, 1970). This raises the question as to whether such a finding indicates an underlying fragmentary organization of the entire behavior system, or whether the neural organization of a system is organized concentrically: the nearer to the centre the higher the chance that stimulation will elicit the whole system. We cannot answer this question at the moment, partly because the organizational structure of the behavior patterns elicited has not been analyzed in detail and partly because we do not know how rigid (or flexible) ethologically defined behavior systems actually are. However, we do know that an individual male rat may start or stop its territorial behavior at any point in the normal sequence and that this depends on which opponent is encountered and where. An intruder who reaches the center of a territory without being perceived will be treated quite differently after being detected, compared to an intruder that is already detected somewhere at the periphery of the territory. It might be that a "fragmentary" organization of behavior at the hypothalamic level has to do with the need of the home defender to adapt its behavior to different territorial situations (cf. section on Behavioral Systems).

AMYGDALA AND MOTIVATED AGONISTIC BEHAVIOR

Kaada (1972), in an extensive review of functional aspects of the amygdala, concludes that this brain area may both facilitate and inhibit larger complexes of behavior, like feeding and mating behavior. At the end of his survey he is inclined to think that "the amygdala adds plasticity to the basic inborn and more fixed reflex mechanisms of the brain stem, possibly by incorporating past experience with the present stimulation". A similar idea is put forward by Gloor (1972) when he writes that: "especially the amygdala provides the link between the master storehouse of information laid down in the neocortex and the fundamental motivational drive mechanisms centered upon in the hypothalamus". The amygdala may play such a role because of its close anatomical relationship with the neocortex, especially with the temporal lobe (Lammers, 1972; Gloor, 1978; Veening, 1978) and with the hypothalamus, by way of the stria terminalis and the ventral amygdalofugal pathway (Lammers, 1972; De Olmos, 1972). This connection is a reciprocal one (cf. Egger, 1972), while (at least in cats: Dreifuss, 1972) amygdala stimulation may either inhibit or excite the same neuron in the median hypothalamus.

Many reports substantiate the idea that for a given environmental constellation the amygdala modulates ongoing behavior on the basis of experience with similar conditions in the past (Fonberg and Delgado, 1961; Rolls and Rolls, 1973; Lepiane and Phillips, 1978; Aronson and Cooper, 1979; Grossman, 1972). The idea that the amygdala really inhibits or facilitates behavior systems has still to be proven. Convincing evidence can be found in the research of Fonberg (1972) with respect to feeding behavior in dogs. She found that bilateral lesions of the dorsomedial amygdala resulted in a long-lasting period of aphagia and hypophagia, while simultaneously the dogs appeared to be completely indifferent to environmental stimuli. On the other hand, bilateral lesions of the lateral amygdala resulted in a strong but transient hyperphagia.

The relationship between territorial agonistic behavior and the amygdala is still unclear. Amygdalectomy reduces intraspecific agonistic behavior in a number of species (in primates: Rosvold et al., 1954; Kling, 1972; in hamster: Bunnell et al., 1970; in rats: Miczek et al., 1974). However, Busch and Barfield (1974) failed to show an effect of amygdaloid lesions on the occurrence of agonistic behavior of male rats in their home cage and directed against a male intruder.

Since in the latter study the lesions comprised large parts of the entire amygdaloid complex and since a functional subdivision of this complex is not unlikely (cf. Fonberg, 1972; Miczek et al., 1974), we repeated the experiment differentiating for corticomedial and basolateral amygdaloid lesions in male rats living in a territorial situation.

The experimental animals, 40 adult males of the WE-zob strain, were housed individually in large wooden cages with a glass front wall. Each of these males lived together with one adult female. Once a day, during the night period of the animals, a strange adult male was put into the home cage mentioned above (after removal of the female) and the behavior was recorded for 10 min. In most cases, much territorial agonistic behavior was initiated and performed by the home male. For each male, 9 observations were made during a period of 2 successive weeks.

Following this, 13 males underwent bilateral lesioning of the corticomedial amygdala, and 13 underwent bilateral lesioning of the basolateral amygdala. In order to destroy these areas sufficiently in the anterior—posterior direction, two lesions, one behind the other, were made. In 7 males electrodes were placed as in the corticomedial group, and in 7 other males as in the basolateral group. In these 14 animals no current was passed through the electrodes,

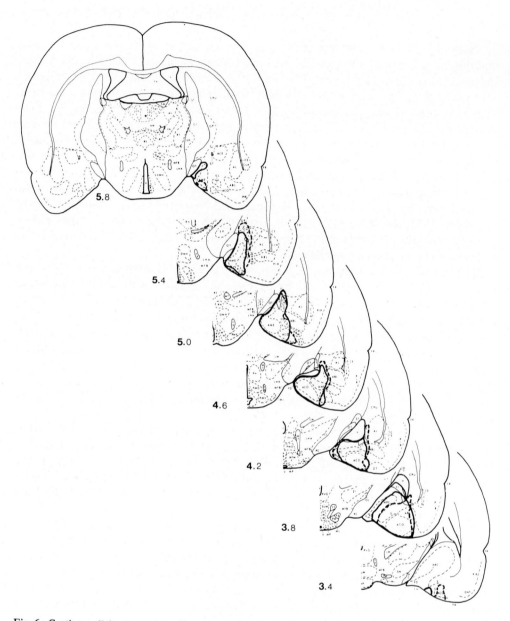

Fig. 6. Corticomedial amygdala lesions. Electrode placements: A 5.2, L ± 4.0, Vert. −2.8 and A 42, L ± 4.2, Vert. −1.8 (according to Pellegrino and Cushman, 1967). Left and right lesions shown on one side.

and the electrodes were removed immediately after placement. In the second and third week after the operation day 9 observations were performed as before. The frequencies (or total durations) of by far the most behavior elements (23 were distinguished) did not differ significantly (Mann–Whitney U-test) between both sham-lesioned groups. Since this was observed during both the pre- and post-operation periods, the behavioral data of both groups will be combined into one control group.

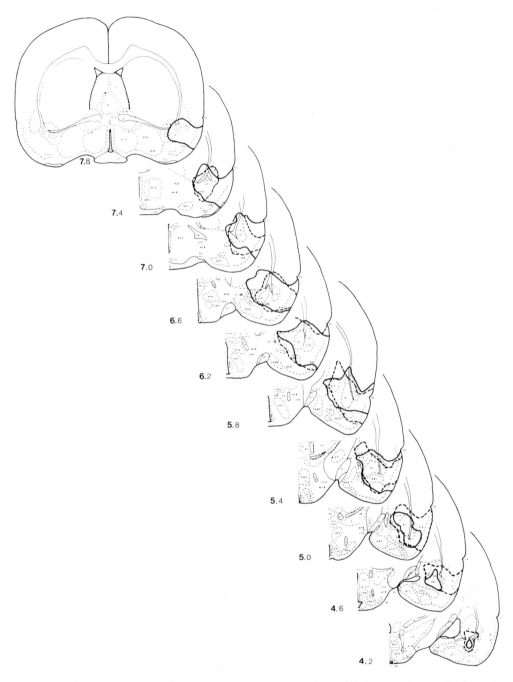

Fig. 7. Basolateral amygdala lesions. Electrode placements: A 5.8, L ± 5.4, Vert. −1.8 and A 4.8, L ± 5.2, Vert. −1.6 (according to Pellegrino and Cushman, 1967). Left and right lesions shown on one side.

Histological examination of the brain areas lesioned (Figs. 6, 7) revealed that in practically all animals of the corticomedial group the n. basalis medialis, n. corticalis and the n. medialis of the amygdala, parts of the stria terminalis and parts of the zona transitionalis

380

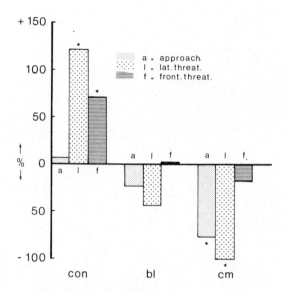

Fig. 8. Effect of sham-lesions (con), basolateral (bl) or corticomedial (cm) lesions of the amygdala on the occurrence of 3 behavioral elements. Ordinate: post-operative level (duration) of 3 behavioral elements (a, l and f) as percentage of their pre-operative levels. Abscissa: the 3 behavioral elements for 3 experimental groups (con, bl, cm) * indicates significant difference between pre- and post-operative level (Wilcoxon matched pairs, $P < 0.05$).

were destroyed bilaterally. In most animals of the basolateral group the following areas were destroyed bilaterally: n. lateralis and n. basalis lateralis of the amygdala, parts of the cortex piriformis and parts of the claustrum (Pellegrino and Cushman, 1967).

Post-operatively, the sham-lesioned males performed lateral threatening and frontal threatening followed by fighting more often than before (Fig. 8). Presumably in the course of the experiment each male became a more experienced defender of its home cage. In the basolateral group (Fig. 8) there was a non-significant tendency to perform less approach and less lateral threatening behavior after the operation. Since also fighting and frontal threatening did not change significantly post-operatively, it might be that the animals of the basolateral group make less use of their pre-operative experience with respect to territorial defence as compared with the control animals.

In contrast, the agonistic behavior of the corticomedial males (Fig. 8) was strongly influenced by the lesion. Post-operatively these males performed significantly less approach and less lateral threatening behavior, while fighting was also strongly reduced. Frontal threatening was at a normal level, while there was an enormous increase in sniffing or investigating the environment.

These data indicate that in the corticomedial group destruction took place of amygdaloid structures (or structures in their immediate vicinity) that normally facilitate territorial agonistic behavior as expressed by the occurrence of approach and lateral threatening behavior followed by fighting.

Moreover, the lesioned structures are less relevant for the occurrence of frontal threatening behavior, which was mainly performed when being investigated by the intruder.

It is interesting to note that these corticomedially lesioned males spent significantly more time in feeding than before, while at the end of the experimental period (3 weeks after the operation day) their body weights were significantly higher than those of the sham-lesioned

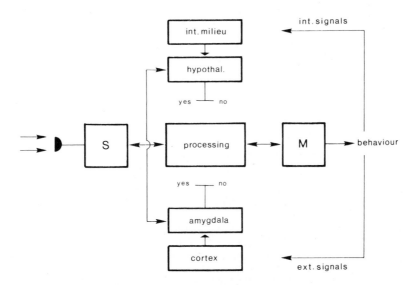

Fig. 9. Summary of possible influence of hypothalamus and amygdala on the connection (processing) of stimulus reception (S) and motoric commands (M). Further explanation in text.

controls. This indicates that the lesions affected an area that normally inhibits food intake behavior. Since Grossman and Grossman (1963) and Box and Mogenson (1975) also found hyperphagia or aphagia in rats depending on the location of the amygdaloid destruction, such data underline that facilitating or inhibiting influences on normal feeding behavior do exist in rats also.

With respect to agonistic behavior, our data only show a facilitating function of corticomedial units of the amygdala, but they stress the need for more specific lesions of the amygdala complex in order to find out whether or not it may also contain inhibiting units. As yet we cannot answer the question whether or not the contribution of the amygdala to territorial agonistic behavior is primarily based on the individual experience of the animal. To investigate that we have to analyze in much more detail the structure of individual agonistic behavior and find out which components of behavior are determined by individual experience. Until now no data are at hand on this point. Only after such individually determined agonistic features have been established may we expect a fruitful analysis with respect to the possible contribution of the amygdala to the occurrence of agonistic behavior.

CONCLUSIONS

At the end of this review of some selected data on the relationship between two brain structures, the hypothalamus and the amygdala, and the occurrence of territorial agonistic behavior, we must admit that the available data do not permit a clear statement on what the behavioral role of both brain structures might be. However, it is clear that an organism, in order to behave adequately in its natural environment, needs to take into account, firstly, whether or not its internal environment permits or asks for a certain behavioral action; this is a first stage at which a whole behavior system might be facilitated or inhibited. Further, the animal may have learned to suppress or to release a certain system under certain external conditions; this individual experience decides at a second stage whether or not a whole

382

behavior system has to be released or not. Perhaps these functions are located in the hypothalamus and amygdala, respectively, (Fig. 9), but this we don't know. What we do know is that this sort of function must exist somewhere in the brain in order to guarantee optimal survival and reproduction of the organism. It is our task to find out where and how these "permissive" functions of the brain are organized. The answer to such questions may make clear what is meant by the title of this chapter, namely, "adaptive aspects of neuronal elements in agonistic behavior".

REFERENCES

Adams, D.B. (1971) Defense and territorial behaviour dissociated by hypothalamic lesions in the rat. *Nature (Lond.)*, 21: 573–574.

Adams, D.B. (1976) The relation of scent-marking, olfactory investigation, and specific postures in the isolation-induced fighting of rats. *Behaviour*, 56: 286–297.

Albert, D.J. and Wong, R.C.K. (1978) Interanimal aggression and hyperreactivity following hypothalamic infusion of local anesthetic in the rat. *Physiol. Behav.*, 20: 755–761.

Alexander, M. and Perachio, A.A. (1973) The influence of target sex and dominance on evoked attack in rhesus monkeys. *Amer. J. Phys. Anthrop.*, 38: 543–547.

Archer, J. (1976) The organisation of aggression and fear in vertebrates. In *Perspectives in Ethology, Vol. 2*, P.P.G. Bateson and P. Klopfer (Eds.), Plenum Press, New York, pp. 231–298.

Aronson, L.R. and Cooper, N.L. (1979) Amygdaloid hypersexuality in male rats re-examined. *Physiol. Behav.*, 22: 257–265.

Baerends, G.P. (1976) The functional organization of behaviour. *Anim. Behav.*, 24: 726–738.

Baerends, G.P. and Kruijt, J.P. (1973) Stimulus selection. In *Constraints on Learning*, R.A. Hinde and J. Stevenson-Hinde (Eds.), Academic Press, New York, pp. 23–50.

Bermond, B. (1978) *Neuro-Hormonal Regulation of Aggressive and Sexual Behaviour in the Rat.* Ph.D. thesis, Amsterdam.

Blanchard, R.J., Blanchard, D.C., Takahashi, T. and Kelley, M.J. (1977) Attack and defensive behaviour in the albino rat. *Anim. Behav.*, 25: 622–634.

Blanchard, R.J., Fukanaga, K., Blanchard, D.C. and Kelley, M.J. (1975) Conspecific aggression in the laboratory rat. *J. comp. physiol. Psychol.*, 89: 1204–1209.

Box, B.M. and Mogenson, G.J. (1975) Alterations in ingestive behaviour after bilateral lesions of the amygdala in the rat. *Physiol. Behav.*, 15: 679–688.

Bunnell, B.N., Sodetz, F.J. and Shalloway, D.T. (1970) Amygdaloid lesions and social behaviour in the golden hamster. *Physiol. Behav.*, 5: 153–161.

Busch, D.E. and Barfield, R.J. (1974) A failure of amygdaloid lesions to alter agonistic behaviour in the laboratory rat. *Physiol. Behav.*, 12: 887–892.

Calhoun, J.B. (1962) *The Ecology and Sociology of the Norway Rat*, United States Dept. of Health, Education and Welfare, Bethesda, Md.

Colgan, P.W. (Ed.) (1978) *Quantitative Ethology*, John Wiley, New York.

Colpaert, F.C. (1975) The ventromedial hypothalamus and the control of avoidance behaviour and aggression: fear hypothesis versus response–suppression theory of limbic system function. *Behav. Biol.*, 15: 27–44.

Dacey, D.M. and Grossman, S.P. (1977) Aphagia, adipsia and sensory-motor deficits produced by amygdala lesions: a function of extra-amygdaloid damage. *Physiol. Behav.*, 19: 389–395.

De Olmos, J.S. (1972) The amygdaloid projection field in the rat as studied with the cupric–silver method. In *The Neurobiology of the Amygdala*, B.E. Eleftheriou (Ed.), Plenum Press, New York, pp. 145–204.

De Ruiter, L. (1967) Feeding behaviour of vertebrates in their natural environment. In *Handbook of Physiology, Section 6: Alimentary Canal, Vol. 1: Food and Water Intake*, Physiological Society, Washington, D.C., pp. 97–116.

Dicks, D., Myers, R.E. and Kling, A. (1969) Uncus and amygdala lesions: effects on social behaviour in the free ranging rhesus monkey. *Science*, 165: 69–71.

Dreifuss, J.J. (1972) Effects of electrical stimulation of the amygdaloid complex on the ventromedial hypothalamus. In *The Neurobiology of the Amygdala*, B.E. Eleftheriou (Ed.), Plenum Press, New York, pp. 295–317.

Egger, M.D. and Flynn, J.P. (1967) Further studies on the effects of amygdaloid stimulation and ablation on hypothalamically elicited attack behaviour in cats. In *Structure and Function of the Limbic System, Progress in Brain Research, Vol. 27*, W.R. Adey and T. Tokizane (Eds.), Elsevier, Amsterdam, pp. 165–182.

Egger, M.D. (1972) Amygdaloid–hypothalamic neurophysiological interrelationships. In *The Neurobiology of the Amygdala*, B.E. Eleftheriou (Ed.), Plenum Press, New York, pp. 319–342.

Flynn, J.P. (1976) Neural basis of threat and attack. In *Biological Foundations of Psychiatry*, R.G. Grenell and S. Gabay (Ed.), Raven Press, New York, pp. 273–295.

Flynn, J.P., Vanegas, H., Foote, W. and Edwards, S. (1970) Neural mechanisms involved in a cat's attack on a rat. In *Neural Control of Behaviour*, R. Whalen, M. Verzeano and N.M. Weinberger, (Eds.), Academic Press, New York, pp. 135–173.

Fonberg, E. (1972) Control of emotional behaviour through the hypothalamus and amygdaloid complex. In *Physiology, Emotion and Psychosomatic Illness*, R. Porter and J. Knight (Eds.), Elsevier, Amsterdam, pp. 131–161.

Fonberg, E. and Delgado, J.M.R. (1961) Avoidance and alimentary reactions during amygdaloid stimulation. *J. Neurophysiol.*, 24: 651–664.

Gloor, P. (1972) Temporal lobe epilepsy: its possible contribution to the understanding of the functional significance of the amygdala and of its interaction with neocortical–temporal mechanisms. In *The Neurobiology of the Amygdala*, B.E. Eleftheriou (Ed.), Plenum Press, New York, pp. 423–457.

Gloor, P. (1978) Inputs and outputs of the amygdala: what the amygdala is trying to tell the rest of the brain. In *Limbic Mechanisms*, K.E. Livingston and O. Horny Kiewicz (Eds.), Plenum Press, New York, pp. 189–209.

Grossman, S.P. (1972) The role of the amygdala in escape–avoidance behaviours. In *The Neurobiology of the Amygdala*, B.E. Eleftheriou (Ed.), Plenum Press, New York, pp. 537–551.

Grossman, S.P. and Grossman, L. (1963) Food and water intake following lesions on electrical stimulation of the amygdala. *Amer. J. Physiol.*, 205: 761–765.

Hazlett, B.A. (Ed.) (1977) *Quantitative Methods in the Study of Animal Behaviour*. Academic Press, New York.

Hess, W.R. and Bruegger, M. (1943) Das subkortikale Zentrum der effektiven Abwehrreaktion. *Helv. physiol. Acta*, 1: 33–52.

Hoebel, B.G. (1976) Satiety: hypothalamic stimulation, anorectic drugs, and neurochemical substrates. In *Hunger: Basic Mechanisms and Clinical Implications*, D. Novin, W. Wyrwicka and G. Bray (Eds.), Raven Press, New York, pp. 33–50.

Hogan, J.A. and Roper, T.J. (1978) A comparison of the properties of different reinforcers. *Advanc. Study Behav.*, 8: 155–254.

Kaada, B.R. (1972) Stimulation and regional ablation of the amygdaloid complex with reference to functional representation. In *The Neurobiology of the Amygdala*, B.E. Eleftheriou (Ed.), Plenum Press, New York, pp. 205–281.

Kling, A. (1972) Effects of amygdalectomy on social-affective behaviour in non-human primates. In *The Neurobiology of the Amygdala*, B.E. Eleftheriou (Ed.), Plenum Press, New York, pp. 511–536.

Kling, A., Lancaster, J. and Benitone, J. (1970) Amygdalectomy in the free-ranging vervet (*Cercopithecus aethiops*). *J. Psychiat. Res.*, 7: 191–199.

Koolhaas, J.M. (1975) *The Lateral Hypothalamus and Intraspecific Aggressive Behaviour in the Rat*, Ph.D. Thesis, Groningen.

Koolhaas, J.M. (1978) Hypothalamically induced intraspecific aggressive behaviour in the rat. *Exp. Brain Res.*, 32: 365–375.

Kruk, M.R., van den Poel, A.M. and De Vos-Frericks, T.P. (1979) The induction of aggressive behaviour by electrical stimulation in the hypothalamus of male rats. *Behaviour*, 70: 292–322.

Lammers, H.J. (1972) The normal connections of the amygdaloid complex in mammals. In *The Neurobiology of the Amygdala*, B.E. Eleftheriou (Ed.), Plenum Press, New York, pp. 123–144.

Lehman, M.N. and Adams, D.B. (1977) A statistical and motivational analysis of the social behaviour of the male laboratory rat. *Behaviour*, 61: 238–274.

Lepiane, F.G. and Phillips, A.G. (1978) Differential effects of electrical stimulation of amygdala, caudate-putamen or substantia nigra pars compacta on taste aversion and passive avoidance in rats. *Physiol. Behav.*, 21: 979–985.

Levison, P.K. and Flynn, J.P. (1965) The objects attacked by cats during stimulation of the hypothalamus. *Anim. Behav.*, 13: 217–220.

Lipp, H.P. and Hunsperger, R.W. (1978) Threat, attack and flight elicited by electrical stimulation of the ventromedial hypothalamus of the Marmoset monkey *Callithrix jacchus*. *Brain Behav. Evol.*, 15: 260–293.

Lore, R.L. and Flanelly, K. (1977) Rat societies. *Scient. American*, 236: 106–116.

Lorenz, K. (1937) Ueber den Begriff der Instinkthandlung. *Folia biotheor.*, 2: 17–50.

Luciano, D. and Lore, R. (1975) Aggression and social experience in domesticated rats. *J. comp. physiol. Psychol.*, 88: 917–923.

MacDonnell, M. and Flynn, J.P. (1966) Sensory control of hypothalamic attack. *Anim. Behav.*, 14: 399–405.

Miczek, K.A., Brykczynski, T. and Grossman, S.P. (1974) Differential effects of lesions in the amygdala, periamygdaloid cortex, and stria terminalis on aggressive behaviours in rats. *J. comp. Physiol. Psychol.*, 87: 760–771.

Mogenson, G.J. and Huang, Y.H. (1973) The neurobiology of motivated behaviour. *Progr. Neurobiol.*, 1: 55–83.

Moyer, K.E. (1968) Kinds of aggression and their physiological basis. *Commun. Behav. Biol.* A, 2: 65–87.

Moyer, K.E. (1980) Biological substrates of aggression. In *Adaptive Capabilities of the Nervous System, Progress in Brain Research, Vol. 53,* M.A. Korner et al. (Eds.), Elsevier, Amsterdam, pp. 359–367.

Olivier, B. (1977a) The ventromedial hypothalamus and aggressive behaviour in rats. *Aggress. Behav.*, 3: 47–56.

Olivier, B. (1977b) *Behavioural Functions of the Medial Hypothalamus in the Rat,* Ph.D. thesis, Groningen.

Panksepp, J. (1971) Aggression elicited by electrical stimulation of the hypothalamus in albino rats. *Physiol. Behav.*, 6: 321–329.

Pellegrino, E.J. and Cushman, A.J. (1967) *A Stereotaxic Atlas of the Rat Brain,* Appleton-Century-Crofts, New York.

Pribram, K.H. (1971) *Languages of the Brain,* Englewood Cliffs, New Jersey.

Prop-van den Berg, C.M., Schuurman, T. and Wiepkema, P.R. (1977) Nembutal treatment of the VMH (rat): effects on feeding and sexual behaviour. *Brain Res.*, 126: 519–529.

Roberts, W.W. (1970) Hypothalamic mechanisms for motivational and species-typical behaviour. In *The Neural Control of Behaviour,* R.E. Whalen, R.F. Thompson, M. Verzeano and N.M. Weinbergen (Eds.), Academic Press, New York, pp. 175–206.

Roberts, W.W., Steinberg, M.L. and Means, L.W. (1967) Hypothalamic mechanisms of sexual, aggressive and other motivational behaviours in the opossum, *Didelphis virginiana*. *J. comp. physiol. Psychol.*, 64: 1–15.

Robinson, B.W., Alexander, M. and Bowne, G. (1969) Dominance reversal resulting from aggressive responses evolved by brain stimulation. *Phyiol. Behav.*, 4: 749–752.

Rolls, B.J. and Rolls, E.T. (1973) Effects of lesions in the basolateral amygdala on fluid intake in the rat. *J. comp. physiol. Psychol.*, 83: 240–247.

Rosvold, H.E., Mirsky, A.F. and Pribram, K.H. (1954) Influence of amygdalectomy on social behaviour in monkeys. *J. comp. physiol. Psychol.*, 47: 173–178.

Schuurman, T. (1980) Hormonal correlates of agonistic behavior in adult male rats. In *Adaptive Capabilities of the Nervous System, Progress in Brain Research, Vol. 53,* M.A. Corner et al. (Eds.), Elsevier, Amsterdam, pp. 415–420.

Telle, H.J. (1966) Beitrag zur Kenntnis der Verhaltensweise von Ratten vergleichend dargestellt bei Rattus norvegicus and Rattus rattus. *Z. angew. Zool.*, 53: 126–196.

Timmermans, P.J.A. (1978) *Social Behaviour in the Rat,* Ph.D. thesis, Nijmegen.

Tinbergen, N. (1950) The hierarchical organization of nervous mechanisms underlying instinctive behaviour. *Symp. Soc. exp. Biol.*, 4: 305–312.

Tinbergen, N. (1951) *The Study of Instinct,* Clarendon Press, Oxford.

Veening, J.G. (1975) *Behavioural Functions of the VMH in the Rat: an Ethological Approach,* Ph.D. thesis, Groningen.

Veening, J.G. (1978) Cortical afferents of the amygdaloid complex in the rat: an HRP study. *Neurosci. Lett.*, 8: 191–195.

Vodegel, N. (1978) A Causal Analysis of the Behaviour of *Pseudotropheus zebra,* Ph.D. thesis, Groningen.

Woodworth, C.H. (1971) Attack elicited in rats by electrical stimulation of the lateral hypothalamus. *Physiol. Behav.*, 6: 345–353.

Is There Evidence for a Neural Correlate of an Aggressive Behavioural System in the Hypothalamus of the Rat?

M.R. KRUK and A.M. VAN DER POEL

Leiden Medical Centre, Sylvius Laboratoria, Department of Pharmacology, Leiden (The Netherlands)

INTRODUCTION

In his introduction to the special issue of Scientific American on the brain, David H. Hubel (1979) writes: "At the present stage, with a reasonable start in understanding the structure and workings of individual cells, neurobiologists are in the position of a man who knows something about the physics of resistors, condensers and transistors and who looks inside a television set. He cannot begin to understand how the machine works as a whole until he learns how the elements are wired together and until he has at least some idea of the purpose of the machine, of its subassemblies and their interactions". The analogy is very useful in behavioural neurobiology. Ideally, the unraveling of the "wiring diagram" of the brain should go together with the testing of intelligent assumptions on the purpose and the functions of its subassemblies and their interactions if we are to clarify the functioning of the brain in behaviour. Naturally, many of these assumptions will have to stem from theories derived from behavioural observations of intact animals. However, even very clear, well-defined behavioural constructs may lack a specific correlate or a distinct localization in the brain. Such constructs may be the consequence of several brain mechanisms, none of which is specifically related to a behavioural phenomenon, each with its own localization and correlates. Or — to extend Hubel's analogy a little further — we may be looking for a word- or a man-generator in a television set, when we search for a representation of behavioural constructs in the brain.

There can be little doubt that neural networks in the brain somehow integrate information concerning internal and external events involved in aggression. But "aggression" is hardly a suitable concept for testing assumptions on brain functions in behaviour. We will have to provide more accurate behavioural constructs. Saying "bite, rage, and attack integrating networks" might be just another way of saying "brain" itself. But even if we could agree on a more precise definition of aggression, i.e. as an "agonistic behavioural system" (Wiepkema et al., 1980), would that allow us to test for functions of the hypothalamus in behaviour? The number of autonomic, endocrine and physiological processes that can be influenced by the hypothalamus suggests that there is more to this structure than behavioural systems alone. Also, anatomical studies reveal many intricate neural networks even within well-defined parts of the hypothalamus (Millhouse, 1973a, b; Saper et al., 1976). All these networks may eventually appear to serve a distinct function of their own. The problem is on which level of complexity of brain organization do we have to test a given behavioural construct?

ATTACKS INDUCED BY ELECTRICAL STIMULATION IN THE HYPOTHALAMUS

An outline of our work on attack behaviour induced by electrical stimulation in the hypothalamus of male CPB-WE rats may help to illustrate the problem. First some results are presented.

(1) CPB-WE rats (WE-zob rats) will attack a weaker albino Wistar rat during stimulation in the hypothalamus. In our test cage these rats did not attack or fight when not stimulated, but engaged in more friendly interactions instead. They did not form a territory during their short stay in the test cage for control or stimulation tests.

(2) At threshold current intensity, the attacks can be classified into two broad categories. In attack *jumps,* the stimulated rat tried to bite the head of its adversary and simultaneously delivered a forceful kick in the belly. In the relatively mild *bite* attack, the head or the back of the neck was simply bitten. Both attacks may be followed by fierce *clinch* fights (Fig. 1). In spontaneous fights between male rats the same types of attacks can be observed.

(3) Stimulation in attack-inducing electrode placements interrupts ongoing sexual activities, eating and drinking. We were not able to modify attack behaviour into sexual behaviour, eating, drinking, carrying or gnawing by stimulation given in the presence of the appropriate objects for releasing such behaviours (Kruk et al., 1979).

(4) Stimulation-induced brain activity is apparently compatible with spontaneous aggression, since CPB-WE rats will fight an intruder in their territory with greater vigour when they are stimulated in the hypothalamus. They also seem to take previous defeats into account during subsequent stimulations (Koolhaas, 1978).

(5) Attack could be induced in about 50% of the 350 electrode implantations tested in our laboratory. The Alloc-3 version of discriminant analysis (Habbema, 1976; Habbema and Hermans, 1978) on the histology of these electrode placements enabled us to delimit an area within the hypothalamus where the chance to induce attacks is greater than 80%.

(6) Other behavioural consequences of stimulation in these electrode implantations are teeth-chattering, pilo-erection and increased locomotion. Rats can also be trained to start or to stop stimulation in many of the electrode placements tested.

Many of the arguments against the localization of behaviourally specific systems in the hypothalamus do not seem to apply in the case of stimulation-induced attacks (Kruk et al., 1979). It is very tempting, therefore, to assume that we are dealing with a neural substrate of an agonistic or aggressive behavioural system in this hypothalamic area. Activation of this area inhibits other behaviours, but is compatible with spontaneous aggression. It induces forward, "appetitive" or "searching" behaviour (locomotion), together with signs of automic

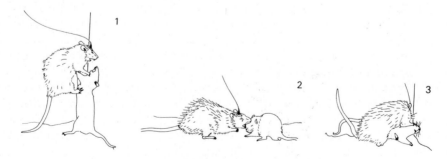

Fig. 1. Attacks induced by electrical stimulation in the hypothalamus of the CPB-WE rat. 1: attack jump. 2: bite attack. 3: start of clinch fight.

arousal (pilo-erection) and teeth-chattering just as in spontaneous aggression. Activation of this substrate will first lead to mild attacks, then to fierce attacks and fights. When the external or internal factors favour aggression, actions increasing the activity may be reinforcing (switch-on). When the internal or external environment is unsuited for aggression, actions decreasing the activity of the substrate may take over (switch-off).

AN "AGGRESSIVE BEHAVIOURAL SYSTEM" IN THE HYPOTHALAMUS?

However, although the concept of a hypothalamic substrate especially subservent to an aggressive behavioural system may seem attractive, the data do not yet justify the acceptance of such an idea.

One major objection is that we do not know whether the area from which attacks can be induced is also involved in spontaneous aggression. The effects of lesions in that area on spontaneous aggression but also on locomotion and the self-stimulation behaviours should give us a clue about the functions of this part of the hypothalamus. But such a study has not yet been done. Ideally, one should like to record — in a variety of behavioural situations — the activity of the cells which during stimulation give rise to attacks. But this would be difficult to accomplish, if only for the fact that we do not know which neuronal elements mediate the aggressive consequences of electrical stimulation in the hypothalamus. After lesioning a little bit of the tissue at the tips of electrodes used for the induction of attacks we found — apart from local degeneration in the hypothalamus — degenerating fibres leading to the central grey of the midbrain, the mammillary bodies and the septum. Thus there are at least 3 possible ways to convey the aggression-inducing neural activity to other parts of the brain. Moreover, we do not even know for certain if the aggressive consequences of stimulation stem from electrical or humoral output of the hypothalamus.

Another objection could be that we arbitrarily fit several behavioural consequences of stimulation into a single conceptual behavioural function. However, these behavioural consequences do not necessarily derive from the activation of only one neural system. Rather, they may stem from the activation of several discrete and unrelated neural systems which overlap within the effective field of the electrode (Roberts, 1969). In many studies of goal-directed behaviours induced by electrical stimulation, current intensities are used which "elicit sufficient locomotory exploration" (Koolhaas, 1978) or forward-moving "searching" behaviour (Valenstein et al., 1969). The underlying assumption presumably is that these locomotor responses derive from the activation of the neural system involved in the goal-directed response. However, there are two types of evidence which suggest that the aggressive consequences and the other behavioural effects of stimulation in fact stem from the activation of different neural systems. In the first place, many of these concomitant behaviours are not limited to the attack-inducing electrode placements, but can also be induced in electrode placements well outside the target area for attack. Secondly, changes in the parameters of the stimulating current affect differentially the distinct behavioural effects, suggesting that either the localization or the excitability of the activated elements differ. We will briefly summarize the evidence for each behavioural consequence of stimulation. For details on methods see Kruk et al. (1978 and 1979).

Locomotion and attack

All electrode placements tested induced locomotion, whether or not they induced attacks.

388

Increasing the current intensity in attack-inducing electrodes increased locomotion in all electrode placements, but aggression only in half of the electrode placements tested.

Threshold current intensities for both attack and locomotion change as a function of the duration of the pulses in the stimulating train. This relation can be adequately described by a hyperbole. According to classical neurophysiology (Lapique, 1926; Blair, 1932) such strength—duration relationships can be defined by their chronaxie and rheobase. The chronaxie obtained for attack behaviour was always shorter than the chronaxie for locomotion. Although such behaviourally derived "chronaxies" may not exactly reflect the properties of the excited membranes, the fact that the strength—duration relations for these behaviours differ systematically, suggests that these behavioural consequences are mediated by different neural elements at the electrode tip (also see Ranck, 1975).

Self-stimulation behaviours and attack

Attack-inducing electrode placements may support either switch-on or switch-off behaviour, support both or support neither. However, the same applies to the electrode placements that do not induce attacks, as has been shown by R.E. Phillips (St. Paul, Minn.) in our laboratory. Similar results have been reported by Herndon et al. (1979) in rhesus monkeys.

Threshold current intensities for attack behaviour depend on the interval between pairs of pulses in the stimulating pulse train. When each second pulse of the pairs comes midway between the preceding and the following pulse, attack thresholds are at their lowest (Fig. 2, control 1). When the interval between the pulse pairs decreases, attack thresholds rise. The maximum is reached at a 0.5—0.8 msec intra-pair interval. This maximum is almost as high as the attack threshold for a stimulating train with only half the pulse frequency (Fig. 2, control 2). At this intra-pair interval, the second pulse of the pairs apparently contributes little to the effect of stimulation. To put it differently, 0.5—0.8 msec after the first pulses of the pairs, the elements mediating the aggressive consequences of stimulation seem to be refrac-

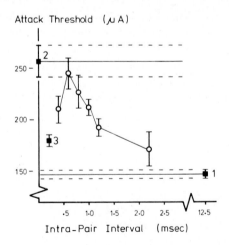

Fig. 2. Intra-pair interval dependent attack threshold changes. The interval is given as the delay between the start of both pulses of the pairs. Thresholds are given as the mean and S.D. of 6 subsequent response changes. Train duration is 10 sec. Control (1) 80 Hz, 0.2 msec pulse duration; control (2) 40 Hz, 0.2 msec duration; control (3) 40 Hz, 0.4 msec pulse duration. Corresponding intra-pair intervals 12.5, 0 and 0.2 msec. Subsequent pairs are of opposite polarity.

tory. At still shorter intra-pair intervals, the attack thresholds decrease again to the threshold value for a train of pulses with twice the pulse duration, but half the pulse frequency of the original train (Fig. 2, control 3). The neural substrate thus increasingly behaves as if it is being stimulated with a train of single pulses of longer duration. This decrease could be due to the summation of latent excitatory effects of the first pulses to the effects of the second pulses in the pairs. Whether refractoriness and latent addition (Lloyd, 1946) in excitable membranes are really at the basis of these attack threshold changes is not clear, but whatever the excitability properties underlying these changes may be, they are probably not the same for stimulation-induced attacks and switch-on behaviour. In 5 electrode placements in which we could demonstrate the effect of intra-pair intervals on attack thresholds, we were unable to detect any significant effect on switch-on behaviour.

Bite attack and attack jump

Why some electrode placements induce bite attacks at threshold current intensity and others attack jumps is not known. But there is evidence to suggest that both forms of attack derive from the activation of the same neural elements.

Electrode placements inducing both attacks seem to cluster in the same hypothalamic area. There is only a slight tendency for bite attack electrodes to lie somewhat more in the periphery of the area for stimulation-induced attack jumps.

Bite attacks can be gradually changed into attack jumps in many, but not all, bite attack electrode placements by increasing the current intensity above threshold.

Attack, pilo-erection and teeth-chattering

Pilo-erection and teeth-chattering are the most elusive concomitant effects of stimulation-induced attack behaviour. Both effects tend to diminish gradually during subsequent stimulation in a given experimental session. Pilo-erection often outlasts stimulation. Electrode placements differ in the extent of teeth-chattering induced at attack threshold current intensity. Quite a few electrodes placed well outside the target area for attack behaviour also induce teeth-chattering. Our records do not permit an assessment of the relationship between stimulation-induced attack behaviour and teeth-chattering or pilo-erection, but it might be that the latter effects do not derive from the activation of the neural elements mediating the aggressive consequences of electrical stimulation in the hypothalamus.

MAKING TOOLS TO MATCH CONCEPTS

None of the concomitant behavioural effects of stimulation-induced attack seems to be either a requirement for, or sufficient for, the induction of attacks. Stimulation-induced attack seems to derive from a substrate on its own. Do these observations allow us to deduce the function of the hypothalamic area involved in stimulation-induced attack? Or less ambitious, do we know something of the function of the neural elements which mediate the aggressive consequences of stimulation? Alas not yet! If nothing else, our very choice of words gives us away. By using imprecise terms like "mediate" and "involved in" we implicitly admit that we do not know which neuronal elements give rise to the behavioural consequences of stimulation. As a consequence we do not know what their function is. However, the available evidence suggests that the concomitant behavioural consequences of electrical stimulation of attack-inducing electrode placements derive from the simultaneous activation of several distinct neural networks. The functional relations of these networks can only be elucidated when the neural elements involved have been identified and when we have developed the tools to determine the normal output of these elements during specific behaviours. In pursuing that objective, our behaviourally derived concepts probably will have to be modified until they ultimately fall apart into hypotheses that can be understood and tested in terms of concepts used in the other brain sciences. In the mean time, we should not jump to conclusions about the localization of behavioural systems in the brain — especially not as concerns aggressive behaviour — as such haste might contribute to clinical applications for which no sound basis in behavioural neurobiology has been demonstrated (Valenstein, 1973). Electrical stimulation and lesioning techniques are not really precise instruments for clarifying the functioning of the brain in behaviour. To invoke Hubel's analogy once more, it is a bit like working on television sets with flint tools.

REFERENCES

Blair, H.A. (1932) On the intensity—time relations for stimulating by electric currents. *J. gen. Physiol.*, 15: 709–729.

Habbema, J.D.F. (1976) A discriminant analysis approach to the identification of human chromosomes. *Biometrics*, 32: 919–928.

Habbema, J.D.F. and Hermans, J.M.H. (1978) *Statistical Methods For Clinical Decision Making*, Ph.D. Dissertion, University of Leiden.

Herndon, J.G., Adrian, A.P. and McCoy, M. (1979) Orthogonal relationship between electrically elicited social aggression and self-stimulation from the same brain sites. *Brain Res.*, 171: 374–380.

Hubel, D.H. (1979) The brain. *Scient. Amer.*, 241: 39–47.

Koolhaas, J.M. (1978) Hypothalamically induced intraspecific aggressive behaviour in the rat. *Exp. Brain Res.*, 32: 365–375.

Kruk, M.R., Kuiper, P. and Meelis, W. (1978) An airpressure-operated commutator system for electrical brain stimulation in a fighting rat. *Physiol. Behav.*, 21: 125–127.

Kruk, M.R., Van der Poel, A.M. and De Vos-Frerichs, T.P. (1979) The induction of aggressive behaviour by electrical stimulation in the hypothalamus of male rats. *Behaviour*, 70: 292–322.

Lapique, L. (1926) *L'Excitabilité en Fonction du Temps*, Hermann, Paris.

Lloyd, D.P.C. (1946) Facilitation and inhibition of spinal motoneurons. *J. Neurophysiol.*, 9: 421–428.

Millhouse, O.E. (1973a) The organization of the ventromedial hypothalamic nucleus. *Brain Res.*, 55: 71–87.

Millhouse, O.E. (1973b) Certain ventromedial hypothalamic efferents. *Brain Res.*, 55: 89–105.

Ranck, J.B. (1975) Which elements are excited in electrical stimulation of mammalian central nervous system: a review. *Brain Res.*, 98: 417–440.

Roberts, W.W. (1969) Are hypothalamic motivational mechanisms functionally and anatomically specific? *Brain Behav. Evol.*, 2: 317–342.

Saper, C.B., Swanson, L.W. and Cowan, W.M. (1976) The efferent connections of the ventromedial nucleus of the hypothalamus of the rat. *J. comp. Neurol.*, 169: 409–442.

Valenstein, E.S. (1973) *Brain Control*, John Wiley, New York.

Valenstein, E.S., Cox, V.C. and Kakolewski, J.W. (1969) The hypothalamus and motivated behaviour. In *Reinforcement and Behaviour*, J. Tapp (Ed.), Academic Press, New York, pp. 242–285.

Wiepkema, P.R., Koolhaas, J.M. and Olivier-Aardema, R. (1980) Adaptive aspect of neuronal elements in agonistic behaviour. In *Adaptive Capabilities of the Nervous System, Progress in Brain Research, Vol. 53*, M.A. Corner et al. (Eds.), Elsevier, Amsterdam, pp. 369–384.

Adaptive Aspects of Hormonal Correlates of Attack and Defence in Laboratory Mice: A Study in Ethobiology

PAUL FRÉDRIC BRAIN

Department of Zoology, University College of Swansea, Swansea, Wales (U.K.)

INTRODUCTION

One should discuss hormonal involvement in agonistic responses (i.e. the full range of conflict behaviour ranging from overt attack to submission and fleeing) rather than limit oneself to "aggression" *or* "submission". Conflict in lower organisms is properly viewed as a continuum in which propensities to attack and flee/submit are intimately mixed.

The modern view is that hormones are not simple behavioural "triggers". Until comparatively recently, however, a rather simplistic view of endocrine involvement in the control of agonistic behaviour tended to dominate clinical and behavioural writing. This held that "aggression" was largely a male characteristic which depended on androgen production in the aggressor and resulted in increased glucocorticoid secretion in the subject of attack. I intend, by describing a diverse variety of studies on laboratory mice, to show that the situation is much more complex than that stated above.

Complex interrelationships are evident between the wide spectrum of interacting hormones (e.g. gonadal steroids and adrenocortical hormones show many subtle influences on each other's activity) and diverse behavioural categories (see recent reviews by Brain, 1979a,b; Leshner, 1978; de Wied et al., 1972). One may also comment that it is often difficult to clearly evaluate hormone/aggression correlations. This problem appears largely a consequence of the following.

(a) *The wide range of situations in which behaviour labelled as "aggression" can be observed (see Moyer, 1980).* It is also apparent that very different measures of attack behaviour are employed by different workers. It seems unlikely, to a majority of workers, that these different "types" of aggression can have common endocrine correlates. Consequently, one must specify particular models of aggression instead of discussing *the* physiological control of aggression. An indication of the range of commonly-employed models of aggression in laboratory mice is provided in Fig. 1.

One must note (cf. Blanchard and Blanchard, 1977; Brain et al., 1979) that the different forms of attack seem to involve different motivations (e.g. the distinction between offensive and defensive biting and between predatory responses and social aggression).

Briefly, studies referred to in this account employ 4 types of murine aggression as shown below.

Self-defensive aggression

Attack on anosmic opponents (rendered so by intranasal perfusion with 4% zinc sulphate

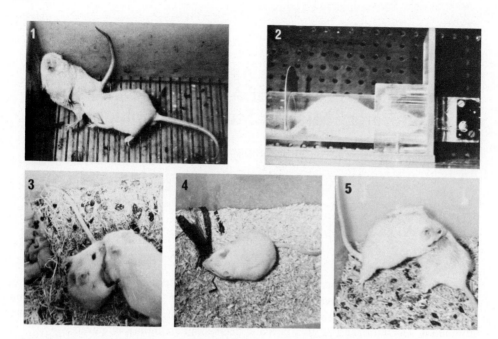

Fig. 1. Some models of aggression employing laboratory mice. 1: self-defensive reflexive fighting in which biting attack is induced by unavoidable electroshock. 2: self-defensive attack on a metal target induced by confining the subject in a narrow tube. Each bite activates a telegraph key. 3: maternal attack by a lactating female (right) on an intruding anosmic male in the presence of the former's litter. 4: predatory aggression by a naive mouse on an introduced locust. 5: social aggression by an individually-housed male mouse (right) on an anosmic opponent.

solution) and biting attacks on an inanimate target can be induced respectively by electroshock and confining the subject within a narrow tube. In the former case, numbers of attacks or bites are usually recorded. Anosmic animals do not fight which means that the intensity of attack can be more easily related to the aggressiveness of the subject. Tests were generally of 10 min duration.

Maternal aggression

This behaviour is fully described in Brain and Al-Maliki (1979). Lactating females were found to reliably attack anosmic, male intruders in the presence of their litters, provided that their own mates had been removed earlier. Again, the total duration of biting attacks can be recorded in a 10 min test.

Predatory aggression

Attack on adult locusts has been fruitfully employed as a model of predatory aggression in laboratory mice (the procedure is described in Al-Maliki and Brain, 1979; Brain and Al-Maliki, 1978, 1979). This model was devised as an alternative to the rat's muricide and ranacide responses. Here, the index of aggression is simply whether or not the mouse kills and consumes the locust within a specified time (up to 6 h).

Social aggression

This model of aggression is the most utilized form of attack in our studies. In this laboratory, aggressiveness has been induced in male mice by individual housing or sexual experience (compared in Brain et al., 1978). Encounters were simplified by employing docile "standard opponents" i.e. group-housed males generally rendered temporarily anosmic or habituated to defeat. These tests were also of 10 min duration. An unusual variant of social aggression was induced in group-housed, intact females or castrated males by using lactating female intruders (Haug and Brain, 1978). In this case, the tests were of 30 min duration.

A battery of measures of attack have been employed including estimation of the accumulated attacking time (AAT: the total number of seconds spent physically biting the opponent) and the number of biting attacks on that animal.

(b) *Comparisons between species.* Comparisons between species sometimes reveal different relationships between specific hormonal changes and attack/defence even when similar contexts are used.

(c) *Endocrine manipulations.* Most produce a spectrum of hormonal consequences, e.g. castration not only removes the *major* source of androgens but results in elevated gonadotrophins and altered adrenocortical activity.

It seems of utility to postulate 3 sources of hormone/agonistic behaviour correlation, as follows.

Maturational influences on subsequent predisposition to show spontaneous or hormonally – mediated attack/defence

These alterations appear to be consequences of changed neural structure (e.g. Raisman and Field, 1973) and/or hormone binding characteristics of the CNS (McEwen et al., 1977a, b). It is not proposed to devote much space to these phenomena but they are adaptive changes in a real and lasting sense. Masculinization/defeminization effects of androgens/oestrogens are actions of this type. Early effects of sex steroid manipulations have been demonstrated in most commonly-utilized laboratory rodents but there is considerable debate concerning the role of oestrogens in such phenomena (reviewed in Brain, 1979c). The effects of neonatally-administered corticosterone (Leshner and Schwartz, 1977) and ACTH (Simon and Gandelman, 1977), respectively decreasing fighting and increasing submissiveness in mice, also belong here.

"Direct" influences on the expression of attack/defence

These effects are presumably mediated by actions of hormones on the CNS. As both fighting and dominance/subordination alter hormonal production, such effects provide a mechanism whereby the predisposition to attack or defend is altered.

"Indirect" influences on the expression of attack/defence

This category may be sub-divided into influences which: (a) appear to be consequences of hormonal actions on "somatic" or "peripheral" targets, producing (in rodents) variations in body size, pelage, pheromone-production, olfactory responsiveness, marking behaviour, etc. (see Brain, 1977); and (b) seem to be due to hormonal actions on activities which are incompatible with attack (e.g. fleeing) or merely compete for available time with this response (e.g. grooming or exploration).

INFLUENCE OF SEX STEROIDS ON TWO FORMS OF SOCIAL ATTACK

The effects of sex steroids on aggressiveness have been predictably intensely researched as the most obvious means of modifying attack behaviour. The situation regarding these effects is, however, surprisingly complex. Common confounding features of studies have been identified (Brain, 1978b) as: (a) failure to discriminate between hormonal influences on central motivational and on peripheral factors; (b) giving repeated injections and testing to subjects which confounds clear interpretation by superimposing variable experiential factors on the physiological manipulations; and (c) use of behavioural tests which may reflect "fear" or predatory responses rather than aggression.

Sex steroids seem particularly important in that variation in these factors may account for the differences in aggressiveness between males and females, dominants and subordinates, etc.

Studies on male mice rendered aggressive by sexual activity

A series of studies in which the above faults were largely eliminated has been described (Bowden, 1979; Bowden and Brain, 1978; Brain, 1978b; Brain and Bowden, 1978). Briefly, mice were rendered aggressive by a single breeding experience which meant that the animals were not hyperreactive at the time of testing. Operation and hormone application durations were rigidly standardized and anosmic opponents were used so that changes in fighting were likely to reflect only alterations in aggressiveness of the treated animal. The aggression was rated by assessing unequivocal biting attack on the opponent.

Conversion of testosterone to oestrogenic metabolites appears important before this androgen can masculinize neonatal rodents or change adult motivation for T-mediated behaviours in some species (including social aggression in mice) (see Table I).

The abilities of a wide range of sex steroids to influence social aggression in castrated TO strain mice were investigated. Daily i.m. injections of oil-based steroid were given 3 days after gonadectomy over a 17-day-period. During this treatment, the animals were individually-housed. Attacks on anosmic "standard opponents" intruded into the test animal's home cage were assessed using a battery of measures under dim red lighting. The effects of these steroids on the weights of sex accessory glands (preputials, seminal vesicles and ventral

TABLE I

LINES OF SUPPORT FOR THE AROMATIZATION HYPOTHESIS

(1) Young female rats and mice can be masculinized by neonatal oestrogen, (Edwards and Herndon, 1970) and neonatal anti-oestrogen feminizes these animals (Booth, 1977).

(2) Ejaculatory behaviour can be restored in castrated rats by combinations of oestrogen and 5α DHT (e.g. Parrott, 1975).

(3) Oestrogens maintain social aggressiveness in castrated male mice at relatively low dosages (Brain and Bowden, 1979).

(4) In some studies, anti-oestrogens appear to block testosterone-maintained behaviour in castrates. Aromatase inhibitors block testosterone but not oestrogen-maintained social aggression in mice (Bowden and Brain, 1978).

(5) The brain binds sex steroids — oestrogens more so than androgens (Morrell et al., 1975).

(6) Neural tissue of a variety of vertebrates has been shown to aromatize convertible androgens to oestrogenic metabolites (Naftolin and Ryan, 1975).

(7) Levels of aromatizing enzymes may be higher in the brains of male rats than in females (Naftolin and Ryan, 1975) but Lupo di Prisco et al. (1978) suggest that this result may be a consequence of housing conditions.

TABLE II

SUMMARY OF THE EFFECTS OF DIFFERENT i.m. DOSES OF SEX STEROIDS ON THE MAIN-
TENANCE OF AGGRESSIVENESS IN CASTRATED MICE RENDERED AGGRESSIVE BY BREED-
ING ACTIVITY

AND, 5α-androstan-3α-ol-17-one; 19-OH DHT, 5α androstan-17β, 19-diol-3-one; 5β DHT, 5β androstan-
17β-ol-3-one; 5α DHT, 5α androstan-17β-ol-3-one; A, androst-4-ene-3, 17 dione; T, 4-androstan-17β,
19-diol-3-one; E1, oestra-1,3,5,(10)-triene-3-ol-17-one; E2, oestra-1,3,5,(10)-triene-3, 17β diol; E3, oestra-
1,3,5,(10)-triene-3, 16α, 17β-triol. ↑, moderate increase; ⇑, marked increase. A moderate increase is a significant elevation, cf. oil-treated castrates, which *does not* exceed values generated for sham-treated,
mock-castrated animals. Marked increases exceed these figures. ns, not significant.

Type of sex steroïd	Compound	Dose/day (µg)									
		0.1	0.5	1	5	25	50	100	500	1000	2000
Non-aromatizable androgens	AND								ns	ns	ns
	19-OH DHT						ns	↑	ns		
	5β-DHT								ns	⇑	ns
	5α-DHT				ns		↑	↑	↑	↑	
Aromatizable androgens	A				ns	↑	↑	ns			
	T			ns	↑	↑	⇑	⇑			
Intermediate	19-OHT						ns	ns	↑		
Oestrogens	E1	ns	↑	⇑	⇑						
	E2	↑	⇑	⇑	⇑						
	E3		⇑	⇑	⇑						

prostates) were assessed in subsequent post-mortem studies. The weights of these androgen-
dependent structures served as an index of the peripheral action of the hormone treatment.

The criterion of effectiveness (in both behavioural and organ weight studies) was the
ability to *maintain* a majority of indices cf. sham-treated controls – i.e. modification of a

TABLE III

SUMMARY OF THE EFFECTS OF DIFFERENT i.m. DOSES OF SEX STEROIDS ON THE WEIGHTS
OF SEX ACCESSORY GLANDS IN CASTRATED MICE

Each accessory gland weight is considered separately in this analysis. ↓, moderate decrease; ↑, moderate
increase; ⇑, marked increase. ns, not siginificant. For abbreviations see Table II.

Type of sex steroid	Compound	Dose/day (µg)									
		0.1	0.5	1	5	25	50	100	500	1000	2000
Non-aromatizable androgens	AND							ns	↑	⇑	
	19-OH DHT						↑	↑	↑		
	5β-DHT								ns	↑	⇑
	5α-DHT				⇑		↑	↑	↑	↑	
Aromatizable androgens	A				↑	ns	↑	↑			
	T			↑	↑	↑	↑	↑			
Intermediate	19-OHT						ns	ns	ns		
Oestrogens	E1	ns	ns	ns	ns						
	E2	ns	ns	↓	ns						
	E3		ns	ns	ns						

single measure of fighting or of a single gland was not regarded as sufficient indication of activity. The influences were held to be maintaining rather than inductive actions as: aggressiveness was elevated prior to castration; and (b) the sex accessories were not allowed to atrophy before treatment.

A synopsis of the behavioural effects of the steroids is presented in Table II and the corresponding influences on sex accessory weights in Table III.

As these studies also suggested that oestrogenic metabolites of testosterone (T) may be more behaviourally potent than the majority of androgens, a further series of studies on the influences of aromatase inhibitors (25–250 μg/day), anti-androgens (0.5–2 mg/day), anti-oestrogens (0.5–2 mg/day) and progesterone (50–1000 μg/day) on T and oestradiol-17β (E2)-treated castrates were carried out using comparable treatment conditions. Actions on both social aggression and weights of sex accessories were examined. A summary of the data from these studies which are detailed elsewhere is provided in Table IV.

Suggestive lines of evidence generated by these studies include observations that in castrates:

(i) oestrogens and aromatizable androgens proved the most effective (on a dose-needed basis) factors regarding their ability to maintain aggressiveness. These effects were *not* dependent on peripheral actions as oestrogens did not augment the weights of sex accessory glands (i.e. no autopheromonal effect) and the opponents were anosmic. A videotape analysis of attacks by T and E2-maintained animals on "standard opponents" suggested that the patterns of behaviour were similar in these two categories, i.e. both hormones generated the same behaviour;

(ii) an aromatase inhibitor (which blocks conversion of T to E2) diminished T's but not E2's effect on social aggression;

(iii) the anti-androgen cyproterone acetate did not markedly alter T-maintained aggression;

TABLE IV

SUMMARY OF ATTEMPTS TO BLOCK TESTOSTERONE (T) OR OESTRADIOL (E2) – MAINTAINED FIGHTING AND ORGAN WEIGHT AUGMENTATION IN "AGGRESSIVE" MICE WITH A VARIETY OF AGENTS

Details of treatments are given in the cited studies. CA, cyproterone acetate or 6-chloro-17-hydroxy 1α, 2α methylene-pregna-4,6-diene-3,20 dione acetate; MER 25, ethamoxytriphetol; anti-aromatase, 4-androsten-3,6,17 trione; progesterone, Δ4-pregnane-3,20 dione.

Compound	Daily dose of maintenance steroid	Behavioural action	Peripheral action	Reference
CA	25 μg T	No effect	Lowers	Brain and Bowden, 1978
	1 μg E2	No effect	Increases	
MER 25	25 μg T	Weak suppression	Low doses increase	Brain and Bowden, 1979
	1 μg E2	Lowers	Lowers	Bowden, 1979
Antiaromatase	25 μg T	Lowers	No effect	Bowden and Brain, 1978
	1 μg E2	No effect	No effect	
Progesterone	25 μg T	Lowers	Increases	Brain and Bowden, 1978
	1 μg E2	No effect	Effect depends on dose	

(iv) the anti-oestrogen MER-25 weakly suppressed T-maintained fighting in some combinations;

(v) large doses of P blocked aggressiveness in mice maintained by testosterone.

These findings provide some general support for the *aromatization hypothesis,* i.e. the view that androgens may have to be neurally converted to oestrogens before altering the motivation for masculine behaviour. This hypothesis is important as: (1) it suggests that changes in the metabolism of hormones may predispose the animal towards behaving in particular ways, e.g. social housing conditions modify T to E2 conversion; (2) it illustrates the fact that the materials do not always influence the animal in the form in which they are administered; and (3) production of a variety of metabolites may enable the animal to separately influence a variety of target organs including the brain.

Careful examination of Tables II–IV will reveal that not all data are apparently in accord with the view that the conversion of T to E2 is essential before testosterone can influence aggressiveness. The "non-aromatizable" androgen 5α DHT seemed, for example, relatively active (see Table II). This compound's intrinsic behavioural effectiveness is also evident in its maintenance of male sexual behaviour in castrates of a variety of species including rats and mice (e.g. Luttge and Hall, 1973). It is suggestive that hypothalamic DHT receptors have been demonstrated in many species (Kato, 1975) and it is known that T is converted to DHT in the hypothalamus of the rat (e.g. Juneja et al., 1976). This localization and conversion may, however, be more concerned with negative feedback inhibition of gonadotrophin release rather than with behavioural activation (although the latter remains a possibility).

The term "non-aromatizable androgen" may be misleading. 5α DHT can be readily metabolized by rat erythrocytes to 3β-androstanediol (Heyns and De Moor, 1974), a metabolite which has a moderate affinity for anterior hypothalamic cytosol E2-receptors and activates mounting in castrated rats (Baum and Vreeburg, 1976). The weak blocking action of MER 25 (see Table IV) may be explained in a similar way, as this "anti-oestrogen" binds to hypothalamic receptors.

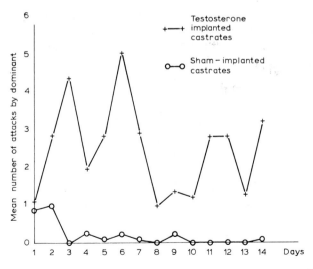

Fig. 2. Mean number of daily attacks in 30 min observation periods by pre-selected dominants on 2 castrated cage-mates s.c. implanted with 25 mg of TP, and 2 castrated sham-implanted cage-mates living as "social" groups (n = 8).

TABLE V

MEDIAN (WITH RANGES) SUMMED AGGRESSION TEST DATA OVER 3 DAYS FOR 3-DAY-ISO-LATED MALE MICE GIVEN ENCOUNTERS WITH SHAM-PREPUTIALECTOMIZED AND PREPU-TIALECTOMIZED "STANDARD OPPONENTS"

Type of intruder	Latency of attack (sec)	Accumulated attacking time	Number of attacks
Sham-preputialectomized	734 (100–1800)	47.9 * (0–110.8)	50 * (0–104)
Preputialectomized	1526 (546–1800)	5.75 (0– 39.6)	6 (0– 33)

* Differs from preputialectomized intruder category $P < 0.05$ (Mann–Whitney U test).

5α-reduction of T and androstenedione seems likely to be important in controlling production of "aggression-modifying pheromones" by a variety of sex accessory glands. Androgenic involvement in the synthesis of these behaviour-modifying odours is emphasized in Fig. 2. Small "social" groups of mice were constituted in rat cages. Groups consisted of one dominant animal (initially rendered highly aggressive by breeding experience) and 4 postpubertal castrates (previously group-housed). Two castrates implanted s.c. with 25 mg T pellets received more daily attacks than two sham-implanted counterparts. One would normally expect the daily incidence of attack to progressively decline in established groups as the "stress" of defeat curtails androgen production in the "subordinates". This reduces their pheromone production without leading to striking changes in behaviour. The effect seems to be pheromonal as similar actions can be induced by marking castrates with the urine of intact males or androgen-treated castrates.

The preputial gland (which is responsive to a wide range of steroids – see Bowden, 1979) has been implicated in the production of these odours. Table V shows that preputialectomy reduces the duration of attack to which "standard opponents" are subjected by individually-housed mice with moderate levels of aggressiveness.

Studies on the response of group-housed mice to lactating female intruders

Use of a term such as "social aggression" implies an unwarranted degree of homogeneity. Accordingly, it is particularly instructive to note a preliminary series of observations on another form of social attack in mice where hormonal influences seem very different to those described above.

Haug (1976) demonstrated that small groups (3s) of habituated Swiss-strain female mice attacked *lactating* (14th day after parturition) intruders more vigorously than other types of "strangers". Subsequently, Haug and Brain (1978) recorded that small groups of castrated *male* mice also evidenced vigorous biting attack on non-habituated lactating but *not* non-lactating intruders. It is interesting to note (Haug and Brain, 1979) that ovariectomized females also generated elevated attack by castrated male residents (see Fig. 3). Implanting ovariectomized female residents 30 days after gonadectomy with 25 mg testosterone propionate (TP) pellets or castrated male residents with either 25 mg TP or 10 mg oestradiol benzoate (OB) reduced their attack on lactating female intruders 14 days later (see Fig. 4).

The suppressive action of TP on this form of attack is opposite to its augmenting effect on social aggression in non-habituated males (see Table II). The fact that OB *and* TP suppressed attack in gonadectomized males whereas only TP had this action in females, is of

Aggression by castrated male residents

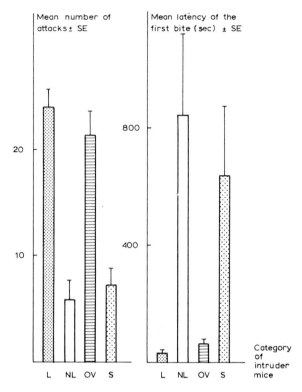

Fig. 3. Mean number of attacks and latencies to first attacks in triads of castrated males in encounters against different types of intruders. L, lactating female; NL, non-lactating female; OV, ovariectomized animals; S, sham-ovariectomized mice. N.B. L and OV categories subject to most attack.

Mean number of attacks directed towards lactating intruders

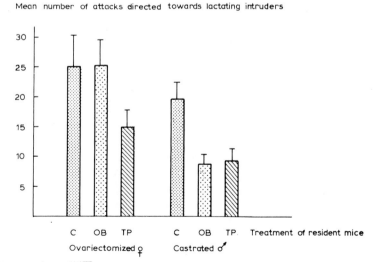

Fig. 4. Mean number of attacks directed towards lactating female intruders by small groups of gonadectomized male and female residents s.c. implanted with C, cholesterol; OB, oestradiol benzoate or TP, testosterone propionate.

400

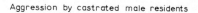

Aggression by castrated male residents

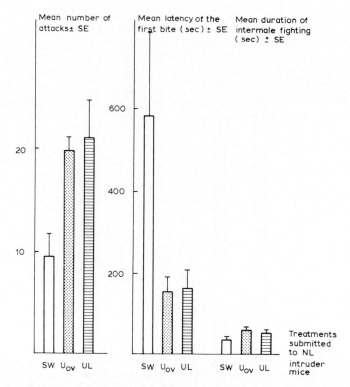

Fig. 5. Mean attack data by castrated male residents on non-lactating female intruders marked with SW, saline; U_{ov}, urine from ovariectomized subjects; UL, urine from lactating females.

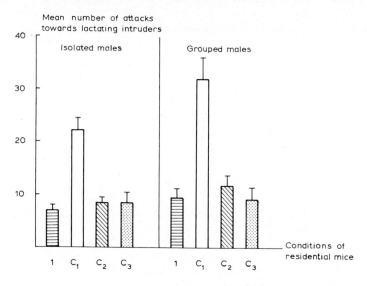

Fig. 6. Mean numbers of attacks by isolated and group (3) – housed males on lactating female intruders. 1, intact; C1, castrated controls; C2, castrated s.c. implanted with E2; C3, castrated s.c. implanted with T.

interest. OB maintains fighting in post-pubertally castrated males (see Table II) whereas only T induced attack by ovariectomized, female isolates on males (Barkley and Goldman, 1978; Simon and Gandelman, 1978). Perhaps the difference between "masculinized" and "feminized" animals is in the brain's response to oestrogen?

Attack by castrated male mice on lactating intruders also seems mediated by urinary pheromones (Brain and Haug, 1979). Triads of castrated male residents showed vigorous attack on non-lactating intruders smeared with the urine of ovariectomized or lactating animals (see Fig. 5). This effect cannot be attributed to increased fighting among members of the triad. Indeed, attack by residents on lactating female intruders is *not* dependent on group-housing (Haug and Brain, in preparation). The response of control intact, castrated and castrated/implanted individually-housed males can be seen to parallel those of group-housed counterparts in Fig. 6 (see below).

Much remains to be learned about the central and peripheral control of this odd form of social aggression. The important point, however, is that these studies emphasize the need to specify the model of aggression used before discussing *the* endocrine control of this behaviour.

EFFECTS OF PITUITARY—ADRENOCORTICAL HORMONES ON AGGRESSIVENESS

Considerable emphasis has been put on the effects of gonadal steroids on attack/defence (Brain, 1979a) but it is now evident that hormones of the pituitary—adrenocortical axis (ACTH and glucocorticoids) exert considerable influences on a variety of behaviours including aggression (reviewed by Brain, 1972, 1979b).

Brain (1971a) postulated affinities between conditioned avoidance reactions, as used by de Wied (1969) in his studies on behaviourally-active peptides, and social aggression. One could argue that in highly-territorial mice, pituitary—adrenocortical hormones may facilitate conditioning of "submissive" status. Stressful attack by the dominant may have affinities with more conventional aversive stimuli (such as electroshock) in conditioned avoidance

TABLE VI

A SYNOPSIS OF THE EFFECTS OF ACUTE (UP TO 12 h) OR CHRONIC (UP TO 17 DAYS) TREATMENTS RELATED TO PITUITARY-ADRENOCORTICAL HORMONES ON SOCIAL AGGRESSION IN "STANDARD OPPONENT" TESTS AND CIRCULATING GLUCOCORTICOID TITRES IN ADULT ISOLATED MALES

Doses and schedules are given in the papers cited in text. ↓, depressed; ↑, augmated; NC, no change.

Treatment	Effects on aggression		Effects on circulating glucocorticoids	
	Acute	Chronic	Acute	Chronic
Adrenalectomy	↓	↓	↓	↓
Glucocorticoids	↑	↑	↑	↑
ACTH 1−24	↑	↓	↑	↑
ACTH 1−10	↑	NC	↑	−
ACTH 11−24	NC	−	↑	−
ACTH 4−10	NC	↓	NC	NC
ACTH 4−10 D-phe	−	NC	NC	−

reactions. It was initially thought to be likely that adrenal hormones generated by defeat promoted the *acquisition of* and retarded the *extinction of* submissiveness. As the natural response of the defeated animal is to flee (an activity prevented by caging) the altered changed incidence of upright posturing may be more accurately regarded as evidence of increased defensiveness (this would also reduce attack). Again, these hormones affect different models of aggression in different ways (see Al-Maliki, 1980). Detail on the involvement of these hormones in social aggression is emphasized by Leshner (1980). However, for comparative purposes, a summary of studies (Brain and Evans, 1977; Brain and Poole, 1974; Brain et al., 1971) on the effects of "stress" hormones on social aggression in isolated male mice is presented in Table VI. This seems appropriate to a full discussion of the adaptive influences of hormones on attack/defence. The first point to note is that acute (within 12 h) effects of i.p. injected ACTH 1–24 (prepared as long-acting solutions) may differ from those apparent chronically (over weeks). Glucocorticoids and steroidogenesis-inducing peptides appear to acutely stimulate social aggression but there is evidence of a chronic (possibly extra-adrenal) suppression of fighting by part of the ACTH molecule. Note that although ACTH 1–10 and ACTH 11–24 are said to have little influence on adrenocortical secretion in rats, they did stimulate corticosterone output in mice.

The acute stimulatory effect of ACTH is not a consequence of altered gonadal function, as this action is evident in gonadectomized males with sexual experience given TP (50 μg/day) or OB (10 μg/day) replacement therapy (see Fig. 7) over 17 days. In this study, ACTH 1–24 was administered 12 h before tests employing standard opponents.

Why are the acute and chronic influences of ACTH 1–24 on social aggression different? Intermittent victory-linked encounters (such as those shown by territorial animals on boundaries) and repeated exposures to defeat (e.g. in a "subordinate" animal within an established "social" group) are qualitatively different, in spite of both being initially stressful. In the first situation, it seems appropriate to respond to attack by fighting back. In the latter

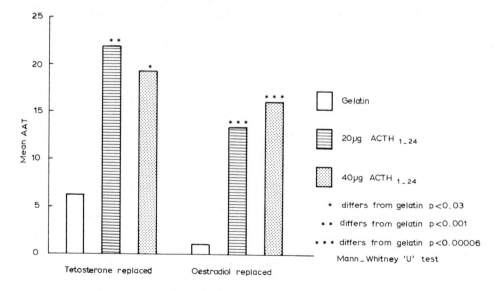

Fig. 7. Acute effects of 2 doses of ACTH 1–24 on social aggression scores over 3 "standard opponent" aggression tests in castrated/sex steroid maintained mice (n = 10).

circumstance, it could be argued that survival is best served if the animal shows a lowered tendency to social aggression and reacts to the approach of the dominant by (if possible) fleeing or taking up a defensive posture. One may also comment that clearly dominant mice generally have lower pituitary–adrenocortical activities than submissive animals forced to remain with them (reviewed in Brain, 1977, 1978a). Therefore the differential effects of short-term and long-term endogenous ACTH would potentiate the establishment of dominance/subordination polarities and reduce energy expenditure. Moreover, one may speculate that increased chronic ACTH/glucocorticoid production in defeated animals would not only change aggressive motivation directly but also indirectly modify fighting by suppressing androgens and associated aggression-promoting pheromone secretion (see earlier).

INVESTIGATIONS ON THE EFFECTS OF FIGHTING EXPERIENCE AND DIFFERENTIAL HOUSING ON HORMONES AND BEHAVIOUR

A thorough understanding of the roles of hormones in the control of attack/defence necessitates a consideration of the effects of these experiences on hormone release. The influences of social aggression on endocrine function have generally involved subjecting relatively docile mice to intermittent periods of defeat (reviewed by Brain, 1977, 1978a, 1979c). Changes in blood levels of LH–RF, TSH, ACTH, LH, FSH, thyroxine, medullary catecholamines, glucocorticoids and androgens have all been described in response to attack in a variety of species, including rodents. It is of particular importance to note that the stress of defeat is correlated with increases in ACTH/glucocorticoids and decreases in circulating androgens (Bronson and Eleftheriou, 1965). As previously noted, those changes would be expected to decrease an animal's social aggressiveness as well as reducing its effectiveness as an attack-releasing stimulus. Hormonal involvement in aggressive responses can also be illustrated by comparing the characteristics of individually-housed (no defeat) and group-housed (where "subordinates" are subjected to repeated defeat) mice. These two approaches are briefly illustrated by reference to the following studies.

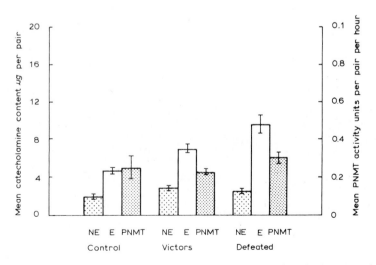

Fig. 8. Adrenomedullary characteristics of isolated, non-fighting "controls" and mice assessed as victors and defeated on the basis of repeated daily encounters.

404

Effects of fighting experience on adrenomedullary activity and its relationship to adrenocortical function

The adrenocortical consequences of defeat in rodents are well-documented (see Brain, 1977). It is consequently proposed to emphasize recent studies on adrenomedullary activity as these: (a) are related to the above; and (b) may be more subtle indicators of adaptive responses. Details of these experiments are provided in Gamal-el-Din (1978) and Huckle-bridge et al. (1980). The studies employed biochemical assays for adrenal norepinephrine (NE), epinephrine (E) and the enzyme phenyl-ethanolamine-N-methyl transferase (PNMT) which converts NE to E.

Effects of the outcome of aggressive encounters

An initial experiment assessed the adrenomedullary characteristics of individually-housed controls and "victors" (animals winning more than 70% of daily encounters given over a 2-week-period) and "defeated" partners from pairings (see Fig. 8). Epinephrine content of the adrenal gland was significantly elevated in victors ($P < 0.05$ compared to controls). A much larger elevation of this hormone was recorded, however, in defeated subjects ($P < 0.01$ compared to controls *and* victors).

A subsequent study employed 9-week-old, individually-housed males subjected daily to: (a) disturbance (removal and replacement of cage top); (b) one defeat by an aggressive "trained fighter"; and (c) two defeats (one in the morning, one in the afternoon) by an aggressive "trained fighter". Each defeat generated at least 5 sec of biting attack in a 15 min observation period. Animals were killed after 3 weeks of such treatment and the adreno-medullary measures for the 3 categories are presented in Fig. 9 (see below). Both one ($P < 0.01$) and two ($P < 0.001$) defeats per day increased PNMT activities compared to controls. Both defeated categories also showed significantly-enhanced adrenal E ($P < 0.01$) contents compared to controls. Adrenal NE content did not differ in these 3 categories.

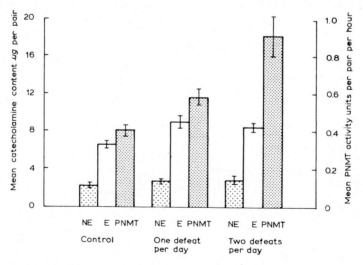

Fig. 9. Adrenomedullary characteristics of undefeated "controls" and mice subjected to one and two defeats per day, respectively.

Predictably, an additional study investigated the effects of repeated "victory", rather than defeat, on adrenomedullary function. Eight-week-old male mice were individually-housed for 3 weeks before being randomly allocated to the following categories subjected daily to: (a) disturbance; (b) one opportunity to defeat an anosmic opponent in their home cage in a 15 min session; and (c) two opportunities to defeat anosmic opponents in their home cage in two 15 min sessions. Treatments were continued over a 3-week-period and a synopsis of the generated adrenomedullary changes is presented in Fig. 10 (see below). Mice experiencing one ($P < 0.05$) and two ($P < 0.01$) victories per day showed elevated PNMT activities compared to controls. Adrenal NE content was elevated in both categories experiencing victory but only reached significance compared to controls in the two victories per day category ($P < 0.02$). Epinephrine did not differ significantly in the 3 categories.

The adrenomedullary consequences of differential fighting experience may be summarized as below. Firstly, PNMT activity generally seemed the most sensitive index of *any* experience. Although this enzyme activity was elevated by both "defeat" and "victory" (independent of whether this experience was once or twice per day), a much more obvious response to "defeat" was evident.

Hormonal factors may have a greater influence than neural factors on PNMT activities (Bhagat and Horenstein, 1976). Indeed, neural stimulation may enhance PNMT synthesis while hormonal stimulation prevents degradation of the enzyme (Ciaranello et al., 1976).

It has been suggested (Henry et al., 1976) that conflicts leading to victory mainly stimulate sympathetic neural activation of adrenocortical function whereas defeat (and its concomitant "depression") activates the adrenocortical axis via ACTH. Glucocorticoids have profound influences on adrenomedullary activity (see Gamal-el-Din, 1978). Ely and Henry (1978) also claim that dominant mice respond to social interaction with a predominantly sympathetic adrenal medullary pattern whereas subordinates respond with a pituitary adrenocortical pattern. Animals forced into different roles show changed activities. Perhaps the elevated PNMT activities of defeated subjects are largely the result of pituitary—adrenocortical stimulation whereas the less marked response in "victors" is a consequence of the less obvious neural activation?

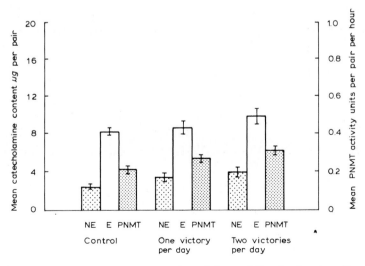

Fig. 10. Adrenomedullary characteristics of inexperienced "controls" and mice given the opportunity to record one and two victories per day on anosmic opponents, respectively.

It is interesting to note that the profound increase in PNMT activity in defeated subjects was accompanied by elevated E concentrations whereas NE accumulated in the adrenals of "victors" with little increase in E. Although PNMT was also elevated in these animals, there is no marked increase in adrenal methylation of NE to E in "victors".

Chronic exposure of male mice to brief periods of fighting results in increased medullary catecholamine content when subjects are sacrificed 24 h after the final session (Hucklebridge, 1973). Adrenal E is depleted in male mice immediately after intense fighting within groups for 60 min (Welch and Welch, 1969). A marked elevation of plasma E is evident in male mice killed 5 min after fighting within groups or defeat by a conspecific with whom they were paired (Hucklebridge et al., 1973). There is consequently an immediate post-fighting release of adrenal catecholamines which may serve to adjust behavioural and metabolic processes. This initial response is followed by an adaptive change in adrenal catecholamine synthesis which maintains the increased demand. Chronic exposure to repeated social stress thus produces an adaptive increase in adrenal biogenic amine storage.

The time course of the adrenomedullary responses to defeat

Knowledge of the time courses of the events described above seems of paramount importance as it is apparent that the period between defeat and sacrifice can have a profound influence on the interpretation of hormone/behaviour relationships. Consequently, adrenal catecholamine content and PNMT activities were measured at 4 intervals (0, 2, 12 and 24 h) after a single (generating 60 sec of biting attack) defeat. The results of this study are presented in Table VII. A second study investigated the time course of the adrenomedullary responses to a series of 3 daily defeats. Here, measurements were made at intervals over the 4-day-period following the last defeat (see Table VIII).

The PNMT response to exposure to a single defeat showed a peak activity after 12 h. Activity then showed a slight decline at 24 h. It is notable that Hoffman et al. (1976) demonstrated a similar time course in PNMT activity response to cold stress in the mouse. The maximal behavioural action of a single ACTH 1–24 injection is also apparent after 12 h (Brain and Evans, 1977).

Adrenal NE and E were both depleted (although not significantly so) when measured immediately after defeat. NE content subsequently increased between 2 and 24 h after this experience. Relatively rapid stimulation of NE synthesis might be expected in a process thought to be largely under sympathetic control. Adrenal E content did not recovery until 24 h after defeat. This suggests that methylation of NE to E does not occur until 12–24 h

TABLE VII

RESULTS OF ADRENOMEDULLARY ANALYSIS OF MICE SACRIFICED AT 4 DIFFERENT INTERVALS AFTER A SINGLE DEFEAT

Mean contents with S.E.s for the paired adrenals are given, PNMT is expressed as units activity/h whereas catecholamines are expressed as μg (n = 10).

Measures	Control	Immediate	2 h	12 h	24 h
PNMT	0.202 ± 0.014	0.197 ± 0.011	0.173 ± 0.010	0.262 ± 0.019	0.244 ± 0.02
E	9.11 ± 0.545	8.494 ± 0.609	7.937 ± 0.887	8.145 ± 0.633	9.096 ± 0.769
NE	2.203 ± 0.304	1.951 ± 0.156	2.650 ± 0.226	2.975 ± 0.221	2.954 ± 0.256

TABLE VIII

THE TIME COURSE OF THE ADAPTIVE RESPONSE TO A SERIES OF 3 CONSECUTIVE DAILY DEFEATS IN MICE

See code used in Table VII. (n = 10).

Measures	Disturbed control	Days after defeat		
		1 day	2 days	4 days
PNMT	0.314 ± 0.021	0.447 ± 0.047	0.414 ± 0.033	0.427 ± 0.042
E	9.734 ± 0.57	10.321 ± 0.772	11.921 ± 0.511	13.794 ± 1.307
NE	2.735 ± 0.253	3.627 ± 0.281	4.608 ± 0.492	4.643 ± 0.326

after defeat as PNMT activity has to be stimulated via the slower glucocorticoid-mediated pathway.

• PNMT activities did not show significant responses to defeat at any of the selected time periods, (1, 2 and 4 days after defeat) in the longer duration study. This finding differed from results presented earlier but it should be noted that the time course obtained following *one* defeat suggested that maximal PNMT elevations were evident after 12 h and returned towards base-line after 24 h. Consequently, the accumulated effect of repeated defeat (as used in the earlier sections) may not be evident after only 3 days of exposure. Alternatively, the lack of a response in the present study may be a consequence of the elevated aggressiveness of all subjects in this experiment. PNMT activity seemed augmented even in control subjects. Perhaps the level is maximal and activity cannot be further enhanced by experience of defeat? Similarly, Maengwyn-Davies et al. (1973) reported that inbred strains of mice that exhibited high levels of aggression did *not* show elevated PNMT activity in response to attack whereas relatively non-aggressive strains did.

Adrenal NE and E contents progressively increased after exposures to defeat were terminated. NE showed the more rapid responses as elevations compared to levels of controls were evident by the second day after defeat. This augmentation persisted until the fourth day. Changes in E content were slower, the increase reaching significance compared to controls only on the fourth day. The different time courses of NE and E can be explained on the basis of the different mechanisms controlling their synthesis and release. Tizabi et al. (1976) demonstrated that, in males of some mouse strains, plasma E and NE returned to control values within 24 h of the final defeat of a series (7 consecutive days).

These data suggest the following pattern of adrenomedullary response to defeat. The exposure causes release of E (and perhaps smaller quantities of NE). An increased rate of catecholamine synthesis is stimulated such that adrenal NE content progressively increases. After approximately 12 h (depending on the strain) PNMT activity is also elevated, enhancing NE methylation and increasing E content. Recovery of E content and adaptive increases (related to the "subordinate" status) are only evident 24 h or longer after defeat. Mice exposed to repeated daily defeat show additive adrenomedullary responses. After fairly long periods of exposure (e.g. 2 weeks), a marked elevation in adrenal E content can be measured 24 h after the final defeat. It must be presumed that stimulation of catecholamine synthesis more than compensates for the loss due to release and adaptive accumulation of E (with associated elevations of PNMT activity) occurs. After only 3 daily exposures, adaptive increases in catecholamine storage are not measurable 24 h after the last defeat but storage continues to increase 2 and 4 days after the final exposure.

Consequently, animal experiments designed to investigate chronic adrenomedullary responses to "stress" of defeat are much influenced by 4 factors, namely: (a) strain of animal employed; (b) duration of the stress provided; (c) frequency of the exposures; and (d) the time interval between the final exposure and sampling. These adrenomedullary changes seem particularly important in that: (a) they occur more quickly than the adreno-cortical changes; and (b) they illustrate that *both* defeated and victorious animals may show biochemical adaptation to experience.

Studies on the effects of differential housing on hormone/aggression correlations

As previously noted, individual housing is a much-utilized means of inducing social aggression in laboratory mice (indeed, this housing condition also augments electroshock-induced defensive aggression and maternal aggression but has no influence on locust-killing). The effects of "isolation" in rats and mice have been systematically investigated in a series of papers (Benton et al., 1978, 1979; Brain, 1971b, 1975a, b; Brain and Benton, 1977, 1979; Brayton and Brain, 1974; Goldsmith et al., 1977, 1978).

There are many conflicting views of the etiology of the profound effects of housing variations. For example, "isolation" can be viewed as stressful "social deprivation" or the least stressed category in crowding studies. A synopsis of some of the behavioural and physiological variations induced by differential housing in male mice is presented in Table IX. This includes a comparison of isolates with dominants and group-housed mice with subordinates.

One must emphasize that:

(a) "isolated" mice generally have visual, olfactory and auditory communication with conspecifics;

(b) the age at and duration of differential housing have profound influences on the changes recorded;

(c) selection of a base-line in differential housing studies is arbitrary. Neither "isolates" nor grouped animals may properly be termed "controls";

(d) erroneous interpretations may be consequences of using batteries of behavioural and physiological tests on the same animals;

(e) "basal" adrenocortical activities of *habituated* individually- and group-housed mice are not very different. Isolates show, however, increased behavioural and adrenocortical *reactivities* to stress and novelty. They also show slower habituation to these factors than

TABLE IX

A COMPARISON OF THE BEHAVIOURAL AND PHYSIOLOGICAL CHARACTERISTICS OF ISO-LATED, GROUPED, DOMINANT AND SUBORDINATE MICE

Subordinate or group-housed mice	Dominant or individually-housed mice
Low "aggressiveness"	High "aggressiveness"
Low gonadal activity	High gonadal activity
Low body weight	High body weight
Low reproductive success	High reproductive success
Poor coat condition	Good coat condition
High adrenocortical reactivity to stress	Low adrenocortical reactivity to stress
Poor immunological responses	Good immunological responses

their group-housed counterparts;

(f) disturbance (including changes in housing conditions) has a greater influence on adrenal/gonadal responses in mice than either isolation or grouping per se;

(g) a detailed videotape analysis of fighting generated by isolation (Childs and Brain, 1979) reveals that the behaviour has obvious affinities with the clear social aggression of dominant animals from groups (i.e. it is social aggression and *not* a "fear-mediated defensive response").

(h) isolates have other affinities with dominants which casts doubt on the evidence for an "isolation stress syndrome" in this species.

BRIEF SYNTHESIS

Emphasis has been directed in our studies to the natural social organization of the laboratory mouse's feral ancestor. Suffice it to say that there is convincing evidence that mature male House mice are generally territorial. Females, however, may form communal nests, generally below the ground. Territorial males appear inhibited in their attack on females or juvenile males. When juvenile males reach puberty, their increased androgen production may generate increased aggression-promoting pheromone production. This, by stimulating the male's attack may encourage migration from the breeding area.

In the laboratory, all-male groups of mice tend to form non-linear hierarchies with one despotic dominant and a number of equally-ranked submissives/defensives in each cage. This may be a consequence of the restricted housing conditions, as the natural response of the defeated "subordinates" seems to be to leave the vicinity of the dominant (i.e. the territory). This reaction may be encouraged by both physical attack and the fact that the dominant's odour assumes aversive characteristics. The submissive show, within these confined conditions, suppressed gonadal function which eventually inhibits both their aggressiveness and

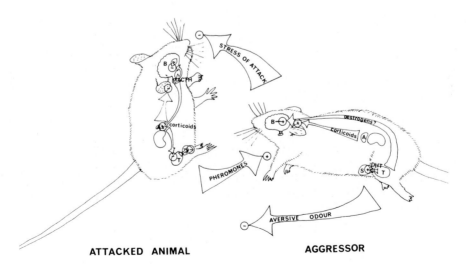

ATTACKED ANIMAL   **AGGRESSOR**

Fig. 11. A summary of the involvement of pituitary adrenocortical and pituitary gonadal factors in dominance/subordination in social aggression. A, adrenal; B, brain; SA, sex accessories; T, testis; ⊖ inhibits; ⊕ augments.

their effectiveness as attack-promoting stimuli (by reducing pheromone production and altering behaviour). These effects are summarized in simplified form in Fig. 11. One should also note that the adrenomedullary changes in response to victory/defeat are also part of this adaptation process. It should also be evident that different forms of aggression are likely to be influenced by very different endocrine factors (e.g. predatory aggression in the mouse appears little altered by adrenal or gonadal hormones).

Perhaps the responses of resident mice to lactating intruders may also be explained by reference to the natural situation? Lactating females generally develop increased maternal aggression in order to protect their young and it may be useful to partially segregate such females at this time. Territorial male mice are likely to be associated with several females plus litters in varying stages of development.

It seems likely that mammals (exemplified by rodents) utilize the subtle relationships between hormonal factors and the CNS to adjust their behavioural/energy utilization characteristics to changes in the environment. An animal's position in a "social organization" is, of course, one such environmental factor. Perhaps hormone-assisted adaptive changes in behaviour rather than selection of favoured genotypes (e.g. Wynne-Edwards, 1962) account for the changing behavioural characteristics of rodents at different stages of their population cycles? Much of the variation may be phenotypic and hormones may be intimately implicated in these responses.

It is almost obligatory to state that much more work needs to be done in this area. In this case, the statement is *not* a modest exaggeration. I would, however, ecourage prospective workers in the area of physiology and behaviour to adopt research strategies that are both systematic and diverse. Some may feel that these two aims are mutually incompatible but narrow specialism, combined with a superficial approach, has generally generated confusion in the area of hormones and aggression and the same may be true of other topics.

SUMMARY

A diverse series of studies on relationships between hormones and attack/defence, largely employing laboratory mice are briefly described. Particular emphasis is directed to the correct identification of the model of "aggression" employed and the site of hormonal action (i.e. central or peripheral). Sex steroids, catecholamines, glucocorticoids and ACTH were all found to correlate with different types of attack behaviour and an attempt was made to relate these relationships to the feral House mouse's territorial habit. It seems likely that rodents make use of hormonal changes consequent to fighting/environmental differences to facilitate adaptation to subsequent pressures.

ACKNOWLEDGEMENTS

I thank Professor E.W. Knight-Jones for facilities in Swansea and the various bodies (the French CNRS, the Italian CNR, the British MRC, Royal Society and SRC) who have (at times) supported the research described here.

Particular thanks are due to my collaborators (and friends) who allowed me to quote conjoint research. They include S. Al-Maliki *, D. Benton *, N. Bowden *, G. Childs *, A. Evans *, C.M. Evans *, M. Homedi *, M. Haug (Université Louis Pasteur), F.H. Hucklebridge (Polytechnic of Central London), L. Gamal-el-Din (Polytechnic of Central London),

---

* Of University College of Swansea, Wales.

J.F. Goldsmith * and S. Parmigiani (Universitá di Parma). My thanks are also due to Drs. A. Brunneman (Schering Ag), H.M. Greven (Organon Ltd) and V. Petrow (Merrill-National Labs.) for provision of chemicals at key points in these studies. I also acknowledge the help of P.J. Llewellyn and C. Stockton with illustrations.

REFERENCES

Al-Maliki, S. (1980) Influences of stress-related hormones on a variety of models of attack behaviour in laboratory mice. In *Adaptive Capabilities of the Nervous System, Progress in Brain Research, Vol. 53,* M.A. Corner et al. (Eds.), Elsevier, Amsterdam, pp. 421–425.

Al-Maliki, S. and Brain, P.F. (1979) Effects of food deprivation on fighting behaviour in "standard opponent" tests by male and female "TO" strain albino mice. *Anim. Behav.,* 27: 562–566.

Barkley, M.S. and Goldman, B.D. (1978) Studies on opponent status and steroid mediation of aggression in female mice. *Behav. Biol.,* 23: 118–123.

Baum, M. and Vreeburg, J.T.M. (1976) Differential effects of the anti-oestrogen MER$_{25}$ and of three 5α-reduced androgens on mounting and lordosis behaviour in the rat. *Horm. Behav.,* 7: 87–104.

Benton, D., Brain, P.F. and Goldsmith, J.F. (1979) Effects of prior housing on endocrine responses to differential caging in male "TO" strain mice. *Physiol. Psychol.,* 7: 89–92.

Benton, D., Goldsmith, J.F., Gamal-El-Din, L., Brain, P.F. and Hucklebridge, F.H. (1978) Adrenal activity in isolated mice and mice of different social status. *Physiol. Behav.,* 20: 459–464.

Bhagat, B.D. and Horenstein, S. (1976) Modulation of adrenal medullary enzymes by stress. In *Catecholamines and Stress,* E. Usdin, R. Kvetnansky and J. Kopin (Eds.), Pergamon Press, New York.

Blanchard, R.J. and Blanchard, D.C. (1977) Aggressive behaviour in the rat. *Behav. Biol.,* 21: 197–224.

Booth, J.E. (1977) Sexual behaviour of male rats injected with the anti-oestrogen MER-$_{25}$ during infancy. *Physiol. Behav.,* 19: 35–39.

Bowden, N.J. (1979) *Studies on the Manner in which Sex Steroids Influence Aggressiveness in Mus musculus.* L., Ph.D. dissertation, University College of Swansea, Wales.

Bowden, N.J. and Brain, P.F. (1978) Blockade of testosterone-maintained intermale fighting in albino laboratory mice by an aromatization inhibitor. *Physiol. Behav.,* 20: 543–546.

Brain, P.F. (1971a) The possible role of the pituitary-adrenocortical axis in aggressive behaviour. *Nature (Lond.),* 233: 489.

Brain, P.F. (1971b) The physiology of population limitation in rodents – a review. *Commun. Behav. Biol.,* 6: 115–123.

Brain, P.F. (1972) Mammalian behavior and the adrenal cortex – a review. *Behav. Biol.,* 7: 453–477.

Brain, P.F. (1975a) What does individual housing mean to a mouse? *Life Sci.,* 16: 187–200.

Brain, P.F. (1975b) Studies on crowding: a critical analysis of the implications of studies on rodents for the human situation. *Int. J. ment. Health,* 4: 15–30.

Brain, P.F. (1977) *Hormones and Aggression, Vol. 1,* Annual Research Reviews, Eden Press, Montreal.

Brain, P.F. (1978a) *Hormones and Aggression, Vol. 2,* Annual Research Reviews, Eden Press, Montreal.

Brain, P.F. (1978b) Steroidal influences on aggressiveness. In *Biological Psychiatry Today,* J. Obiols et al. (Eds.), Elsevier/North-Holland, Amsterdam.

Brain, P.F. (1979a) Effects of the hormones of the pituitary–gonadal axis on behaviour. In K. Brown and S.J. Cooper (Eds.), *Chemical Influences on Behaviour,* Academic Press, pp. 255–328.

Brain, P.F. (1979b) Effects of the hormones of the pituitary–adrenocortical axis on behaviour. In *Chemical Influences on Behaviour,* K. Brown and S.J. Cooper (Eds.), Academic Press, pp. 329–371.

Brain, P.F. (1979c) *Hormones, Drugs and Aggression, Vol. 3,* Annual Research Reviews, Eden Press, Montreal.

Brain, P.F. and Al-Maliki, S. (1978) A comparison of "intermale fighting" in "standard opponent" tests and attack directed towards locusts by "TO" strain mice: effects of simple experimental manipulations. *Anim. Behav.,* 26: 723–737.

---

* Of University College of Swansea, Wales.

Brain, P.F. and Al-Maliki, S. (1979) A comparison of effects of simple experimental manipulations on fighting generated by breeding activity and predatory aggression in "TO" strain mice. *Behaviour,* 69: 183–200.

Brain, P.F. and Benton, D. (1977) What does individual housing mean to a research worker? *IRCS J. Med. Sci.,* 5: 459–463.

Brain, P.F. and Benton, D. (1979) The interpretation of physiological correlates of differential housing in laboratory rats. *Life Sci.,* 24: 99–116.

Brain, P.F. and Bowden, N.J. (1978) Studies on the blockade of testosterone or oestradiol − 17β maintained fighting in castrated "aggressive" mice. *J. Endocr.,* 77: 37–38P.

Brain, P.F. and Bowden, N.J. (1979) Sex steroid control of intermale fighting in albino laboratory mice. In *Current Developments in Psychopharmacology,* Vol. 5, W.B. Essman and L. Valzelli (Eds.), Spectrum, pp. 403–465.

Brain, P.F. and Evans, A.E. (1977) Acute influences of some ACTH-related peptides on fighting and adrenocortical activity in male laboratory mice. *Pharmacol. Biochem. Behav.,* 7: 425–433.

Brain, P.F. and Haug, M. (1979) Implication of urinary pheromones in the attack directed by groups of castrated male mice towards female intruders. *J. Endocr.,* 83: 40.

Brain, P.F. and Poole, A.E. (1974) The role of endocrines in isolation-induced intermale fighting in albino laboratory mice. 1. Pituitary-adrenocortical influences. *Aggress. Behav.,* 1: 39–69.

Brain, P.F., Al-Maliki, S. and Childs, G. (1979) Videotape studies on different forms of murine aggression. *Exp. Brain. Res.,* 36: R6.

Brain, P.F., Nowell, N.W. and Wouters, A. (1971) Some relationships between adrenal function and isolation-induced intermale aggression in albino mice. *Physiol. Behav.,* 6: 27–29.

Brain, P.F., Benton, D. and Bolton, J.C. (1978) A comparison of agonistic behavior in individually housed male mice and those cohabiting with females. *Aggress. Behav.,* 4: 201–206.

Brayton, A.R. and Brain, P.F. (1974) Effects of "crowding" on endocrine function and retention of the digenean parasite *Microphallus pygmaeus* in male and female albino mice. *J. Helminth.,* 48: 99–106.

Bronson, F.H. and Eleftheriou, B.E. (1965) Behavioural, pituitary and adrenal correlates of controlled fighting (defeat) in mice. *Physiol. Zool.,* 38: 406–411.

Childs, G. and Brain, P.F. (1979) A videotape analysis of biting targets employed in intraspecific fighting encounters in laboratory mice from four treatment categories. *ICRS Med. Sci.,* 7: 44.

Ciaranello, R.D., Wooten, G.F. and Axelrod, J. (1976) Regulation of rat adrenal dopamine β-hydroxylase. II. Receptor interaction in the regulation of enzyme synthesis and degradation. *Brain Res.,* 113: 349–362.

De Wied, D. (1969) Effects of peptide hormones on behaviour. In *Frontiers in Neuroendocrinology,* W.F. Ganong and L. Martini (Eds.), Oxford University Press, London, pp. 97–140.

De Wied, D., van Delft, A.M.L., Gispen, W.H., Weijnen, J.A.W.M. and van Wimersma-Greidanus, Tj.B. (1972) The role of pituitary–adrenal system hormones in active-avoidance conditioning. In *Hormones and Behavior,* S. Levine (Ed.), Academic Press, New York, pp. 135–171.

Edwards, D.A. and Herndon, J. (1970) Neonatal estrogen stimulation and aggressive behavior in female mice. *Physiol Behav.,* 5: 993–995.

Ely, D.L. and Henry, J.P. (1978) Neuroendocrine response patterns in dominant and subordinate mice. *Horm. Behav.,* 10: 156–169.

Gamal-el-Din, L.A. (1978) *Some Aspects of Adrenomedullary Function in Relation to Agonistic Behaviour in the Mouse (Mus musculus),* Ph.D. dissertation, Polytechnic of Central London, U.K.

Goldsmith, J.F., Brain, P.F. and Benton, D. (1977) Effects of age at differential housing and the duration of individual housing/grouping on intermale fighting behavior and adrenocortical activity in "TO". strain mice. *Aggress. Behav.,* 2: 307–323.

Goldsmith, J.F., Brain, P.F. and Benton, D. (1978) Effects of the duration of individual or group housing on behavioral and adrenocortical reactivity in male albino mice. *Physiol. Behav.,* 21: 757–760.

Haug, M. (1976) *Etude d'un Comportement d'Aggression de Souris Femelles vis-à-vis de Congénères Allaitantes: Analyse du Mécanisme,* Doctorat de 3° Cycle Université Louis Pasteur, Strasbourg, France.

Haug, M. and Brain, P.F. (1978) Attack directed by groups of castrated male mice towards lactating or non-lactating intruders: a urine-dependent phenomenon? *Physiol. Behav.,* 21: 549–552.

Haug, M. and Brain, P.F. (1979) Effects of treatments with testosterone and oestradiol on the attack directed by groups of gonadectomized male and female mice towards lactating intruders. *Physiol. Behav.,* 23: 397–400.

Henry, J.P., Kross, M.E., Stephens, P.M. and Watson, F.M.C. (1976) Evidence that differing psychosocial stimuli lead to adrenal cortical stimulation by autonomic or endocrine pathways. In *Hypertension and Brain Mechanisms, Progress in Brain Research, Vol. 47,* W. de Jong, A.P. Provoost and A.P. Shapiro (Eds.), Elsevier, Amsterdam, pp. 263–276.

Heyns, W. and De Moor, P. (1974) A 3(17)β-hydroxysteroid dehydrogenase in rat erythrocytes: conversion of 5α-dihydrotestosterone into 5α-androstane-3β, 17β-diol and purification of the enzyme by affinity chromatography. *Biochim. biophys. Acta (Amst.),* 358: 1–13.

Hoffman, A., Harbough, R., Erdelyi, E., Dornbush, J., Ciaranello, R. and Barchas, J. (1976) Delayed increase of adrenal TH and PNMT activities following cold stress in the mouse. *Life Sci.,* 17: 557–562.

Hucklebridge, F.H. (1973) *Some Relationships between Adrenomedullary Function and Social Stress in the Laboratory Mouse,* Ph.D. dissertation, University of Hull, U.K.

Hucklebridge, F.H., Gamal-el-Din, L. and Brain, P.F. (1980) Social status and the adrenal medulla in the House mouse (*Mus musculus* L). In preparation.

Hucklebridge, F.H., Nowell, N.W. and Dilks, R.A. (1973) Plasma catecholamine response to fighting in male albino mice. *Behav. Biol.,* 8: 785–800.

Juneja, H., Vasconti, F., Motta, M. and Martini, L. (1976) Effect of testosterone and of its 5α-reduced metabolites on L.H. secretion. In *Vth Int. Congr. Endocrinol. (Hamburg),* Abstr. 283.

Kato, J. (1975) The role of hypothalamic and hypophyseal 5α-dihydrotestosterone, estradiol and progesterone receptors in the mechanism of feedback action. *J. steroid Biochem.,* 6: 979–987.

Leshner, A.I. (1978) *An Introduction to Behavioral Endocrinology,* Oxford University Press, New York.

Leshner, A.I. (1980) The interaction of experience and neuroendocrine factors in determining behavioral adaptations to aggression. In *Adaptive Capabilities of the Nervous System, Progress in Brain Research, Vol. 53,* Elsevier, Amsterdam, pp. 427–438.

Leshner, A.I. and Schwartz, S.M. (1977) Neonatal corticosterone treatment increases submissiveness in adulthood in mice. *Physiol. Behav.,* 19: 163–166.

Lupo di Prisco, C., Lucarini, N. and Dessi-Fulgheri, F. (1978) Testosterone aromatization in rat brain is modulated by social environment. *Physiol. Behav.,* 20: 345–348.

Luttge, W.G. and Hall, N.R. (1973) Androgen-induced agonistic behavior in castrate male Swiss–Webster mice: comparison of four naturally occurring androgens. *Behav. Biol.,* 8: 725–732.

Maengwyn-Davies, G.D., Johnson, D.G., Thoa, N.B., Weise, V.K. and Kopin, I.J. (1973) Influence of isolation and of fighting on adrenal tyrosine hydroxylase and phenylethanolamine-N-methyl-transferase activities in three strains of mice. *Psychopharmacologia (Berl.),* 28: 339–350.

McEwen, B.S., Lieberburg, I., Chaptal, C. and Krey, L.C. (1977a) Aromatization: important for sexual differentiation of the neonatal rat brain. *Horm. Behav.,* 9: 249–263.

McEwen, B.S., Lieberburg, I., Maclusky, N. and Plapinger, L. (1977b) Do estrogen receptors play a role in the sexual differentiation of the rat brain? *J. steroid Biochem.,* 8: 593–598.

Morrell, J.I., Kelley, D.B. and Pfaff, D.W. (1975) Sex steroid binding in the brains of vertebrates. In *Brain – Endocrine Interaction II. The Ventricular System,* Karger, Basel, pp. 230–256.

Moyer, K.E. (1980) Biological substrates of aggression. In *Adaptive Capabilities of the Nervous System, Progress in Brain Research, Vol. 53,* M.A. Corner et al. (Eds.), Elsevier, Amsterdam, pp. 359–367.

Naftolin, F. and Ryan, K.J. (1975) The metabolism of androgens in central neuroendocrine tissues. *J. steroid Biochem.,* 6: 993–997.

Parrott, R.F. (1975) Aromatizable and 5α-reduced androgens: differentiation between central and peripheral effects on male rat sexual behavior. *Horm Behav.,* 6: 99–108.

Raisman, G. and Field, P.M. (1973) Sexual dimorphism in the neuropil of the preoptic area of the rat and its dependence on neonatal androgen. *Brain Res.,* 54: 1–29.

Simon, N.G. and Gandelman, R. (1977) Decreased aggressive behavior in the offspring of ACTH-treated mice. *Behav. Biol.,* 21: 478–488.

Simon, N.G. and Gandelman, R. (1978) The estrogenic arousal of aggressive behavior in female mice. *Horm. Behav.,* 10: 118–127.

Tizabi, Y., Kopin, I.J., Maengwyn-Davies, G.D. and Thoa, N.B. (1976) Attack-induced changes in response to decapitation of plasma catecholamine of victim mice. *Psychopharmacol. Commun.,* 2: 391–402.

Welch, B.L. and Welch, A.S. (1969) Fighting: preferential lowering of norepinephrine and dopamine in the brainstem, concomitant with a depletion of epinephrine from the adrenal medulla. *Commun. Behav. Biol.,* 3: 125–130.

Wynne-Edwards, V.C. (1962) *Animal Dispersion in Relation to Social Behaviour,* Oliver and Boyd, London.

Hormonal Correlates of Agonistic Behavior in Adult Male Rats

T. SCHUURMAN

Department of Zoology, State University of Groningen (The Netherlands)

INTRODUCTION

Most studies of the hormonal correlates of agonistic behavior in adult animals have been performed in mice (see Brain, 1980; Leshner, 1980), and only a few in rats. In the following pages I shall briefly report on my (as yet unpublished) experiments in adult male rats.

Two themes were investigated: (a) relationships between hormone levels and agonistic behavior; and (b) hormonal and behavioral changes after agonistic experience.

The experimental animals were Tryon Maze Dull S-3 rats, which show a high level of aggressive behavior, as do wild rats. Twenty behavioral elements of the experimental rats were registered, either during tests in which a male stimulus rat (WEzob strain) was placed into the home cage of the experimental rat, or in a cage that was strange to both rats. During certain behavioral tests, blood samples for hormone assays were taken by means of an indwelling jugular vein cannula, according to Steffens (1969).

GONADAL HORMONES AND AGONISTIC BEHAVIOR

Relationships between hormone levels and agonistic behavior

Many studies have revealed that androgens can maintain and facilitate inter-male aggression in mice (e.g. Beeman, 1947; Leshner and Moyer, 1975). Androgens that can be aromatized in the brain seem to be especially important (see Brain, 1980). Only Barfield (1972) has previously reported the effects on inter-male aggression in rats of manipulating baseline androgen levels. Like Barfield, I studied the effects of castration and subsequent testosterone propionate treatment on agonistic behavior in adult male rats. Special attention was given to the latency of the behavioral effect after a changed baseline androgen level. Fig. 1 shows that the amount of aggressive behavior directed towards a male opponent in an unfamiliar cage decreased strongly after castration. During testosterone propionate treatment, pre-castration levels of aggressive behavior were regained. Plasma testosterone levels of the rats were very low after castration, while at the end of the hormone treatment these levels were similar to pre-castration ones. In fact, as early as two days after castration the rats behaved significantly less aggressively, whereas the sham-operated rats did not behave any differently from in the pre-operation tests (Fig. 2). Surprisingly, these same castrates maintained a rather high level of aggressive behavior in the home cage for weeks, and only in the second post-operative test period (42–51 days after castration) did they show a significant decrease of aggressive behavior towards an intruder in this situation. A rapid effect was also observed

416

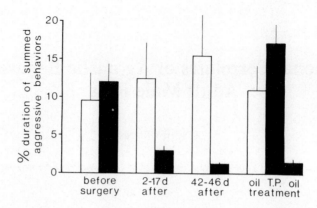

Fig. 1. Effect of castration and subsequent testosterone propionate (T.P.) treatment on inter-male aggression tested in an unfamiliar cage. Each rat was tested at least 6 times in each condition. Each test lasted 10 min. Aggressive behaviors: lateral threat, chase, fight and keep down. Bars: S.E.M. ■, castrated rats (n = 9); □, sham-operated rats (n = 5). After the second post-operative test period 6 out of 9 castrated rats received T.P. treatment (0.75 mg s.c. for 18 days), the remaining 3 and the sham-operated rats received daily oil injections.

during testosterone propionate treatment, in that pre-castration aggression levels were regained by the second day of the treatment. Thus there were rapid as well as slow effects of manipulating plasma testosterone level on aggression.

Most attempts to relate plasma testosterone levels of intact mice to differences in aggressiveness have failed (e.g. Selmanoff et al., 1977; Dessi-Fulgheri et al., 1976). Rose et al. (1971) found such a correlation in rhesus monkeys. No such correlation has yet been reported in rats. One reason for this failing might be the pulsatile nature of the testosterone secretion in rats and mice (Bartke et al., 1973; Bartke and Dalterio, 1975; Keating and Tcholakian, 1979; Mock et al., 1978). This phenomenon makes it necessary to take many

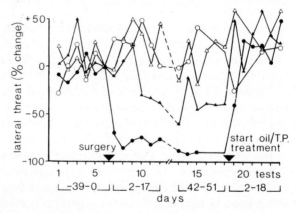

Fig. 2. Effect of castration and subsequent testosterone propionate (T.P.) treatment on the amount of lateral threat during tests in the home cage and in an unfamiliar cage. The baseline was based on the last pre-operative test. ●———●, castrated rats (n = 9), tests in an unfamiliar cage; ▲———▲, home cage tests on the same rats; ○———○, sham-operated rats (n = 5), tests in an unfamiliar cage; △———△, home cage tests. Fifty-one days after surgery 6 out of 9 castrated rats received T.P. treatment (0.75 mg s.c. for 18 days) while the sham-operated rats received daily oil injections.

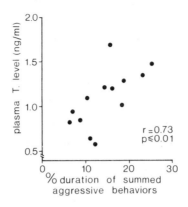

Fig. 3. Correlation between baseline plasma testosterone (T.) level and inter-male aggression. % Durations of aggressive behaviors (see Fig. 1) were measured during a 15 min test 1 or 2 days before, and on the day of blood sampling. At least 25 blood samples per rat were taken to determine baseline plasma T. level, peak concentrations >3 ng T./ml (see text) were excluded. Statistics: Spearman rank correlation.

blood samples in order to determine overall plasma testosterone concentration. In most studies, however, only a single sample was taken per animal.

In my experiments adult male S-3 rats showed a rather constant baseline plasma testosterone level, alternated with short-lasting (maximum 1 h) high testosterone concentrations up to 20 ng/ml (blood sampling every 15 min for at least 8 h per rat). Baseline plasma testosterone levels differed between individuals (range 0.5–2 ng/ml). These differences were correlated with individual differences in aggressiveness (Fig. 3).

Although rats were less aggressive following castration, they never behaved defensively or submissively during the tests. Therefore a low performance of aggressive behavior together with low plasma testosterone levels are not necessarily associated with a high degree of defensive and submissive behavior. This agrees with results of Barfield (1972), who saw no loss of dominance in his castrated rats. This suggests that aggressiveness and defense/submission belong to different behavioral systems which, moreover, are probably affected by different hormones (see Leshner, 1980).

Hormonal and behavioral changes after agonistic experience

It appeared that rats behaved significantly less aggressively and more defensively after suffering a serious defeat. These behavioral changes manifested themselves more obviously when the rats were tested in an unfamilar cage than when tested in the home cage. These defeated rats also showed lowered plasma testosterone levels (Fig. 4). On the other hand, rats that won serious encounters showed neither behavioral changes nor decreased plasma–testosterone levels (Fig. 4). Bronson and Eleftheriou (1964) reported that seminal vesicle weight of mice was inversely correlated with the number of defeats, suggesting a lowered testosterone secretion. Bronson et al. (1973) measured lower plasma LH and plasma FSH concentrations in defeated mice as compared to dominant mice. Similarly, Rose et al. (1972) reported lowered plasma testosterone concentrations after defeat in rhesus monkeys.

The finding that castrated rats continued defending their home cages against male intruders for weeks, whereas they almost immediately stopped attacking opponents in an

418

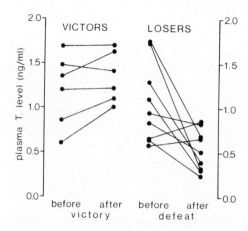

Fig. 4. Plasma testosterone (T.) levels of winners and losers 1 or 2 days before, and 1 or 2 days after a 1 h aggressive encounter. Each point represents mean plasma T. level of a rat. At least 20 blood samples per rat in each condition were taken.

unfamiliar cage, indicates that maintenance of the former type of aggression is much less testosterone-dependent than is maintenance of the latter one. Moyer (1968) had already distinguished between territorial defense and inter-male aggression which was not specifically related to a particular area, and he predicted that experimental manipulations would probably differentially affect the two types of aggression. Presumably the presence of a male intruder in the home cage is a stronger stimulus for attack. Chronically lowered plasma testosterone level, however, does affect aggression in the home cage.

Decreased testosterone secretion contributes to the behavioral changes seen after defeat, as is suggested by the rapid fall of aggressive behavior in an unfamiliar cage after castration. Experiments are in progress to test this hypothesis.

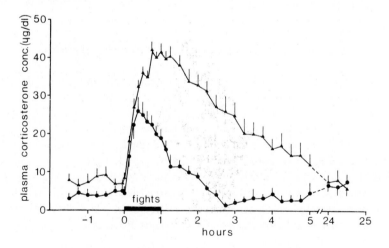

Fig. 5. Pituitary–adrenal response of winners (●———●) (n = 6), and losers (▲———▲) (n = 9) during and after a 1 h aggressive encounter. Bars: S.E.M.

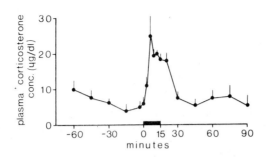

Fig. 6. Pituitary–adrenal response of rats (n = 8) that had experienced a serious defeat 1 or 2 days previously, when meeting a non-aggressive male opponent (from 0–15 min). Bars: S.E.M.

PITUITARY–ADRENAL HORMONES AND AGONISTIC BEHAVIOR

Relationships between hormone levels and agonistic behavior

In mice, long-lasting high pituitary–adrenal activity suppresses aggression towards conspecifics, ACTH probably being the relevant hormone (see Brain, 1980). In addition, this hormonal state facilitates submissive behavior, in which case corticosterone is probably the relevant hormone (see Leshner, 1980). Because all rats showed the same baseline corticosterone levels in my studies, it was impossible to correlate individual differences in aggressiveness with individual differences in basal pituitary–adrenal activity.

Hormonal and behavioral changes after agonistic experience

Rats that had experienced a serious defeat one or two days earlier, had normal baseline plasma corticosterone levels, just like winners of serious fights. Yet, two differences between losers and winners must be mentioned.

(1) During the aggressive encounter and for some hours afterwards, defeated rats showed a very high plasma corticosterone level. Winners too showed elevated plasma corticosterone levels, but they regained their resting level soon after removal of the defeated opponent (Fig. 5). Comparable differences between losers and winners of encounters have been described in mice (Bronson and Eleftheriou, 1964; Leshner, 1980).

(2) One or two days after a defeat, rats showed an exaggerated pituitary–adrenal response when meeting a (non-aggressive) male opponent, despite the absence of fights (Fig. 6). Undefeated controls showed only minor plasma corticosterone elevations in such a situation (data not shown here).

It is now being investigated whether these differences are related to the behavioral changes after defeat.

ACKNOWLEDGEMENTS

This work was (in part) supported by the Netherlands Organization for the Advancement of Pure Research (ZWO).

REFERENCES

Barfield, R.J., Busch, D.E. and Wallen, K. (1972) Gonadal influence on agonistic behavior in the male domestic rat. *Horm. Behav.,* 3: 247–259.

Bartke, A. and Dalterio, S. (1975) Evidence for episodic secretion of testosterone in laboratory mice. *Steroids,* 26: 749–756.

Bartke, A., Steele, R.E., Musto, N. and Caldwell, B.V. (1973) Fluctuations in plasma testosterone levels in adult male rats and mice. *Endocrinology,* 92: 1223–1228.

Beeman, E.A. (1947) The effect of male hormone on aggressive behavior in mice. *Physiol. Zool.,* 20: 373–405.

Brain, P.F. (1980) Adaptive aspects of hormonal correlates of attack and defence in laboratory mice: a study in ethobiology. In *Adaptive Capabilities of the Nervous System, Progress in Brain Research, Vol. 53,* M.A. Corner et al. (Eds.), Elsevier, Amsterdam, pp. 391–413.

Bronson, F.H. and Eleftheriou, B.E. (1964) Chronic physiological effects of fighting in mice. *Gen. comp. Endocr.,* 4: 9–14.

Bronson, F.H., Stetson, M.H. and Stiff, M.E. (1973) Serum FSH and LH in male mice following aggressive and non-aggressive interaction. *Physiol. Behav.,* 10: 369–372.

Dessi-Fulgheri, F., Lucarini, N. and Lupo di Prisco, C. (1976) Relationships between testosterone metabolism in the brain, other endocrine variables and intermale aggression in mice. *Aggress. Behav.,* 2: 223–231.

Keating, J. and Tcholakian, R.K. (1979) In vivo patterns of circulating steroids in adult male rats. I. Variations in testosterone during 24- and 48-hour standard and reverse light/dark cycles. *Endocrinology,* 104: 184–189.

Leshner, A.I. (1980) The interaction of experience and neuroendocrine factors in determining behavioral adaptations to aggression. In *Adaptive Capabilities of the Nervous System, Progress in Brain Research, Vol. 53,* M.A. Corner et al. (Eds.), Elsevier, Amsterdam, pp. 427–438.

Leshner, A.I. and Moyer, J.A. (1975) Androgens and agonistic behavior in mice: relevance to aggression and irrelevance to avoidance-of-attack. *Physiol. Behav.,* 15: 695–699.

Mock, E.J., Norton, H.W. and Frankel, A.I. (1978) Daily rhythmicity of serum testosterone concentration in the male laboratory rat. *Endocrinology,* 103: 1111–1121.

Moyer, K.E. (1968) Kinds of aggression and their physiological basis. *Commun. Behav. Biol.,* 2: 65–87.

Rose, R.M., Gordon, T.P. and Bernstein, I.S. (1972) Plasma testosterone levels in the male rhesus: influences of sexual and social stimuli. *Science,* 178: 643–645.

Rose, R.M., Holaday, J.W. and Bernstein, I.S. (1971) Plasma testosterone, dominance rank and aggressive behaviour in male rhesus monkeys. *Nature (Lond.),* 231: 366–368.

Selmanoff, M.K., Goldman, B.D. and Ginsburg, B.E. (1977) Serum testosterone, agonistic behavior, and dominance in inbred strains of mice. *Horm. Behav.,* 8: 107–119.

Steffens, A.B. (1969) A method for frequent sampling of blood and continuous infusion of fluids in the rat without disturbing the animal. *Physiol. Behav.,* 4: 883–896.

Influences of Stress-Related Hormones on a Variety of Models of Attack Behaviour in Laboratory Mice

SAMI AL-MALIKI

Department of Zoology, University College of Swansea, Swansea, Wales (U.K.)

INTRODUCTION

Different forms of fighting behaviour are said to have different physiological bases (Moyer, 1968; Brain, 1979) which may be indicated by simple experimental manipulations (e.g. Brain and Al-Maliki, 1978). "Stress-related" (i.e. pituitary—adrenocortical) hormones have recently been shown to influence social aggression in laboratory mice (reviewed by Brain, 1979). It was consequently thought to be of interest to study the effects of acutely-administered ACTH and/or glucocorticoids on different types of murine aggression in TO strain mice, especially as Brain (1980) has emphasized the importance of hormonal adaptations in modulating aggression in this strain.

EFFECTS OF CORTROPHIN/ZN AND DEXAMETHASONE ON SOCIAL AGGRESSION AND LOCUST KILLING BEHAVIOUR IN MALE MICE

Ninety-six naive and ninety-six sexually-experienced males were used in this experiment. Naive subjects were allocated to individual housing at approximately 18 weeks of age,

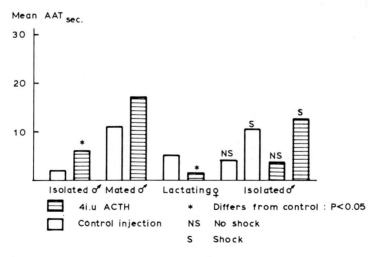

Fig. 1. Acute effects of injection with 4 IU of ACTH/Zn on social aggression in isolated and sexually-experienced males; maternal aggression in lactating females and shock-induced aggression in isolated male mice.

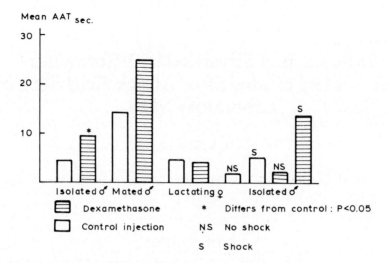

Fig. 2. Acute effects of injection with 200 μg dexamethasone on social aggression in isolated and sexually-experienced males, maternal aggression in lactating females and shock-induced aggression in male mice.

whereas mated males were separated from their mates and housed individually for only one day prior to testing. Categories (n = 24) were injected i.p. with one of the following materials 12 h before behavioural testing: (1) r IU. ACTH (Cortrophin/Zn, Organon Labs); (2) a zinc-containing control injection; (3) 200 μg of dexamethasone (Dexadreson, Organon Labs); or (4) saline controls for dexamethasone.

Half of the animals in each experimental category received a single 10 min aggression test with an anosmic "standard opponent" in their cleaned home cage. "Standard opponents" were rendered anosmic by nasal perfusion with 4% zinc sulphate solution. The remainder of each category was then assessed for locust-killing behaviour by introducing an adult locust for 6 h into the cleaned home cage. Simple "alive" or "killed and consumed" data were

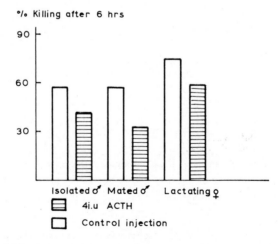

Fig. 3. Acute effects of injection with 4 IU ACTH/Zn on locust-killing in isolated males, sexually-experienced males and lactating female mice.

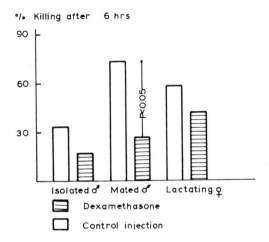

Fig. 4. Acute effects of injection with 200 μg dexamethasone on locust-killing behaviour in isolated males, sexually-experienced males and lactating female mice.

recorded at intervals during the 6 h after the introduction of the locust (Brain and Al-Maliki, 1978). Eventually, results were presented as the percentage of mice which killed the locust. The behavioural tests are described in more detail by Brain (1980).

The social aggression results are presented in Figs. 1 and 2, and demonstrate that both ACTH and dexamethasone significantly enhance this form of attack in the naive, individually-housed male mice (cf. Brain and Evans, 1977; Brain et al., 1971). These treatments also increased social aggression in mated males, but the augmentations did not reach significance in this case. This might be due to the high base line of aggression in mated males, which would make it relatively difficult to show augmentation effects on fighting. The effects of these hormones on locust-killing are illustrated in Figs. 3 and 4. ACTH and dexamethasone had little influence on this response, confirming that social aggression and locust-killing are likely to have different physiological bases.

INFLUENCE OF ACTH AND DEXAMETHASONE INJECTIONS ON MATERNAL ATTACK ON A CONSPECIFIC INTRUDER AND ON LOCUST-KILLING BEHAVIOUR IN FEMALE MICE

Ninety-six lactating female mice were employed in this experiment. These females were allocated to mated pairs at 9 weeks of age with males of the same age. Males were removed when their mates became notably pregnant, and the females were then provided with shredded paper to facilitate nest construction. Litters were adjusted to 6 pups on the day of parturition. One week later, these animals were allocated to 4 experimental categories (n = 24) which were treated, 12 h prior to behavioural testing, with the same materials and doses as employed in the first experiment. Half of the animals in each experimental category received a single 10 min test with an anosmic male 'standard opponent' intruder whilst the remainder received a single 6 h locust-killing test. Tests were carried out in the lactating female's home cage in the presence of that animal's litter.

Maternal aggression data are also presented in Figs. 1 and 2, and locust-killing material in Figs. 3 and 4. The results indicate that ACTH, but not dexamethasone, reduced maternal attack on male intruders, but that neither ACTH nor dexamethasone consistently influenced locust-killing in these animals.

EFFECTS OF ACTH AND DEXAMETHASONE INJECTIONS ON SELF-DEFENSIVE AGGRESSION IN MALE MICE

Eighty-eight naive male mice, individually-housed for 3 days at approximately 18 weeks of age, were used in this study. After initial isolation, mice were allocated to categories (n = 22) and injected i.p., 12 h prior to behavioural testing, with the same materials and doses that were employed in experiments 1 and 2. Half of the subjects in each treatment category received a single 10 min encounter with an anosmic 'standard opponent' in a shock box (converted mouse box) — 0.8 mA current was applied to the grid floor of the apparatus every 5 sec. The remainder experienced similar encounters without the current being applied. Electroshock-induced fighting in rats and mice has been described as "self-defensive" aggression (see Brain, 1980).

Data for this experiment are presented in histogram form in Figs. 1 and 2. ACTH and dexamethasone produced a slight increase in self-defensive aggression but this trend did not reach statistical significance. The non-shocked controls in this experiment showed consistent but low levels of fighting.

CONCLUSION

The results from these experiments provide further support for the view that aggression is not a unitary concept, and suggest that stress-related hormones alter different forms of attack in different ways. Perhaps essentially *offensive* responses (i.e. social aggression) are influenced by stress-related hormones in a fundamentally different way from forms of aggression that are more obviously *defensive* (as in maternal attack and electroshock-induced fighting).

ACKNOWLEDGEMENTS

Professor E.W. Knight-Jones is thanked for the use of facilities at Swansea, and Dr. Paul Brain for supervising this work. The help of Dr. David Benton in preparing the manuscript for publication is acknowledged.

REFERENCES

Brain, P.F. (1979) *Hormones, Drugs and Aggression., Vol. 3., Annual Research Reviews*, Eden Press, Montreal.

Brain, P.F. (1980) Adaptive aspects of hormonal correlates of attack and defence in laboratory mice: a study in ethobiology. In *Adaptive Capabilities of the Nervous System, Progress in Brain Research, Vol. 53*, M.A. Corner et al. (Eds.), Elsevier, Amsterdam, pp. 391–413.

Brain, P.F. and Al-Maliki, S. (1978) A comparison of "intermale" fighting in 'standard opponent' tests and attack directed towards locusts by "TO" strain mice: effects of simple experimental manipulations. *Anim. Behav.*, 26: 723–737.

Brain, P.F., Nowell, N.W. and Wouters, A. (1971) Some relationships between adrenal function and the effectiveness of a period of isolation in inducing intermale aggression in albino mice. *Physiol. Behav.*, 6: 27–29.

Brain, P.F. and Evans, A.E. (1977) Acute influences of some ACTH-related peptides on fighting and adrenocortical activity in male laboratory mice. *Pharmacol. Biochem. Behav.*, 7: 425–433.

Moyer, K.E. (1968) Kinds of aggression and their physiological basis. *Commun. Behav. Biol.*, 2: 65–87.

The Interaction of Experience and Neuroendocrine Factors in Determining Behavioral Adaptations to Aggression

ALAN I. LESHNER

Department of Psychology, Bucknell University, Lewisburg, Pa. 17837 (U.S.A.)

INTRODUCTION

Throughout recorded history, scholars have been concerned with the origins of our competitive tendencies. During the past 50 years, that interest has been expressed in a large amount of experimental attention devoted to what are now called the *agonistic behaviors,* which include both aggressive and submissive groups of responses. The central question seems to have remained "why do individuals fight?", and a variety of theories has been proposed to account for fighting. These theories have focused on the internal impetus to aggression (e.g. Lorenz, 1966), the environmental conditions which elicit this behavior (e.g. Hutchinson, 1972), and the consequences to the animal of behaving in an aggressive manner (e.g., Baenninger, 1974; Leshner and Nock, 1976). The issue of why animals fight has not been resolved, and the debate continues. In the process of asking that general question, however, much has been learned about agonistic responding. Included in the information accumulated has been the important fact that an individual's experiences in an agonistic encounter have major consequences for its behavior in future competitive situations, and some of those experiential effects are the topic of this discussion.

In any instance of competition, there is both a winner and a loser. To date, most investigators have focused on the consequences of fighting for the winner (e.g., Johnson, 1972; Montagu, 1974; Scott, 1971). In contrast, most of our recent work has been directed towards the case of the loser. Our research is concerned with the factors that determine behavioral adaptations to being aggressed upon, in particular the quality of *submissiveness,* or the readiness to surrender following an attack by an opponent animal. Our studies focus on the interaction between experiential and physiological factors in determining submissiveness in mice.

SOME PRELIMINARY COMMENTS ON THE NATURE OF SUBMISSIVENESS

The submissive behaviors include a wide range of behavior patterns, such as flight, passivity, avoidance, and the stereotyped postures exhibited by defeated or subordinate individuals (Grant and Mackintosh, 1963; Leshner, 1975). These behaviors seem to be adaptations of the loser to the stresses of being defeated, because they can serve as mechanisms for terminating or preventing attack by the opponent, either by providing a mechanism for escape or by signalling surrender to the victor (Eibl-Eibesfeldt, 1975; Wilson, 1975).

Virtually all species exhibit submissive or appeasement postures of one kind or another,

428

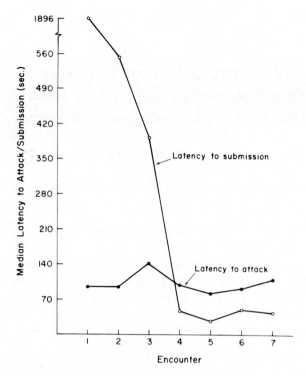

Fig. 1. The median latency to attack or submit in winning and losing mice, respectively, over consecutive encounters.

and these gestures are species-specific in form (Eibl-Eibesfeldt, 1975). That is, each species has its characteristic set of behavior patterns that can serve appeasement or surrender functions. Therefore, these behavior patterns may be unlearned or "pre-programmed" into the organism. But, it is important that although an animal may not need to learn *how* to act submissively, it clearly does have to learn *when* to be submissive. Virtually no animal surrenders before some experience with defeat, and in successive encounters involving defeat experiences, the loser surrenders more and more quickly. This point is emphasized by a study summarized in Fig. 1, where Nock and I showed that in successive encounters between the same two mice, the loser surrendered more and more readily, until it finally submitted before the opponent had even attacked. But, that point where surrender preceded the opponent's attack came only after repeated experiences of defeat. One might draw an analogy here to traditional shock-mediated avoidance learning situations, where an animal learns over repeated trials to avoid an aversive stimulus by engaging in a specific behavior pattern. Therefore, we argue that *when* to be submissive must in fact be learned.

An important point that should be included in any discussion of submissiveness is that this quality is not simply the opposite of aggressiveness. It is true that highly aggressive animals are rarely submissive, and that highly submissive animals are rarely aggressive; these behaviors may be exclusive in their extremes. However, an animal can be nonaggressive but not particularly submissive. Therefore, these traits of nonaggressiveness and submissiveness are dissociable. This kind of separation has been carried out primarily using physiological manipulations, including modifying neural states (e.g. Lau and Miczek, 1977) and modifying the endocrine characteristics of the individual (e.g. Leshner and Moyer, 1975; Leshner and

Politch, 1979; Maruniak et al., 1977). Using both of these kinds of manipulations one can produce animals that are nonaggressive but not particularly submissive.

Whether an individual is behaving submissively has been determined in a variety of ways, including the number of submissive postures displayed (Brain and Poole, 1974; Nock and Leshner, 1976). In the work to be discussed here, an animal is considered to be submissive only when it has effectively "surrendered" to the opponent. Submission is defined as occurring when the test animal: (1) exhibits the classical rigid upright submissive posture; and (2) fails to fight back when subsequently attacked by the opponent (Ginsburg and Allee, 1942; Nock and Leshner, 1976; Scott, 1946). Thus, in our studies, submissiveness is measured in terms of the amount of aggression by an opponent needed to induce submission in the test mouse. The smaller the number of distinct aggressive bouts needed to induce submission, the more submissive the test mouse is considered.

HORMONAL CONTROL OF SUBMISSIVENESS

Some indirect tests

Our first studies concerned with the role of endocrine factors in behavioral adaptations to aggression examined a behavior assumed to be an indirect measure of an animal's submissiveness, the tendency to avoid attack from a trained fighter mouse. In those studies, we examined the roles of both the androgens and the hormones of the pituitary–adrenocortical axis on behavior in a passive avoidance situation where the aversive stimulus was attack by a trained fighter mouse. That series of studies on avoidance-of-attack showed, first, that although the androgens are important to one agonist behavior, aggression, they seem unimportant to the tendency to avoid attack; castration did not affect avoidance-of-attack (Leshner and Moyer, 1975). This finding, in combination with some other studies (Barfield et al., 1972; Maruniak et al., 1977), suggested indirectly that the androgens also would be irrelevant to submissiveness. This suggestion was supported by our later direct tests (Leshner and Politch, 1979).

Most of our efforts in studying the tendency to avoid attack were focused on the pituitary–adrenocortical hormones, ACTH and corticosterone. Studies relating those hormones to avoidance-of-attack showed that corticosterone plays an important role in determining this behavior, whereas ACTH levels are relatively unimportant (Leshner, Moyer and Walker, 1975; Moyer and Leshner, 1976). These studies provided indirect evidence suggesting a role for this adrenal steroid in the control of submissiveness.

Direct tests of pituitary–adrenal effects on submissiveness

More recently, we have examined pituitary–adrenal effects on submissiveness directly. In these and the later studies to be discussed, submissiveness is measured in encounters with "opponent" mice. The opponents also are male, adult CD-1 mice, but in contrast to the experimental animals, the opponents had all been isolated for at least 6 weeks prior to their use, in order to facilitate their aggressiveness (Sigg, 1969; Valzelli, 1969). The test for submissiveness consists simply of placing the two mice (one test animal and one opponent) into a wooden arena, and allowing them to interact until one submits. The measure of submissiveness used is the number of aggressions by the opponent needed to induce submission in the test animal, with submission defined as stated above. An aggression is defined as a

430

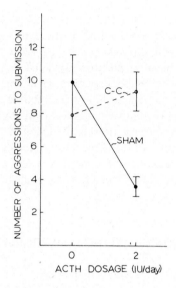

Fig. 2. Mean ± S.E. number of aggression to submission in intact mice (sham) and mice with controlled corticosterone levels (C–C) treated with either a placebo or 2 IU/day ACTH. (Modified from Leshner and Politch, 1979.)

distinct bout of biting. The smaller the number of aggressions needed to induce submission, the more submissive the test animal is considered. The encounter is terminated when the test animal has submitted.

The first study of that series (Leshner and Politch, 1979) accomplished two goals. It showed: (1) that generally increasing pituitary–adrenal hormone levels by ACTH treatment increases submissiveness; and (2) that this facilitation of submissiveness by the pituitary–adrenal hormones is dependent on the animal's being able to respond to ACTH treatment with increases in corticosterone levels; the submissiveness of mice with controlled levels of

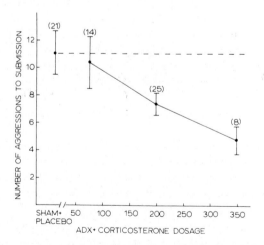

Fig. 3. Dose–response relationship between corticosterone dosages and mean ± S.E. number of aggressions to submission in adrenalectomized mice. The number in parentheses indicates the number of mice in each independent group.

corticosterone is not affected by exogenous ACTH. The findings of that study are reproduced in Fig. 2, which shows the effects of ACTH versus placebo treatment on the submissiveness of intact mice (sham) and mice which had been adrenalectomized and treated with a fixed replacement dosage (200 μg/day) of corticosterone (controlled-corticosterone, CC). These findings support the suggestion from our studies of avoidance-of-attack that corticosterone levels are important to submissiveness.

All of the evidence discussed so far has really only indirectly pointed to corticosterone as a controller of submissiveness. The studies on the relationship of the pituitary—adrenal hormones to the tendency to avoid attack used an indirect behavioral measure of submissiveness. In addition, the studies just discussed of ACTH treatment manipulated pituitary—adrenal hormone levels generally and deduced an effect of corticosterone by subtraction of effects: elevations in both ACTH and corticosterone had effects on submissiveness, whereas elevations of ACTH only had no effect. Therefore, we conducted another group of studies examining directly the effects of corticosterone on submissiveness.

The findings from these studies combined are presented in Fig. 3, which shows a dose—response relationship between chronic (3 weeks long) corticosterone dosages and levels of submissiveness in independent groups of adrenalectomized mice. These levels were compared to those of sham-operated animals treated with a placebo. Statistical examination of these data showed, first, that mice adrenalectomized and treated for 3 weeks with 75 μg/day corticosterone were as submissive as sham-operated controls. Second, there was a progressive increase in submissiveness in the groups treated with higher dosages. These findings support all of the earlier indirect evidence which suggested a role for corticosterone in determining submissiveness, and they argue that corticosterone's effects are exerted in a dose—response manner.

It should be mentioned here that we have not always found a statistically reliable (at or near the 0.05 level) facilitation of submissiveness within the dosage range of 100—300 μg/day (e.g. Leshner et al., in press). Reliable effects are observed in the intermediate dosage ranges only when very large numbers of subjects are used. Therefore, one would have to say that although very high dosages (e.g. 350 μg/day) of corticosterone do reliably increase submissiveness, the effects at more intermediate dosages are weaker. This, of course, might be expected when observing a dose—response relationship.

HORMONAL MEDIATION OF THE EFFECTS OF DEFEAT ON SUBMISSIVENESS: THE INTERACTION OF EXPERIENTIAL AND ENDOCRINE FACTORS

During the past 10 years, it became apparent that there is a striking similarity between the form of the behavioral and hormonal responses to defeat and the behavioral effects of the hormonal states that seem most effective in modifying agonistic response patterns. First, both victorious and defeated mice show post-competition elevations in circulating corticosterone levels, and the loser's response is significantly greater and lasts longer than that of the victor. The effects of competition on plasma corticosterone levels in both winners and losers are shown in Fig. 4. Second, the experience of defeat leads to decreases in aggressiveness and increases in submissiveness (Ginsburg and Allee, 1942; Kahn, 1951; Scott and Marston, 1953). Third, experimentally producing the hormonal characteristics of defeated mice — increased ACTH and corticosterone levels — in naive mice leads to decreases in aggressiveness and increases in submissiveness (Brain et al., 1971; Leshner et al., 1973; Leshner and Politch, 1979). In fact, a dosage of ACTH effective in modifying submissiveness (2 IU/day) produces

432

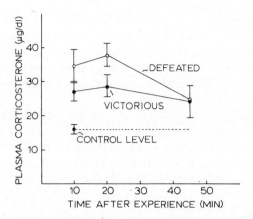

Fig. 4. Mean ± S.E. corticosterone levels of defeated and victorious mice at different times following a single agonistic encounter.

plasma corticosterone levels equal to those of defeated mice (Fig. 5). Thus, defeated mice have elevated pituitary—adrenal hormone levels, reduced levels of aggressiveness and increased levels of submissiveness, and naive mice with these same hormonal characteristics are less aggressive and more submissive than normal animals.

This similarity led to the proposition that experiential and endocrine factors interact in determining an animal's behavioral adaptations to the stresses of defeat. The specific hypothesis was that the hormonal responses to defeat play a role in mediating the effects of that experience on ongoing and future agonistic responding (Leshner, 1975). Cast another way, it was suggested that defeated animals become less aggressive and more submissive, in part because they respond to defeat with increases in pituitary—adrenal activity levels.

We have used two kinds of approaches to study the interaction between experiential and endocrine factors in submissive responding. Both involve manipulation of the hormonal

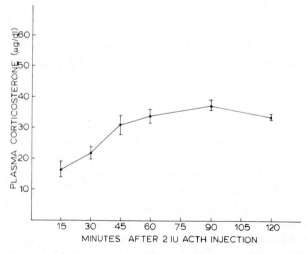

Fig. 5. Mean ± S.E. plasma corticosterone levels at different times following a single injection with 2 IU ACTH.

responses to defeat. The first approach involves preventing those endocrine responses, and the second involves exaggerating those responses.

The effects of preventing the hormonal responses to defeat

If it is true that the hormonal responses to defeat facilitate the behavioral responses to that experience, then preventing those endocrine responses should decrease and/or delay the behavioral changes that normally follow defeat. In 1976, we published a series of studies using this approach (Nock and Leshner, 1976). In those studies, we removed the gland producing the response being studied, and then treated the animals with a fixed replacement dosage of the test hormone(s). For example, in one study, we compared the agonistic behavior of hypophysectomized mice treated with 0.75 IU/day ACTH and 150 μg/day testosterone with that of intact mice throughout an initial agonistic encounter. The findings from that study are reproduced in Fig. 6, which shows the amount of aggressive and submissive behavior shown by intact (SH) and controlled hormone (CH) mice vincentized into halves of the encounter. As can be seen from this figure, mice which could not respond to defeat with the usual increase in ACTH and decrease in androgen levels became nonaggressive and submissive later in the encounter than did intact animals. Thus, preventing the normal hormonal responses to defeat delayed the onset of the behavior patterns typical of defeated mice. (As a side note, preventing the hormonal responses to victory had no effect.)

Later studies in that same series (Nock and Leshner, 1976), showed that the effects of generally preventing hormonal responses to defeat, through hypophysectomy and replacement with both ACTH and testosterone, were in fact due to having modified the pituitary—adrenal responses. Therefore, these studies provided the first evidence for the hypothesis that neuroendocrine, particularly adrenocortical, factors mediate the effects of defeat on agonistic response patterns.

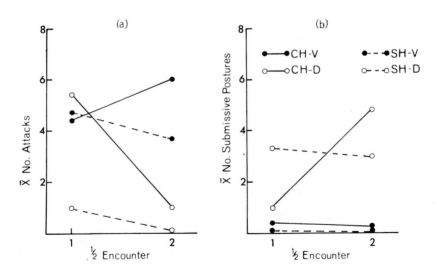

Fig. 6. Mean number of attacks (a) and submissive postures (b) displayed by victorious (V) and defeated (D) mice in each half of a single agonistic encounter. CH animals were hypophysectomized and treated with both ACTH and testosterone, and SH mice were sham-hypophysectomized and treated with two placebos. (From Nock and Leshner, 1976.)

The effects of exaggerating the hormonal responses to defeat

The series of studies just discussed employed one approach to the hormonal mediation hypothesis, preventing hormonal responses. The second approach we used was to exaggerate the normal hormonal responses to defeat. If the hypothesis is true, then exaggerating pituitary—adrenal responses should increase the effects of defeat on submissive responding.

The paradigm used in the studies to be discussed in this section involves treating mice around the time of a defeat with the test hormone and then examining levels of submissiveness at some later time. Because we are in effect manipulating both defeat and hormone treatment simultaneously, two facts must first be established in order to interpret these studies accurately: (1) that the experience of defeat does in fact increase later submissiveness; and (2) that the hormone treatment used does not affect later submissiveness independently of the defeat experience. Having established these facts, we would be certain that what we are studying is an interaction between experiential and endocrine factors.

Fig. 7 presents the results of a study establishing the first point, that a prior experience of defeat (Test I, Fig. 7) leads to an increase in later submissiveness (Test II). This finding is not at all surprising, since earlier studies (e.g. Ginsburg and Allee, 1942; Scott and Marston, 1953) have made the same point, although using different techniques for assessing submissiveness.

Fig. 8 shows the effects of a single injection of either a placebo, 2 IU ACTH, or 300 μg corticosterone on submissiveness tested either 24 h, 48 h, or 7 days after that injection. Each point represents an independent group of at least 10 mice. This study showed no effects of any hormone treatment at any time, thereby establishing the second point: that the hormone treatments to be used in later studies have no effects by themselves on later submissiveness.

Having established these two facts, we turned to the examination of the effects of exaggerating the normal hormonal responses to defeat on later submissiveness. We began

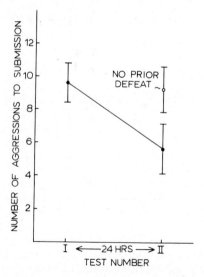

Fig. 7. Mean ± S.E. number of aggression to submission during an initial defeat (Test I) and a second defeat 24 h later (Test II).

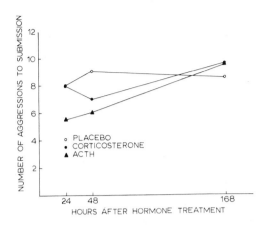

Fig. 8. Mean number of aggression to submission in mice treated with either a placebo, corticosterone, or ACTH and tested either 24 h, 48 h, or 7 days after the hormone treatment.

with producing general increases in pituitary—adrenal activity levels by injecting 2 IU ACTH immediately after an initial defeat. The results of that study (Roche and Leshner, 1979) are reproduced in Fig. 9. As the figure shows, ACTH treatment immediately after an initial defeat increased submissiveness when subjects were tested either 24 or 48 h later, but not 7 days later. Thus, this study supports the hypothesis that the normal pituitary—adrenal responses to defeat facilitate later submissiveness, since exaggerating those hormonal responses increased later submissiveness.

The next study in this series examined the effects of exaggerating the adrenocortical responses to defeat with corticosterone treatments. We turned here to corticosterone, because all of our earlier studies (e.g. Leshner and Politch, 1979, and studies discussed above) had suggested that the critical pituitary—adrenal hormone in submissiveness was corticosterone, and that the effects of ACTH are really due to its trophic actions on the

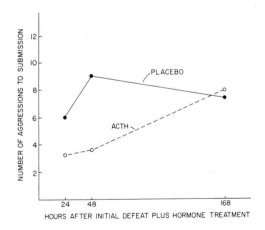

Fig. 9. Mean number of aggressions to submission in mice treated with either a placebo or 2 IU ACTH immediately after an initial defeat and tested for submissiveness either 24 h, 48 h, or 7 days after the initial defeat plus hormone treatment. All points represent independent groups. (From Roche and Leshner, copyright 1979 by the American Association for the Advancement of Science.)

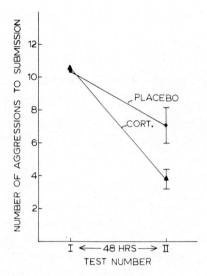

Fig. 10. Mean ± S.E. number of aggression to submission in mice treated with either a placebo or 300 μg corticosterone (cort.) prior to an initial defeat experience (Test I) and tested againt 48 h later (Test II).

adrenal cortex. Therefore, in this study, mice were treated with a single injection of 300 μg corticosterone or a placebo 1 h before an initial encounter and tested again for submissiveness in a second test conducted 48 h later. The results of this study, summarized in Fig. 10, revealed that treatment before the first encounter had no effect on submissiveness during that encounter, but that treatment before Test I did affect submissiveness during the second test, 48 h later. Thus, this corticosterone treatment produced no effect on initial submissiveness, but when the hormone treatment had been coupled with the experience of defeat, subsequent submissiveness was increased. This finding is basically the same as the findings of the previous study, where coupling an initial defeat with increased pituitary—adrenal hormone levels increased future submissiveness. This study extends those earlier findings, however, by establishing that increasing corticosterone levels alone has the same effect as does generally increasing pituitary adrenal hormone levels by ACTH treatment.

CONCLUDING COMMENTS

The studies described here show clearly that the adrenal glucocorticoid corticosterone is involved in the control of submissiveness in mice. However, that control is not exclusive, since, in fact, the primary controller of submission is the experience of defeat. Defeat can induce submission totally independently of corticosterone levels, and no hormonal manipulation can elicit submissive behaviors in the absence of that critical experience. Therefore, one can only argue that changes in corticosterone levels interact with the experience of defeat to affect submissiveness.

The studies discussed here show, further, that the form of corticosterone's interaction with defeat is probably sequential. That is, the most likely explanation of corticosterone's effects is that defeat first leads to an increase in corticosterone levels, which, then, facilitates the occurrence of submission. The greater the corticosterone response to the experience of defeat, the more readily the animal will surrender, and the lesser the response, the less readily the animal will submit. The existence of this sequence shows that experiential and hormonal factors do in fact interact to determine behavioral adaptations to aggression.

SUMMARY

A series of studies was described which examined the interaction between experiential and neuroendocrine, particularly pituitary—adrenal, factors in determining the readiness of mice to submit in aggressive encounters with other mice. A variety of approaches was discussed, all pointing to the adrenal hormone corticosterone as an important controller of submissive responding. Some studies focused on the tendency to avoid attack, as studied in a laboratory—specific situation resembling more traditional kinds of avoidance situations. Other studies examined submissive behaviors in more natural situations, simple encounters between two opponents. Further studies examining the interaction between experiential and adrenocortical factors in submissiveness suggested that the most likely sequence of events in losing animals is that the experience of defeat leads to an increase in corticosterone levels, which, then, facilitates the occurrence of the behavioral adaptations to aggression, specifically submission.

ACKNOWLEDGEMENTS

This work was supported by U.S.P.H.S. Grant MH 31086.

In addition to the collaborators mentioned in the text and bibliography, A. Besser, S. Korn, J.Mixon, C. Prindle and C. Rosenthal participated in this work. I am very grateful to N. Cain and O. Floody for their constructive criticisms on earlier versions of this manuscript.

REFERENCES

Baenninger, R. (1974) Some consequences of aggressive behavior: a selective review of the literature on other animals. *Aggress. Behav.*, 1: 17—37.
Barfield, R.J., Busch, D.E. and Wallen, K. (1972) Gonadal influences on agonistic behavior in the male domestic rat. *Horm. Behav.*, 3: 247—259.
Brain, P.F., Nowell, N.W. and Wouters, A. (1971) Some relationships between adrenal function and the effectiveness of a period of isolation in inducing intermale aggression in albino mice. *Physiol. Behav.*, 6: 27—29.
Brain, P.F. and Poole, A.E. (1974) The role of endocrines in isolation-induced intermale fighting in albino laboratory mice. I. Pituitary—adrenocortical influences. *Aggress. Behav.*, 1: 39—69.
Eibl-Eibesfeldt, I. (1975) *Ethology: The Biology of Behavior*, Holt, Rinehart and Winston, New York.
Ginsburg, B. and Allee, W.C. (1942) Some effects of conditioning on social dominance and subordination in inbred strains of mice. *Physiol. Zool.*, 15: 485—506.
Grant, E.C. and Mackintosh, J.H. (1963) A comparison of the social postures of some common laboratory rodents. *Behaviour*, 21: 246—259.
Hutchinson, R.R. (1972) The environmental causes of aggression. In *Nebraska Symposium on Motivation*, J.K. Cole and D.D. Jensen (Eds.), Univ. Nebraska Press, Lincoln, pp. 155—181.
Johnson, R.N. (1972) *Aggression in Man and Animals*, W.B. Saunders, Philadelphia.
Kahn, M.W. (1951) The effect of severe defeat at various age levels on the aggressive behavior of mice. *J. genet. Psychol.*, 79: 117—130.
Lau, P. and Miczek, K.A. (1977) Differential effects of septal lesions on attack and defensive—submissive reactions during intraspecies aggression in rats. *Physiol. Behav.*, 18: 479—485.

438

Leshner, A.I. (1975) A model of hormones and agonistic behavior. *Physiol. Behav.,* 15: 225–235.

Leshner, A.I., Korn, S.J., Mixon, J.F., Rosenthal, C. and Besser, A.K. (1980) Effects of corticosterone on submissiveness in mice: some temporal and theoretical considerations. *Physiol. Behav.,* 24: 283–288.

Leshner, A.I. and Moyer, J.A. (1975) Androgens and agonistic behavior in mice: relevance to aggression and irrelevance to avoidance-of-attack. *Physiol. Behav.,* 15: 695–699.

Leshner, A.I., Moyer, J.A. and Walker, W.A. (1975) Pituitary–adrenocortical activity and avoidance-of-attack in mice. *Physiol. Behav.,* 15: 689–693.

Leshner, A.I. and Nock, B.L. (1976) The effects of experience on agonistic responding: an expectancy theory interpretation. *Behav. Biol.,* 17: 561–566.

Leshner, A.I. and Politch, J.A. (1979) Hormonal control of submissiveness in mice: irrelevance of the androgens and relevance of the pituitary–adrenal hormones. *Physiol. Behav.,* 22: 531–534.

Leshner, A.I., Walker, W.A., Johnson, A.E., Kelling, S.J., Kreisler, S.J. and Svare, B.B. (1973) Pituitary adrenocortical activity and intermale aggressiveness in isolated mice. *Physiol. Behav.,* 11: 705–711.

Lorenz, K. (1966) *On Aggression,* Bantam Books, New York.

Maruniak, J.A., Desjardins, C. and Bronson, F.H. (1977) Dominant–subordinate relationships in castrated male mice bearing testosterone implants. *Amer. J. Physiol.,* 233: E495–E499.

Montagu, A. (1974) Aggression and the evolution of man. In *The Neuropsychology of Aggression,* R.E. Whalen (Ed.), Plenum Press, New York, pp. 1–29.

Moyer, J.A. and Leshner, A.I. (1976) Pituitary–adrenal effects on avoidance-of-attack in mice: separation of the effects of ACTH and corticosterone. *Physiol. Behav.,* 17: 297–301.

Nock, B.L. and Leshner, A.I. (1976) Hormonal mediation of the effects of defeat on agonistic responding in mice. *Physiol. Behav.,* 17: 111–119.

Roche, K.E. and Leshner, A.I. (1979) ACTH and vasopressin treatments immediately after a defeat increase future submissiveness in mice. *Science* 204: 1343–1344.

Scott, J.P. (1946) Incomplete adjustment caused by frustration of untrained fighting mice. *J. comp. Psychol.,* 39: 379–390.

Scott, J.P. (1971) Theoretical issues concerning the origin and causes of fighting. In *The Physiology of Aggression and Defeat,* B.E. Eleftheriou and J.P. Scott (Eds.), Plenum Press, New York, pp. 11–41.

Scott, J.P. and Marston, M.W. (1953) Nonadaptive behavior resulting from a series of defeats in fighting mice. *J. abnorm. soc. Psychol.,* 48: 417–428.

Sigg, E.B. (1969) Relationship of aggressive behavior to adrenal and gonadal function in male mice. In *Aggressive Behaviour,* S. Garattini and E.B. Sigg (Eds.), John Wiley, New York, pp. 143–149.

Valzelli, L. (1969) Aggressive behaviour induced by isolation. In *Aggressive Behaviour,* S. Garattini and E.B. Sigg (Eds.), John Wiley, New York, pp. 70–76.

Wilson, E.O. (1975) *Sociobiology: The New Synthesis,* Harvard University Press, Cambridge.

Subject Index

440